Integration of Palliative Care in Chronic Conditions:
An Interdisciplinary Approach

Edited by
Kim Kuebler, DNP, APRN, ANP-BC

Oncology Nursing Society
Pittsburgh, Pennsylvania

ONS Publications Department
Publisher and Director of Publications: William A. Tony, BA, CQIA
Managing Editor: Lisa M. George, BA
Assistant Managing Editor: Amy Nicoletti, BA, JD
Acquisitions Editor: John Zaphyr, BA, MEd
Copy Editors: Vanessa Kattouf, BA, Andrew Petyak, BA
Graphic Designer: Dany Sjoen
Editorial Assistant: Judy Holmes

Library of Congress Cataloging-in-Publication Data

Names: Kuebler, Kim K., editor. | Oncology Nursing Society, issuing body.
Title: Integration of palliative care in chronic conditions : an
   interdisciplinary approach / edited by Kim Kuebler.
Description: Pittsburgh, Pennsylvania : Oncology Nursing Society, [2016] |
   Includes bibliographical references and index.
Identifiers: LCCN 2016030745 | ISBN 9781935864899
Subjects: | MESH: United States. Patient Protection and Affordable Care Act.
   | Hospice and Palliative Care Nursing | Chronic Disease–nursing |
   Palliative Care–legislation & jurisprudence | Chronic Pain–nursing |
   Patient-Centered Care | Case Reports
Classification: LCC RA999.H66 | NLM WY 152.3 | DDC 362.17/56–dc23 LC record available at https:// lccn.loc.gov/2016030745

Publisher's Note

This book is published by the Oncology Nursing Society (ONS). ONS neither represents nor guarantees that the practices described herein will, if followed, ensure safe and effective patient care. The recommendations contained in this book reflect ONS's judgment regarding the state of general knowledge and practice in the field as of the date of publication. The recommendations may not be appropriate for use in all circumstances. Those who use this book should make their own determinations regarding specific safe and appropriate patient care practices, taking into account the personnel, equipment, and practices available at the hospital or other facility at which they are located. The editor and publisher cannot be held responsible for any liability incurred as a consequence from the use or application of any of the contents of this book. Figures and tables are used as examples only. They are not meant to be all-inclusive, nor do they represent endorsement of any particular institution by ONS. Mention of specific products and opinions related to those products do not indicate or imply endorsement by ONS. Websites mentioned are provided for information only; the hosts are responsible for their own content and availability. Unless otherwise indicated, dollar amounts reflect U.S. dollars.

ONS publications are originally published in English. Publishers wishing to translate ONS publications must contact ONS about licensing arrangements. ONS publications cannot be translated without obtaining written permission from ONS. (Individual tables and figures that are reprinted or adapted require additional permission from the original source.) Because translations from English may not always be accurate or precise, ONS disclaims any responsibility for inaccuracies in words or meaning that may occur as a result of the translation. Readers relying on precise information should check the original English version.

Printed in the United States of America

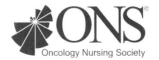

Innovation • Excellence • Advocacy

Contributors

Editor

Kim Kuebler, DNP, APRN, ANP-BC
Director, Multiple Chronic Conditions Resource Center
CEO, Advanced Disease Concepts LLC
Adjunct Professor, South University School of Nursing and Health Professions
Medical Leader, Ortho Sport and Spine Physicians
Savannah, Georgia

Chapter 1. Overview; Chapter 2. The Patient Protection and Affordable Care Act; Chapter 5. Care of Multiple Chronic Conditions; Chapter 6. Comparative Effectiveness Research; Chapter 7. Health Policy and the Role of Advanced Practice Nurses; Chapter 12. Cardiovascular Disease; Chapter 14. Chronic Obstructive Pulmonary Disease; Chapter 20. Chronic Nonmalignant Pain

Authors

Kristi A. Acker, DNP, FNP-BC, AOCNP®, ACHPN
Assistant Professor, Graduate Nursing
University of Alabama Capstone College of Nursing
Tuscaloosa, Alabama
Advanced Oncology/Hematology and Hospice and Palliative Nurse Practitioner
Oncology Associates of West Alabama
Tuscaloosa, Alabama
Chapter 1. Overview; Chapter 19. Anxiety

Adegoke O. Adeniji, RPh, PhD
Assistant Professor of Pharmaceutical Sciences
South University School of Pharmacy
Savannah, Georgia
Chapter 8. Metabolism and Excretion in Disease; Chapter 9. Cytochrome P450 in Palliative Care; Chapter 10. Drug–Drug Interactions in Palliative Care

Terry A. Badger, PhD, PMHCNS-BC, FAAN, FAPOS
Professor
University of Arizona College of Nursing
Tucson, Arizona
Chapter 25. Depression

Stephanie Banasik, MSN, RN, ANP-BC
DaVita
Hilton Head Island, South Carolina
Chapter 13. Chronic Kidney Disease

Kimberly L. Barefield, PharmD, BCPS, CDE
Associate Professor
South University School of Pharmacy
Savannah, Georgia
Chapter 11. Palliative Care and Concomitant Medications

Debi Boyle, MSN, RN, AOCNS®, FAAN
Oncology Clinical Nurse Specialist/Palliative
    Care Nurse Lead
University of California Irvine Medical Center,
    Chao Family Comprehensive Cancer Center
Orange, California
*Chapter 43. Compassionate Self-Care: An Interdisciplinary
Approach*

Kelly Browning, MSN, RN, FNP
Registered Nurse
Bluffton-Okatie Outpatient Center
Okatie, South Carolina
Chapter 23. Dehydration

Rosanne Burson, DNP, ACNS-BC, CDE, FAADE
Associate Professor
University of Detroit Mercy
Detroit, Michigan
Chapter 4. Self-Management in Chronic Disease

Nancy Jo Bush, RN, MN, MA, AOCN®, FAAN
Lecturer/Oncology Nurse Practitioner
University of California, Los Angeles School of
    Nursing
Los Angeles, California
*Chapter 43. Compassionate Self-Care: An Interdisciplinary
Approach*

Craig S. Conoscenti, MD, FCCP
Principal Expert, Clinical Development and
    Medical Affairs
Pulmonary Fibrosis Program Area Lead
Boehringer Ingelheim Pharmaceuticals
Ridgefield, Connecticut
Chapter 22. Cough; Chapter 26. Dyspnea

Peg Esper, DNP, MSN, MSA, ANP-BC, AOCN®
Oncology Nurse Practitioner
South Lyon, Michigan
Chapter 16. General Oncology

Christine Estabrook, DNP, MSN, ANP-BC, AOCNP®
Assistant Professor
University of South Alabama
Mobile, Alabama
Chapter 40. Cultural Considerations

Janice Firn, PhD, LMSW
Clinical Social Worker
Division of Geriatric and Palliative Medicine
University of Michigan Health System
Ann Arbor, Michigan
*Chapter 38. Patient and Family Goal Setting; Chapter
39. Interdisciplinary Team Collaboration, Continuity, and
Communication*

**Jennifer Fournier, MSN, APRN-CNS, ACNS-BC,
    AOCN®, CHPN**
Clinical Special Services Manager
Nancy N. and J.C. Lewis Cancer & Research
    Pavilion at St. Joseph's/Candler
Savannah, Georgia
*Chapter 33. Communicating With the Patient and Family;
Chapter 34. Preparing the Patient and Family for End of
Life; Chapter 35. Advance Care Planning; Chapter 36.
Preparation Versus Crisis Approach to Care*

Catherine Fowler, DHSc, RN
Faculty
Georgia College and State University
Milledgeville, Georgia
Chapter 17. Musculoskeletal Disorders: Osteoarthritis

**Sheri D. Froelich, DNP, MSBA, ANP-BC, ACHPN,
    PMHNP-BC**
Nurse Practitioner
Alcona Health Center
Alpena, Michigan
Chapter 1. Overview

Ami K. Goodnough, DNP, NP-C, ACHPN
Assistant Professor
University of South Alabama
Mobile, Alabama
Palliative Nurse Practitioner
University of Alabama School of Medicine
Birmingham, Alabama
Chapter 40. Cultural Considerations

Denise Soltow Hershey, PhD, FNP-BC
Assistant Professor
College of Nursing, Michigan State University
East Lansing, Michigan
Chapter 15. Endocrine Disorders

Mary Margaret Hillstrand, DNP, ANP
Owner, Mary Margaret Hillstrand DNP, LLC
Anchorage, Alaska
Adjunct Faculty
University of Alaska School of Nursing
Anchorage, Alaska
Adjunct Faculty
Vanderbilt University
Nashville, Tennessee
Chapter 18. Neurologic Conditions

Helene M. Holbrook, DNP, FNP-C
Virtual Faculty, Contributing
Walden University
Minneapolis, Minnesota
Chapter 24. Dementia

Marcelle Kaplan, MS, RN, CBCN®, CNS
Oncology Nursing Consultant
Merrick, New York
Chapter 29. Hypercalcemia of Malignancy; Chapter 30. Malignant Pleural Effusion; Chapter 31. Spinal Cord Compression; Chapter 32. Superior Vena Cava Syndrome

Nicole Peters Kroll, PhD, RN, ANP-C
Nurse Practitioner and Occupational Health
    Director
University Occupational Health Partners
College Station, Texas
Assistant Professor/Assistant Program Director
College of Nursing and Public Health
South University Online
Savannah, Georgia
Chapter 3. Patient-Centered Outcomes of Care

Mark Lazenby, PhD, APRN, AOCNP®, FAPOS
Associate Professor of Nursing and Divinity
Yale University
New Haven, Connecticut
Chapter 25. Depression

Rebecca Lichwala, MSN, ARNP, AOCNP®, NP-C
Advanced Registered Nurse Practitioner, Adult
    Hematology/Oncology
St. Joseph's Hospital, Cancer Institute
Tampa, Florida
Chapter 41. Spiritual and Religious Care; Chapter 42. Hope and Loss

Launa M.J. Lynch, PhD
Assistant Professor
South University School of Pharmacy
Savannah, Georgia
Chapter 8. Metabolism and Excretion in Disease; Chapter 9. Cytochrome P450 in Palliative Care; Chapter 10. Drug–Drug Interactions in Palliative Care

Jackie Matthews, RN, MS, AOCN®, ACHPN, CNS
Vice President, Palliative and Supportive Care
Hospice of Dayton
Dayton, Ohio
Chapter 28. Pruritus

Laura McRee, DNP, ACNP-BC
Clinical Assistant Professor, Specialty Coordi-
    nator—Adult Gerontology Acute Care Nurse
    Practitioner
University of Arizona
Tucson, Arizona
Chapter 25. Depression

Vicky V. Mody, PhD
Associate Professor of Pharmaceutical Sciences
Philadelphia College of Osteopathic Medicine
    School of Pharmacy
Suwanee, Georgia
Chapter 8. Metabolism and Excretion in Disease; Chapter 9. Cytochrome P450 in Palliative Care; Chapter 10. Drug–Drug Interactions in Palliative Care

Katherine Moran, DNP, RN, CDE, FAADE
Associate Professor
University of Detroit Mercy
Detroit, Michigan
Chapter 4. Self-Management in Chronic Disease

Mary E. Murphy, MS, AOCN®, ACHPN, CNS
Chief Nursing and Care Officer
Hospice of Dayton
Dayton, Ohio
Chapter 28. Pruritus

Francois Prizinski, DPT, OCS, COMT, FAAOMPT
Vice President and Administrator
NxtGen Institute of Physical Therapy
PT Center, Director of Clinical Education
Physicaltherapycenter.org
Snellville, Georgia
Chapter 20. Chronic Nonmalignant Pain

Christopher Schuetz, DPT
Physical Therapist
OSTI Physical Therapy
McHenry, Illinois
Chapter 20. Chronic Nonmalignant Pain

Mary Atkinson Smith, DNP, FNP-BC, ONP-C, RNFA, CNOR
Nurse Practitioner and RNFA
Starkville Orthopedic Clinic
Starkville, Mississippi
Education and Programs Director
Mississippi Rural Health Association
Madison, Mississippi
Assistant Professor/Assistant Program Director
College of Nursing and Public Health
South University Online
Savannah, Georgia
Chapter 3. Patient-Centered Outcomes of Care; Chapter 7. Health Policy and the Role of Advanced Practice Nurses; Chapter 20. Chronic Nonmalignant Pain

Suzette Walker, DNP, FNP-BC, AOCNP®
Nurse Practitioner
McKenzie Health System
Sandusky, Michigan
Chapter 21. Constipation; Chapter 27. Insomnia; Chapter 37. Identifying Team Disciplines

Myrshia L. Woods, MHS, PA-C
Physician Assistant–Certified
Department of Cardiology
MD Anderson Cancer Center
Houston, Texas
Chapter 12. Cardiovascular Disease

Disclosure

Editors and authors of books and guidelines provided by the Oncology Nursing Society are expected to disclose to the readers any significant financial interest or other relationships with the manufacturer(s) of any commercial products.

A vested interest may be considered to exist if a contributor is affiliated with or has a financial interest in commercial organizations that may have a direct or indirect interest in the subject matter. A "financial interest" may include, but is not limited to, being a shareholder in the organization; being an employee of the commercial organization; serving on an organization's speakers bureau; or receiving research funding from the organization. An "affiliation" may be holding a position on an advisory board or some other role of benefit to the commercial organization. Vested interest statements appear in the front matter for each publication.

Contributors are expected to disclose any unlabeled or investigational use of products discussed in their content. This information is acknowledged solely for the information of the readers.

The contributors provided the following disclosure and vested interest information:

Kim Kuebler, DNP, APRN, ANP-BC: Multiple Chronic Conditions Resource Center, stock ownership

Rosanne Burson, DNP, ACNS-BC, CDE, FAADE: My Self-Management Team, Inc., employment or leadership position

Ami K. Goodnough, DNP, NP-C, ACHPN: Aspire Health, Central Alabama Chapter of Hospice and Palliative Nurses Association, employment or leadership position

Mary Margaret Hillstrand, DNP, ANP: Biogen Idec, Genzyme, consultant or advisory role; Accordia, Biogen Idec, Genzyme, honoraria

Katherine Moran, DNP, RN, CDE, FAADE: My Self-Management Team, Inc., employment or leadership position

Table of Contents

Preface

Integration of Palliative Care in Chronic Conditions: An Interdisciplinary Approach is written by and for interdisciplinary healthcare professionals managing patients with symptomatic chronic conditions. The 2010 passage of the largest and most complex legislation in U.S. healthcare history, the Patient Protection and Affordable Care Act, has promoted massive changes. These innovative changes are directly linked to a new system that provides incentives for quality patient-centered outcomes that adhere to the three tenets of the Affordable Care Act: better health, better care, and cost-effectiveness.

The new era of clinical transparency and quality metrics requires the application and implementation of evidence-based practice. The purpose of this textbook is to provide interdisciplinary healthcare teams with a road map to ensure best practices in the care and management of the largest, fastest growing, and costliest U.S. patient population—those with multiple chronic conditions.

This textbook provides an overview of the current legislative influence that has created a shift in clinical paradigms to meet the nation's escalating patient population. Detailed, specific, and succinct information directs healthcare professionals on the evidence used to integrate symptom management or palliative care interventions to promote optimal patient-centered outcomes.

In 2012, the National Quality Forum separated palliative care from end-of-life care. Palliative care is primarily the relief of symptoms through an interdisciplinary or team approach to care. The Affordable Care Act's influence on team-based comprehensive care and the shift toward community-driven services provide an ideal opportunity to use this resource to address the clinical demands and reduce the economic burden generated by the growing population of patients with multiple chronic conditions. Maintaining physical function, reducing symptoms, and preventing disease exacerbation promote patient quality of life. This informative text is a collection of the current evidence used to improve the quality of care for the tsunami of an aging society.

Foreword

This text, edited by Dr. Kim Kuebler, offers countless insights and evidence-based discussions on how to practice and integrate palliative care into systems care, particularly with chronic and life-threatening conditions. I have known Dr. Kuebler for more than 24 years. I have watched her practice and teaching of palliative care resonate from rural Michigan to many fine academic and hospital settings in our country. Dr. Kuebler is a champion of the integration of palliative care with chronic or life-threatening conditions, and her editing of this text is a harbinger of the future. This text will leapfrog palliative care to its rightful place in healthcare delivery systems and offer support to those who desire justification and enhancement of their skills. It also tells a powerful story to the policy makers and insurance companies that determine benefit and reimbursement packages.

Dr. Kuebler has taken the justification of palliative care integration into chronic disease management to a new level with this superb tapestry of chapters. This comprehensive text brings excitement to the reader and offers a much-needed clarity that palliative care advocates and practitioners have been seeking. Each chapter details the depth and scope of how to provide an interdisciplinary practice to chronic conditions and palliative care.

The chapters offer a path to the type of palliative care acceptance that has frustrated so many for so long. The reader will have access to a collection of the best writers and practitioners in the field of chronic conditions and palliative care in this one comprehensive text. Its practical approach is refreshing.

We read and hear much about the cost of care, the experience of care, and the need for healthy outcomes. If we are committed to the treatment of chronic conditions, then palliative care must be part of an interdisciplinary approach. We also hear that change takes place when the process is disrupted. For far too long, the health industrial complex has focused on the sickness model of health care. It is time to put an increased focus on preventive care, curative care, and palliative care.

Traditional models of health care have been reluctant to champion the consumer choice model or consumers' participation in their own healthcare delivery. We are entering an exciting era of healthcare enlightenment, where the decision makers and funders will realize that consumers and their families have a rightful role in the decisions that affect them as a diagnosis is rendered. Who better to partner with consumers and families than palliative care professionals, where all involved can collectively find a process that they can respect and accept? Moving forward, choice, self-management, and participation should be the norm when it comes to treating a chronic condition that warrants palliative care.

I have a friend who has been through a year of surgeries and radiation therapy for cancer. He has had setbacks with various infections and has been in and out of three hospitals for the past three months. He is now home. His doctors are recommending 40 days of daily radiation treatments; however, in talking with him the other day, he had a different attitude. He was not talking about the 40 days of radiation therapy, but rather about visiting his in-laws and family who live 700 miles away. He was connecting with work friends. He was talking about experiencing a quality of life with those he loved.

After spending time with those most important to him, he reconsidered radiation therapy. What happened during this time? What altered his view of the future? It is clear he decided to stop listening to those who were trying to just keep him alive, as what they were doing was cutting him off from what was important to him. I believe he experienced firsthand what this text is sharing with the reader. He now has some mastery over what is happening to him. He now has choices and options as he faces his chronic conditions. He is upbeat about life and has accepted the reality that extraordinary medical intervention in the last months of one's life has little apparent benefit.

What a powerful text Dr. Kuebler has edited advocating for the full integration of palliative care into our system of health care. For too long, health professionals and advocates have championed full palliative care acceptance only to receive marginal recognition and acceptance. As populations continue to age, the number of patients with chronic or life-threatening conditions will only increase. In the United States, it is estimated that more than 75% of health expenditures are for chronic health conditions. For many, being sick with a chronic condition is a full-time job. This text offers the hope that the healthcare system of the future will be easier to navigate and offer personalized and respectful interventions. This is the definitive text on palliative care, so enjoy it to its fullest.

James K. Haveman
Retired Director of the Michigan Department of Community Health
January 2016

CHAPTER 1

Overview

Kim Kuebler, DNP, APRN, ANP-BC, Kristi A. Acker, DNP, FNP-BC, AOCNP®, ACHPN, and Sheri D. Froelich, DNP, MSBA, ANP-BC, ACHPN, PMHNP-BC

I. Definition
  A. The World Health Organization (WHO, n.d.) defines palliative care as an interdisciplinary approach of care used to improve the quality of life for patients and families living with and dying from advanced disease through the prevention and relief of symptoms by the impeccable assessment and management of pain and other problems, physical, psychosocial, and spiritual.
  B. Palliative care
    1. Provides skilled, evidence-based symptom management
    2. Promotes quality of life throughout the disease trajectory—up to and including the time of death
    3. Recognizes the debility and decline from the burden of disease, symptoms, and age in the dying process
    4. Integrates expertise from all disciplines (e.g., medicine, nursing, social work, spiritual providers) to address and individually manage the myriad of issues associated with complex disease management
    5. Offers a support system to help patients live as actively as possible until death
    6. Implements a team approach to address the needs of patients and families, including bereavement preparation and follow-up
    7. Is integrated earlier in the course of disease and used concomitantly with medical modalities intended to prolong life, including chemotherapy, radiation, and surgery (WHO, n.d.). Prudent diagnostics should be used to investigate underlying causes of symptoms.
  C. The Center to Advance Palliative Care (CAPC) influences the national direction, integration, and implementation of palliative care in the United States and endorses the WHO definition, purpose, and function of palliative care. Primary care providers in the routine management of patients with multiple chronic conditions (MCCs) are expected to provide the basic elements of palliative care, such as pain and symptom assessment and management and advance care planning (National Consensus Project for Quality Palliative Care [NCP], 2013).
  D. The Institute of Medicine* (IOM, 2014) defines *palliative care* as an umbrella term that encompasses a spectrum of approaches in delivering care for people

---

On March 15, 2016, the Institute of Medicine (IOM) of the National Academies of Sciences, Engineering, and Medicine was renamed the Health and Medicine Division (HMD). Reports issued prior to this change will continue to be cited as IOM reports throughout this book.

with advanced conditions. Various organizations have developed conceptual or functional definitions of palliative care, suggesting that it aims to prevent, relieve, reduce, or soothe the symptoms of diseases or disorders without producing a cure (IOM, 2014).

1. In 2013, WHO further elaborated on the definition and role of palliative care to include a broader concept that involves all care systems, including hospice, that prioritize symptom control and do not necessarily require the presence of an imminently terminal condition or a time-limited prognosis and therefore may extend beyond six months (Connor & Bermedo, 2014).

2. Palliative care should include a balance of comfort measures and curative interventions that vary across a wide spectrum of healthcare delivery systems (Connor & Bermedo, 2014).

3. Palliative care should focus on achieving the best possible quality of life for patients and caregivers based on patient and family needs and goals and independent of a prognosis.

4. Interdisciplinary palliative care teams assess and treat symptoms, support decision making, and help match treatments through shared decision making between the patient and family.

5. Patient and family goals should drive the patient-specific plan of care and mobilize practical support for the patient and caregivers.

6. The Centers for Medicare and Medicaid Services (CMS, 2008) describe palliative care as patient- and family-centered care that optimizes quality of life by anticipating, preventing, and treating poorly managed symptoms.

E. Palliative care throughout the continuum or trajectory of disease involves addressing physical, intellectual, emotional, social, and spiritual needs and facilitating patient autonomy, access to information, and choice (CMS, 2008).

1. CMS (2008) changed its definition of palliative care and for the first time did not provide specific language on prognostic indicators or time specificity (e.g., implemented in the last six months of life) (see Figure 1-1).

2. The National Quality Forum (NQF) described palliative care as patient- and family-centered care that optimizes quality of life by anticipating, preventing, monitoring, and managing suffering.

   a) In 2012, NQF separated palliative care from end-of-life care and developed hospice measurements for evaluation and determination of quality measurements (see Figure 1-2).

   b) Beginning in 2014 and for each year thereafter, a hospice program's failure to submit required quality data will result in a reduction of two per-

---

Figure 1-1. New Centers for Medicare and Medicaid Services (CMS) Definition of Palliative Care

New CMS Definition of Palliative Care Does Not Mention Prognosis
"Palliative care means patient- and family-centered care that optimizes quality of life by anticipating, preventing, and treating suffering. Palliative care throughout the continuum of illness involves addressing physical, intellectual, emotional, social, and spiritual needs and to facilitate patient autonomy, access to information, and choice" (p. 32204).

Note. Based on information from Centers for Medicare and Medicaid Services, 2008.

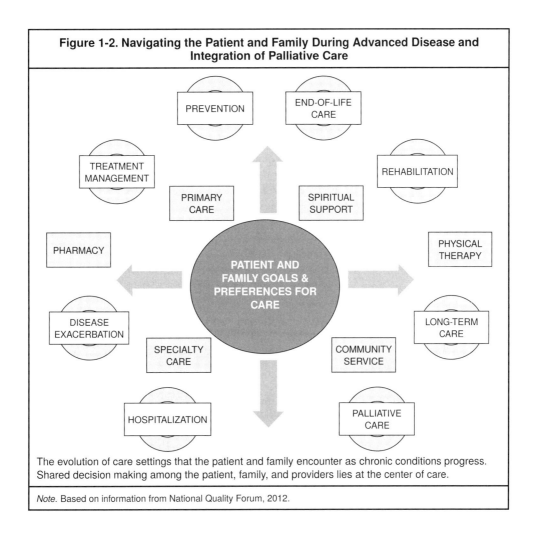

Figure 1-2. Navigating the Patient and Family During Advanced Disease and Integration of Palliative Care

The evolution of care settings that the patient and family encounter as chronic conditions progress. Shared decision making among the patient, family, and providers lies at the center of care.

Note. Based on information from National Quality Forum, 2012.

centage points to the market basket percentage increase for that fiscal year (NQF, 2012).

c) The data submitted by individual hospice programs must be made publicly available, with hospice programs having an opportunity to review the data prior to their release. No date has been specified to begin public reporting of hospice quality data (NQF, 2015).

d) CMS finalized the Hospice Item Set (HIS) in the 2014 rule to meet the quality reporting requirements for hospices for the 2016 payment determination (NQF, 2015).

e) All Medicare-certified hospices are required to submit an HIS-Admission record and HIS-Discharge record for each patient admission to specific hospice programs (NQF, 2015).

3. NQF (2015) measures applicable to palliative care include the following:

a) Patients treated with an opioid are equally prescribed a bowel regimen.

b) Pain screening is performed using psychometric pain evaluation and assessment tools.

c) Dyspnea treatment is identified.

  d) Dyspnea screening and the use of evidence-based interventions are insti-
tuted.

  e) Beliefs and values are uniquely addressed and evaluated (if desired by the
patient).

 4. Previous NQF (2012) recommendations included in the 2015 measurements
include goal attainment, patient engagement, care coordination, depression
assessment and management, the caregiver role, and timely referral to hospice (NQF, 2015).

 5. The NQF (2015) measures require that hospice programs in the United States
identify a future direction for their program that includes the following:

  a) Develop an outcome measure addressing evidence-based pain management.

  b) Select measures that address care coordination, communication, timeliness and responsiveness of care, and 24-hour access to the healthcare
team.

II. Key aspects

 A. Since the recognition of the Medicare hospice benefit in 1982, the emergence
of palliative care has taken time to differentiate from hospice or end-of-life
care. These terms often are used synonymously by healthcare professionals and
the public. Despite the current initiative for earlier integration of palliative care
interventions into the trajectory of disease, barriers remain because of nomenclature and understanding the differences between palliative care, hospice, and
end-of-life care.

  1. Barriers include limitations of current evidence-based guidelines that identify
and inform providers on the integration of skilled palliative care interventions
in advanced symptomatic disease.

  2. The Agency for Healthcare Research and Quality (2015) implemented SHARE
decision making between providers and patients. This approach is essential as
the patient and family proactively plan for palliative care.

  3. Proactive patient-centered palliative care communication reduces delays in opti-
mally managing the complex care needs of the patient and family (Callaway, 2012).

  4. Studies examining earlier integration of palliative care principles have demonstrated improved patient adherence to treatment modalities, along with
improved management of psychological stressors, greater quality of life, and
improved survival rates (Bakitas et al., 2009; Temel et al., 2010).

  5. Escalating costs, along with the growing burden of symptomatic MCCs, provider shortages, and an expanding aging population, have resulted in policy
makers and healthcare administrators turning to palliative care models that
have demonstrated past success and are forecasted to deliver future promise.

  6. Many initiatives for advancing and improving palliative care originate from
partnerships. The following are exemplars of such collaborations:

   a) A multifaceted coalition including the American Academy of Hospice
and Palliative Medicine, CAPC, the Hospice and Palliative Nurses Association, the Last Acts Partnership, and the National Hospice and Palliative Care Organization convened to develop NCP. This coalition sought
to reach a consensus in defining palliative care and outlining its philosophy and principles.

   b) The NCP clinical practice guidelines were first released in 2004 and revised
in 2009 and 2013. For a complete review of this palliative care resource
and to download the guidelines, see www.nationalconsensusproject.org.

       c) In 2006, NQF, a private, nonprofit organization, released *A National Framework and Preferred Practices for Palliative and Hospice Care Quality.* Together, NCP and NQF have collaborated to advance palliative care.

       d) After a thorough review, NQF endorsed the following eight domains for palliative care outlined from the *Clinical Practice Guidelines for Quality Palliative Care* (NCP, 2013):

          (1) Domain 1: Structure and Processes of Care

          (2) Domain 2: Physical Aspects of Care

          (3) Domain 3: Psychological and Psychiatric Aspects of Care

          (4) Domain 4: Social Aspects of Care

          (5) Domain 5: Spiritual, Religious, and Existential Aspects of Care

          (6) Domain 6: Cultural Aspects of Care

          (7) Domain 7: Care of the Patient at the End of Life

          (8) Domain 8: Ethical and Legal Aspects of Care

B. The Robert Wood Johnson Foundation (RWJF) brought attention to end-of-life conversations for seriously ill and dying patients.

   1. RWJF released a groundbreaking report emphasizing the need for improved communication at the end of life in *JAMA* in November 1995 (Connors et al., 1995). Shortcomings surrounding healthcare delivery and patient preferences in advanced disease helped RWJF to identify a need for research in palliative care.

   2. RWJF helped to establish the following programs and initiatives:

       a) Last Acts®, a consumer organization formed as an end-of-life awareness campaign (De Milto, 2002)

       b) Promoting Excellence in End-of-Life Care, which highlighted the need for physicians to become competent in providing high-quality health care to patients in noncurative situations

       c) Education in Palliative and End-of-Life Care, an important program in which the American Medical Association designed a "train the trainer" course to educate physicians in end-of-life care and provided the model of curriculum used today for training physicians, nurses, and other palliative care professionals

       d) Advanced Practice Nursing: Pioneering Practices in Palliative Care

   3. For more information on RWJF, see www.rwjf.org.

C. Key drivers for quality palliative care access and integration

   1. American Society of Clinical Oncology (ASCO): ASCO is a nonprofit physician organization dedicated to issues unique to clinical oncology and provides clinical opinions based on emerging palliative care data. For more information, see www.asco.org.

   2. The Joint Commission (TJC)

       a) TJC provides palliative care certification designed to recognize hospital inpatient programs that demonstrate high-quality interdisciplinary palliative care.

       b) TJC certifies hospital compliance with relevant standards for the effective use of evidence-based clinical practice guidelines, along with quality improvement performance measures.

       c) For more information on TJC palliative care certification, see www.jointcommission.org/certification/palliative_care.aspx.

   3. Health and Medicine Division (HMD, formerly IOM) of the National Academies of Sciences, Engineering, and Medicine

        a) HMD's aim is to help individuals in government and the private sector make informed health decisions, including palliative care issues, by providing reliable evidence.

        b) For more information, see www.nationalacademies.org/hmd/About -HMD.aspx.

    4. CAPC

        a) CAPC remains the leading source for resources in palliative care program development with established tools and educational preparation for providers and agencies.

        b) In addition, CAPC releases a state-by-state report card and rankings in state and regional access to palliative care in hospitals.

        c) For more information, see www.capc.org/about/capc.

    5. The Quality Oncology Practice Initiative (QOPI®)

        a) QOPI is a quality improvement program for outpatient hematology and oncology practices.

        b) The initiative provides data-driven quality improvement and promotes self-examination and improvement in practice.

        c) For more information, see www.instituteforquality.org/qopi-qcp.

  D. The IOM (2014) report *Dying in America: Improving Quality and Honoring Individual Preferences Near the End of Life* highlighted the crucial and often stressful decision making that has become increasingly more complex in today's healthcare delivery system by doing the following:

    1. Underscoring the national priority to improve end-of-life care through improved communication, advance care planning, and increased institutional accountability through development of quality measures

    2. Recognizing that patient-centered care is the cornerstone for the delivery of palliative care

  E. Quality improvement in patient care continues to emerge as a national priority.

    1. The escalating Medicare population dying from MCCs is compounded with poorly managed symptoms, exacerbations in disease, prevalence of polypharmacy, and the complexities that occur from an uncoordinated healthcare delivery system.

    2. Quality should begin to increase with adherence to the NQF measurements and public transparency requirements—all a direct result of the Patient Protection and Affordable Care Act (ACA).

III. Current findings

  A. Within recent years, research interests in palliative care issues have gained momentum.

    1. Although much of the palliative care literature to date has originated from oncology settings, favorable outcomes have helped to propel interests for research inquiries outside of oncology and into other specialties such as cardiology, pulmonary, and neurology.

    2. As expected, research findings demonstrate that earlier palliative care integration helps to improve overall patient outcomes.

  B. Most palliative care evidence has originated from oncology settings, and elements of clinical palliative care remain less developed than other well-established medical specialties (Norris et al., 2008).

  C. A landmark 1995 study by Connors et al. has been credited for launching investigational interests in end-of-life communications, patient goals of care, caregiver distress, and healthcare delivery.

1. The Study to Understand Prognoses and Preferences for Outcomes and Risks of Treatment (SUPPORT) was a randomized controlled clinical trial conducted over 10 years that yielded startling findings.
    a) Significant deficits in physician knowledge or understanding of individual patient healthcare preferences, including advance care planning and physical symptom management
    b) Inadequate communication between healthcare providers and seriously ill patients and discrepancies between patient care delivery and individual patient preferences and goals
2. The SUPPORT study proved monumental in advancing the need for further palliative care research and served as a driving force behind the development of palliative care as a specialty within the United States (Connors et al., 1995).

D. Two out of three Medicare beneficiaries are diagnosed with MCCs (U.S. Department of Health and Human Services [DHHS], 2010, 2016). The integration of palliative care can be used to decrease the excessive costs of care burdening the current healthcare system (Ward, Schiller, & Goodman, 2014) (see Table 1-1).

IV. Relevance to practice
A. The largest U.S. patient population is those who are living with and dying from MCCs (U.S. DHHS, 2010). This patient population uses the majority of healthcare resources and requires full collaboration with multiple disciplines to ensure optimal patient outcomes (see Table 1-2).
B. Improving symptom management in patients with MCCs reduces disease exacerbation, which helps to prevent and reduce admission into hospital and decrease cost of care (IOM, 2014).
    1. Preventing symptoms through skilled palliative care helps patients to maintain physical functioning and reduce deconditioning and debility.
    2. Integrating pertinent disciplines into the management of patient care can help to ensure that all patient issues are addressed and appropriately managed, including physical, psychological, emotional, spiritual, and rehabilitation (WHO, n.d.).
    3. The integration of palliative care should begin at the onset of a confirmed diagnosis of a chronic condition and used throughout the disease trajectory up to and including the time of death (IOM, 2014).
    4. Interdisciplinary palliative care interventions increase in intensity in the presence of symptoms, exacerbations, debility, and approaching death.
    5. Symptom management is palliative care, and knowledge and understanding of the pharmacologic and nonpharmacologic interventions and collaboration with the interdisciplinary healthcare team can be combined to ensure supportive, coordinated, and comprehensive care for patients and their families in the last years of life.
    6. Providers prescribing medications require knowledge and skill in understanding drug–drug interactions because 95% of medications prescribed in the palliative setting go through the cytochrome P450 enzyme system and increase the propensity for adverse reactions in the setting of more than five concomitant medications (U.S. DHHS, 2010).
    7. Clinical care plans should be used and routinely updated based on patient and family needs.
    8. As the disease trajectory progresses, the care plan requires modification and is used to guide the interdisciplinary team to support the multiple dimensions of the patient.

Table 1-1. Cost Savings Attributed to Palliative Care Access		
Study	**Methods**	**Results**
May et al. (2015)	Prospective, observational design using clinical and cost data collected for patients with advanced cancer in the United States from 2007–2011	Earlier palliative care consultation within 6 days of admission was associated with an estimated reduction by $1,312 (14%) in total direct costs in hospital stay compared with no intervention. Furthermore, palliative care intervention within 2 days yielded a cost reduction of $2,280 (24%). The authors concluded that earlier palliative care consultation is associated with lower cost of hospital stay for patients with advanced cancer.
McCarthy et al. (2015)	Analysis matching palliative care patients to nonpalliative care patients using propensity score methods	Overall cost savings from palliative care were $3,426 per patient for those patients dying in the hospital. The authors concluded that appropriately selected and timed palliative care consults result in hospital cost savings.
Morrison et al. (2008)	Analysis matching palliative care to usual care using administrative data from 8 hospitals from 2002–2004	Palliative care patients who were discharged alive had an adjusted net savings of $1,696 in direct costs per admission, including reduction in laboratory and intensive care costs, compared to usual care patients. Palliative care patients who died had an adjusted net savings of $4,908 in direct costs per admission compared to usual care patients.
Starks et al. (2013)	Analysis of data for 1,815 palliative care patients and 1,790 comparison patients from 2 academic hospitals from 2005–2008 matched on discharge dispositions, length of stay (LOS), and propensity for palliative care consultation	Significant savings per admission were associated with shorter LOS. LOS of 1–7 days indicated lower palliative care patient costs by 13% ($2,141) and for survivors by 19.1% ($2,946). Stays of 8–30 days were associated with reductions in cost for palliative care patients by 4.9% ($2,870) and for survivors by 6%. Extrapolating the per-admission cost across the palliative care patient groups with lower costs showed savings of about $1.46 million for LOS under a week and about $2.5 million for LOS of 8–30 days. There was no difference in costs for patients with LOS > 30 days, suggesting that earlier involvement in palliative care results in cost savings.

9. No hierarchy of care exists in the palliative care setting—the patient and family are at the core and are central in the shared decision making of the patient's care.

10. Shared decision making among the patient, family, and healthcare team should be an ongoing dialogue to ensure comprehensive, coordinated, and cost-effective care that demonstrates patient-centered outcomes (Agency for Healthcare Research and Quality, 2015).

11. Members of the interdisciplinary team should integrate and apply real-life data gained from comparative effectiveness research to determine best patient outcomes.

12. Management of symptoms, promotion of ongoing physical functioning, and tailoring of the patient's care plan should accommodate the physical, emotional, and spiritual changes that occur along the trajectory of MCCs.
13. The chronic care reimbursement model in the primary care setting is an ideal opportunity to integrate the use and implementation of palliative care into the management of patients with MCCs.
14. Collecting outcomes through the use of psychometrically sound assessment tools is key in determining value versus volume as the United States moves toward a non–fee-for-service healthcare delivery model.

C. Individualized patient care plans that focus on effective palliative care are used to reduce a crisis-like approach to dying and use a coordinated approach to support the patient and family in the face of advanced disease and ensuing death.
1. The patient's care plan should accommodate disease management based on the patient's physical changes and presenting symptoms.
2. The interdisciplinary healthcare team should rely on patient self-report of symptoms versus diagnostic criteria explicitly.
3. The healthcare team should implement advance directives long before the patient begins to dramatically decline. Advance care planning should be an ongoing discussion and perpetually updated to meet the care needs of the patient and family as disease progresses.
4. The healthcare team also should engage the patient and family in shared decision making about advanced disease goals and approaching debility and death.

D. The IOM (2014) report *Dying in America: Improving Quality and Honoring Individual Preferences Near the End of Life* recognized the high cost of care in patients aged 65 years and older and the economic burden that this will have on the American population.
1. The burden of serious illnesses among the nation's Medicare-eligible (65 and older) and old-old (85 and older) populations has risen markedly.
2. Currently, two-thirds of people aged 65 years and older suffer from serious MCCs (Centers for Disease Control and Prevention, 2013).
3. By contrast, 31% of those aged 45–64 years and only 6% of those aged 18–44 years were treated for two or more chronic conditions in 2009 (Machlin & Soni, 2013).

Table 1-2. Average Medicare Expenditures per Fee-for-Service Beneficiary by Number of Chronic Conditions, 2010

Number of Chronic Conditions	Cost of Care
0–1	$2,025
2–3	$5,698
4–5	$12,174
6 or more	$32,658

The 15 chronic conditions included in this analysis are high blood pressure, high cholesterol, ischemic heart disease, arthritis, diabetes, heart failure, chronic kidney disease, depression, chronic obstructive pulmonary disease, Alzheimer disease, atrial fibrillation, cancer, osteoporosis, asthma, and stroke.

Note. Based on information from Centers for Medicare and Medicaid Services, 2012; Institute of Medicine, 2014.

4. Medicare spending rises dramatically with increases in the number of chronic conditions. Medicare beneficiaries with five or more such conditions accounted for nearly two-thirds of Medicare dollars spent in 2007 (Anderson, 2010).

V. Role of the advanced practice registered nurse (APRN)

A. In combination with our nation's aging crisis, the prevalence of MCCs continues to increase.

1. This combination provides opportunities to demonstrate improved patient outcomes.

2. Close to half of Americans aged 65 years or older have three or more chronic conditions, with slightly more than 20% suffering with five or more chronic conditions (Norris et al., 2008).

B. In 2000, 24.5% of hospitals with more than 50 beds reported having a palliative care program, whereas in 2013, that number had grown to 72.3% (CAPC, 2015). Based on this growth, the realization of palliative care programs is primarily identified in the acute care setting.

C. APRNs understand the clinical value of keen assessment and the use and implementation of best evidence to direct a standard of care that promotes optimal patient-centered outcomes.

D. According to the *Clinical Practice Guidelines for Quality Palliative Care* (NCP, 2013), current palliative care delivery models limit the ability to integrate palliative care into the management of common chronic conditions but have separated and specialized routine interdisciplinary care and management into isolated settings to include the following:

1. Hospice care—a program to provide end-of-life care for patients with terminal illness with a life expectancy of six months or less

2. Palliative care—institution-based programs that provide skilled physical, psychosocial, and spiritual distress management for patients with serious or life-threatening illnesses that can include consultative services, fixed-bed units, or swing beds

3. Outpatient palliative care—programs that provide continuity of care to patients in ambulatory care settings

4. Community palliative care—programs consisting of consultant teams who collaborate with hospice and home health agencies to support seriously ill patients who are not enrolled in hospice services

E. The critical decision making that is required in the patient's care management along the trajectory of disease, such as determining physical performance status, performing concomitant disease and symptom management, understanding complex pathophysiology, interfacing with different disciplines, and using specialized referrals, sets APRNs in the primary care setting apart from those with specialized focus on only palliative care.

F. Existing barriers to implementing palliative interventions

1. Health professionals' understanding of palliative care as separate and different than end-of-life care

2. Acceptance and understanding of implementing sound symptom management based on current evidence-based practice

3. Patient–caregiver willingness or understanding

4. Access to palliative care resources or interdisciplinary team accessibility

5. Association of palliative care with end-of-life care and dying

6. Poor reimbursement for lengthy patient–provider communication

G. Examples of outcomes that palliative care APRNs are uniquely positioned to provide
   1. Has an advanced understanding of MCCs, pathophysiology, associated symptoms, and diagnostics to determine disease progression
   2. Is skilled in implementing best evidence to promote optimal outcomes for symptomatic conditions that interfere with physical functioning
   3. Demonstrates knowledge of drug–drug interactions and the implications of ethnicity on the cytochrome P450 enzyme system, which is responsible for metabolizing the majority of medications used in the palliative care setting
   4. Understands and appreciates the role of coordinated care for the patient and family
   5. Provides a conduit for the patient to ensure appropriate referrals and management from multiple health professional disciplines
   6. Participates in demonstrating optimal patient-centered outcomes that will and can be used for reimbursement mechanisms
   7. Recognizes the dynamics of health policy on the changing landscape of patient care and remains flexible and dynamic in the era of the ACA

H. NQF provides quality measures designed to measure the quality of care provided by nurses who work in hospitals. The National Database of Nursing Quality Indicators® provides the largest nursing registry for measuring and comparing data for hospital performance and provides an incentive for continuous quality improvement.

Case Study

L.J., a 62-year-old woman, comes to the clinic with complaints of progressive dyspnea and exercise intolerance. She has a past medical history of hypertension, hyperlipidemia, chronic obstructive pulmonary disease (forced expiratory volume in one second, or FEV_1, less than 70% predicted), sleep apnea, morbid obesity (body mass index greater than 35), type 2 diabetes, depression, and osteoporosis. She complains of peripheral edema, productive cough, and lethargy. Her symptoms have worsened over the past two days and she is having difficulty sleeping in her bed.

On physical examination, L.J. appears morbidly obese, deconditioned, and dyspneic while ambulating in orthopneic position and using pursed-lip breathing. She has dry oral mucosa, crowded uvula 3+, and bilateral cervical lymphadenopathy and is febrile with a temperature of 101.5°F (38.6°C). She is tachycardic with a heart rate of 112 and irregular thready pulse. Examination also found bilateral diminished lower lung sounds, rales and rhonchi bilateral mid and upper lobes, increased anterior and posterior diameter, and increased jugular vein distension bilaterally. Her abdomen was too obese to examine. Peripheral extremities show brisk patellar reflexes bilaterally 3/4 and symmetrical. Office diagnostics showed pulse oximetry in room air of 87% and nonfasting glucose finger stick of 288 mg/dl.

The differentials from this clinical encounter include chronic obstructive pulmonary disease exacerbation, dehydration, hyperglycemia, fever, hypoxemia, morbid obesity, dyspnea, exercise intolerance, orthopnea, productive cough, and lethargy. The ARPN recognizes the fragile status of this patient and institutes the following interventions: oxygen at 2 L per nasal cannula, IV hydration of normal saline, azithromycin, and 3 units of regular insulin subcutaneous injection.

During the clinical encounter, the APRN learns that the patient has not been adherent with her home medications and diabetic management. She provides the patient with information on the importance of maintaining her medication regimen (long-acting anticholinergic and short-acting beta-2 agonist, metformin 1,000 mg every 12 hours, bupropion extended release 150 mg daily, celecoxib 200 mg daily, lisinopril 20 mg daily, and simvastatin 20 mg at bedtime) and the pulmonary symptoms that lead to an exacerbation.

The APRN stabilized L.J. in the clinic and sent her home with APRN home visits to ensure that she stabilizes and regains her medical management. L.J. was referred to a community-based self-management program to help reinforce and empower her disease management practices. The APRN ensured that L.J. was scheduled for a clinic appointment at the end of the week and encouraged her to contact the clinic if her symptoms worsen. L.J. will continue to receive symptom management to reduce exacerbation development and will work with her healthcare team in shared decision making to ensure that she reduces the physical and psychological burdens associated with her concomitant conditions influenced largely by lifestyle.

References

Agency for Healthcare Research and Quality. (2015, September). The SHARE approach. Retrieved from http://www.ahrq.gov/professionals/education/curriculum-tools/shareddecisionmaking/index.html

Anderson, G. (2010). *Chronic care: Making the case for ongoing care.* Retrieved from http://www.rwjf.org/content/dam/farm/reports/reports/2010/rwjf54583

Bakitas, M., Lyons, K.D., Hegel, M.T., Balan, S., Brokaw, F.C., Seville, J., … Ahles, T.A. (2009). Effects of a palliative care intervention on clinical outcomes in patients with advanced cancer: The Project ENABLE II randomized controlled trial. *JAMA, 302,* 741–749. doi:10.1001/jama.2009.1198

Callaway, C. (2012). Timing is everything: When to consult palliative care. *Journal of the American Academy of Nurse Practitioners, 24,* 633–639. doi:10.1111/j.1745-7599.2012.00746.x

Center to Advance Palliative Care. (2015). The growth of palliative care in U.S. hospitals: 2015 snapshot (2000–2013). Retrieved from https://media.capc.org/filer_public/34/77/34770c03-a584-4079-a9ae-edb98dab6b20/growth_snapshot_2016_final.pdf

Centers for Disease Control and Prevention. (2013). *The state of aging and health in America 2013.* Retrieved from http://www.cdc.gov/features/agingandhealth/state_of_aging_and_health_in_america_2013.pdf

Centers for Medicare and Medicaid Services. (2008). Center for Clinical Standards and Quality Survey and Certification Group. Retrieved from https://www.gpo.gov/fdsys/pkg/FR-2008-06-05/pdf/08-1305.pdf

Centers for Medicare and Medicaid Services. (2012). *Chart book: Chronic conditions among Medicare beneficiaries, 2012 edition.* Retrieved from https://www.cms.gov/Research-Statistics-Data-and-Systems/Statistics-Trends-and-Reports/Chronic-Conditions/2012ChartBook.html

Connor, S.R., & Bermedo, M.C.S. (Eds.). (2014). *Global atlas of palliative care at the end of life.* Retrieved from http://www.who.int/nmh/Global_Atlas_of_Palliative_Care.pdf

Connors, A.F., Jr., Dawson, N.V., Desbiens, N.A., Fulkerson, W.J., Jr., Goldman, L., Knaus, W.A., … Ransohoff, D. (1995). A controlled trial to improve care for seriously ill hospitalized patients: The Study to Understand Prognoses and Preferences for Outcomes and Risks of Treatments (SUPPORT). *JAMA, 274,* 1591–1598. doi:10.1001/jama.1995.03530200027032

De Milto, L. (2002, October 1). Assessment of Last Acts Program provides recommendations for future direction: Assessing progress and opportunities for the Last Acts initiative. Retrieved from http://www.rwjf.org/en/library/research/2002/10/assessment-of-last-acts-r--program-provides-recommendations-for-.html

Institute of Medicine. (2014). *Dying in America: Improving quality and honoring individual preferences near the end of life.* Washington, DC: National Academies Press.

Machlin, S.R., & Soni, A. (2013). Health care expenditures for adults with multiple treated chronic conditions: Estimates from the Medicare Expenditure Panel Survey, 2009. *Preventing Chronic Disease, 10,* 120172. doi:10.5888/pcd10.120172

May, P., Garrido, M.M., Cassel, J.B., Kelley, A.S., Meier, D.E., Normand, C., … Morrison, R.S. (2015). Prospective cohort study of hospital palliative care teams for inpatients with advanced cancer: Earlier consultation is associated with larger cost-saving effect. *Journal of Clinical Oncology, 33,* 2745–2752. doi:10.1200/JCO.2014.60.2334

McCarthy, I.M., Robinson, C., Huq, S., Philastre, M., & Fine, R.L. (2015). Cost savings from palliative care teams and guidance for a financially viable palliative care program. *Health Services Research, 50,* 217–236. doi:10.1111/1475-6773.12203

Morrison, R.S., Penrod, J.D., Cassel, J.B., Caust-Ellenbogen, M., Litke, A., Spragens, L., & Meier, D. (2008). Cost savings associated with US hospital palliative care consultation programs. *Archives of Internal Medicine, 168,* 1783–1790. doi:10.1001/archinte.168.16.1783

National Consensus Project for Quality Palliative Care. (2013). *Clinical practice guidelines for quality palliative care* (3rd ed.). Retrieved from http://www.nationalconsensusproject.org/NCP_Clinical_Practice_Guidelines_3rd _Edition.pdf

National Quality Forum. (2006). *A national framework and preferred practices for palliative and hospice care quality: A consensus report.* Retrieved from https://www.qualityforum.org/Publications/2006/12/A_National _Framework_and_Preferred_Practices_for_Palliative_and_Hospice_Care_Quality.aspx

National Quality Forum. (2012). NQF endorses palliative and end-of-life care measures. Retrieved from https:// www.qualityforum.org/News_And_Resources/Press_Releases/2012/NQF_Endorses_Palliative_and_End -of-Life_Care_Measures.aspx

National Quality Forum. (2015). *MAP 2015 considerations for selection of measures for federal programs: Post-acute care/long-term care.* Retrieved from http://www.qualityforum.org/Setting_Priorities/Partnership/MAP_PAC -LTC_Programmatic_Deliverable_-_Final_Report.aspx

Norris, S.L., High, K., Gill, T.M., Hennessy, S., Kutner, J.S., Reuben, D.B., ... Landefeld, C.S. (2008). Health care for older Americans with multiple chronic conditions: A research agenda. *Journal of the American Geriatrics Society, 56,* 149–159. doi:10.1111/j.1532-5415.2007.01530.x

Starks, H., Wang, S., Farber, S., Owens, D.A., & Curtis, J.R. (2013). Cost savings vary by length of stay for inpatients receiving palliative care consultation services. *Journal of Palliative Medicine, 16,* 1215–1220. doi:10.1089/jpm.2013.0163

Temel, J.S., Greer, J.A., Muzikansky, A., Gallagher, E.R., Admane, S., Jackson, V.A., ... Lynch, T.J. (2010). Early palliative care for patients with metastatic non–small-cell lung cancer. *New England Journal of Medicine, 363,* 733–742. doi:10.1056/NEJMoa1000678

U.S. Department of Health and Human Services. (2010). *Multiple chronic conditions: A strategic framework: Optimum health and quality of life for individuals with multiple chronic conditions.* Retrieved from http://www .hhs.gov/ash/initiatives/mcc/mcc_framework.pdf

U.S. Department of Health and Human Services. (2016). About the multiple chronic conditions initiative. Retrieved from http://www.hhs.gov/ash/about-ash/multiple-chronic-conditions/about-mcc/index.html

Ward, B.W., Schiller, J.S., & Goodman, R.A. (2014). Multiple chronic conditions among US adults: A 2012 update. *Preventing Chronic Disease, 11,* 130389. doi:10.5888/pcd11.130389

World Health Organization. (n.d.). WHO definition of palliative care. Retrieved from http://www.who.int/ cancer/palliative/definition/en

Section I.

Use of Palliative Care in Chronic Conditions and the Affordable Care Act

CHAPTER 2

The Patient Protection and Affordable Care Act

Kim Kuebler, DNP, APRN, ANP-BC

I. Definition
   A. The Patient Protection and Affordable Care Act (ACA) was signed by President Obama in March 2010 and includes multiple provisions that will take effect over several years.
      1. This legislation includes Medicaid expansion and eligibility, the establishment of health insurance exchanges, and prohibitions of health insurers from denying coverage for preexisting conditions.
      2. The ACA is a once-in-a-generation change to the familiar U.S. health system (Kocher, Emanuel, & DeParle, 2010).
         a) Guarantees access to health care for all Americans
         b) Creates new incentives to make needed changes in clinical practice
         c) Focuses on improved coordination and quality health care
         d) Gives providers more information to make informed decisions together with the patient and family through shared decision making
         e) Changes the reimbursement system to value versus volume
   B. Key provisions are intended to extend coverage to millions of uninsured Americans, implement measures that will lower healthcare costs, and improve system efficiency.
   C. The ACA assures Americans better health security by putting in place comprehensive health insurance reforms that will accomplish the following:
      1. Expand coverage
      2. Hold insurance companies accountable
      3. Lower healthcare costs
      4. Provide more choices
      5. Enhance the quality of care for all Americans
      6. Close the "donut hole" in Medicare
      7. Ensure quality health system performance
      8. Provide funding for workforce training
   D. The ACA contains two separate pieces of legislation—the Patient Protection and Affordable Care Act and the Health Care and Education Reconciliation Act of 2010. Together these acts expanded Medicaid coverage to millions of low-income Americans and made numerous changes to both Medicaid and the Children's Health Insurance Program (Centers for Medicare and Medicaid Services [CMS], n.d.-a).
   E. Table 2-1 identifies the ACA's provisions and respective description.

Table 2-1. Provisions of the Patient Protection and Affordable Care Act	
Provisions	**Description**
Eligibility	Provisions fill in current gaps in coverage for the poorest Americans by creating a minimum Medicaid income eligibility level across the country.
Financing	Beginning in 2014, coverage for newly eligible adults will be fully funded by the federal government for three years. It will phase down to 90% by 2020.
Information technology systems and data	Policy and financing structure is designed to provide states with tools needed to achieve the immediate and substantial investment in information technology systems that is needed to ensure that Medicaid systems will be in place in time for the January 1, 2014, launch date or the new Affordable Insurance Exchanges as well as the expansion of Medicaid eligibility.
Coordination with affordable insurance exchanges	This system enables individuals and families to apply for coverage using a single application and have their eligibility determined for all insurance affordability programs through one simple process.
Benefits	People newly eligible for Medicaid will receive a benchmark benefit or benchmark equivalent package that includes the minimum essential benefits provided in the Affordable Insurance Exchanges.
Community-based long-term services and supports	These provisions include a number of program and funding improvements to help ensure that people can receive long-term care services and supports in their home or the community.
Quality of care and delivery systems	Improvements will be made in the quality of care and the manner in which that care is delivered while at the same time reducing costs.
Prevention	The legislation promotes prevention, wellness, and public health and supports health promotion efforts at the local, state, and federal levels.
Children's Health Insurance Program (CHIP)	Provisions extend funding for CHIP through fiscal year 2015 and continue the authority for the program through 2019.
Dual eligible	A new office will be created within the Centers for Medicare and Medicaid Services to coordinate care for individuals who are eligible for both Medicaid and Medicare ("dual eligible" or Medicare-Medicaid enrollees).
Provider payments	States will receive 100% federal matching funds for the increase in payments.
Program transparency	Promotes transparency about Medicaid policies and programs, including establishing meaningful opportunities for public involvement in the development of state and federal Medicaid waivers.
Program integrity	Numerous provisions are designed to increase program integrity in Medicaid, including terminating providers from Medicaid that have been terminated in other programs, suspending Medicaid payments based on pending investigations or credible allegations of fraud, and preventing inappropriate payment or claims under Medicaid.

Note. From "The Affordable Care Act," by Centers for Medicare and Medicaid Services, n.d.-a. Retrieved from http://medicaid.gov/affordablecareact/affordable-care-act.html.

II. Key aspects
   A. Title IV—Prevention of Chronic Disease and Improving Public Health—of the ACA promotes disease prevention, wellness, and public health initiatives and supports health promotion efforts within local communities and at the state and federal levels.
   B. The ACA has appropriated unprecedented funding to these areas (CMS, n.d.-b).
      1. The act mandated creation of a national prevention and health promotion strategy that incorporates effective and achievable methods to improve the health status of Americans.
      2. The ACA empowers individuals to take charge of their health through self-management practices and promotes health prevention and screenings as a priority by waving co-payments for patients with Medicare and Medicaid.
   C. Subtitles and sections in Title IV of the ACA that are pertinent to multiple chronic conditions
      1. Subtitle A—Modernizing disease prevention and public health systems
         a) Sec. 4001—National Prevention, Health Promotion and Public Health Council
         b) Sec. 4003—Clinical and community preventive services
         c) Sec. 4004—Education and outreach campaign regarding preventive benefits
      2. Subtitle B—Increasing access to clinical preventive services
         a) Sec. 4103—Medicare coverage of annual wellness visit providing a personalized prevention plan
         b) Sec. 4104—Removal of barriers to preventive services in Medicare
         c) Sec. 4105—Evidence-based coverage for preventive services in Medicare
         d) Sec. 4106—Improving access to preventive services for eligible adults in Medicaid
         e) Sec. 4108—Incentives for prevention of chronic diseases in Medicaid
      3. Subtitle C—Creating healthier communities
         a) Sec. 4202—Healthy aging, living well; evaluation of community-based prevention and wellness programs for Medicare beneficiaries
         b) Sec. 4204—Immunizations
         c) Sec. 4205—Nutrition labeling of standard menus items at chain restaurants
III. Medicaid grants
   A. Medicaid Incentives for Prevention of Chronic Disease Grants is a new program established by the ACA and administered by CMS (2015b), with $85 million in funding to extend over a five-year period.
   B. Ten states (Wisconsin, Minnesota, New York, Nevada, New Hampshire, Montana, Hawaii, Texas, California, and Connecticut) receive these grants, which are subject to annual renewal (CMS, 2015b).
   C. The grant requirements include promoting tobacco cessation, reducing obesity, lowering cholesterol, reducing hypertension, and avoiding the onset of diabetes or improving the management of this condition.
   D. These grants are advancing the goals of Million Hearts, a national public–private initiative to prevent one million heart attacks and strokes over the next five years by addressing and reducing major cardiovascular risk factors, including the following measures (CMS, 2015b):
      1. Aspirin for patients at risk
      2. Blood pressure control
      3. Cholesterol management
      4. Smoking cessation

IV. Patient's Bill of Rights
  A. The ACA puts consumers back in charge of their health care. The new "Patient's Bill of Rights" provides Americans with the stability and flexibility to make informed choices about their own health (CMS, 2015a).
  B. Provisions in the Patient's Bill of Rights
    1. Insurers can no longer cancel a patient's insurance if a mistake was made on the application.
    2. Americans now have a right to appeal a health insurance company's decision to deny payment for a claim or to terminate a specific health coverage plan.
    3. The ACA has banned health plans from putting annual or lifetime dollar limits on any health plan or insurance policy.
    4. Recommended preventive care will be covered at no cost to the patient.
    5. The ACA helps to preserve patients' choices of providers and allows for open access to out-of-network emergency services.
    6. Insurance company barriers to necessary immediate or emergent care will be removed.
V. Overview of the ACA
  A. The ACA addresses two major barriers to the provision of consistent and standardized delivery of high-quality care: information and incentives (Kocher et al., 2010).
    1. The American Recovery and Reinvestment Act of 2009 has provided more than $25 billion toward incentives for providers and health systems to use electronic health records.
    2. The ACA provides long-term funding for patient-centered outcomes research to give providers and patients the clinical information needed to make better informed and personal decisions about their health care.
    3. The ACA will provide healthcare providers with the financial support for making these changes while discouraging fee-for-service for ordering unnecessary diagnostics and interventions (Kocher et al., 2010).
    4. By removing barriers, the ACA allows providers to modify their practices through incentives that focus on coordinated preventive care and reduce chronic condition complications (Kocher et al., 2010).
  B. ACA summary points
    1. Key points of the ACA and the American Recovery and Reinvestment Act of 2009 that will affect healthcare delivery in the United States (Kocher et al., 2010)
      a) Focus care on patient experiences and shared decision making.
      b) Expand the use of electronic health records with the capacity of drug–drug interactions, guideline recommendations, alerts, and other decision support tools.
      c) Redesign the care system to include a team of non-physician providers such as nurse practitioners, physician assistants, care coordinators, registered dietitians, and physical therapists.
      d) Establish patient care teams that use bundled payments and incentive programs such as accountable care organizations and patient-centered medical homes.
      e) Prioritize and proactively manage preventive care to ensure routine screening and identification of high-risk patients.
      f) Reduce hospital readmission rates for chronic conditions and reduce hospital-acquired infections.

        g) Engage and facilitate shared decision making and self-management inter-
         ventions among the patient, family, and providers.

        h) Simplify medical office administration processes for captured cost savings

        i) Employ patient engagement and monitoring through technology, home
         visits, and interdisciplinary support.

        j) Implement comparative effectiveness research to tailor individualized
         patient care.

C. Current findings: The ACA promotes prevention of disease and encourages Americans to reach their full potential of health and wellness (Koh & Sebelius, 2010).

   1. The legislation has removed barriers to accessing clinical preventive services.

   2. The legislation has removed cost as a barrier to preventive services (Koh & Sebelius, 2010).

   3. Providers and payers adhere to the rated A (strongly recommended) and B (recommended) preventive health screenings made by the U.S. Preventive Services Task Force (USPSTF).

D. The ACA established the National Prevention, Health Promotion and Public Health Council, which includes more than a dozen additional federal agencies to develop a prevention and health strategy for the country (Koh & Sebelius, 2010).

   1. The council will build on the 30-year foundation initiatives of Healthy People, USPSTF, Community Prevention Services Task Force, and the Advisory Committee on Immunization Practices.

   2. Appropriations for the newly formed Prevention and Public Health Fund grew from $500 million in 2010 to $2 billion in fiscal year 2015 and were used to invest in a wide range of prevention and wellness programs administered by the U.S. Department of Health and Human Services (DHHS) (Koh & Sebelius, 2010).

   3. The ACA appropriated $1.5 billion for the National Health Service Corps between 2011 and 2015 to integrate health professionals in underserved areas through Health Resources and Services Administration–funded community health centers (Koh & Sebelius, 2010).

   4. The ACA also established the National Health Care Workforce Commission to analyze the needs to guide future healthcare professional placements throughout the United States.

VI. Center for Medicare and Medicaid Innovation (CMMI)

A. Congress established the CMMI in the ACA to test and evaluate new payment and delivery models.

B. CMMI is charged with identifying, developing, assessing, supporting, and disseminating new care models that reduce expenditures under Medicare, Medicaid, or the Children's Health Insurance Program while improving or maintaining care quality.

C. The ACA suggests that the Innovation Center explore multipayer initiatives to address the Triple Aim to (a) improve the individual experience of care, (b) improve the health of populations, and (c) reduce per capita costs of care for populations (Berenson & Cafarella, 2012).

D. The ACA appropriated $10 billion for CMMI every 10 years, into perpetuity. Although $10 billion per decade represents a major spending commitment, it is still only about 0.1% of Medicare and Medicaid spending (Berenson & Cafarella, 2012).

E. CMMI model areas of funding pertinent to chronic conditions (CMS, n.d.-c)

   1. New care models: Accountable care organizations and similar care models are being designed to incentivize healthcare providers to become accountable

for a patient population and to invest in a healthcare infrastructure and redesigned care processes that provide patients with coordinated care and high-quality, efficient service delivery.

2. Bundled payments for care improvement: Medicare currently makes separate payments to individual providers for the services furnished to the same beneficiary for a single illness or course of treatment (an episode of care). Offering these providers a single, bundled payment for an episode of care will require joint accountability for the patient's care outcomes.

3. Primary care transformation: This transformation will place primary care providers as the key point of contact for a patient's healthcare needs. Strengthening and increasing access to primary care is critical in promoting health and reducing overall healthcare costs.

4. Advanced primary care practices called "medical homes": These care models use a team-based interdisciplinary approach while emphasizing prevention, health information technology, care coordination, and shared decision making between patients and the healthcare team.

5. Initiatives focused on dual Medicare and Medicaid enrollees: Patients enrolled in both Medicare and Medicaid (the "dual eligible") account for a disproportionate share of the programs' expenditures. A fully integrated, person-centered system of care that ensures comprehensive care will better serve this population in a high-quality, cost-effective manner.

6. Initiatives to speed the adoption of best practices: Recent studies indicate that it takes nearly 17 years on average before best practices backed by research are incorporated into widespread clinical practice, and even then, the application of the knowledge is unpredictable. The Innovation Center is partnering with a broad range of healthcare providers, federal agencies, professional societies, and other experts and stakeholders to test new models for disseminating evidence-based best practices and significantly increasing the speed of adoption.

7. Initiatives to accelerate the development and testing of new payment and service delivery models: Currently, multiple innovations are underway that can be used as models to improve the healthcare system. Healthcare delivery models will come from local communities and healthcare leaders from across the nation. Partnership with these local and regional stakeholders will allow CMS to accelerate the testing of models today that may be the next breakthrough tomorrow.

VII. Health Care Payment Learning and Action Network (HCPLAN)

A. In March 2015, President Obama announced the establishment of the HCPLAN to achieve better care, smarter spending, and healthier Americans (CMS, 2016a).

1. DHHS is collaborating with partners in the private, public, and nonprofit sectors to transform the nation's health system to emphasize value over volume.

2. DHHS has reached its goal of tying 30% of Medicare fee-for-service payments to quality or value through alternative payment models by 2016. DHHS hopes to increase this number to 50% by 2018 (CMS, 2015a, 2016a; U.S. DHHS, 2016).

3. DHHS also has set a goal of tying 85% of all Medicare fee-for-service payments to quality or value by 2016 and 90% by 2018 (CMS, 2015a, 2016).

4. HCPLAN's objectives (CMS, 2015a, 2016a)

   a) Offer a convening body to facilitate joint implementation of new payment models of healthcare delivery *b)* Identify areas of agreement and move toward alternative payment models and determine how best to analyze data and report on these new payment models

        c) Collaborate to generate evidence, share approaches, and remove barriers to new models of healthcare delivery

        d) Develop common approaches to core issues such as beneficiary attribution, financial models, benchmarking, quality and performance measurement, risk adjustment, and other pertinent topics

        e) Create implementation guides for payers, purchasers, providers, and consumers

B. The CMS Alliance to Modernize Healthcare (CAMH), operated by the MITRE Corporation, convened the Guiding Committee to provide executive leadership for the HCPLAN.

    1. The 24 Guiding Committee members are influential leaders in their fields and represent diverse stakeholder groups, including providers; health plans; purchasers/employers; consumers/patients; and state, regional, and federal representatives (CMS, 2016a).

    2. The Guiding Committee will begin its work by identifying priorities of the HCPLAN and will provide practical assistance to the achievable fields in 2016 and lay out a strategy for aligning members and achieving the network's goals (CMS, 2016a).

C. Funding of $800 million to support this initiative is designed to support more than 150,000 clinician practices over the next four years in sharing, adapting, and further developing comprehensive quality improvement strategies (U.S. DHHS, 2014).

D. Strategies of the initiative

    1. Promote broad payment and practice reform in primary care and specialty care

    2. Promote care coordination between providers of services and suppliers

    3. Establish community-based health teams to support chronic care management

    4. Promote improved quality and reduced cost by developing a collaborative of institutions that support practice transformation

VIII. Health information technology

A. The Office of the National Coordinator for Health Information Technology (ONC) released *Connecting Health and Care for the Nation: A Shared Nationwide Interoperability Roadmap* in January 2015.

B. ONC laid out a vision for a future health information technology ecosystem where electronic health information is appropriately and readily available to empower consumers and support clinical decision making, inform the American population and public health with value-based payment, and advance the science of information technology use (ONC, 2015).

    1. ONC is committed to leading and collaborating with the health information technology and healthcare sector to define a shared roadmap for achieving interoperable health information technology that will support a broadscale learning health system by 2024 (ONC, 2015).

    2. This roadmap reflects the result of collaborative work among federal, state, community, and private partners. It provides a plan for what needs to happen, by when, and by what responsible entity to see that electronic health information is available to serve the American population (ONC, 2015).

IX. Relevance to practice

A. Between 2009 and 2012, the federal government recorded the largest budget deficit relative to the size of the economy since 1946, causing the U.S. debt to escalate (Lynn & Montgomery, 2015).

B. More rigorous and far-reaching analyses are needed to demonstrate the effectiveness of reforms in the U.S. healthcare delivery system that can produce high-quality results similar to those used in lean manufacturing processes (Womack, Jones, & Roos, 2007).

C. The baby boomers began to turn 65 in 2011; by 2020, the United States will be experiencing a demographic shift in demand for healthcare and long-term care services that will challenge communities, states, and the federal government as never before seen (Lynn & Montgomery, 2015).

D. Every day, 10,000 baby boomers are entering into the Medicare system, and for the first time in history, tens of millions of Americans, including boomers, gen Xers, millennials, and beyond, are on track to become octogenarians and nonagenarians (Montgomery & Lynn, 2014).

   1. It is the dawn of global longevity—Americans are living 20–30 years after the traditional age of retirement (Montgomery & Lynn, 2014).

   2. Before boomers begin to reach old age in 2030, the existing healthcare system cannot meet the needs of middle-aged Americans concerned about the cost and availability of surgical procedures. This misalignment gravely affects the individual care needs of frail elders (Montgomery & Lynn, 2015).

   3. Approximately 5 million Americans were frail elders in 2010, and this is expected to grow to more than 20 million by 2050 (Montgomery & Lynn, 2014).

E. The Center for Elder Care and Advanced Illness at the Altarum Institute has developed the MediCaring® model as a modified Medicare accountable care organization (Lynn, 2013). MediCaring proposes the following elements for reform:

   1. Frail elders who are living with disabilities and lack of physical reserve from advanced age form a special patient population cohort. This is a time to rearrange services and focus on individual patient needs (Lynn, 2013).

   2. Healthcare providers need to comprehensively understand individual patient needs, priorities, and situations and develop longitudinal care planning through interdisciplinary teams (Montgomery & Lynn, 2014).

   3. Long-term care services and supports, such as housing, nutrition, social supports, safety, transportation, personal care needs, and caregiver support, should be broadened and reconfigured. Patients and their caregivers will require support and preparation as they age and disabilities become burdensome (Montgomery & Lynn, 2014).

   4. Healthcare programs should provide local monitoring and management and not rely on state and federal services. Communities need to come together to support the myriad services required of this aging and growing patient population, such as coalitions of healthcare providers, civic leaders, and public government (Montgomery & Lynn, 2014). MediCaring suggests the reorganization of health and social services to create a local entity to monitor and manage this community-based system (Lynn, 2013).

   5. MediCaring requires individualized care plans that reflect elder patients' strengths and needs throughout the trajectory of their life (Lynn, 2013).

X. Supreme Court ruling

  A. A June 22, 2015, United States Supreme Court ruling upheld a critical part of the ACA's confirmation ruling that low- and middle-income residents in the 34 states without healthcare exchanges can continue to receive the federal tax credits that can lower health insurance premiums (Clark, 2015).

B. The 6.4 million Americans who receive subsidies through the federal marketplace are in the conservative Southern states governed by Republican politics (Barnes, 2015).

C. Subsidies can now be allowed for residents of Florida, Georgia, North Carolina, and Texas, where elected officials oppose the healthcare law and have not set up state exchanges (Barnes, 2015).

D. The second largest cohort of Americans to receive healthcare subsidies live in the Midwest and include Illinois, Indiana, Ohio, and Wisconsin (Barnes, 2015).

E. In the 6–3 decision, the justices were asked to interpret a passage in the ACA that said tax credits are authorized for those who buy insurance on marketplaces that are established by the state (Barnes, 2015).

F. Federal exchanges were authorized for states that did not set up their own, and the Obama administration argued that millions of people served by a federal marketplace were entitled to the subsidies (Barnes, 2015).

G. A panel of the U.S. Court of Appeals for the Fourth Circuit previously ruled unanimously that the Internal Revenue Service was within its authority to interpret the law to mean that all Americans should receive the subsidies. The ACA statute authorized the federal healthcare exchange to step in for states that did not establish their own (Barnes, 2015).

XI. Role of the advanced practice registered nurse (APRN)

A. Graduate nurse education demonstration

1. Clinical education for APRNs: The ACA funded $10 million to five hospitals with the requirement that 50% of funding is allocated to community-based education and APRN practice.

2. The primary goal of this demonstration is to increase the provision of qualified training for APRN students, including clinical skills to provide primary care, preventive care, transitional care, chronic care management, and other services appropriate for Medicare beneficiaries (Health Resources and Services Administration, 2012).

B. Independence at Home Demonstration Program

1. This program was created by the ACA and conducted by CMMI to test a home service and payment incentive model that uses home-based primary care teams designed to improve healthcare delivery and payment incentives to improve health outcomes and reduce expenditures for Medicare beneficiaries with multiple chronic conditions.

2. The home-based primary care teams are directed by physicians and nurse practitioners. CMS awards incentive payments to providers who succeed in reducing costs and meeting specific quality measures (CMS, 2016).

C. APRNs are key providers under the ACA and will require a strong understanding and adaptation of the myriad changes unfolding in a healthcare climate that will reimburse for value versus volume or traditional fee-for-service.

1. Remaining current and proactive about the ACA's mandates will promote the potential for reform while recognizing the professional need for significant transformation (Davis, Abrams, & Stremikis, 2011).

2. APRNs will have to understand the role of new payment models such as accountable care organizations, patient-centered medical homes, and bundled care and how these new healthcare models will affect patient care and provider reimbursement.

3. The ACA promotes health prevention and promotion, an ideal position for APRNs, whose primary function is to improve patient-centered outcomes through the implementation of best evidence.
4. Use and implementation of evidence-based interventions can help to reduce hospital admissions, thereby reducing administrative responsibilities and burdens, and to facilitate interdisciplinary coordination across the continuum of care (Davis et al., 2011).
5. The ACA has the potential to realign incentives within the healthcare system and create opportunities for providers to be rewarded for delivering high-value, patient-centered primary care (Davis et al., 2011).
6. Transformation from the ACA will lead to better outcomes for patients, increase job satisfaction among providers, and encourage more sustainable levels of health spending for the nation (Davis et al., 2011).

D. APRNs understand the value of the interdisciplinary team and are the cogs-in-the-wheel who can sort and organize the primary care needs of the patient and family. Competent and skilled APRNs understand how to work with the team and what discipline can support the best interventions in specific clinical situations.

E. APRNs are skilled and knowledgeable about chronic conditions, how symptoms occur throughout the trajectory of disease and debility, and how to effectively assess and evaluate the patient's physical, emotional, social, and spiritual needs through interdisciplinary partners.

F. APRNs are required to stay current with health policy and the issues affecting patient-centered outcomes through the use of comparative effectiveness research to achieve cost-effective comprehensive care.

G. APRNs demonstrate leadership through the use of evidence to direct the clinical care needs of patients with concomitant chronic conditions and do not rely on anecdotal and culture-centric practices that promote costly off-label uses or interventions that are outside of current guidelines.

H. APRNs recognize that USPSTF is the federal entity that directs healthcare screenings and standards of care associated with health promotion and prevention.

I. To effectively practice and meet the medical management needs of America's largest patient population, APRNs require knowledge of the roles and responsibilities of the various entities under DHHS, including the Agency for Healthcare Research and Quality, the Patient-Centered Outcomes Research Institute, the National Quality Forum, the Centers for Disease Control and Prevention, CMMI, and the National Heart, Lung, and Blood Institute, among others, who direct and define specific practice patterns that influence optimal outcomes.

J. APRNs will remain current and trained in new technology associated with electronic health record and technology devices used to support patients and their families in the communities.

K. APRNs will participate in shared decision making between providers and patient family needs, using and implementing self-management practices to empower patients to take accountability for their own health and quality of life.

XII. Interface to palliative care

A. Title IV of the ACA is focused on effective management of chronic conditions, and the newly formed CMS chronic care reimbursement model provides patients and families with 24/7 access to his or her primary care providers to ensure coordinated and comprehensive healthcare management throughout the disease trajectory from diagnosis to death.

1. Palliative care interventions that have a primary focus on symptom management should be integrated at the onset of a diagnosis of symptomatic conditions and not reserved for end-of-life care (Kuebler, 2012).
2. The intensity of palliative care interventions is heightened as the patient approaches end of life when symptoms are escalated.
3. Evidence-based interventions should be implemented to support the value versus volume criteria of the ACA to ensure patient-centric outcomes.
4. The use and implementation of practice or cultural-centric interventions that are not based on current evidence is discouraged, and the use of guideline recommendations is encouraged.
5. Healthcare providers should rely on sufficient evidence to support off-label use of any intervention that has not been approved by the U.S. Food and Drug Administration (FDA) to ensure safety and efficacy for the patient population living with and dying from symptomatic chronic conditions.
6. Healthcare providers should recognize the FDA's position statement on the use of compounded medications that have not undergone FDA approval testing for safety and efficacy (U.S. FDA, 2016).

B. The use of shared decision making and self-care management initiatives that are integral components of Title IV of the ACA should be implemented in the care plan for patients in the palliative care setting.
1. The interdisciplinary team should collaborate and work together with the patient and family to address and effectively manage the myriad needs associated with the advancing stages of chronic conditions.
2. Discussions on advance care planning should remain dynamic and occur frequently to ensure that patient and family needs are continuously assessed and evaluated.
3. Use of shared decision making and self-management allows the patient and family to be actively involved in the patient's care and become adequately prepared to meet the physical, emotional, social, and spiritual demands associated with advancing disease and a poor prognosis.
4. Encouraging shared decision making and self-management practices will reduce a crisis-like approach to end-of-life care and help to reduce associated costs from an uncoordinated care delivery system of multiple providers.

C. Accountable care organizations, medical home models, and bundled services will need to demonstrate the coordination and inclusion of palliative care in the optimal management of patients with symptomatic chronic conditions and not perpetuate the uncoordinated and costly approach that currently exists for this patient population.
1. Patient-centered outcomes generated from comparative effectiveness research will provide the direction for the best approach to ensure individualized patient-centric care.
2. The community-centered approach to care that comes from the ACA models encourages multiple stakeholders to ensure best care and services for the frail elderly and those who are dwindling and require extensive support services to address and meet the care needs of this growing U.S. patient population.
3. The ACA has created several opportunities to partner with multiple disciplines within a community to demonstrate a collaborative commitment to meet the individualized care of patients living with and dying from symptomatic chronic conditions.

Case Study

M.K. is a 79-year-old homebound Caucasian woman who lives with multiple chronic conditions, including congestive heart failure, chronic obstructive pulmonary disease, osteoarthritis, obesity, and depression. Because of her homebound status, she has difficulty accessing medical care, getting groceries, banking, and attending her Sunday church services. M.K. does not have a support system in her community, and her two children live a full-day plane trip away.

M.K. fell in her home and was able to access her phone to call 911. She was taken to the emergency department and admitted to the hospital with a diagnosis of a fractured right hip requiring immediate surgery, anemia, dehydration, and urinary tract infection. Following surgical repair of her hip, she was transferred for six weeks of rehabilitation to strengthen and increase her physical functioning.

Her two children were worried about M.K. returning to her home and being physically functional. Homecare services will follow M.K. for a short period of time. M.K.'s children quickly learned about her primary care provider (PCP), who participates in the chronic care reimbursement model. M.K. now pays her PCP $8 a month to gain access to her physician's office 24 hours a day, seven days a week. Medicare reimburses her PCP a little more than $40 a month to provide a minimum of 20 minutes a month by directly calling her to check in and make sure that she is maintaining her physical functioning and evaluating the need for further services. M.K.'s children feel much better leaving her in her home knowing that she has a direct line to her PCP's office for any emergent needs she might encounter.

References

American Recovery and Reinvestment Act, Pub. L. No. 111-5, 123 Stat. 115. (2009). Retrieved from https://www.whitehouse.gov/recovery/about

Barnes, R. (2015, April 5). Supreme Court hears lots of interpretations of what it just said. *Washington Post*. Retrieved from https://www.washingtonpost.com/politics/courts_law/supreme-court-hears-lots-of-interpretations-of-what-it-just-said/2015/04/05/8af13aaa-d9a2-11e4-b3f2-607bd612aeac_story.html

Berenson, R.A., & Cafarella, N. (2012). The Center for Medicare and Medicaid Innovation: Activity on many fronts. Retrieved from http://www.rwjf.org/en/library/research/2012/02/the-center-for-medicare-and-medicaid-innovation.html

Centers for Medicare and Medicaid Services. (n.d.-a). The Affordable Care Act. Retrieved from http://medicaid.gov/affordablecareact/affordable-care-act.html

Centers for Medicare and Medicaid Services. (n.d.-b). The Affordable Care Act in action at CMS. Retrieved from https://www.cms.gov/about-cms/aca/affordable-care-act-in-action-at-cms.html

Centers for Medicare and Medicaid Services. (n.d.-c). Center for Medicare and Medicaid Innovation. Retrieved from https://innovation.cms.gov

Centers for Medicare and Medicaid Services. (2015a, January 26). Better care, smarter spending, healthier people: Paying providers for value, not volume. Retrieved from https://www.cms.gov/Newsroom/Media ReleaseDatabase/Fact-sheets/2015-Fact-sheets-items/2015-01-26-3.html

Centers for Medicare and Medicaid Services. (2015b, August 6). Medicaid incentives for the prevention of chronic diseases model. Retrieved from https://innovation.cms.gov/initiatives/mipcd

Centers for Medicare and Medicaid Services. (2016a, March 3). Health Care Payment Learning and Action Network. Retrieved from https://innovation.cms.gov/initiatives/Health-Care-Payment-Learning-and-Action-Network

Centers for Medicare and Medicaid. (2016b). Independence at home demonstration. Retrieved from https://innovation.cms.gov/initiatives/independence-at-home

Clark, P. (2015, June 25). Upholding affordable health care [Infographic]. *Washington Post*. Retrieved from https://www.washingtonpost.com/national/health-science/upholding-affordable-health-care/2015/06/25/23ffb50c-1b46-11e5-93b7-5eddc056ad8a_graphic.html

Davis, K., Abrams, M., & Stremikis, K. (2011). How the Affordable Care Act will strengthen the nation's primary care foundation. *Journal of General Internal Medicine, 26,* 1201–1203. doi:10.1007/s11606-011-1720-y

Health Resources and Services Administration. (2012, December 13). Advanced Nursing Education Program (ANE): Fiscal year 2013 technical assistance webinar. Retrieved from http://bhpr.hrsa.gov/nursing/grants/anetawebinarslides12132012.pdf

Kocher, B., Emanuel, E.J., & DeParle, N.-A.M. (2010). The Affordable Care Act and the future of clinical medicine: The opportunities and challenges. *Annals of Internal Medicine, 153,* 536–539. doi:10.7326/0003 -4819-153-8-201010190-00274

Koh, H.K., & Sebelius, K.G. (2010). Promoting prevention through the Affordable Care Act. *New England Journal of Medicine, 363,* 1296–1300. doi:10.1056/NEJMp1008560

Kuebler, K. (2012). Implications for palliative care nursing education. *Clinical Scholars Review, 5,* 86–90.

Lynn, J. (2013). Reliable and sustainable comprehensive care for frail elderly people. *JAMA, 310,* 1935–1936. doi:10.1001/jama.2013.281923

Lynn, J., & Montgomery, A. (2015). Creating a comprehensive care system for frail elders in "age boom" America. *Gerontologist, 55,* 278–285. doi:10.1093/geront/gnu175

Montgomery, A., & Lynn, J. (2014). The MediCaring™ model: Best plan for frail elders in the longevity era. *Public Policy and Aging Report, 24,* 112–117. doi:10.1093/ppar/pru020

Office of the National Coordinator for Health Information Technology. (2015). *Connecting health and care for the nation: A shared nationwide interoperability roadmap* (Final version 1.0). Retrieved from https://www.healthit.gov/sites/default/files/hie-interoperability/nationwide-interoperability-roadmap-final-version-1.0.pdf

Patient Protection and Affordable Care Act, 42 U.S.C. § 18001 et seq. (2010). Retrieved from http://www.hhs.gov/healthcare/about-the-law/read-the-law/index.html

U.S. Department of Health and Human Services. (2014, October 23). HHS secretary announces $840 million initiative to improve patient care and lower costs. Retrieved from http://www.hhs.gov/about/news/2014/10/23/hhs-secretary-announces-840-million-initiative-improve-patient-care-and-lower-costs.html

U.S. Department of Health and Human Services. (2016, March). HHS reaches goal of tying 30 percent of Medicare payments to quality ahead of schedule. Retrieved from http://www.hhs.gov/about/news/2016/03/03/hhs-reaches-goal-tying-30-percent-medicare-payments-quality-ahead-schedule.html

U.S. Food and Drug Administration. (2016, April 15). Compounding Quality Act: Title I of the Drug Quality and Security Act of 2013. Retrieved from http://www.fda.gov/drugs/GuidanceComplianceRegulatoryInformation/PharmacyCompounding

Womack, J.P., Jones, D.T., & Roos, D. (2007). *The machine that changed the world.* New York, NY: Free Press.

CHAPTER 3

Patient-Centered Outcomes of Care

Mary Atkinson Smith, DNP, FNP-BC, ONP-C, RNFA, CNOR,
and Nicole Peters Kroll, PhD, RN, ANP-C

I. Definition
   A. Outcomes of care are described as a patient's state of health that results from receiving health care (National Quality Measures Clearinghouse, 2015). Patient-centered outcomes (PCOs) are derived from a partnership between healthcare providers, patients, and family members and focus on patient preferences, needs, education, and support in a manner that enhances informed decision making and participation in self-management among patients (Institute of Medicine, 2001).
   B. In 1988, the Pickler/Commonwealth Patient-Centered Care Program used the term *patient-centered care* to highlight the charge by healthcare providers, systems, and staff to move the focus from diagnosis and management of diseases to a patient-centered approach to care that identifies patient and family (Allshouse, 1993).
   C. PCOs emerged from section 6301 of the Patient Protection and Affordable Care Act (ACA) and have guided the development of the Patient-Centered Outcomes Research Institute (PCORI) (U.S. Government Accountability Office, 2010).
   D. The 2010 National Healthcare Disparity Report emphasized the important role of patient-centered care in improving patient-centric outcomes that reduce morbidity and mortality (Agency for Healthcare Research and Quality [AHRQ], 2011).
II. Key aspects
   A. PCORI highlights a national agenda to establish priorities for patient-centered outcomes research (PCOR) by producing data generated from comparative effectiveness research (CER) to better inform patients, healthcare providers, payers, and policy makers on effective and cost-effective treatments (PCORI, 2014). PCORI aims to improve quality of care and outcomes by collecting patient-reported outcomes (PROs) data (Snyder, Jensen, Segal, & Wu, 2013).
   B. PROs data comprise the patient's perspective.
      1. PROs are defined as self-reports of health status provided directly from a patient without the patient's response being interpreted by a healthcare provider or another individual (National Quality Forum [NQF], n.d.-b; U.S. Food and Drug Administration, 2009).
      2. Using available innovative technologies to assist with data collection methods can serve as a facilitator to electronically collect PROs, allowing the perspective of patients to be included in PCOR (Snyder et al., 2013).

3. PROs are beneficial from three points of data collection: population health surveillance, individualized patient–provider communication, and research (Lipscomb, Donaldson, & Hiatt, 2004).
   a) PROs population health surveillance data can be collected from disease registry databases, health-related surveys, and health insurance claims and incorporated into PCOR.
   b) PROs pertaining to individual patient–provider communication can be used in the clinical setting to screen for certain medical conditions, observe progress of patients over a span of time, and aid decision making and can be linked to electronic health records (Greenhalgh, 2009).
   c) In research studies such as clinical trials and observational studies, PROs are used as outcome measures or to provide answers for defined questions (Bing et al., 2000).
C. Patient-reported outcome measures (PROMs) are used to gauge the quality of health care from the patient perspective. Data can be used to close the gap between the healthcare provider and the patient when determining best outcomes. This information is used to guide patient-specific plans of care (Barry & Edgman-Levitan, 2012; Hostetter & Klein, 2012).
D. PROMs are tools developed to standardize the measurement of PROs and assist healthcare providers in understanding, for example, the influence chronic disease has on a patient's life (Nelson et al., 2015).
   1. Standardization of PROMs will provide more objective measures for quality improvement when assessing and determining successful measures.
   2. Patients, providers in clinical practice, researchers, and healthcare organizations can use PROMs to evaluate the quality of provided services (Nelson et al., 2015).
      a) Healthcare organizations may use PROMs for assessing performance, determining value for cost, benchmarking, or guiding quality improvement modalities.
      b) Researchers can use PROMs in clinical trials for screening purposes and evaluation of treatment outcomes.
      c) PROMs will play an integral role in the work produced by PCORI regarding the identification of measures required for CER.
      d) Healthcare providers can use PROMs in clinical practice in assisting a diagnosis and monitoring patient progress.
      e) Patients can benefit from PROMs when choosing a provider or deciding on a specific treatment.
E. The Patient-Reported Outcomes Measurement Information System (PROMIS) is a program established in 2004 and funded by the National Institutes of Health. Its goal is to develop more accurate PROMs and minimize the quantity of inquiries required, which will allow easier PROMs use in clinical practice.
   1. PROMIS collects, measures, and analyzes data pertaining to PCOs to assist researchers, clinicians, and patients in collaboratively defining and validating PROMs pertaining to various diseases, allowing the development of more precise measures (Hostetter & Klein, 2012).
   2. PROMIS has united healthcare providers, patients, and research scientists, enabling these groups to define and endorse PROMs pertaining to the care provided for patients with various disabilities, cancer, or chronic medical conditions (e.g., chronic obstructive pulmonary disease, HIV).

    F. NQF is a nonpartisan, nonprofit organization that focuses on quality improvement in health care by endorsing solidarity standards pertaining to the measurement of performance and ensuring high-quality public reporting of performance (NQF, n.d.-a).

        1. NQF (n.d.-b) promotes high-quality, affordable health care through performance improvement and accountability.

        2. NQF (2013) identified three key clinical aspects to promote PCOs, including health-related quality of life (HRQOL), reduction of symptoms, and engagement in self-management practices that promote healthy lifestyle changes.

    G. The Institute for Healthcare Improvement (IHI) is a nonprofit, independent organization and a leading worldwide innovator in healthcare improvement.

        1. IHI establishes partnerships with healthcare leaders, visionaries, and providers in clinical practice to improve the health status of individual patients and populations (IHI, 2016).

        2. IHI recognizes that PCOs are a mechanism to capture direct reporting from the patient and assist healthcare organizations in transforming into value-based systems of care (IHI, 2016).

III. Current findings

    A. Since the ACA's inception, changes that have occurred have empowered patients through shared decision making and self-management, allowing them to be responsible for their own health outcomes (Sacristán, 2013).

    B. The ACA calls for new "Shared Decisionmaking Resource Centers" (section 3506) to initiate shared decision making into practice. In addition, the Center for Medicare and Medicaid Innovation (section 3021) examines how support tools can be used to improve patient understanding of treatment options (U.S. Government Accountability Office, 2010).

    C. AHRQ, a part of the U.S. Department of Health and Human Services, was funded by ACA to implement PCOR.

        1. AHRQ provides clinician research summaries, consumer research summaries, and online interactive tools to aid patients in the decision-making process as well as tools and data for use by healthcare professionals and policy makers (AHRQ, 2015b).

        2. PCOR promotes quality of care, patient experience, and patient satisfaction with health care, while simultaneously improving health outcomes and decreasing costs (AHRQ, 2015b).

    D. A systematic review of 115 randomized clinical trials compared customary care to decision aids used in direct care for specific disorders. These aids increased patient knowledge and management of their specific diseases by 13%, precipitating an increase in patient involvement by 34% (Stacey et al., 2014).

    E. The use of decision aids when compared to usual care resulted in increased communication between patients and healthcare providers, reduced patients' feelings of being uninformed, decreased the number of people who were passive in making healthcare choices, and lowered the proportion of patients who remained undecided after research intervention. Patient groups receiving decision aids did not differ from the comparison cohort in terms of health outcomes, adherence to choices made, or resources used (Stacey et al., 2014).

    F. Providers, hospitals, and health systems are now being held responsible for patient outcomes. Accountable care organizations (ACOs) are groups of physicians, hospitals, and other healthcare providers that merge together to coordinate quality medical care to Medicare patients.

1. The goals for ACOs are to ensure patients receive the correct care at the correct time, avoid duplication and medical errors, and increase provider accountability and cost containment.
2. When an ACO is successful in supplying quality health care and decreasing spending, it will receive a share of the Medicare savings (Centers for Medicare and Medicaid Services [CMS], 2015b).
3. In contrast, when quality measures are not met and negative patient outcomes occur, risk-bearing ACOs will be assessed a reduction in payment.
4. The original ACOs offered by Medicare included a Medicare Shared Savings Program (MSSP), Advance Payment (AP), and Pioneer.
   a) MSSP assists Medicare fee-for-service providers in becoming ACOs.
   b) AP is a supplementary incentive program for medical providers in the Shared Savings Program (SSP).
   c) The Pioneer model is a program designed for initial adopters of coordinated care; however, it is no longer accepting applications.
5. In 2015, CMS announced the Next Generation (NG) ACO Model and the Comprehensive End-Stage Renal Disease (CESRD) Care Model as benchmarking methods related to expenditures, risks, and quality (CMS, 2015b).
6. Of 353 ACOs that participated in MSSP and Pioneer programs in 2014, CMS reported a total net program savings of $411 million (CMS, 2015b).
   a) The 2014 quality and financial performance results for SSP ACOs that began the program in 2012 and reported in both 2013 and 2014 indicated improvement in 27 of 33 quality measures (CMS, 2015b).
   b) Since the inception of the ACO program, almost 8.9 million combined beneficiaries have been served by the models (CMS, 2015b).
   c) Currently, 477 ACOs exist across the SSP, Pioneer, NG, and CESRD models. Of these, 64 are in risk-bearing tracks (CMS, 2015b).
IV. Relevance to practice
   A. In an attempt to control healthcare expenses, there is movement to change payment models from patient focused to population based, which reward providers who successfully manage the majority of a patient's health care (Alternative Payment Model [APM] Framework and Progress Tracking Work, 2016). This paradigm shift has allowed greater focus on clinical practice modalities that promote more positive PCOs and improve quality of life through maintaining physical function, minimizing chronic disease exacerbations, and preventing emergency department visits and hospitalizations (Kuebler, 2015).
   B. Scoring systems such as the Hospital Consumer Assessment of Healthcare Providers and Systems are used to influence payment within Medicare's Value-Based Purchasing Program. In 2015, scores were allocated with 30% based on the patient experience and 70% allotted to patient outcomes, core measures, and efficiency (Capko, 2014).
   C. CMS has implemented the Physician Quality Reporting System (PQRS), which uses a combination of incentive payments and payment adjustments to promote quality reporting of information (CMS, 2015b). In 2015, PQRS began applying negative payment adjustments to providers who did not appropriately report transparent quality measures for Medicare Physician Fee Schedule services covered by Medicare (CMS, 2015a, 2015b).
   D. The APM Framework and Progress Tracking Work Group advocates a paradigm shift to shared-risk, population-based payments. APM modified and refined the

payment model originally created by CMS, recognizing that ACOs may use an SSM for several years and transition into a shared-risk model (APM, 2016).

    E. CMS is implementing policies to reward providers financially for offering better coordination of care for Medicare patients.

    F. Patient-centered care based on an interdisciplinary approach has been found to have better patient outcomes. PCORI places the patient at the core of the healthcare team and uses patient involvement in CER, believing the patient is a fundamental team member and affects overall outcomes (PCORI, 2013).

V. Role of the advanced practice registered nurse (APRN)

    A. APRNs play a vital role in highlighting and promoting positive PCOs.

       1. APRNs promoting positive PCOs can only come from exemplar clinical practice, education, leadership, mentoring, understanding and developing health policy, and demonstrating quality measures (Kuebler, 2015).

       2. APRNs can promote and demonstrate innovation, focus on patient engagement, encourage interdisciplinary collaboration, use risk assessment strategies, and implement best evidence to enhance the quality of patient-centered care.

          a) Promoting patient engagement used to enhance PCOs will include educating and empowering patients to take ownership of their own self-management for best outcomes (Kuebler, 2015).

          b) Encouraging patients to use support tools such as AHRQ contributes to promoting their wellness, planning their health care, and understanding their diagnosis (AHRQ, 2015a).

          c) APRNs need to be familiar with their referral sources and their community resources.

          d) Implementation of best care models can assist APRNs in improving patient outcomes.

          e) APRNs must know where to access current clinical guidelines and how to implement them in practice.

       3. Quality guidelines for patient care include but are not limited to those from AHRQ, the U.S. Preventive Services Task Force, PCORI, and the Multiple Chronic Conditions Resource Center, in addition to the U.S. Food and Drug Administration Medication Updates and American Association of Nurse Practitioners SmartBrief Clinical Updates.

       4. Performing risk assessments and patient profiling to determine patients who are at high risk for experiencing negative outcomes (e.g., exacerbations, hospitalizations, hospital readmissions, poor quality of life) is becoming very important in the current healthcare landscape.

          a) Unplanned 30-day risk-standardized readmission rate to hospitals began to receive a 3% penalty in late 2014 (CMS, 2015b).

          b) APRNs can be vital in decreasing readmissions in acute care hospitals by preventing disease exacerbations through prudent symptom management.

       5. Education is an important role for APRNs in the promotion of PCOs.

          a) Remaining current regarding state-of-the-art patient treatments, advances in science and technology, and current medication use is key in the approach to improved health care and will benefit the population.

          b) Continued education allows APRNs to develop or participate in developing evidence-based clinical practice guidelines that promote timely, appropriate, effective, and efficient delivery of healthcare services.

    B. APRNs serve as effective leaders in transforming clinical practice in ways that focus on PCOs. APRNs also are seen as key members of interdisciplinary care teams.

        1. APRNs must grow into leaders by supporting adaptation to current practice changes. These changes inspire and motivate others to achieve a higher level of performance (Smith, 2011).

        2. A priority for APRNs should be to drive the development and implementation of digital technology with the intent and purpose of improving PCOs.

        3. APRNs should strive to participate in and promote innovative practice changes based on PCOs and data results produced from PROMs.

        4. APRNs are leading interdisciplinary teams in clinical practice. Interdisciplinary approaches to patient care improve patient outcomes as well as influence the patient's ability to make better healthcare decisions (Medical Practice Insider, 2012).

    C. APRNs should be available to mentor fellow nurses and APRNs, students, and other professionals in delivering and measuring patient-centered care.

    D. It is imperative that APRNs participate and lead policy-related agendas that focus on evidence-based practice recommendations and advocate for positive outcomes and desirable quality of life for patients with multiple chronic conditions.

        1. Nurses are the largest body of healthcare professionals in the United States and need to harness the collective power that can be used to influence and shape health policy initiatives.

        2. APRNs in independent practice can meet the requirements to be included in an ACO. Current legislation limits the assignment of patients receiving care in an ACO to primary care physicians. Medicare patients who would like to glean benefits from an ACO cannot be assigned to an APRN (American Association of Nurse Practitioners, 2012).

    E. Participating in and supporting the collection and analysis of data to assist with the evaluation and measurement of PCOs is an important component of the APRN role.

    F. PCORI is committed to addressing the questions and concerns most relevant to patients and families.

    G. PCORI funds CER, which presents providers and patients with comparative data suggesting that one intervention is better than another. CER provides important direction to produce improved PCOs (PCORI, 2014).

  VI. Interface to palliative care

    A. Palliative care providers, as with other healthcare disciplines, are focusing on improving quality of life, assisting in decision making, and controlling costs (Antunes, Harding, & Higginson, 2014; McKinney, 2013).

        1. PCOs are important in providing significance to palliative care; however, current findings are limited (Etkind et al., 2015).

        2. A Michigan-based ACO focusing on outcomes of patients with late-stage chronic diseases showed significant patient-centered cost savings, a decrease in the number of days spent in the intensive care unit, and a reduction in hospital admissions (McKinney, 2013).

    B. The term *patient-centered outcome measures* (PCOMs) encompasses both patient- and proxy-reported measures with an emphasis on concerns important to the patient (Etkind et al., 2015).

        1. This is especially important for patients with multiple chronic diseases who are unable to speak for themselves and need family or caregivers to speak for them.

    2. Palliative care was one of the early disciplines to begin to adopt PCOMs, as literature focusing on PCOs dates back as early as 1985 (Etkind et al., 2015).

    3. Strong evidence supports that PCOM feedback on the healthcare process permits increased responsiveness and holistic care in the following ways (Etkind et al., 2015):

        a) Heightened awareness of symptoms

        b) Elevated communication concerning HRQOL

        c) Increased referrals from providers based on patients' HRQOL

    4. Statistics suggest moderate evidence that PCOM data have a positive effect on emotional and psychological HRQOL. However, some indication exists that PCOMs do not improve overall HRQOL in palliative care (Etkind et al., 2015).

    5. Routine use of PCOMs in palliative care practices has been slow and challenging to execute (Antunes et al., 2014).

    6. Online PCOMs and training in palliative care resources are becoming more readily available (Antunes et al., 2014).

C. Specific healthcare decision aids for palliative care patients and caregivers are available online. Some organizations that provide these tools include the Center to Advance Palliative Care, the National Hospice and Palliative Care Organization, the National Institute of Nursing Research, and AHRQ.

D. To foster quality palliative care and encourage consistent high standards and continuity across the palliative care continuum, clinical guidelines have been established. Guidelines can be obtained specifically related to palliative care from the National Consensus Project for Quality Palliative Care, the Multiple Chronic Conditions Resource Center, the Centre for Palliative Care, and the National Comprehensive Cancer Network®.

Case Study

X.P. is an 80-year-old woman who is a retired school teacher with a medical history of hypertension, dementia, and depression. She was diagnosed with colorectal cancer in the past year and has recently become homebound. She occasionally takes acetaminophen 1,000 mg every four hours, as needed, for minor aches and pains. She has a prescription for tramadol 50 mg PO every eight hours for pain, as needed. Over the past year, X.P. has been hospitalized eight times because of her physical decline from managing her malignancy.

The APRN makes a house call after learning from X.P.'s daughter that her mother had become progressively agitated, with several episodes of urinary incontinence and a dramatic change in her cognitive status. The daughter is concerned her mother is in pain. The APRN performs a dipstick of the patient's urine and finds it positive for nitrates, trace blood, and leukocytes. The APRN recognizes the multiple issues that can be contributing to X.P.'s presenting symptoms and sudden changes.

Based on the physical examination, the APRN determines that X.P. is dehydrated and has somatic pain with movement of her bilateral hips that is exacerbated with position changes and when attempting to ambulate. X.P. has continued to take her daily lisinopril 20 mg, despite having a blood pressure of 146/88 mm Hg. She has been taking amitriptyline 20 mg at bedtime for the depression and neuropathy that she developed following chemotherapy.

Based on the most current evidence-based guidelines, the APRN recognizes that the majority of the patient's problems can easily be resolved by modifying her medications and infusing IV fluids for fluid and volume replacement. The APRN provides the daughter with the following information and changes in X.P.'s plan of care:

- Discontinue all use of tramadol and acetaminophen, as both of these medications stimulate the central nervous system and can create cognitive changes, complicated further by her urinary tract infection.
- Prescribe sulfamethoxazole-trimethoprim 500 mg BID for three days.
- Recommend celecoxib 200 mg daily to control her somatic musculoskeletal pain.
- Discontinue lisinopril, as the guidelines from the Eighth Joint National Committee (James et al., 2014) increased the normal range of blood pressure (e.g., 140/90 mm Hg).
- Discontinue the amitriptyline because of its anticholinergic side effects and place X.P. on duloxetine for her chemotherapy-related neuropathy and to manage her depression.

The APRN recognizes the value of implementing best practices through the use of current guidelines taken from AHRQ representing standard of care. Accessing and implementing guidelines in the clinical management of X.P. will assist in promoting improved PCOs.

References

Agency for Healthcare Research and Quality. (2011). *2010 national healthcare disparities report.* Retrieved from http://archive.ahrq.gov/research/findings/nhqrdr/nhdr10/nhdr10.pdf

Agency for Healthcare Research and Quality. (2015a). Patients and consumers. Retrieved from http://www.ahrq.gov/patients-consumers/index.html

Agency for Healthcare Research and Quality. (2015b). Surveys and tools to advance patient-centered care: Shared decision-making. Retrieved from http://www.ahrq.gov/cahps/quality-improvement/improvement-guide/6-strategies-for-improving/communication/strategy6i-shared-decisionmaking.html

Allshouse, K.D. (1993). Treating patients as individuals. In M. Gerteis, S. Edgman-Levitan, L. Daley, & T. Delbanco (Eds.), *Through the patient's eyes: Understanding and promoting patient-centered care* (pp. 19–27). San Francisco, CA: Jossey-Bass.

Alternative Payment Model Framework and Progress Tracking Work Group. (2016). *Alternative payment model (APM) framework: Final white paper.* Retrieved from https://hcp-lan.org/workproducts/apm-whitepaper.pdf

American Association of Nurse Practitioners. (2012, June). Fact sheet: Accountable care organizations (ACO). Retrieved from https://www.aanp.org/legislation-regulation/federal-legislation/medicare/68-articles/343-accountable-care-organizations

Antunes, B., Harding, R., & Higginson, I.J. (2014). Implementing patient-reported outcome measures in palliative care clinical practice: A systematic review of facilitators and barriers. *Palliative Medicine, 28,* 158–175. doi:10.1177/0269216313491619

Barry, M.J., & Edgman-Levitan, S. (2012). Shared decision making—The pinnacle of patient-centered care. *New England Journal of Medicine, 366,* 780–781. doi:10.1056/NEJMp1109283

Bing, E.G., Hays, R.D., Jacobson, L.P., Chen, B., Gange, S.J., Kass, N.E., ... Zucconi, S.L. (2000). Health-related quality of life among people with HIV disease: Results from the Multicenter AIDS Cohort Study. *Quality of Life Research, 9,* 55–63. doi:10.1023/A:1008919227665

Capko, J. (2014). The patient-centered movement. *Journal of Medical Practice Management, 29,* 238–242.

Centers for Medicare and Medicaid Services. (2015a, December 2). Shared Savings Program. Retrieved from https://www.cms.gov/Medicare/Medicare-Fee-for-Service-Payment/sharedsavingsprogram/index.html

Centers for Medicare and Medicaid Services. (2015b). *2015 Physician Quality Reporting System (PQRS): Implementation guide.* Retrieved from http://www.cms.gov/Medicare/Quality-Initiatives-Patient-Assessment-Instruments/PQRS/Downloads/2015_PQRS_ImplementationGuide.pdf

Etkind, S.N., Daveson, B.A., Kwok, W., Witt, J., Bausewein, C., Higginson, I.J., & Murtagh, F.E.M. (2015). Capture, transfer, and feedback of patient-centered outcomes data in palliative care populations: Does it make a difference? A systematic review. *Journal of Pain and Symptom Management, 49,* 611–624. doi:10.1016/j.jpainsymman.2014.07.010

Greenhalgh, J. (2009). The applications of PROs in clinical practice: What are they, do they work, and why? *Quality of Life Research, 18,* 115–123. doi:10.1007/s11136-008-9430-6

Hostetter, M., & Klein, S. (2012). Using patient-reported outcomes to improve health care quality. *Quality Matters.* Retrieved from http://www.commonwealthfund.org/publications/newsletters/quality-matters/2011/december-january-2012/in-focus

Institute for Healthcare Improvement. (2016). About us. Retrieved from http://www.ihi.org/about/Pages/default.aspx

Institute of Medicine. (2001). *Envisioning the national health care quality report.* Washington, DC: National Academies Press.

James, P.A., Oparil, S., Carter, B.L., Cushman, W.C., Dennison-Himmelfarb, C., Handler, J., … Ortiz, E. (2014). 2014 evidence-based guideline for the management of high blood pressure in adults: Report from the panel members appointed to the Eighth Joint National Committee (JNC 8). *JAMA, 311,* 507–520. doi:10.1001/jama.2013.284427

Kuebler, K. (2015). Federal initiatives in self-management for patients with multiple chronic conditions: Implications for the doctor of nursing practice. *Clinical Scholars Review, 8,* 139–144. doi:10.1891/1939-2095.8.1.139

Lipscomb, J., Donaldson, M.S., & Hiatt, R.A. (2004). Cancer outcomes research and the arenas of application. *Journal of the National Cancer Institute Monographs, 2004,* 1–7. doi:10.1093/jncimonographs/lgh038

McKinney, M. (2013). Beyond hospice: New models of care focus on advanced illnesses. *Modern Healthcare, 43*(17), 14–15.

Medical Practice Insider. (2012, April). Interprofessional care teams improve clinical outcomes [Press release]. Retrieved from http://www.medicalpracticeinsider.com/press-release/interprofessional-care-teams-improve-clinical-outcomes

National Quality Forum. (n.d.-a). About us. Retrieved from http://www.qualityforum.org/story/About_Us.aspx

National Quality Forum. (n.d.-b). Patient-reported outcomes. Retrieved from http://www.qualityforum.org/Projects/n-r/Patient-Reported_Outcomes/Patient-Reported_Outcomes.aspx

National Quality Forum. (2013, December). *Patient-reported outcomes in performance measurement.* Retrieved from http://www.qualityforum.org/Publications/2012/12/Patient-Reported_Outcomes_in_Performance_Measurement.aspx

National Quality Measures Clearinghouse. (2015). Selecting health outcome measures for clinical quality measurement. Retrieved from http://www.qualitymeasures.ahrq.gov/tutorial/HealthOutcomeMeasure.aspx

Nelson, E.C., Eftimovska, E., Lind, C., Hager, A., Wasson, J.H., & Lindblad, S. (2015). Patient reported outcome measures in practice. *BMJ, 350,* g7818. doi:10.1136/bmj.g7818

Patient-Centered Outcomes Research Institute. (2014). Why PCORI was created. Retrieved from http://www.pcori.org/about-us/why-pcori-was-created

Sacristán, J.A. (2013). Patient-centered medicine and patient-oriented research: Improving health outcomes for individual patients. *BMC Medical Informatics and Decision Making, 13,* 6. doi:10.1186/1472-6947-13-6

Smith, M.A. (2011). Are you a transformational leader? *Nursing Management, 42*(9), 44–50. doi:10.1097/01.NUMA.0000403279.04379.6a

Snyder, C.F., Jensen, R.E., Segal, J.B., & Wu, A.W. (2013). Patient-reported outcomes (PROs): Putting the patient perspective in patient-centered outcomes research. *Medical Care, 51,* S73–S79. doi:10.1097/MLR.0b013e31829b1d84

Stacey, D., Légaré, F., Col, N.F., Bennett, C.L., Barry, M.J., Eden, K.B., … Wu, J.H.C. (2014). Decision aids for people facing health treatment or screening decisions. *Cochrane Database of Systematic Reviews, 2014*(1). doi:10.1002/14651858.CD001431.pub4

U.S. Food and Drug Administration. (2009). *Guidance for industry: Patient-reported outcome measures: Use in medical product development to support labeling claims.* Retrieved from http://www.fda.gov/downloads/Drugs/Guidances/UCM193282.pdf

U.S. Government Accountability Office. (2010). Subtitle D—Patient-centered outcomes research. Retrieved from http://www.gao.gov/about/hcac/pcor_sec_6301.pdf

CHAPTER 4

Self-Management in Chronic Disease

Rosanne Burson, DNP, ACNS-BC, CDE, FAADE,
and Katherine Moran, DNP, RN, CDE, FAADE

I. Definitions
  A. Self-management is defined as an individual's capability to detect and manage the symptoms, treatments, physical and psychosocial consequences, and lifestyle changes inherent in living with multiple chronic conditions (MCCs) (Barlow, Wright, Sheasby, Turner, & Hainsworth, 2002).
    1. Self-management occurs in the context of everyday life.
    2. This includes development of patient confidence to deal with medical, role, and emotional management associated with MCCs.
      a) Medical management includes taking medications as prescribed and attending medical and therapeutic appointments.
      b) Role management allows for adapting to changes in lifestyle, behavioral management, and life roles.
      c) Learning to live with MCCs and evolving health status changes can affect perceived quality of life.
      d) Incorporating needed lifestyle changes for each condition can result in complex regimens.
      e) Life roles in work, the family, and society may be affected, which can change the way patients are viewed by themselves and others.
      f) Emotional management includes processing emotions that arise from living with debilitating or symptomatic MCCs (Schulman-Green et al., 2012).
    3. Self-management is a process of patients and families enhancing knowledge and beliefs (e.g., self-efficacy, outcome expectations), self-regulation skills and abilities (e.g., goal setting, self-monitoring, decision making, planning and action, emotional control), and social facilitation (e.g., support, collaboration) to achieve both proximal and distal health-related outcomes (Ryan, 2009; Ryan & Sawin, 2009; Schulman-Green et al., 2012; Self-Management Science Center, n.d.).
    4. Outcomes for self-management behaviors and costs of healthcare services
      a) Proximal outcomes include patients who self-manage and are empowered to monitor and preemptively manage symptoms that can precipitate disease exacerbations through behavioral change activities (e.g., dietary

changes, correct medication use, open and ongoing communication with their healthcare team).

b) Distal outcomes evaluate health status, quality of life, and cost of health.

c) Self-management applies to MCC management, prevention, and optimal health promotion.

5. With MCCs, multiple providers and care settings exist, which may lead to poor coordination or collaboration of care. The lack of care coordination and the added burdens of personal care may interfere with patients' ability to self-manage.

6. Additional factors affecting self-management include patient demographics (e.g., age, socioeconomic status, education, culture, disease burden, intensity of medical management, support system) and system factors (e.g., communication with providers, ability to engage in shared decision making [SDM] with healthcare provider) (Schulman-Green et al., 2012).

B. Self-management support includes interventions and education within systems by healthcare providers that serve to strengthen patient abilities in managing health problems (Brady, 2011).

1. Success requires ongoing assessment and evaluation of progress through setting goals and determining problem-solving support.

2. Self-management support is recognized as a key component in improving the overall health of a population (Liddy, Blazkho, & Mill, 2014).

C. Self-management education requires interactive educational interventions specifically designed to enhance individual patient engagement.

1. Self-management education is patient specific and focuses on building and developing skills that include goal setting, SDM, problem solving, and self-monitoring (Brady, 2011).

2. The ability to succeed in solving patient-identified problems increases self-efficacy (Bodenheimer, Lorig, Holman, & Grumbach, 2002).

D. SDM occurs when a healthcare provider and a patient work together to make the best healthcare decisions for the patient at the clinical encounter (Gionfriddo et al., 2014).

1. Decisions should take into account evidence-based information about available options. The clinician and the patient share their knowledge, values, and preferences together.

2. The benefit of SDM is that the patient will have an increased knowledge of the options available with an accurate expectation of benefits and risks.

a) The decision that is made is consistent with the patient's values and increases patient participation.

b) This method has been shown to reduce decision conflict and the proportion of patients who are passive in the decision-making process, which may improve clinical outcomes.

3. Clinician satisfaction also is improved when this approach is used in the care of patients with chronic conditions. This is a patient-centered approach to practice, where whole-person knowledge and respect for patient preferences and relationships are valued (Ferrer & Gill, 2013).

II. Key aspects

A. Self-management is a popular subject and is used to promote health and wellness in patients living with MCCs.

1. Health behavior theories are used by providers to better understand a patient's ability to self-manage chronic conditions.

2. Theories such as the ecological theory of health behavior, the health belief model, the social cognitive theory, and the transtheoretical model (stages of change) all explore internal and external factors that can influence a patient's ability to implement and maintain healthy behaviors (Evans, 2013). For example, a patient's external factors may include pressure from family members to stop smoking in order to improve health. Internal factors may include a feeling of accomplishment when quitting smoking.

B. The understanding of concepts related to self-management has evolved to include self-efficacy, empowerment, and therapeutic relationships. The transition of self-management has moved from a perspective of compliance to one of adherence. This adherence goes from and through the patient, then to the provider, and finally to SDM that considers all aspects important to the patient (Agency for Healthcare Research and Quality [AHRQ], 2015; Burson & Moran, 2015).

    1. Empowering patients suggests that patients make their own healthcare choices from available therapeutic options.

    2. Criteria for optimal patient-centered outcomes are met through the use and implementation of self-management.

    3. A collaborative partnership exists between providers, patients, and the healthcare team.

    4. Patients are informed, motivated, and involved as partners in their own health care.

C. Self-determination theory has been used to better understand patient motivation.

    1. Motivation is driven by an individual's basic psychological need for autonomy (to be in control or given a choice), competence (through mastery over challenges), and relatedness (by connecting with others).

    2. When these three conditions occur, individuals have what is referred to as *intrinsic motivation* to pursue things meaningful to them (Ryan & Deci, 2000).

    3. The key to achieving intrinsic motivation is supportive coaching with evaluation of patient readiness to change.

D. Self-management requires a process that eventually empowers patients to take charge of their healthcare management.

    1. Historically, patients are provided treatment plans versus being actively engaged in the process of self-management.

    2. Patients, when first exposed to the concept of self-management, may not understand its basic premise and the importance of active participation and implementation to alter unhealthy behaviors.

    3. Patients will require interdisciplinary healthcare support during this transition.

    4. Patients should be viewed as the experts in their own health care and empowered to manage the challenging and complex care needs associated with MCCs.

    5. Tasks for healthcare team members to complete to effectively offer optimal self-management support include the following:

        a) Perform an assessment of their own personal and professional attitudes for the implementation of SDM between patients and the healthcare team that directs and empowers patient self-management.

        b) Identify professional skills to implement when approaching patients and encouraging engagement in self-management.

        c) Participate in SDM with patients to determine a specific and dynamic patient-centered care plan to ensure success in patient implementation and engagement.

III. Current findings
   A. Self-management can be used to reduce risk factors that precipitate disease exacerbations, promote adherence to medication and therapy, increase physical activity, and reduce hospital admission rates (Kuebler, 2015).
   B. Self-management has gained national prominence as a broader concept in patient healthcare education. Governments in many developed countries have successfully demonstrated how to manage the escalating costs of chronic disease in aging populations by shifting healthcare responsibilities to patients and families (Redman, 2013).
   C. Healthcare policy is influencing self-management.
      1. The Patient Protection and Affordable Care Act (ACA) has influenced massive initiatives in self-management in an era of value over volume and quality measures (U.S. Department of Health and Human Services [DHHS], 2016).
      2. The MCC Strategic Framework has identified self-management as one of four key directives in the care and management of patients living with and dying from more than two concomitant conditions (Centers for Medicare and Medicaid Services [CMS], 2016). The MCC Strategic Framework directs the following strategies:
         a) Develop and improve evidence-based self-care management activities and programs.
         b) Develop systems to promote models that address common risk factors and challenges associated with many chronic conditions.
         c) Enhance sustainability of evidence-based self-management activities and programs.
         d) Improve the efficiency, quality, and cost-effectiveness of evidence-based self-management activities and programs.
   D. The majority of self-management programs and current initiatives in the United States occur as community- and home-based services. Using these systems would accomplish the following (U.S. DHHS, 2010):
      1. Improve access to effective community- and home-based services for the MCC population through information and referral, options counseling, and smooth care transitions between healthcare settings.
      2. Provide training and information on evidence-based self-management and improve support for family caregivers.
      3. Improve infrastructure (e.g., telemonitoring, shared information services) and promote educational and technological innovations that permit people with MCCs to remain maximally functional and independent, understand and better manage their conditions, and reside safely in their homes or other settings.
   E. The Patient-Centered Outcomes Research Institute (PCORI) was authorized by Congress to fund comparative effectiveness research (PCORI, 2014).
      1. Focuses on outcomes that matter to the patient
      2. Compares benefits and harms of interest, such as quality of life, mobility, ability to carry out tasks, ability to focus, return to work, side effects, symptoms, and survival
      3. Aims to inform patients and providers as they make decisions
      4. Compares and weighs the options
      5. Provides decision aids that can be used to facilitate SDM. *Decision aids* are "tools designed to help people participate in decision-making about two or more healthcare options.... [They] provide information about the options and

help patients to clarify and communicate the personal values that they associate with different features of the options" (Volk & Llewellyn-Thomas, 2012, p. 2).

F. Stanford's Chronic Disease Self-Management Program is the largest federal project in the country and is used to spread self-management programs throughout the United States (Stanford Medicine, n.d.).

1. This project is led by the U.S. Administration on Aging, with participation from the Centers for Disease Control and Prevention and CMS.
2. The program enables older Americans with chronic diseases to learn how to self-manage and take control of their health.
3. Content includes stress management, the benefits of physical activity and good nutrition, and communication with healthcare providers. Action plans are developed through planning and feedback (Kuebler, 2015).
4. People with different chronic health problems attend together.
5. Workshops are facilitated by two trained leaders, one of whom has a chronic disease.

G. The Self-Management Alliance (http://ncoa_archive.ncoa.org/improve-health/center-for-healthy-aging/national-self-management.html) is a collaboration between nonprofits, businesses, and government dedicated to achieving the second goal of the MCC Strategic Framework. Goals of the Self-Management Alliance include the following:

1. Establish a shared measurement framework for self-management.
2. Leverage resources to build a national network.
3. Increase awareness and activate people with MCCs.
4. Develop and maintain a skilled workforce.
5. Address critical gaps in knowledge.
6. Create a national dialogue on medication management.
7. Develop a supportive policy environment.

H. CMS has a chart book on chronic conditions among Medicare beneficiaries, which includes state reports on prevalence of MCCs and utilization/spending (see www.cms.gov/Research-Statistics-Data-and-Systems/Statistics-Trends-and-Reports/Chronic-Conditions/index.html).

I. AHRQ's SHARE program offers webinars related to SDM (see www.ahrq.gov/professionals/education/curriculum-tools/shareddecisionmaking/index.html).

IV. Relevance to practice

A. Consider the patient's perspective as a unique individual. Identify individual patient internal challenges related to MCCs.

B. Patients can feel overwhelmed or resilient and determined to persevere. Understanding patients' current perspective will give the team insight into their changing needs and their ability to self-manage.

C. Physical and emotional symptoms and impaired physical functioning can prevent patients from completing self-management tasks.

1. Examples include depression and pain, which can decrease motivation and energy or increase anxiety, sleep disturbances, and worry (Liddy et al., 2014).
2. Cognitive strategies that can help patients overcome barriers include prioritizing conditions, reframing and regulating the amount of attention given to each condition, encouraging patients to engage in life and body listening, or relinquishing control to another source (e.g., a doctor, God).
3. Linking to other existing self-management practices can accommodate additional conditions. For instance, some of the same skills used by a patient suc-

cessfully incorporating dietary changes in the management of hypercholesterolemia also can be used to self-manage dietary changes for diabetes.

D. Social support can be a barrier to self-management. Both lack of support and too much family or friend interference can be viewed as barriers.

E. Lack of financial resources can contribute to barriers in self-management (e.g., no insurance, expensive medications, inability to access health care) as well as changes in work abilities that affect financial status.

   1. Myriad factors can influence a patient's ability to engage in self-management practices, including culture, gender, age, literacy levels, and readiness to change.

   2. The successful implementation of self-management will require an individualized approach with SDM that focuses on patient-specific goals working within the health system.

F. Patients report that they do not always have a therapeutic relationship with their provider.

   1. This may be related to current healthcare systems set up from an acute care rather than chronic care approach, or it may be related to specific care providers.

   2. Issues that have been identified (Liddy et al., 2014)

      a) Contradictory knowledge and instructions

      b) Poor access—in relation to convenience and urgent concerns

      c) Challenges with medication, such as issues related to side effects, coordination, and overreliance

G. To overcome these barriers, providers should adopt strategies that foster shared power and responsibility: Develop a therapeutic environment that includes truly listening to the patient, focus on providing simple information, use integrated care plans that are individualized, and take time to clarify conflicting treatment.

H. Provider/healthcare team perspective

   1. An assessment of the provider/healthcare team's knowledge and skills concerning self-management is essential to a successful therapeutic relationship. Consider the provider/healthcare team's values, attitudes, and judgments toward those with chronic disease.

      a) Is there a sense of blame toward those who have been unable to make lifestyle changes or participate in self-management?

      b) Is there a commitment to SDM rather than a view of the need for adherence to a prescribed behavior?

      c) Self-reflection is important to identify any bias that may be preventing the provider from developing an environment that can be helpful for the patient.

      d) If the provider feels that something is a waste of time or takes too long, the patient will feel judged.

      e) It is important to address negative beliefs.

      f) The provider will set the stage with the patient, opening up opportunities for collaboration that will empower the patient to participate in self-management.

   2. It is only with shared knowledge, power, and autonomy that the patient–provider partnership will develop.

      a) Understanding what the patient and provider each bring to the table is critical in the development of the partnership, where honesty and respect are demonstrated as information is shared, consensus is built, and plans are made.

  b) While clinicians bring knowledge about treatment options, experience, and an open, nonjudgmental attitude, patients bring knowledge about themselves, their preferences, and their experiences.
3. Identify the skill level the provider has in building a therapeutic relationship and initiating an SDM framework.
4. Steps of the SHARE approach
  a) Seek the patient's participation. Explain the need for potential treatment options.
  b) Help the patient explore and compare treatment options.
  c) For informed decision making to occur, the provider must present quantified risk information in a way the patient can understand.
  d) Describe the alternatives in detail using decision support tools.
  e) Help the patient explore the options, taking values and preferences into consideration.
  f) Reach decisions with the patient. Solutions are seen "in harmony with larger patterns of patient lives and clinical practice" (Ferrer & Gill, 2013, p. 303).
  g) Evaluate the patient's decision.
5. Different situations will require unique approaches.
6. Having a toolbox of skills used at the right time with the right person will increase the confidence of the provider, the experience for the patient, and ultimately, the success of the encounter.
7. Motivational interviewing is an evidence-based communication approach.
  a) The goal is to support patients' self-determined goals rather than to impose goals.
  b) The motivational interviewing approach explores an individual's commitment to changing a behavior, while respectfully encouraging goals that will help the individual achieve identified goals (Elwyn et al., 2014).
  c) Steps of motivational interviewing
    (1) Affirming: Provide authentic support for what the patient is accomplishing. This genuine approach engages the patient and begins the relationship.
    (2) Active listening: Identify barriers and work collaboratively with patients.
      (a) Active listening with reflections and support is therapeutic.
      (b) Reflection leads to insight, which leads to change.
      (c) Psychosocial issues are the main barriers to self-management (Funnell, 2015).
      (d) Active listening enables identification of a focus and a direction for change.
    (3) Engaging the patient: Focus on collaboration, not confrontation. This step develops patient motivation.
    (4) Helping patients become involved in their own care: Develop a plan that fosters commitment to change based on the patient's solution to the identified problem.
    (5) Promoting self-motivation
8. Another technique used to develop a therapeutic relationship and foster SDM is the ALE Model (Davis & Pierre-Louis, 2015).
  a) Ask open-ended questions (e.g., tell me more, how, explain, clarify).
  b) Listen to the patient.

    c) Empathize/empower with solicited information.
      (1) Give advice by asking for permission.
      (2) Connect to the patient's own concerns.
      (3) Follow up with the teach-back method ("What was the most important thing we discussed today?").
        (a) Once the patient has identified an area of concern, solicit and discuss the patient's self-generated solutions and offer information collaboratively.
        (b) Assessing needs, preferences, behaviors, readiness, and barriers to self-management engages the patient and develops a therapeutic relationship.
        (c) This information directs patient-specific behavior changes, interventions, collaborative care planning, and problem solving (Battersby et al., 2010).

9. Identify areas for self-management that directly affect the patient's area of concern. For example, if fatigue is identified, what aspects of physical activity, nutrition, and sleep could influence the symptom of fatigue?

10. Determine the patient's educational needs.
    a) Information alone is insufficient.
    b) Together, determine what knowledge, skills, and coping mechanisms are needed for the patient to be successful.
    c) Determine how this education will be provided. Many formats are available to address these educational needs, ranging from individual, group, and self-instruction to telehealth.
    d) Steps in collaborative problem solving
      (1) Define the problem.
      (2) Brainstorm solutions.
      (3) Address barriers.
      (4) Choose a strategy.
      (5) Try it.
      (6) Evaluate it.
    e) Each step is important, but understanding the problem is key to success.
    f) The focus should be on choices and consequences, not adherence or compliance.
      (1) Identify a healthy behavioral change the patient can readily address. Once this is determined, a goal can be set.
      (2) For instance, the healthy change is to lose weight, while the goal is to lose four pounds in the next month.
    g) Identify realistic behaviors that will be steps to reach the goals.
      (1) Behaviors that will assist in reaching the identified goal should be specific, measurable, attainable, realistic, and time sensitive (SMART). An example would be "to meet the goal of losing four pounds in the next month, I will eat carrots for a snack instead of the ice cream that I usually eat."
      (2) Personalize the goal with a written action plan that includes self-monitoring by the patient with regular follow-up.
    h) Assess readiness for self-management.
      (1) On a scale of 1–10, how confident is the patient that he or she will be able to do this behavior?

          (2) If the patient does not choose a 10, help identify the patient's barriers.

          (3) Identifying barriers prior to initiation can ensure the development of a more appropriate plan.

          (4) By helping the patient understand the areas that he or she has already been self-managing, self-efficacy can be increased.

    i) Problem solve with the patient to resolve any barriers. The patient should be verbalizing these issues and designing the solution. The provider should be asking questions to help the patient in identifying the plan.

    j) Use stress reduction and mindfulness techniques to help the patient relax and move forward. *Mindfulness* is a meditation technique that allows one to focus on the present experience without judgment.

    k) Identify resources.

          (1) Consider all community and individual resources needed and available.

          (2) Multifaceted interventions are usually required and include spiritual, social, and transportation services to assist in managing medical, psychosocial, spiritual, and financial aspects (Schulman-Green et al., 2012).

          (3) Specific resources needed should be individualized to the patient's preferences, which can change over time as self-management skills evolve and as illness and other changes occur.

I. Patient perspective

  1. Self-management is a skill that patients with chronic disease need in order to live well with their condition.

    a) Both patients and providers need to develop skills in identifying the best application of evidence for SDM to occur in each unique individual.

    b) Federal initiatives and policies can help drive the achievement of self-management development that is supported by frameworks and reimbursement.

  2. Managing a chronic condition day after day is a lot of work. Patients become overwhelmed, frustrated, or disengaged or even ignore their healthcare needs for long periods of time.

  3. When patients experience poor outcomes, healthcare professionals caring for these patients also can become frustrated. While the reasons for treatment failure often are multifactorial, helping patients to improve health outcomes can be accomplished by starting with what is important to them.

  4. Simply telling patients what to do does not motivate them toward desired behavioral changes. In fact, in many cases, patients become defensive and are less likely to integrate healthy behaviors.

  5. Personal motivation drives behavioral change. Patients need to be the center of the healthcare team and active participants in their own health care (Funnell, 2000).

  6. Practitioners that exemplify the role of a healthcare partner—someone who empowers patients through education and support—help patients make decisions about their health that lead to improved outcomes. In this type of *patient–provider partnership*, in which patients are provided with effective options instead of simply being told what to do, patients have more confidence in their ability to reach self-management goals (Williams et al., 2006; Williams, McGregor, Zeldman, Freedman, & Deci, 2004).

  7. In addition to developing an effective patient–provider partnership, practitioners need to understand what motivates patients toward self-management.

        a) Self-determination theory has been used to better understand patient motivation.

        b) What motivates patients to make behavioral changes to improve their health can be influenced by internal factors (feeling of accomplishment), external factors (pressure from others), or a combination of both (Schatell & Alt, 2008).

        c) According to self-determination theory, motivation is driven by an individual's basic psychological need for autonomy (in control; given a choice), competence (through mastery over challenges), and relatedness (by connecting with others).

           (1) Intrinsic motivation stems from these three conditions, enabling individuals to pursue things meaningful to them (Ryan & Deci, 2000).

           (2) The key to achieving intrinsic motivation is support.

    8. It is important that patients understand that their condition is serious; however, it also is important for them to recognize that their condition is one that is primarily self-managed and that they have options that will allow them to do something about it (Funnell, 2000).

    9. A good place to start is by having a meaningful conversation with patients to better understand what is important to them, thoroughly understanding their perceived barriers to self-management, and assessing their readiness to change.

    10. Once a relationship and trust are established, provide condition-specific education that focuses on patients' self-identified areas.

    11. Finally, work with patients to develop personally meaningful self-management goals.

  V. Role of the advanced practice registered nurse (APRN)

    A. Collaborative roles exist within the SDM Model.

      1. Decision coach: Nurse, social worker, health educator. Decision coaches can provide evidence-based information and education.

      2. Support staff: Manager of clinical processes and resources

      3. Family: Lends support and clarification

      4. Medical treatment specialist: Physician, APRN

    B. Self-management needs are unique to each individual and change over time.

      1. Understanding the roles of other providers, including social workers, psychologists, psychiatrists, chaplains, nutritionists, and educators, is critical and can assist the patient through the process.

      2. The APRN must look at the patient as a whole.

        a) What self-management activities is the patient engaged in that can affect other activities?

        b) Currently, how important is each activity to the patient (Schulman-Green et al., 2012)?

      3. Continued communication with the patient will allow understanding of how the person's needs change over time.

    C. APRNs who are aware of federal initiatives and evidence-based interventions can promote self-management and participate in the collection of measurable outcomes (Kuebler, 2015).

  VI. Interface to palliative care

    A. Advance care planning takes into consideration patient goals and preferences for future care by creating a plan for when illness or injury impedes the ability to think or communicate about health decisions (Butler, Ratner, McCreedy, Shippee, & Kane, 2014).

B. Less than 50% of patients with advanced disease have an advance directive in their medical record (Kass-Bartelmes & Hughes, 2003).

C. Patient preferences will include religious or spiritual values, quality of life, and other facets used to make decisions.

D. Process for advance care planning
   1. Learning about the anticipated condition and the options for care
   2. Considering the options
   3. Choosing a plan that is consistent with the patient's values and wishes
   4. Communicating preferences (oral or written)
   5. SDM may include family, caregivers, attorneys, or other professionals.

E. Decision aids for advance care planning could be helpful in SDM.

F. Patients with established conditions need to have knowledge of their prognosis and the potential implications of decisions.

G. Providers need more concrete information as to what and when to talk about in the course of a patient's trajectory.

H. Advance care planning should be an ongoing process that is revised as the patient lives with the condition.

I. Research efforts need to support advance care planning decision aids (Butler et al., 2014).
   1. The effectiveness of current aids should be studied.
   2. Tools should be easily accessible, readable, and understandable.

Case Study

R.P. is a 65-year-old man who has been living with type 2 diabetes for the past five years. He is married, has two grown children, and plans on retiring within the next year. His daughter is going through a divorce and has recently moved in (along with her two children) with R.P. and his wife. R.P. has a demanding job as the chief financial officer for a local manufacturing company and works long hours, including many weekends. His long work hours have caused a strain on his marriage. R.P. struggles with his diet and often forgets to take his medications. He was recently diagnosed with proliferative retinopathy and has an ulcer on his right foot that is not responding well to treatment. He has been under the care of a wound care specialist for the past nine months. He has been hospitalized twice in the past six months related to uncontrolled blood glucose.

The best approach to addressing his uncontrolled diabetes is to start with the development of a therapeutic relationship through active listening, open-ended questions, authentic support, and engagement through collaboration. The goal is to identify the patient's personal issues related to diabetes control.

As an opening question, the APRN asks, "What is your biggest concern related to your ability to manage your health?" R.P. could respond in many ways—perhaps his biggest concern is related to finances and how this has interrupted his work life, his relationship with his wife, his feelings of loss of control, his concerns about his retinopathy, or his fear of blindness. This single question can lead to the primary concern for the patient and increase the potential for the patient to be motivated and committed to begin working on self-determined goals and behavior changes.

R.P. responds that he is concerned that his wound has not been healing and perhaps he will lose his leg. The APRN's second question is designed to move the conversation forward:

"Can I tell you about a few areas that might help to improve the chances of your wound healing?" By staying focused on what is of interest and importance to the patient, the nurse improves the chance of being heard and for the patient to improve self-management abilities. The patient affirms that he is very interested in this information. The APRN shares evidence that improved blood glucose and nutrition may increase his body's ability to heal the wound. In fact, improved blood glucose also may delay the progression of retinopathy and other complications of diabetes.

The APRN then asks, "Do you see any components of your current diabetes management that could improve and affect your blood glucose control?" R.P. identifies that he could improve taking his blood glucose medication regularly and would be willing to focus more on nutrition. So, the healthy change is to affect blood glucose by taking medication regularly. At this point, it is important to identify the barriers to taking medication in order to develop realistic behaviors to reach the goal of improved blood glucose. R.P. states that he remembers to take his morning insulin but forgets to take it at lunch and dinner. Rather than jumping in to develop a plan for him, the APRN helps the patient determine how he will address this. The nurse develops a written action plan that is based on what the patient plans to accomplish. The action plan includes self-monitoring of his success and a follow-up plan with the APRN.

Finally, the APRN asks, "How confident are you that you will be able to accomplish this behavior on a scale of 1–10, with 10 being most confident?" R.P. states he is at a 5 in his confidence level. The nurse then asks, "How can you move your confidence from a 5 to an 8 or a 10?" This question will assist R.P. in identifying potential barriers and discern a solution. Solutions may include stress reduction techniques, mindfulness, or the identification of resources from his family, friends, and community. The key is to help R.P. identify specific resources individualized to his preferences and current needs.

References

Agency for Healthcare Research and Quality. (2015, June). Self-management support. Retrieved from http://www.ahrq.gov/professionals/prevention-chronic-care/improve/self-mgmt/index.html

Barlow, J., Wright, C., Sheasby, J., Turner, A., & Hainsworth, J. (2002). Self-management approaches for people with chronic conditions: A review. *Patient Education and Counseling, 48,* 177–187. doi:10.1016/S0738-3991(02)00032-0

Battersby, M., Von Korff, M., Schaefer, J., Davis, C., Ludman, E., Greene, S.M., … Wagner, E.H. (2010). Twelve evidence-based principles for implementing self-management support in primary care. *Joint Commission Journal on Quality and Patient Safety, 36,* 561–570.

Bodenheimer, T., Lorig, K., Holman, H., & Grumbach, K. (2002). Patient self-management of chronic disease in primary care. *Journal of the American Medical Association, 288,* 2469–2475. doi:10.1001/jama.288.19.2469

Brady, T.J. (2011, May). *Sorting through the evidence for the Arthritis Self-Management Program and the Chronic Disease Self-Management Program: Executive summary of ASMP/CDSMP meta-analyses.* Retrieved from http://www.cdc.gov/arthritis/marketing-support/self-management/docs/pdf/asmp-executive-summary.pdf

Burson, R., & Moran, K.J. (2015). Empowerment and engagement. *Home Healthcare Now, 33,* 49–50. doi:10.1097/NHH.0000000000000178

Butler, M., Ratner, E., McCreedy, E., Shippee, N., & Kane, R.L. (2014). Decision aids for advance care planning: An overview of the state of the science. *Annals of Internal Medicine, 161,* 408–418. doi:10.7326/M14-0644

Centers for Medicare and Medicaid Services. (2016). Chronic conditions overview. Retrieved from https://www.cms.gov/Research-Statistics-Data-and-Systems/Statistics-Trends-and-Reports/Chronic-Conditions/index.html

Davis, E.D., & Pierre-Louis, M. (2015). Communicating with patients with diabetes: A paradigm shift. *Practical Diabetology, 34*(1), 17–21.

Elwyn, G., Dehlendorf, C., Epstein, R.M., Marrin, K., White, J., & Frosch, D.L. (2014). Shared decision-making and motivational interviewing: Achieving patient-centered care across the spectrum of health care problems. *Annals of Family Medicine, 12,* 270–275. doi:10.1370/afm.1615

Evans, M.W. (2013). Understanding health behavior. In C. Hawk & W. Evans (Eds.), *Health promotion and wellness: An evidence-based guide to clinical preventive services* (pp. 4–13). Philadelphia, PA: Lippincott Williams & Wilkins.

Ferrer, R.L., & Gill, J.M. (2013). Shared decision-making, contextualized. *Annals of Family Medicine, 11,* 303–305. doi:10.1370/afm.1551

Funnell, M.M. (2000). Helping patients take charge of their chronic illnesses. *Family Practice Management,* 7(3), 47–51. Retrieved from http://www.aafp.org/fpm/2000/0300/p47.html

Funnell, M.M. (2015). Supporting effective self-management from the clinic to the community [Webcast]. *American Diabetes Association 62nd Annual Advanced Postgraduate Course.* Retrieved from http://www .healthmonix.com/adawebcast62/login.aspx

Gionfriddo, M.R., Leppin, A.L., Brito, J.P., LeBlanc, A., Boehmer, K.R., Morris, M.A., … Montori, V.M. (2014). A systematic review of shared decision making interventions in chronic conditions: A review protocol. *Systematic Reviews, 3,* 38. doi:10.1186/2046-4053-3-38

Kass-Bartelmes, B.L., & Hughes, R. (2003). *Advance care planning: Preferences for care at the end of life. Research in action* (Research in Action Issue No. 12, AHRQ Pub. No. 03-0018). Rockville, MD: Agency for Healthcare Research and Quality.

Kuebler, K. (2015). Federal initiatives in self-management for patients with multiple chronic conditions: Implications for the doctor of nursing practice. *Clinical Scholars Review, 8,* 139–144. doi:10.1891/1939-2095.8.1.139

Liddy, C., Blazkho, V., & Mill, K. (2014). Challenges of self-management when living with multiple chronic conditions: Systematic review of the qualitative literature. *Canadian Family Physician, 60,* 1125–1133. Retrieved from http://www.cfp.ca/content/60/12/1123.long

Patient-Centered Outcomes Research Institute. (2014). About us. Retrieved from http://www.pcori.org/about-us

Redman, B.K. (2013). *Advanced practice nursing ethics in chronic disease self-management.* New York, NY: Springer.

Ryan, P. (2009). Integrated theory of health behavior change: Background and intervention development. *Clinical Nurse Specialist, 23,* 161–170. doi:10.1097/NUR.0b013e3181a42373

Ryan, P., & Sawin, K.J. (2009). The individual and family self-management theory: Background and perspectives on context, process, and outcomes. *Nursing Outlook, 57,* 217–225.e6. doi:10.1016/j.outlook.2008.10.004

Ryan, R.M., & Deci, E.L. (2000). Self-determination theory and the facilitation of intrinsic motivation, social development, and well-being. *American Psychologist, 55,* 68–78. doi:10.1037/0003-066X.55.1.68

Schatell, D., & Alt, P.S. (2008). How understanding motivation can improve dialysis practices. *Nephrology News and Issues,* pp. 32–36. Retrieved from http://lifeoptions.org/catalog/pdfs/news/ru0908.pdf

Schulman-Green, D., Jaser, S., Martin, F., Alonzo, A., Grey, M., McCorkle, R., … Whittemore, R. (2012). Processes of self-management in chronic illness. *Journal of Nursing Scholarship, 44,* 136–144. doi:10.1111/j.1547 -5069.2012.01444.x

Self-Management Science Center at University of Wisconsin–Milwaukee. (n.d.). The individual and family self-management theory. Retrieved from http://uwm.edu/nursing/about/centers-institutes/self-management/theory

Stanford Medicine. (n.d.). Chronic Disease Self-Management Program (Better Choices, Better Health® Workshop). Retrieved from http://patienteducation.stanford.edu/programs/cdsmp.html

U.S. Department of Health and Human Services. (2010, December). Multiple chronic conditions—A strategic framework: Optimum health and quality of life for individuals with multiple chronic conditions. Retrieved from http://www.hhs.gov/ash/initiatives/mcc/mcc_framework.pdf

U.S. Department of Health and Human Services. (2016). Prevention and Public Health Fund. Retrieved from http://www.hhs.gov/open/prevention

Volk, R., & Llewellyn-Thomas, H. (2012). The 2012 IPDAS background document: An introduction. In R. Volk & H. Llewellyn-Thomas (Eds.), *2012 update of the International Patient Decision Aids Standards (IPDAS) Collaboration's background document.* Retrieved from http://ipdas.ohri.ca/IPDAS-Introduction.pdf

Williams, G.C., McGregor, H.A., Sharp, D., Levesque, C., Kouides, R.W., Ryan, R.M., & Deci, E.L. (2006). Testing a self-determination theory intervention for motivating tobacco cessation: Supporting autonomy and competence in a clinical trial. *Health Psychology, 25,* 91–101. doi:10.1037/0278-6133.25.1.91

Williams, G.C., McGregor, H.A., Zeldman, A., Freedman, Z.R., & Deci, E.L. (2004). Testing a self-determination theory process model for promoting glycemic control through diabetes self-management. *Health Psychology, 23,* 58–66. doi:10.1037/0278-6133.23.1.58

CHAPTER 5

Care of Multiple Chronic Conditions

Kim Kuebler, DNP, APRN, ANP-BC

I. Definition
  A. Multiple chronic conditions (MCCs) are concomitant medical conditions that occur in patients with one or more chronic diseases (U.S. Department of Health and Human Services [DHHS], 2010).
    1. Chronic conditions are those that persist for longer than one year, require ongoing medication attention, and often limit patient activities of daily living and interfere with patient-perceived quality of life (Centers for Medicare and Medicaid Services [CMS], 2012; U.S. DHHS, 2010).
    2. An example of a patient with MCCs is a patient who is currently living with a confirmed diagnosis of congestive heart failure (CHF), arthritis, hypertension, obesity, and type 2 diabetes mellitus.
  B. As the patient's number of chronic conditions increases, so too do the effects of increased morbidity and mortality, cost of care, hospitalization, confusing or conflicting advice from multiple physicians and other healthcare providers, and use of more than five concomitant medications (National Quality Forum [NQF], 2012; U.S. DHHS, 2010).
  C. Patients with MCCs experience poor day-to-day functioning, which contributes to deconditioning, frailty, and disability (U.S. DHHS, 2010). The decline in functional status contributes to limited access to health care, inability to self-manage, and an untoward reliance on caregiver support and demand (U.S. DHHS, 2010).
  D. More than one-fourth of the American population has more than one chronic condition, and more than two-thirds of Medicare beneficiaries have MCCs, with approximately 14% having more than six concomitant chronic conditions (Medicare Payment Advisory Commission [MedPAC], 2014; Ward & Schiller, 2013).
    1. This is the largest, fastest-growing, and costliest U.S. patient population (Goodman, Posner, Huang, Parekh, & Koh, 2013).
    2. By 2020, it is expected that more than 81 million Americans will have MCCs (Partnership to Fight Chronic Disease, n.d.).
  E. Treatment of chronic conditions such as heart disease, diabetes, and cancer, to name a few, now accounts for almost 93% of Medicare spending.
    1. Beneficiaries with six or more chronic conditions accounted for 46% of all Medicare spending in 2010 (MedPAC, 2014).

2. In 2010, the traditional Medicare fee-for-service program spent an average of $32,658 per beneficiary with six or more chronic conditions compared to an average of $9,738 for all other beneficiaries (MedPAC, 2014).
3. Because of this public healthcare burden, DHHS announced a public call for comments pertaining to patients who are living with and dying from MCCs.

II. Key aspects
   A. DHHS administers a significant number of federal programs that are directed toward the prevention and optimal management of chronic conditions that include financing healthcare services, delivering health care to patients with MCCs, conducting basic intervention and systems research, and implementing programs to prevent and manage chronic disease while ensuring safe and effective medications for chronic disease (Parekh, Goodman, Gordon, & Koh, 2011).
      1. DHHS convened a departmental work group on patients with MCCs. The group established the following priorities (Parekh et al., 2011):
         a) Create an inventory of existing DHHS programs, activities, and initiatives with a focus on improving the health of patients with MCCs
         b) Develop a strategic framework that could be used as a map for improving the health and well-being of patients with MCCs
      2. The work group included high-level individuals from every agency under the DHHS umbrella.
      3. The draft framework was announced in the *Federal Register* in May 2010, along with a request for feedback.
      4. Comments from approximately 250 stakeholder organizations and others were used to shape the final version of the strategic framework (Parekh et al., 2011).
   B. The strategic framework is titled *Optimum Health and Quality of Life for Individuals With Multiple Chronic Conditions* (U.S. DHHS, 2010).
      1. The four interdependent goals identified in the framework include the following:
         a) Foster healthcare and public health systems changes to improve the health of patients with MCCs.
         b) Maximize the use of proven self-care management and other services by patients with MCCs.
         c) Provide better tools and information to healthcare, public health, and social service workers who deliver care to patients with MCCs.
         d) Facilitate research to fill knowledge gaps and identify interventions and systems to benefit individuals with MCCs.
      2. Each of these goals within the framework includes key objectives and strategies that DHHS, in conjunction with stakeholders, will use to guide initiatives, innovation, and policy supporting the care needs of patients with MCCs.
   C. The Agency for Healthcare Research and Quality (AHRQ) has funded the AHRQ MCC Research Network, which aligns with DHHS's effort to address MCC issues.
      1. AHRQ's focus is to implement a key goal of the DHHS's strategic framework to increase clinical, community, and patient-centered health research on MCCs.
      2. The AHRQ MCC Research Network aims to provide a source for understanding specific interventions that provide the greatest benefit for patients with MCCs with attention to safety and effectiveness (AHRQ, 2015).
      3. The AHRQ MCC Research Network advances the field of MCC research, provides evidence-based guidance for clinicians and patients, and advises policy makers about improved methods to measure and promote quality care for the complex needs of this patient population (AHRQ, 2015).

D. NQF, under contract with DHHS, convened a steering committee of multiple stakeholders in June 2010 to develop a measurement framework for evaluating care for patients with MCCs (NQF, 2012).

1. The steering committee's work was influenced and informed by several important national initiatives promoted by DHHS as well as public–private sector initiatives (NQF, 2012).

2. The NQF steering committee focused on the following aspects related to patients with MCCs:

   a) Establish a shared definition of MCCs that can be used to effectively measure the quality of care for patients with MCCs

   b) Develop and identify high-leverage measurement areas for the U.S. population of patients with MCCs in an effort to mitigate unintended consequences and measurement burden

   c) Establish a conceptual model that serves as an organizing structure for identifying and prioritizing quality measures

   d) Design guiding principles to address the methodologic and practical measurement issues

3. The steering committee report identified opportunities for applying the framework relevant to current policy context and for including a coordinated approach for filling measure gaps, including establishing a common data platform to collect information ranging from healthcare records to patient-reported data (NQF, 2012).

4. The committee's selection criteria for measurement were based on identifying cross-cutting areas that offer the greatest potential for reducing disease burden and cost while improving well-being, which was reported as being valued most by patients and their families (NQF, 2012).

5. The final measure concepts

   a) Optimizing function, maintaining function, or preventing further decline in function

   b) Creating seamless transitions among multiple providers and sites of care

   c) Recording patient-important outcomes (including patient-reported outcomes) and relevant outcomes (disease-specific outcomes)

   d) Avoiding inappropriate, nonbeneficial care, particularly at the end of life

   e) Providing access to a usual source of care

   f) Reporting transparency of cost (total cost)

   g) Developing shared accountability across patients, families, and providers

   h) Implementing shared decision making

E. In 2011, CMS released a report titled *Multiple Chronic Conditions Among Medicare Beneficiaries: State-Level Variations in Prevalence, Utilization, and Cost* (Lochner, Goodman, Posner, & Parekh, 2013).

1. CMS administrative data collected from beneficiaries with MCCs in 2011 were calculated by tabulating the number of conditions from a set of 15 through the use of diagnosis codes from clinical encounter claims (Lochner et al., 2013).

   a) Thirty-one million beneficiaries were fee-for-service U.S. residents residing in all 50 states and Washington, DC.

   b) Among beneficiaries with six or more chronic conditions, prevalence rates were lowest in Alaska and Wyoming at 7% and highest in Florida and New Jersey at 18%.

    c) Readmission rates into hospitals were lowest in Utah at 19% and highest in Washington, DC, at 31%. The number of emergency department visits per beneficiary was lowest in New York and Florida at 1.6% and highest in Washington, DC, at 2.7%.

    d) Medicare spending per beneficiary was lowest in Hawaii ($24,086) and highest in Maryland, Washington, DC, and Louisiana (more than $37,000).

    e) Medicare spending is expected to continue to escalate until 2050, with 10,000 beneficiaries currently entering into the Medicare system daily (see Figure 5-1).

2. This study has identified key knowledge gaps on the burden of MCCs in this patient population.

3. The results directly address the fourth goal of the DHHS strategic framework, supporting targeted research on patients living with symptomatic MCCs (U.S. DHHS, 2010).

4. The findings from this study expand prior research on MCCs among Medicare beneficiaries at the national level and identify state-level variations in the prevalence of healthcare utilization and Medicare spending for beneficiaries with MCCs. Having pertinent state-level data is important for decision making aimed at improved program planning, financing, and delivery of care management for patients with MCCs (Lochner et al., 2013).

III. Current findings

    A. The 2015 White House Conference on Aging was titled "21st Century Challenge for Healthy Aging: Balancing Living Well With the Reality of Multiple Chronic Conditions" (Parekh, 2014).

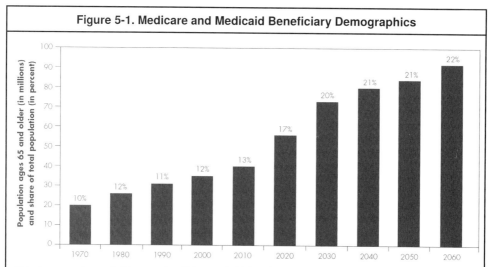

Figure 5-1. Medicare and Medicaid Beneficiary Demographics

The sheer numbers of older people will be much higher than in prior years, as will the older population's share of the total population.

Note. Based on information from U.S. Census Bureau, 2015a, 2015b.

From *Report to the Congress: Medicare and the Health Care Delivery System* (p. 39), by Medicare Payment Advisory Commission, 2015. Retrieved from http://www.medpac.gov/-documents-/reports.

    1. Select DHHS activities based on the strategic framework on MCCs that are currently being implemented and highlighted by the White House Conference.

        a) Payment for chronic care management services, initially introduced in the July 2013 *Federal Register*, began in October 2015.

        b) CMS will reimburse primary care practices a capitated amount for managing the care needs of patients with more than one chronic condition.

        c) This is the first non–fee-for-service model guaranteed to provide patients access to care 24 hours a day, 7 days a week.

    2. CMS is testing a new care model through the Independence at Home Demonstration, which is currently providing 8,000 frail Medicare beneficiaries with MCCs and functional limitations with access to home-based primary care (CMS, n.d.).

B. Evidence-based community programs have worked in conjunction with 200,000 older U.S. residents with MCCs to complete a Chronic Disease Self-Management Education program through the Administration for Community Living programs (Parekh, 2014).

    1. The Health Resources and Services Administration is creating an interprofessional curriculum for MCC education and training intended to be disseminated to providers (Parekh, 2014).

    2. The U.S. Food and Drug Administration announced a policy to more closely examine populations included in clinical trials of new drug applications to discourage the exclusion of patients with MCCs (Parekh, 2014).

    3. Patient-centered outcomes research—AHRQ created a nationwide MCC Research Network, and the National Institutes of Health has issued seven new funding opportunities for patients with MCCs since 2010 (Parekh, 2014).

C. The strategic framework has provided the tool to measure and evaluate the effect on current initiatives funded by the Patient Protection and Affordable Care Act (ACA) of 2010 (U.S. DHHS, 2010).

    1. The framework helps promote and implement community-based programs to establish partnerships among interdisciplinary providers who share mutual goals of promoting healthy aging and preventing the development of frailty, disability, and functional limitations (Schreiber, 2014).

    2. A paradigm shift needs to occur in the culture of care provided for the largest and fastest-growing U.S. patient population with a focus on health, prevention, and safety while decreasing costs of care (Schreiber, 2014).

IV. Relevance to practice

A. Systems of care delivery need to shift from a healthcare system that traditionally has been incentivized to care for acute illness and to manage chronic disease exacerbations to a system that is focused on preventing disease and promoting wellness (Schreiber, 2014).

B. The reactive medical care approach that is both familiar and prevalent among U.S. healthcare systems has resulted in the medicalization of healthcare delivery, creating an isolated approach to care that exists in silos and is separate from the community-based organizations that provide care and services outside of acute medical management (Schreiber, 2014).

C. Newer models of care utilize community agencies that can promote proactive, preventive intervention based within a patient's community.

    1. An example would be an agency focused on aging.

2. This type of community agency centers on the needs and wants of the individualized patient within a home setting and focuses on what matters most to the patient and caregiver (Kleinman & Foster, 2011; Schreiber, 2014).

D. A 2011 Robert Wood Johnson Foundation survey of more than 1,000 primary care providers recognized that individual patients' social needs determined their healthcare outcomes. Of the physicians surveyed, 85% did not feel confident that they could help to meet the social needs of their patients.

E. Area agencies on aging can provide the conduit needed between providers and the community for patients with MCCs by working among providers, social services, and community-based organizations, resulting in improved health and patient independence within the community (Schreiber, 2014).

F. CMS has funded multiple community-based programs occurring in many different settings. The diversification of these programs has been funded to ensure sustainability by integrating them into medical homes, accountable care organizations (ACOs), dual-eligible plans, and other shared-risk pilots (CMS, n.d.; Schreiber, 2014).

G. Since the ACA became law, there has been an increased focus on alternative payment models such as ACOs, medical homes, and care bundling. Recent ACO demonstration data have shown promise; yet, these models are relatively new and no significant data exist to suggest that the manner in which these care models are structured will improve quality and significantly reduce Medicare spending long term (U.S. Senate Committee on Finance, 2015).

H. A white paper by the Partnership to Fight Chronic Disease (2013) identified a healthcare delivery system that has become disconnected between medical care, public health, and community services.

1. Rather than collaborating to promote disease prevention and patient education, the healthcare delivery system described in the white paper took a reactive approach, focusing instead on acute care needs and lacking the evaluation of socioeconomic issues confronting patients that would lead to the patient population adopting healthy behaviors.

2. Prevention and wellness should be the primary outcomes in the complex management of MCCs.

I. The Chronic Care Model is a core concept of the Robert Wood Johnson Foundation national program Improving Chronic Illness Care (ICIC, n.d.). Funding availability ended in 2011 (see Figure 5-2).

1. Studies that have evaluated the use of the Chronic Care Model suggest lack of care coordination as one of the major deficiencies in the optimal management of MCCs.

2. Deficiencies included the following (ICIC, n.d.):
   a) Practitioners who are rushed during evaluation and treatment and, as a result, do not follow established practice guidelines
   b) Lack of coordinated care and use of multiple providers
   c) Lack of proactive follow-up to ensure positive outcomes
   d) Patients who are not well educated on how to successfully manage their chronic conditions

J. The ACA identified an emphasis on team-based care and collaboration among multiple providers and disciplines and established the Patient-Centered Outcomes Research Institute (PCORI, 2014).

K. PCORI provides funding sources for comparative effectiveness research (CER) with a mandate from Congress to improve the quality of evidence available to

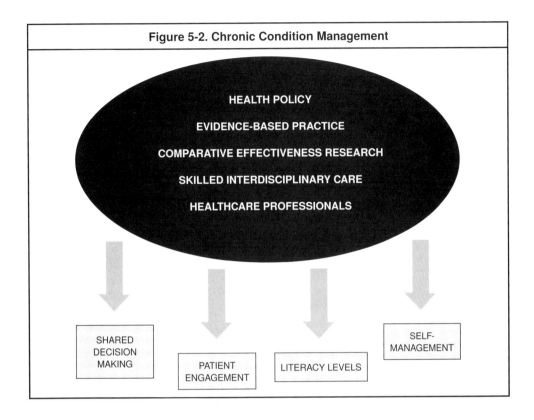

Figure 5-2. Chronic Condition Management

HEALTH POLICY

EVIDENCE-BASED PRACTICE

COMPARATIVE EFFECTIVENESS RESEARCH

SKILLED INTERDISCIPLINARY CARE

HEALTHCARE PROFESSIONALS

SHARED DECISION MAKING

PATIENT ENGAGEMENT

LITERACY LEVELS

SELF-MANAGEMENT

patients, caregivers, clinicians, employers, insurers, and policy makers with access to pertinent, real-world information to help them make informed health decisions (PCORI, 2014).

    1. The importance of including research for MCCs was included in the development of PCORI's National Priorities for Research and Research Agenda (PCORI, 2012).

    2. This agenda recognized that research is needed to improve patient-centered care and evaluate quality outcomes.

    3. CER is research that compares one intervention or treatment to another, determining which specific intervention can be used to promote optimal patient-centered outcomes (PCORI, 2014).

V. Role of the advanced practice registered nurse (APRN)

  A. APRNs are required to be familiar with and proficient in how the ACA will influence clinical practice for the care and management of patients with MCCs.

  B. Responsibilities of APRNs

    1. Acquire the clinical knowledge and skills gained from the implementation of evidence-based practice guidelines to ensure optimal patient outcomes and future reimbursement for the largest U.S. patient population.

    2. Be proactive in preventing chronic disease, reducing disease exacerbations, lowering hospital admission and readmission rates, maintaining patients' physical functioning, and engaging patients in self-management practices.

    3. Become proficient in understanding the use of CER in the clinical setting to influence patient-centered outcomes and its relevance to patients with MCCs.

4. Recognize how the Chronic Care Model can be implemented in practice to utilize community resources, pertinent disciplines, and education through engagement among patients, families, and providers in shared health decision making (ICIC, n.d.).
5. Recognize the paradigm shift from fee-for-service clinical encounters to capitated rates based on around-the-clock availability and ongoing communication with patients by email, text messaging, and telephone conversations (CMS, 2014).
   a) The new program will pay physicians for managing Medicare patients with two or more chronic conditions, even when contacts are made by telephone or email rather than face-to-face.
   b) To qualify for the program, physicians need to have electronic health record systems and be able to exchange information on patients with other caregivers.
   c) Physicians or their staff must be available to communicate with, receive, and treat patients around the clock.
   d) To accommodate this level of availability, Medicare has loosened its "incident to" rule, which requires doctors to directly supervise staff. Under the new requirements, practices can outsource the coverage.
   e) The final ruling, released by CMS on October 31, 2014, allows physicians to be paid $40.39 per patient per month. In return, patients must agree to enter the program, which requires an $8 copay each month (CMS, 2014).
6. Maintain a relevant and dynamic evidence-based practice through the use of current and credible sources that direct exemplar disease and symptom management practices.
7. Use an interdisciplinary approach of care to address the complex care needs of patients living with and dying from MCCs.

VI. Interface to palliative care
   A. The integration of palliative care into the management of MCCs, symptoms, and associated consequences is essential. The concomitant association of multiple diseases, symptoms, psychological influence, alterations in functional status, and poor quality of life requires the knowledgeable use of palliative interventions.
   B. Palliative care is synonymous with symptom management and should not be reserved for the last months, weeks, or days of life.
   C. NQF (2012) separated palliative care from end-of-life care. This suggests that better patient outcomes from palliative care should be implemented earlier in the chronic disease trajectory, including rehabilitation.
   D. Palliative interventions focus on the management of common symptoms (physical, emotional, spiritual) that accompany chronic conditions from an interdisciplinary approach.
   E. Palliative care employs the best evidence to support the use of concomitant medications to ensure optimal patient outcomes, with an understanding of cytochrome P450 enzyme incompatibilities, and selecting a single medication that has multiple indications.
   F. Primary care providers using the Chronic Care Model will provide palliative care and management for patients with symptomatic chronic conditions throughout the patient's disease trajectory until death.
   G. Optimal symptom management reduces the incidence of disease exacerbations, reduces hospital admission rates, and helps to maintain physical functioning.

Case Study

J.H. is a 72-year-old Caucasian man with a 48-pack-year history of smoking. He has a forced expiratory volume in one second, or FEV_1, of less than 65% predicted, confirming stage 3 chronic obstructive pulmonary disease (COPD). He has a body mass index of 42, confirming morbid obesity, and a confirmed diagnosis of CHF with an ejection fraction of 35%. J.H. has been diagnosed with type 2 diabetes from a recent hemoglobin A1c of 8.1%. He presents to the clinic with complaints of dyspnea, cough, purulent mucus, fatigue, insomnia, fever, and exercise intolerance.

The APRN's objective in managing this patient is to prevent exacerbation of his COPD and CHF by prescribing either a macrolide or quinolone based on current guideline recommendations. The APRN maximizes bronchodilator management by adding an inhaled long-acting beta-2 agonist and combined corticosteroid to his long-acting anticholinergic broncho-dilator (tiotropium) and instructed him to use his short-acting beta-2 agonist (albuterol) every four hours to reduce his dyspnea and exercise intolerance. The APRN educates the patient on adequate hydration to reduce the viscosity of his mucus and to prevent the development of pneumonia. To get his symptoms under control from his COPD exacerbation, J.H. is scheduled to return to the clinic at the end of the week. The APRN instructs the patient to use his home-delivered oxygen by nasal cannula at 2 L continuously and to use inhaled nasal saline as directed. The APRN recommends the use of acetaminophen 500 mg every six hours as needed for fever. J.H. is encouraged to check his fasting glucose every morning and each evening prior to sleep and to bring a record of his dietary intake and glucose readings with him when he returns to the clinic. He has been informed that the inhaled corticosteroid may increase his glucose readings. The APRN obtained a finger-stick glucose reading of 220 mg/dl during his clinic visit.

From this clinical encounter, the APRN documents follow-up in four days to evaluate patient symptoms. If the patient becomes more symptomatic, he is instructed to contact the APRN immediately for consideration of a systemic corticosteroid. The APRN understands that J.H.'s symptoms must be controlled before the additional issues associated with his newly diagnosed diabetes can be addressed. The APRN plans to draw a fasting comprehensive metabolic profile, lipids, and complete blood count with differential on his next visit because he was nonfasting on presentation. The APRN will consider referring the patient to a registered dietitian so he can adopt a self-management program to ensure his adherence to diet, exercise, and disease management. The nurse also will consider referring the patient back to his pulmo-nologist for a repeat spirometry to evaluate any changes in pulmonary function through monitoring of his FEV_1. The nurse's assessment findings for this clinical encounter include COPD exacerbation, CHF, type 2 diabetes, dyspnea, cough, mucus, fever, exercise intolerance, and dehydration.

References

Agency for Healthcare Research and Quality. (2015, September). Multiple chronic conditions. Retrieved from http://www.ahrq.gov/professionals/prevention-chronic-care/decision/mcc/index.html

Centers for Medicare and Medicaid Services. (n.d.). The Center for Medicare and Medicaid Innovation. Retrieved from https://innovation.cms.gov

Centers for Medicare and Medicaid Services. (2012). *Multiple chronic conditions: A strategic framework.* Retrieved from http://www.hhs.gov/ash/initiatives/mcc/mcc_framework.pdf

Centers for Medicare and Medicaid Services. (2014, November 13). Medicare program; revisions to payment policies under the Physician Fee Schedule, Clinical Laboratory Fee Schedule, access to identifiable data for the Center for Medicare and Medicaid Innovation models and other revisions to part B for CY 2015. *Federal Register, 79*, 67548–68010.

Goodman, R.A., Posner, S.F., Huang, E.S., Parekh, A.K., & Koh, H.K. (2013). Defining and measuring chronic conditions: Imperatives for research, policy, program, and practice. *Preventing Chronic Disease, 10*, 120239. doi:10.5888/pcd10.120239

Improving Chronic Illness Care. (n.d.). The Chronic Care Model. Retrieved from http://www.improvingchronic care.org/index.php?p=The_Chronic_Care_Model&s=2

Kleinman, R., & Foster, L. (2011, July). *Multiple chronic conditions among OAA title III program participants* (Administration on Aging Research Brief No. 4). Retrieved from http://www.aoa.acl.gov/Program_Results/docs/2011/AoA4_Chronic_508.pdf

Lochner, K.A., Goodman, R.A., Posner, S., & Parekh, A. (2013). Multiple chronic conditions among Medicare beneficiaries: State-level variations in prevalence, utilization, and cost, 2011. *Medicare and Medicaid Research Review, 23*(3), E1–E10. doi:10.5600/mmrr.003.03.b02

Medicare Payment Advisory Commission. (2014, March). *Report to the Congress: Medicare payment policy.* Retrieved from http://www.medpac.gov/documents/reports/mar14_entirereport.pdf

National Quality Forum. (2012, May). *Endorsement summary: Multiple chronic conditions measurement framework.* Retrieved from http://www.qualityforum.org/Projects/Multiple_Chronic_Conditions_Measurement_Framework.aspx

Parekh, A.K. (2014, December 11). 2015 White House Conference on Aging webinar: 21st century challenge for healthy aging: Balancing living well with the reality of multiple chronic conditions. Retrieved from http://www.hhs.gov/ash/initiatives/mcc/final-whcoa-mcc-slides-remediated.pdf

Parekh, A.K., Goodman, R.A., Gordon, C., & Koh, H.K. (2011). Managing multiple chronic conditions: A strategic framework for improving health outcomes and quality of life. *Public Health Reports, 126*, 460–471. Retrieved from http://www.ncbi.nlm.nih.gov/pmc/articles/PMC3115206/pdf/phr126000460.pdf

Partnership to Fight Chronic Disease. (n.d.). About the Partnership to Fight Chronic Disease. Retrieved from http://www.fightchronicdisease.org/about

Partnership to Fight Chronic Disease. (2013). *Implications of growing prevalence of multiple chronic conditions: Needs great, evidence lacking* [White paper]. Retrieved from http://www.fightchronicdisease.org/resources/implications-growing-prevalence-multiple-chronic-conditions-needs-great-evidence-lacking

Patient-Centered Outcomes Research Institute. (2012). *National priorities for research and research agenda.* Retrieved from http://www.pcori.org/sites/default/files/PCORI-National-Priorities-and-Research-Agenda.pdf

Patient-Centered Outcomes Research Institute. (2014, October 6). Comparative effectiveness research projects for patients with multiple chronic conditions. Retrieved from http://www.pcori.org/about-us

Patient Protection and Affordable Care Act, 42 U.S.C. § 18001 et seq. (2010). Retrieved from http://www.hhs.gov/healthcare/about-the-law/read-the-law/index.html

Robert Wood Johnson Foundation. (2011, December). *Health care's blind side: The overlooked connection between social needs and good health.* Retrieved from http://www.rwjf.org/content/dam/farm/reports/surveys_and_polls/2011/rwjf71795

Schreiber, R. (2014). Fighting chronic illnesses with evidence-based programs. Retrieved from https://mahealthyagingcollaborative.org/fighting-chronic-illnesses-with-evidence-based-programs

U.S. Census Bureau. (2015a). Population estimates. Retrieved from http://www.census.gov/popest/data/historical/index.html

U.S. Census Bureau. (2015b). Population projections. Retrieved from https://www.census.gov/population/projections/data/national/index.html

U.S. Department of Health and Human Services. (2010, December). *Multiple chronic conditions—A strategic framework: Optimum health and quality of life for individuals with multiple chronic conditions.* Retrieved from http://www.hhs.gov/ash/initiatives/mcc/mcc_framework.pdf

U.S. Senate Committee on Finance. (2015, May 14). A pathway to improving care for Medicare patients with chronic conditions [Video]. Retrieved from http://www.finance.senate.gov/hearings/hearing/?id=da0dc749-5056-a032-52db-7b58f5d1c8b

Ward, B.W., & Schiller, J.S. (2013). Prevalence of multiple chronic conditions among US adults: Estimates from the National Health Interview Survey, 2010. *Preventing Chronic Disease, 10*, 120203. doi:10.5888/pcd10.120203

CHAPTER 6

Comparative Effectiveness Research

Kim Kuebler, DNP, APRN, ANP-BC

I. Definition
   A. Comparative effectiveness research (CER) is the direct comparison between existing healthcare interventions or evidence on the effectiveness, benefits, and harms of different treatment options (Agency for Healthcare Research and Quality [AHRQ], 2014).
   B. The National Institutes of Health (NIH) in 2010 defined CER as "the conduct and synthesis of systematic research comparing different interventions and strategies to prevent, diagnose, treat, and monitor health conditions" (U.S. National Library of Medicine, 2016).
   C. The American Recovery and Reinvestment Act of 2009 provided $1.1 billion for patient-centered research, also known as CER. Specifically, the act directed $400 million to NIH, $400 million to the U.S. Department of Health and Human Services (DHHS), and $300 million to AHRQ (U.S. Food and Drug Administration [FDA], 2010).
      1. CER evidence is generated from research studies that compare drugs, medical devices, tests, surgeries, or ways to deliver health care (AHRQ, 2014).
      2. Two types of CER exist: research that evaluates and compares existing evidence, and the research designed to generate new comparative evidence.
         a) CER researchers evaluate available evidence about the benefits and harms of specific interventions for various patient populations.
         b) The evidence comes from existing randomized clinical trials, nonrandomized trials, observational studies, and other types of research.
         c) This information or evidence is viewed as a research review because this process is a systematic review of the most current evidence (AHRQ, 2014).
      3. CER methodology generates new comparative evidence to promote patient-centered outcomes.
      4. CER requires the development, expansion, evaluation, and use of a variety of data sources and methods that conduct timely and relevant research that is promptly disseminated (AHRQ, 2014).
      5. CER data are useful for clinicians, patients, policy makers, and health plans to discern what is in the best interest for patients. CER is real time and reflects the needs of a specific patient population.
      6. Seven steps involved with CER (AHRQ, 2014)

       a) Identify new and emerging clinical interventions.

       b) Review and synthesize current medical research.

       c) Identify gaps between existing medical research and the needs of clinical practice.

       d) Promote and generate new scientific evidence and analytic tools.

       e) Train and develop CER researchers.

       f) Translate and disseminate research findings to diverse stakeholders.

       g) Reach out to stakeholders through public forums.

II. Key aspects

  A. AHRQ is the lead federal agency under the U.S. DHHS charged with improving the quality, safety, efficiency, and effectiveness of health care for all Americans (AHRQ, 2014).

  B. AHRQ oversees the Effective Health Care Program (EHC) and funds individual researchers, research centers, and academic organizations that will work directly with AHRQ to produce CER and effectiveness data (AHRQ, 2013).

    1. EHC partners with multiple networks of researchers and clinical teams across the United States, utilizing stakeholder input when conducting research; performing systematic reviews; and translating, disseminating, and implementing research findings (AHRQ, 2013).

    2. Under the EHC, several groups participate in specific aspects of CER, including the following:

      a) Healthcare Horizon Scanning System, which is a system for identifying new and emerging areas of health care that may require comparative effectiveness review and funding

      b) Evidence-Based Practice Centers, which scan and perform in-depth reviews of emerging health technologies and innovation to better inform and direct patient-centered outcomes research. The centers were initially developed through the American Recovery and Reinvestment Act of 2009, and in December 2014, AHRQ awarded five-year contracts to 13 centers.

      c) Centers for Education and Research on Therapeutics, which is a new national program and initiative to increase awareness and reduce the harm of new, existing, or combined medications, medical devices, and biologic interventions. Six centers currently exist (AHRQ, 2013).

      d) Scientific Resource Center, which is housed at the Portland, Oregon, Veterans Administration Center and ensures that scientific rigor and peer review are consistent for the mission and purpose of the EHC (AHRQ, 2013)

    3. The EHC works with many agencies and affiliations to support the dissemination, translation, and implementation of CER information and data. Several of these entities completed their assignments in 2013 and 2014 (AHRQ, 2013).

  C. The Patient-Centered Outcomes Research Institute (PCORI) was created to provide reliable CER data to promote trustworthy clinical choices when patients, families, and clinicians face a wide range of complex and often confusing medical data (PCORI, 2014).

    1. In 2012, PCORI began funding patient-centered CER. The funding is guided by the *National Priorities for Research and Research Agenda* and managed by PCORI's established scientific programs to track and evaluate effectiveness (PCORI, 2014).

    2. Five national priorities (PCORI, 2012)

      a) Assessing prevention, diagnosis, and treatment options: Focuses on the clinical aspects of safety and efficacy of prevention, diagnosis, and treatment options that work best for different patients with a specific health condition

      b) Improving healthcare systems: Involves the comparison of health system approaches to improve access to care, use of self-management interventions, innovation in technology, coordination of complex chronic conditions, and creation of an informed and skilled healthcare workforce

      c) Communicating and disseminating research: Reviews comparisons of best approaches for providing CER information, dissemination of results, and the use of the information that is used in shared decision making between providers and patients

      d) Addressing disparities: Identifies any differences in prevention, diagnosis, or treatment effectiveness across ethnic populations and best practices used to achieve the best outcomes

      e) Accelerating patient-centered outcomes research and methodologic research: Provides the infrastructure to hold data that are used to improve the analytic methods of CER that promote patient-centered outcomes and to train researchers, patients, and other stakeholders to participate in CER

   3. PCORI is charged with the scientific development and methods used in CER and the production and dissemination of valid, reliable, trustworthy data that provide useful information when making healthcare decisions (PCORI, 2013). The Methodology Committee oversees CER design and implementation.

   4. PCORI's emphasis on "real-world" data involves the engagement of patients and the broader community to participate in CER studies and to help disseminate important and meaningful information that can be used to inform and promote optimal outcomes (PCORI, 2013).

D. Funded projects must fall under one of the five priority areas and include patient and community stakeholders involved in the application, CER design, implementation, and dissemination of data (PCORI, 2013).

   1. PCORnet, the National Patient-Centered Clinical Research Network, is a resource established to provide a representative network for conducting CER.

   2. This network provides a wide range of "real-time" and "real-world" observational and experimental data collected in clinical settings (PCORI, 2013).

   3. CER data are collected and stored under rigorous security protocols and can be shared across networks (PCORI, 2013).

      a) FDA, under the guidance of DHHS, is and will continue to use CER data to answer and inform healthcare priorities through the infrastructure development of repositories to hold large study data (U.S. FDA, 2010).

      b) Current work of FDA in CER (U.S. FDA, 2010)

         (1) Enable pilots of CER and other complex research findings through the agency's untapped massive stores of patient safety and clinical efficacy data

         (2) Develop expertise across FDA and develop collaboration among the CER-funded agencies (e.g., NIH, AHRQ) to seek guidance. in the use, development, participation, and evaluation of CER data

         (3) Develop and refine agency policies in the use of CER data and of existing FDA-approved data when comparing one intervention to another.

(4) Inform and improve medical and regulatory decision making that can best improve patient-centered outcomes

III. Current findings
    A. The current clinical guidelines are primarily based on disease-specific outcomes.
        1. These guidelines may not be relevant for patients with multiple chronic conditions (MCCs) (Maciejewski & Bayliss, 2014).
        2. Applying disease-specific guidelines may lead to poor outcomes, such as treatment–treatment and treatment–condition interactions and consequences that can lead to inefficient management and impede the ability to engage in patient–provider shared decision making (Maciejewski & Bayliss, 2014).
    B. A paucity of current evidence exists to direct and inform the care of patients with MCCs. Experts suggest a significant need exists for epidemiologic, health delivery, and intervention studies that can adequately address the complex care needs for patients with MCCs (Maciejewski & Bayliss, 2014).
    C. Healthcare organizations, quality assessment organizations, funders, payers, patient advocates, professional societies and organizations, and policy makers all recognize the knowledge gaps required to address the largest and fastest growing U.S. patient population (Maciejewski & Bayliss, 2014).
    D. CER is recognized as the number-one solution for generating evidence to inform the care and management of patients with MCCs (AHRQ, 2014; Maciejewski & Bayliss, 2014).
        1. One of the most challenging barriers for CER in patients with MCCs is to ensure heterogeneity of the study population (Maciejewski & Bayliss, 2014).
        2. Chronic conditions occur in various combinations. These conditions carry distinct effects on individual patients, thereby making study population generalizability difficult to obtain in CER methods (Maciejewski & Bayliss, 2014; Smith, 2013).
        3. Determinants for relevant outcomes in the MCC patient population have not been well defined, and CER studies will require rigorous methods to account for the individual variations that occur in this patient population (Maciejewski & Bayliss, 2014).
    E. The Institute of Medicine (IOM) was charged by DHHS to form a consensus committee and solicit stakeholder input that would be used to identify and direct national priorities for spending the $400 million designated for the DHHS secretary (IOM, 2009).
        1. The committee's principal task was to prepare a list of national priorities for CER funding and solicit a wide array of public input and deliberation over a list of nominated research topics (IOM, 2009).
        2. Given the information from stakeholders and the general public, the committee developed the infrastructure to sustain a long-term national CER agenda. Economic and benefit considerations took precedence (IOM, 2009).
        3. The committee developed a broad-based portfolio of high-priority topics based on the following criteria:
            a) Clinical category
            b) Study population
            c) Categories of interventions
            d) Research methodology
        4. The IOM committee sought balance across these categories. Balance among the categories establishes a portfolio of studies of diseases and conditions that

have the greatest effects on the health of Americans, as well as rare diseases and conditions that severely affect subgroups of the U.S. population (IOM, 2009).

5. The committee recognized the value of extending the practice of drug-to-drug comparisons to various routinely used interventions, including diagnostics, surgical techniques, and therapeutic alternatives (IOM, 2009).

6. CER studies also should examine the quality of different means of delivering care (IOM, 2009).

   a) The committee strongly recommended that the CER priorities involve balanced methodologies when researchers conduct systematic reviews, randomized trials, observational studies, and database research (IOM, 2009).

   b) The $400 million that was dispersed to DHHS from the Patient Protection and Affordable Care Act of 2010 (ACA) is being used to build this national portfolio with important data that can be used in the clinical setting between providers and patients (IOM, 2009).

IV. Relevance to practice

   A. The challenge for health professionals when effectively managing patients with MCCs, which is America's largest patient population, is to find nonbiased data to promote optimal outcomes (Tinetti & Studenski, 2011).

   B. Considering the infinite combinations of concomitant conditions, interventions, and other factors that significantly affect patient outcomes will create a challenge when identifying representative study populations for CER in the MCC patient population (Tinetti & Studenski, 2011).

   C. CER is predicted to accelerate the movement toward outcome-driven decision making, reimbursement, quality assessment, and cost-effectiveness (Tinetti & Studenski, 2011).

   1. Patient-reported outcomes that promote quality of life and subjective self-reporting on disease and symptom burden, as well as patient-individualized goals of care, are highly relevant for the MCC population (Wu, Snyder, Clancy, & Steinwachs, 2010).

   2. Challenges facing rigorous research to assess patient-centered outcomes in patients with MCCs have been widely recognized, and leaders at the Centers for Medicare and Medicaid Services, the National Quality Forum, the National Committee for Quality Assurance, and others are encouraging the development of quality measures that reflect real-world situations for this patient population (Maciejewski & Bayliss, 2014; Smith, 2013).

   3. Quality measures in the MCC population must be based on outcomes that are valid for heterogeneous populations and demonstrate sensitivity to intervention and change over time (Maciejewski & Bayliss, 2014).

   D. PCORI (2013) established standards when funding CER projects to focus on patient-centered outcomes.

   1. These standards represent "best practice" recommendations for improving the quality and value of patient-centered outcomes and CER methodology.

   2. The standards aim to promote transparency, rigor, and other scientific improvements to strengthen the science and methods of both patient-centered outcomes and CER (PCORI, 2013).

   E. The ACA's funding on CER data requires that methodologic standards provide specific criteria for the following:

   1. Internal validity—generate robust data to make comparisons of interventions

   2. Timeliness—are quickly applicable to meet the demands of patients with MCCs

      3. Generalizability—are relevant to clinical practice and patient preference

  F. For CER data to be meaningful and useful to patients, providers, policy makers, and payers when making specific health decisions and developing research proposals and protocols, it is important for researchers to ask the right questions, which include the following:

      1. Describe the specific health decision that CER data are intended to inform.

      2. Identify and describe the specific population whom the question will benefit.

      3. Explain how the study results can be used to inform the health decision.

  G. Methods of CER should be used to inform the question, which is different from what has been traditionally practiced.

  H. CER results should be used to inform health decisions through comparisons (Selby, Hickam, Mittman, & Tunis, 2013; Smith, 2013).

V. Role of the advanced practice registered nurse (APRN)

  A. The National Institute of Nursing Research (NINR, 2010), in collaboration with the American Association of Colleges of Nursing (AACN), produced *Promoting America's Health Through Nursing Science*, which highlights the role of CER.

      1. NINR has invested funding in CER to demonstrate optimal health prevention and promotion strategies or interventions that can bring about system-wide improvements in patient outcomes (NINR, 2011).

      2. CER is a critical area of inquiry at a time when consumers requiring health care obtain quality care focused on prevention that is affordable and accessible to all Americans (NINR, 2011).

      3. "What is efficacious in randomized clinical trials is not always effective in the real world of day-to-day practice. . . . Practice-based research [CER] provides the laboratory that will help generate new knowledge and bridge the chasm between recommended care and improved health" (Westfall, Mold, & Fagnan, 2007, pp. 402, 406).

  B. Evidence-based medicine is what drives evidence-based practice and predominantly includes data that come from randomized clinical trials (RCTs) and meta-analysis. RCTs are important when confirming if a treatment causes a desired effect and/or is less likely to reveal combinations of interventions or practice patterns that are effective, efficient, and cost-effective in routine care (Horn & Gassaway, 2007).

  C. CER can help to determine best interventions and treatments for a specific patient population.

      1. Engaging in CER will promote competition for investigation at the level of specific diseases, concomitant conditions, and specific types of patients, which in turn will speed the development of the right kind of information and improve value, or what can be measured as cost-effective patient-centered outcomes (care versus cost) (Horn & Gassaway, 2007).

      2. Researchers and users of CER appreciate the scientific rigor that answer real-world questions about its use in daily practice and applicability to a specific patient population (e.g., patients with more than one chronic condition) (Horn & Gassaway, 2007).

      3. RCTs do not routinely have primary endpoints that align with real-world practice and can prevent the use of evidence by clinicians who might not have the time to utilize, for example, a psychometric evaluation tool to assess or measure a condition in the clinical encounter.

      4. Clinicians, patients, and policy makers want to know if the intervention caused an effect and how or why it worked.

     5. RCTs are designed to maximize the chance of a positive effect from a new or current treatment and to confirm analysis of the original study hypothesis without taking into account relevant to real-world needs and practice (Horn & Gassaway, 2007).

     6. RCTs focus on meeting primary endpoints and assessing the hypothesis, which is not always relevant for clinicians and patients.

  D. APRNs in clinical settings require relevant data that can be used to make comparisons between interventions and patient populations.

     1. CER is ideal for real-world comparisons and is used in patient and family communications about efficacy and safety.

     2. APRNs in the wake of the ACA will be required to possess the skill set necessary to ensure optimal patient-centered outcomes with cost-effective and competent care that prevents patients from seeking costly acute care management.

     3. The use and implementation of CER data enables APRNs and patients to engage in shared decision-making conversations about what is in their best interest when comparing one intervention to another.

     4. APRNs should recognize the scientific changes that were established by the ACA and refine a new practice paradigm to embrace an understanding and implementation of CER data in clinical practice.

     5. CER is real-world, real-time, and real-life information that is relevant and current, and its use by APRNs in clinical practice is consistent with meeting patients and families where they are and with what they need.

     6. APRNs should use current resources to guide the development and implementation of CER projects (see Figure 6-1).

VI. Interface to palliative care

  A. Because of its real-world methodology, analysis, and implementation, CER data provide relevancy in palliative care or in the management of the myriad symptoms that occur in the presence of MCCs throughout the disease trajectory.

  B. Comparisons between drug classes to effectively manage specific symptoms and in various ethnic patient populations can provide APRNs with important

---

Figure 6-1. Resources for Comparative Effectiveness Research Information

AcademyHealth—Comparative Effectiveness Research: www.academyhealth.org/content.cfm?Item Number=2841&

Agency for Healthcare Research and Quality—What Is Comparative Effectiveness Research: http://effectivehealthcare.ahrq.gov/index.cfm/what-is-comparative-effectiveness-research1

Brigham and Women's Hospital—Patient-Centered Comparative Effectiveness Research Center: www.brighamandwomens.org/research/centers/pcerc/default.aspx

Comparative Effectiveness Research (journal): www.dovepress.com/comparative-effectiveness -research-journal

Health Services Research Information Central—Comparative Effectiveness Research: www.nlm.nih .gov/hsrinfo/cer.html

Institute of Translational Health Sciences—Institute for Comparative Effectiveness Research: www .iths.org/education/sdlc/research-initiation/comparative-effectiveness-research-training

Kaiser Family Foundation—Explaining Health Care Reform: What Is Comparative Effectiveness Research? http://kff.org/health-costs/issue-brief/explaining-health-care-reform-what-is-comparative

The Lewin Group—Center for Comparative Effectiveness Research: www.lewin.com/cer

National Information Center on Health Services Research and Health Care Technology: www.nlm.nih .gov/hsrinfo/cer.html

National Pharmaceutical Council—Comparative Effectiveness Research: www.npcnow.org/issues/ comparative-effectiveness-research

and timely information to promote best outcomes in individual patients who often suffer the consequences of poorly managed symptoms and combinations of medications.

C. CER data that can be used to determine disease management interventions based on where patients are in the trajectory of their illness can prevent the under- or overuse of diagnostics and interventions. CER data are applicable to patients living with symptomatic chronic conditions where little evidence is currently available, as RCTs primarily populate clinical trials with homogenous subjects.

D. APRNs are ideal investigators and partners in developing and participating in CER studies by interfacing with interdisciplinary partners to ensure that optimal patient-centric outcomes are obtained through real patient encounters.

1. APRNs are accountable stewards in the management of the patient with progressive, symptomatic, and chronic conditions.
2. APRNs use best available evidence to guide cost-effective clinical management of patients with MCCs.
3. APRNs must remain current and relevant in the dynamic changes of new evidence.
4. APRNs must rely on current data to guide practice and recognize the differences between evidence and anecdote when promoting optimal patient-perceived quality of life.

Case Study

O.N. is a 78-year-old Irish retired priest with a 92-pack-year smoking history, aortic aneurysm repair, hyperlipidemia, and obesity. He comes to the clinic today with complaints of dyspnea, chest tightness, cough, increased mucus production, daytime somnolence, and feelings of depression. The APRN learns that he was the rector of a huge cathedral for more than 30 years and has recently retired. He tells the nurse he is embarrassed when he gives mass because he loses his breath and has to stop in the middle of his sentences to cough and try to regain his breath. He no longer smokes and underwent an aortic aneurysm repair six months ago overseas.

His biggest concern is his shortness of breath during mass and his daytime somnolence. Together the nurse and O.N. review the recent CER data on the use of long-acting anticholinergics as maintenance therapy for chronic obstructive pulmonary disease combined with a short-acting beta-agonist as rescue. The nurse is familiar with a recent meta-analysis on the use of corticosteroids and the propensity for pneumonia. Based on a full evaluation of O.N.'s recent pulmonary function test and forced expiratory volume in one second, or FEV_1, of 66%, predicted, CER data suggest that the patient would benefit best from a long-acting anticholinergic (tiotropium) every day and the use of a beta-2 agonist (albuterol) for rescue therapy versus a long-acting beta-2 agonist combined with a corticosteroid. The APRN prescribes the recommended therapy for O.N. and refers him to a pulmonologist for sonography to evaluate for sleep apnea and repeat spirometry; a registered dietitian for weight loss; and a behavioral health counselor for evaluation of his depression and recent life change associated with retirement.

References

Agency for Healthcare Research and Quality. (2013). Comparative effectiveness reviews. Retrieved from http:// www.ahrq.gov/professionals/systems/long-term-care/reviews/index.html

Agency for Healthcare Research and Quality. (2014). *Methods guide for effectiveness and comparative effectiveness reviews.* Retrieved from http://www.effectivehealthcare.ahrq.gov/ehc/products/60/318/CER-Methods-Guide-140109.pdf

Horn, S.D., & Gassaway, J. (2007). Practice-based evidence study design for comparative effectiveness research. *Medical Care, 45*(10), S50–S57. doi:10.1097/MLR.0b013e318070c07b

Institute of Medicine. (2009). *Initial national priorities for comparative effectiveness research.* Washington, DC: National Academies Press.

Maciejewski, M.L., & Bayliss, E.A. (2014). Approaches to comparative effectiveness research in multimorbid populations. *Medical Care, 52*(3, Suppl. 2), S23–S30. doi:10.1097/MLR.0000000000000060

National Institute of Nursing Research. (2010). Promoting America's health through nursing science. Retrieved from http://www.aacn.nche.edu/government-affairs/archives/NINR_Factsheet.pdf

National Institute of Nursing Research. (2011). *Bringing science to life: NINR strategic plan* (NIH Publication No. 11-7783). Retrieved from https://www.ninr.nih.gov/sites/www.ninr.nih.gov/files/ninr-strategic-plan-2011.pdf

Patient-Centered Outcomes Research Institute. (2012). Methodological standards and patient-centeredness in comparative effectiveness research: The PCORI perspective. *JAMA, 307,* 1636–1640. doi:10.1001/jama.2012.466

Patient-Centered Outcomes Research Institute. (2013). Improving our national infrastructure to conduct comparative effectiveness research. Retrieved from http://www.pcori.org/research-results/pcornet-national-patient-centered-clinical-research-network/improving-our-national

Patient-Centered Outcomes Research Institute. (2014, April 28). Research methodology. Retrieved http://www.pcori.org/research-results/research-methodology

Patient Protection and Affordable Care Act, 42 U.S.C. § 18001 et seq. (2010). Retrieved from http://www.hhs.gov/healthcare/about-the-law/read-the-law/index.html

Selby, J.V., Hickam, D., Mittman, B., & Tunis, S. (2013). Using the PCORI methodology standards to generate robust, relevant, and timely evidence for patient-centered outcomes research [Webinar]. Retrieved from http://www.academyhealth.org/Training/ResourceDetail.cfm?ItemNumber=11023

Smith, S.R. (2013). Introduction to developing a protocol for observational comparative effectiveness research: A user's guide. In P. Velentgas, N.A. Dreyer, P. Nourjah, S.R. Smith, & M.M. Torchia (Eds.), *Developing a protocol for observational comparative effectiveness research: A user's guide* (pp. 1–6). Rockville, MD: Agency for Healthcare Research and Quality.

Tinetti, M.E., & Studenski, S.A. (2011). Comparative effectiveness research and patients with multiple chronic conditions. *New England Journal of Medicine, 364,* 2478–2481. doi:10.1056/NEJMp1100535

U.S. Food and Drug Administration. (2010, November 15). *Comparative effectiveness research plan.* Retrieved from http://www.fda.gov/downloads/AdvisoryCommittees/CommitteesMeetingMaterials/ScienceBoardtotheFoodandDrugAdministration/UCM233255.ppt

U.S. National Library of Medicine. (2016). Comparative effectiveness research (CER). Retrieved from https://www.nlm.nih.gov/hsrinfo/cer.html

Westfall, J.M., Mold, J., & Fagnan, L. (2007). Practice-based research—"Blue Highways" on the NIH roadmap. *JAMA, 297,* 403–406. doi:10.1001/jama.297.4.403

Wu, A.W., Snyder, C., Clancy, C.M., & Steinwachs, D.M. (2010). Adding the patient perspective to comparative effectiveness research. *Health Affairs, 29,* 1863–1871. doi:10.1377/hlthaff.2010.0660

CHAPTER 7

Health Policy and the Role of Advanced Practice Nurses

Kim Kuebler, DNP, APRN, ANP-BC,
and Mary Atkinson Smith, DNP, FNP-BC, ONP-C, RNFA, CNOR

I. Definition
   A. The World Health Organization (WHO, n.d.) defines health policy as "decisions, plans, and actions that are undertaken to achieve specific health care goals within a society."
   B. An explicit health policy can accomplish several things (WHO, n.d.):
      1. Define a vision for the future that helps to establish targets and points of reference for the short and medium term
      2. Outline priorities and the expected roles of different groups
      3. Build consensus and informs people
   C. The Centers for Disease Control and Prevention (2015) define health policy to include the development, implementation, and direction for law affecting public health and regulation and practices that influence healthcare systems, promote organizational change, and influence professional behaviors to promote optimal health outcomes.
   D. The health of the American population is influenced by public health policies to promote health and prevent disease.
   E. National health strategies, plans, and initiatives, such as Healthy People 2020, have policy implications (Centers for Disease Control and Prevention, 2015).
   F. Population health is a comprehensive and coordinated framework used to better understand and improve the health and well-being of a specific population (Weiner, 2008).
      1. Public health can be defined as societal actions and collaboration used to improve and promote health; its core functions relate to assessment, assurance, and health policy (Weiner, 2008).
      2. Medical care is defined as healthcare management and services provided to patients experiencing acute or chronic conditions (Weiner, 2008).
      3. Health policy includes "the planning, development, and implementation of interventions designed to maintain and improve the health of a group of individuals" (Weiner, 2008, Slide 6).
      4. Health policy determines the direction of clinical practice, where funding is needed for research, and reimbursement for clinical care and services and is

used to direct and influence the development of evidence-based clinical practice guidelines.

II. Key aspects
    A. State and federal branches of government regulate the organization, financing, and delivery of health care in the United States.
        1. State and federal lawmakers work closely with state and federal health agencies to develop health policy.
        2. Governmental health policies often serve as the guiding force for the development of policies in public and private healthcare organizations (D'Antonio, Fairman, & Lewenson, 2016).
        3. The federal and state governmental structure includes three branches: executive, legislative, and judicial.
    B. Individual states play a major role in the financing and organizing of healthcare delivery through health policy.
    C. State governments are structured according to state constitutions and are modeled after the structure of the federal government (Porche, 2012).
        1. Powers that are not granted to the federal government are reserved for the individual states and their people and are divided into state and local branches of government (Whitehouse.gov, n.d.).
        2. State-level distribution of governmental structure includes the executive, legislative, and judicial branches.
        3. The U.S. Constitution says that all states must uphold a republican form of government, which means that the power rests in and is exercised directly by the state's citizens or through representatives who are chosen by the state's citizens.
        4. The governor, who is directly elected by the state's citizens, directs the executive branch of state government.
        5. The additional leaders of a state's executive branch are directly elected as well and include the lieutenant governor, the attorney general, the secretary of state, auditors, and commissioners.
        6. States may vary in their executive structure.
        7. State agencies and departments are under the direct supervision of the governor. Certain state agencies, divisions, or departments are key players in health policy, such as the state departments of health, Medicaid divisions, department of human services, department of mental health, and regulatory agencies such as the medical board, pharmacy board, and nursing board.
        8. The legislative branch of state governments is made up of elected representatives who address topics introduced by the governor or by other legislative members.
            a) In most states, the legislature is divided into two houses, or chambers: the senate (a smaller upper chamber) and the house of representatives (a larger lower chamber). Nebraska is the exception with only one chamber in its legislature (Whitehouse.gov, n.d.).
            b) The legislative branch (state senators and representatives) may author and introduce bills that may become law, if passed. A state's legislature is also responsible for approving a state's budget, in addition to the initiation of tax legislation.
        9. A state's judicial branch is most often led by the state's supreme court, which handles the correction of errors in lower-level state courts. However, errors can be appealed to the U.S. Supreme Court.
    D. The U.S. federal government is located in Washington, DC.

1. The federal government has 10 regional offices.
2. The federal government consists of the same three branches as in the states: executive, legislative, and judicial.
3. The federal government also includes independent establishments and government corporations.
4. The executive branch of the federal government includes the president, vice president, the president's cabinet, and the executive branch agencies.
    a) The executive branch agency that is most involved in health policy is the U.S. Department of Health and Human Services (DHHS).
    b) DHHS's mission is to protect and enhance the well-being and health of Americans by supporting advancements in public health, medicine, and social services (U.S. DHHS, n.d.).
    c) DHHS consists of the following 11 divisions, of which eight are part of the U.S. Public Health Service and three are human service agencies that may serve to direct policy pertaining to clinical practice:
        (1) Administration for Children and Families
        (2) Administration for Community Living
        (3) Agency for Healthcare Research and Quality (AHRQ)
        (4) Agency for Toxic Substances and Disease Registry
        (5) Centers for Disease Control and Prevention
        (6) Centers for Medicare and Medicaid Services (CMS)
        (7) Food and Drug Administration
        (8) Health Resources and Services Administration (HRSA)
        (9) Indian Health Service
        (10) National Institutes of Health (NIH)
        (11) Substance Abuse and Mental Health Services Administration
5. The legislative branch of federal government is referred to as Congress.
    a) Congress comprises the Senate and the House of Representatives.
    b) Each state has two elected senators in Congress. The number of elected representatives per state is based on the state's population.
    c) Federal senators and representatives are often referred to as a congressman or congresswoman.
    d) However, the term *congressman* or *congresswoman* is most often used when referring to a representative.
    e) The role of senators and representatives in Congress in health policy includes financing, structuring, and distributing health care.
6. The judicial branch of the federal government consists of the U.S. Supreme Court, the U.S. courts of appeals, and the U.S. district courts.
E. Nongovernmental healthcare organizations
    1. Examples of nongovernmental healthcare organizations that serve to direct health policy in public and private sectors of the United States
        a) The Health and Medicine Division of the National Academies of Sciences, Engineering, and Medicine (formerly the Institute of Medicine [IOM])
        b) National Quality Forum
        c) Robert Wood Johnson Foundation
        d) Commonwealth Fund
    2. Private businesses also play a role in shaping health policy on state and national levels as purchasers of health insurance and providers in healthcare delivery. An example of this is the market-based model of managed care (Barr, 2011).

F. Individual state licensure regulates advanced practice registered nurse (APRN) practice through the state board of nursing and is considered a barrier to APRNs being able to practice to the full extent of their formal education (American Association of Nurse Practitioners [AANP], 2015a).

III. Current findings

A. Various organizations have released policy reports and recommendations pertaining to the barriers of APRN practice over the past few years.

1. AANP advocates for full practice authority (FPA) for APRNs, which is "the collection of state practice and licensure laws that allow for all nurse practitioners to evaluate patients, diagnose, order and interpret diagnostic tests, initiate and manage treatments—including prescribing medications—under the exclusive licensure authority of the state board of nursing" (AANP, 2015a, p. 1).

2. The National Council of State Boards of Nursing (NCSBN) has initiated the Campaign for APRN Consensus, which consists of promoting the Consensus Model for APRN Regulation among all states.

   a) It is an initiative that serves to facilitate the alignment of APRN regulations in individual states in a way that promotes uniformity of APRN practice among all states (NCSBN, n.d.-b).

   b) NCSBN (n.d.-a) recognizes the four roles of the APRN to be the clinical nurse specialist, the certified nurse practitioner, the certified registered nurse anesthetist, and the certified nurse midwife.

   c) Individual state boards of nursing should consider adopting the APRN consensus model to create uniformity pertaining to education, credentialing, licensing, and clinical practice for APRNs and removal of barriers that lead to limited APRN practice (Sullivan-Marx, 2015).

3. In 2011, IOM published a report called *The Future of Nursing: Leading Change, Advancing Health.*

   a) IOM recommended that APRNs play an active role in and lead interprofessional teams in health care.

   b) During this time of healthcare reform with rapidly changing healthcare environments, nurse practitioners (NPs) should have the ability to focus on outcome-driven approaches to the delivery of health care through innovative models of care delivery that support positive patient outcomes (Hain & Fleck, 2014).

   c) A key recommendation of the IOM report is to dissolve barriers that prevent NPs from practicing to the full extent of their education and training, which will serve to improve access to high-quality care among all individuals, especially those residing in rural and underserved areas.

4. The National Governors Association (NGA, 2012) published a position statement on the role of nurse practitioners in meeting the increasing demand for primary care, as a result of the IOM (2011) report on nursing and the Patient Protection and Affordable Care Act (ACA) of 2010.

   a) NGA reviewed the health services research literature and concluded that APRNs are well qualified to deliver certain elements of primary care.

   b) In light of the research evidence, states might consider changing scope of practice restrictions and ensuring adequate reimbursement for APRN services as a way of encouraging and incentivizing greater APRN involvement in the provision of primary health care for the nation's fastest growing patient population (NGA, 2012).

5. In March 2014, the Federal Trade Commission (FTC) released a policy report titled *Policy Perspectives: Competition and the Regulation of Advanced Practice Nurses.*

    a) In this policy analysis, FTC reported that mandated collaborative agreements between APRNs and physicians are not needed when it comes to achieving positive outcomes from physician–APRN care coordination. In addition, excessive regulations pertaining to supervision of APRNs by physicians may serve to increase the cost and prices of health care.

    b) This report also discusses the point that fixed regulations pertaining to APRN supervision may lead to constraints in innovative models of healthcare delivery, in addition to ignoring concerns of competition in health care in ways that will impede the use of more competitive models of quality improvement, increase prices, and minimize access to healthcare services (FTC, 2014).

6. HRSA (2013) reports an estimated shortage of 20,400 primary care physicians by 2020 and that this projected shortage can be avoided by fully integrating APRNs into all models of healthcare delivery. HRSA attributes this expected increasing demand in primary care services to be due to an increase in the aging population, general population growth, and the expected growth of health insurance coverage resulting from the ACA and the assumed expansion of Medicaid among the individual states (HRSA, 2013).

B. Currently, seven states have passed laws granting FPA to APRNs, making it a total of 22 states providing similar laws for APRN practice. Other states have passed laws to lessen restrictions on NP practice (AANP, 2015b).

C. The Frontlines to Lifelines Act (S. 297) was introduced in January 2015 and proposes timely access to healthcare services for veterans by granting FPA to nurse practitioners who are practicing with the Veterans Health Administration system regardless of their state-specific scope of practice.

IV. Relevance to practice

A. The passage of the ACA creates many opportunities for APRNs to be involved in health policy initiatives and demonstrate leadership and innovation to improve patient-centric care for patients with chronic conditions.

1. The ACA allows APRNs to be active players in the new reimbursement models of care that include nurse-managed health centers, accountable care organizations, patient-centered medical homes, and patient-centered outcomes research (Sullivan-Marx, 2015).

2. The ACA reduces barriers that interfere with APRN prescribing of class II medications, which often are required to ensure optimal symptom management. In states with significant practice barriers, APRNs can communicate with their legislators to address practice issues that prevent optimal patient care management.

B. The lack of FPA among APRNs leads to limitations in policy, limited scope of practice, lack of or limited prescriptive authority, restricted clinical privileges, constraints in credentialing, and lower reimbursement rates (Russell, 2012).

C. Opportunities for APRNs to demonstrate leadership and improve patient care

1. Participate as a member of an expert panel to update, revise, and develop clinical evidence-based practice guidelines for patients with multiple chronic conditions (MCCs).

2. Collaborate with all disciplines in the care and management of patients living with and dying from more than one chronic condition and begin to collect pertinent data that demonstrate positive patient-centric outcomes.
3. Demonstrate accountability on the appropriate use of healthcare resources through implementation of best evidence.
4. Utilize comparative effectiveness research to engage in important shared decision-making conversations with patients and their families.

V. Role of the APRN
   A. APRNs who are interested in health policy have to remain current on specific policy agendas for community, state, and federal initiatives.
   B. APRNs represent a large and escalating population of professionals who can play a proactive role in influencing legislation on relevant, important, and timely healthcare topics.
   C. Membership in professional nursing organizations provides a collective voice and discipline representation at key policy tables such as the National Quality Forum, IOM, the Institute for Healthcare Improvement, AANP, and the American Nurses Association (Sullivan-Marx, 2015).
   D. APRNs can be represented in governmental agencies under DHHS, such as HRSA, AHRQ, NIH, and CMS.
      1. Opportunities for APRNs in HRSA that may serve to develop future policy pertaining to advanced practice nursing include applying and participating in grant-funded opportunities that focus on distribution of APRNs in underserved areas to increase access to care for patients with MCCs.
      2. Funding opportunities also exist that focus on the future development of APRNs to better prepare them to meet the expanded needs of patients with MCCs.
      3. AHRQ has initiatives that APRNs can participate in that serve to improve quality of care and promote patient-centered care and shared decision making as healthcare transformation from the ACA ensues.
      4. NIH has opportunities for APRNs to be involved in research that focuses on the primary care workforce shortages and ways APRNs are able to alleviate this shortage by investigating existing APRN scope of practice laws.
      5. APRNs can collaborate with CMS on various demonstrations pertaining to innovative care delivery models that can lead to revision of current reimbursement policies to improve payment to APRNs that is more consistent with the amount of time required to effectively manage patients with MCCs.
   E. Informed and articulate APRNs should keep their legislators informed about pertinent healthcare issues.
   F. APRNs can serve as advocates by running for and being elected to public office; lobbying for specific political action; and advocating for patients through practice, education, and research.
      1. APRNs can serve to effectively analyze policy in a way that clearly identifies specific healthcare issues and are well informed and prepared to engage in clear and concise communication with key legislators to influence policy changes or development.
      2. APRNs should recognize the reimbursement changes mandated by the ACA and participate in the requirement for collecting patient outcomes to support best practices.

G. APRNs can participate in the goals of the ACA by engaging patients in shared decision making and encouraging self-management interventions to promote improved health and well-being.

VI. Interface to palliative care

    A. Providers who remain informed and prepared for the massive changes generated from the ACA will be ready to modify their practice from fee-for-service to value-based care.

    B. The chronic care reimbursement model is the first non–fee-for-service model where APRNs can demonstrate leadership by coordinating comprehensive primary care for patients living with and dying from symptomatic chronic conditions, thus reducing fragmented and costly care.

    C. Proactively managing exacerbations in chronic conditions such as congestive heart failure and chronic obstructive pulmonary disease will reduce admission into hospital and help to prevent the CMS readmission 30-day penalty (CMS, 2016).

        1. Patients and families will require ongoing shared decision-making discussions in the setting of progressive disease and increased debility.

        2. End-of-life discussions are billed and add value to patient preparation.

    D. The ACA promotes coordinated cost-effective care that is focused on each individual patient and demonstrated through outcome measurements that quantify value versus volume. Focusing on individualized patient outcomes promotes coordinated care for this patient population.

    E. Providers who are informed and trained on effective symptom management can integrate the use of palliative interventions into the care of patients who are living with more than one chronic condition, which will reduce disease exacerbations and hospital admissions and readmissions and promote physical functioning and improved quality of life in a cost-effective manner that represents the goals and direction of community, state, and federal healthcare initiatives in chronic care.

Case Study

K.L. is a 47-year-old APRN who is passionate about the legislative issues targeting the care of patients with MCCs. In 2010, she found a call from DHHS seeking testimony on new care models proposed for the management of patients with MCCs. K.L. submitted one of 500 testimonies and consequently became a stakeholder. She has been following the innovation that has occurred from ACA funding for the various agencies under DHHS. Because of K.L.'s clinical work with patients with MCCs, she has scheduled appointments with her state representative, congressman, and U.S. senator to inform them of important aspects of her practice.

She became aware of train-the-trainer opportunities on shared decision making through AHRQ and attended one of 10 federally funded meetings. K.L. is now a fully trained trainer and has begun to train some of her colleagues. Together, they are planning to implement this intervention into several senior-living high rises in her local community.

K.L. understands the value of supporting patients with MCCs to engage in shared decision-making practices that promote the use of self-management interventions to reduce disease exacerbations. She recognizes the new changes unfolding in her practice as she implements new ideas and approaches for her patients. K.L. is prepared to provide outcome measurements from her interventions and embrace a new payment system where she will be reimbursed for her value to the patient rather than the volume of patients she encounters within a clinic day.

References

American Association of Nurse Practitioners. (2015a). Issues at-a-glance: Full practice authority. Retrieved from https://www.aanp.org/images/documents/policy-toolbox/fullpracticeauthority.pdf

American Association of Nurse Practitioners. (2015b). State practice environment. Retrieved from https://www.aanp.org/legislation-regulation/state-legislation/state-practice-environment

Barr, D.A. (2011). *Introduction to U.S. health policy: The organization, financing, and delivery of health care in America* (3rd ed.). Baltimore, MD: Johns Hopkins University Press.

Centers for Disease Control and Prevention. (2015). Definition of policy. Retrieved from http://www.cdc.gov/policy/analysis/process/definition.html

Centers for Medicare and Medicaid Services. (2016). Readmissions Reduction Program (HRRP). Retrieved from https://www.cms.gov/Medicare/medicare-fee-for-service-payment/acuteinpatientPPS/readmissions-reduction-program.html

D'Antonio, P., Fairman, J., & Lewenson, S.B. (2016). An historical perspective on policy, politics, and nursing. In D.J. Mason, D.B. Gardner, F.H. Outlaw, & E.T. O'Grady (Eds.), *Policy and politics in nursing and health care* (7th ed., pp. 22–29). St. Louis, MO: Elsevier.

Federal Trade Commission. (2014). *Policy perspectives: Competition and the regulation of advanced practice nurses.* Retrieved from https://www.ftc.gov/system/files/documents/reports/policy-perspectives-competition-regulation-advanced-practice-nurses/140307aprnpolicypaper.pdf

Frontlines to Lifelines Act of 2015, S. 297, 114th Cong. (2015). Retrieved from https://www.congress.gov/bill/114th-congress/senate-bill/297

Hain, D., & Fleck, L.M. (2014). Barriers to NP practice that impact healthcare redesign. *Online Journal of Issues in Nursing, 19*(2), Manuscript 2. Retrieved from http://www.nursingworld.org/MainMenuCategories/ANAMarketplace/ANAPeriodicals/OJIN/TableofContents/Vol-19-2014/No2-May-2014/Barriers-to-NP-Practice.html

Health Resources and Services Administration. (2013). *Projecting the supply and demand for primary care practitioners through 2020.* Retrieved from http://bhpr.hrsa.gov/healthworkforce/supplydemand/usworkforce/primarycare

Institute of Medicine. (2011). *The future of nursing: Leading change, advancing health.* Washington, DC: National Academies Press.

National Council of State Boards of Nursing. (n.d.-a). APRN campaign for consensus: Moving toward uniformity in state laws. Retrieved from https://www.ncsbn.org/738.htm

National Council of State Boards of Nursing. (n.d.-b). APRNs in the U.S. Retrieved from https://www.ncsbn.org/aprn.htm

National Governors Association. (2012). *The role of nurse practitioners in meeting increasing demand for primary care.* Retrieved from http://www.nga.org/files/live/sites/NGA/files/pdf/1212NursePractitionersPaper.pdf

Porche, D.J. (2012). *Health policy: Application for nurses and other healthcare professionals.* Burlington, MA: Jones & Bartlett Learning.

Russell, K.A. (2012). Nurse practice acts guide and govern nursing practice. *Journal of Nursing Regulation, 3*(3), 36–42. doi:10.1016/S2155-8256(15)30197-6

Sullivan-Marx, E.M. (2015). Navigating the political system. In R.M. Patton, M.L. Zalon, & R. Ludwick (Eds.), *Nurses making policy: From bedside to boardroom* (pp. 77–101). New York, NY: Springer.

U.S. Department of Health and Human Services. (n.d.). About HHS. Retrieved from http://www.hhs.gov/about/index.html

Weiner, J.P. (2008). *Health policy and the delivery of health care: Introduction and private health plan case study* [Lecture slides]. Johns Hopkins University Bloomberg School of Public Health. Retrieved from http://ocw.jhsph.edu/courses/IntroHealthPolicy/PDFs/IHP_lec7_weiner.pdf

Whitehouse.gov. (n.d.). State and local government. Retrieved from https://www.whitehouse.gov/1600/state-and-local-government

World Health Organization. (n.d.). Health policy. Retrieved from http://www.who.int/topics/health_policy/en

Section II.

Pharmacology of Palliative Care

CHAPTER 8

Metabolism and Excretion in Disease

Adegoke O. Adeniji, RPh, PhD, Launa M.J. Lynch, PhD, and Vicky V. Mody, PhD

I. Definitions
   A. *Pharmacokinetics* is the study of a drug's absorption, distribution, metabolism, and excretion inside the body. It studies the movement of the drug within the body from the moment it enters the body to the time it is excreted and is commonly described as what the body does to the drug.
   B. *Pharmacodynamics* is the study of the biochemical and physiologic effects of drugs on the body and the mechanisms through which the drugs elicit these effects.
   C. *Bioavailability* is the fraction of a parent drug that reaches the systemic circulation following administration by any route. The value ranges from zero to one (0–1).
   D. *Metabolism* is the enzyme-catalyzed conversion of a parent drug into one or more chemical analogs within the body.
   E. The liver is the primary site for biotransformation of drugs within the body, although other sites such as the blood, kidney, and gut are also involved in the metabolism of drugs.
   F. *First-pass metabolism* is the biotransformation of a drug by the liver following absorption from the gut prior to reaching the systemic circulation. First-pass metabolism leads to a reduction in the bioavailability of a drug.
   G. *Elimination half-life* ($t_{1/2}$) is the time required to remove 50% of a compound or drug from the systemic circulation.
   H. *Renal clearance of a drug* is the volume of plasma from which a drug is completely removed by the kidney in a given amount of time.
II. Key aspects
   A. The course of drug action is often altered in disease conditions, leading to changes in a patient's drug exposure.
   B. Drugs are primarily metabolized in the liver by enzymes that catalyze conjugation (phase II) and nonconjugation (phase I) reactions. The parent drug and the metabolites are subsequently excreted by the kidney.
   C. Changes in hepatic and renal function can lead to changes in the metabolism and excretion of drugs.
   D. The effect of hepatic and renal diseases on metabolism and excretion differs from drug to drug and is dependent on the specific pathway of a drug's elimination.
   E. Renal disease decreases glomerular filtration and tubular secretion and also affects the nonrenal clearance of drugs.

F. Hepatic diseases impair blood flow to the liver, reduce the expression and activity of metabolizing enzymes, and alter plasma protein binding of drugs.

G. An understanding of how the pharmacokinetics of a drug changes in disease conditions is essential to optimize drug therapy and minimize adverse events. This information guides the choice of drug used and the appropriate dose required.

H. The pathway of a drug from the time it is administered to the time it leaves the body (excretion) involves transit across multiple physiologic membranes and an intricate sequence of biochemical processes.

1. This pathway is often referred to as the pharmacokinetics of a drug (i.e., what the body does to the drug) in contrast to pharmacodynamics (i.e., what the drug does to the body).

2. Pharmacokinetics provides information that is used in drug dosing and serves as a guide in assessing the optimal clinical context in which the drug should be used.

I. An orally administered drug is absorbed from the gastrointestinal tract by traversing the enterocytes either by passive diffusion or carrier-mediated transport into the hepatic portal system, where it may undergo biotransformation by the liver (see Figure 8-1).

1. This phenomenon, referred to as first-pass metabolism, is extensive in some drugs and can significantly reduce the concentration of drugs that reaches the systemic circulation. Once in the systemic circulation, the drug is distributed to the whole body during which it interacts with the cognate receptor, enzyme, ion channel, or other biomolecules to elicit the desired therapeutic effects as well as adverse side effects.

2. The drug is distributed to the liver, where it may undergo cytochrome P450 (CYP) and non-CYP enzyme-mediated biotransformation (metabolism), or to the kidney, where it is excreted from the body via the urine.

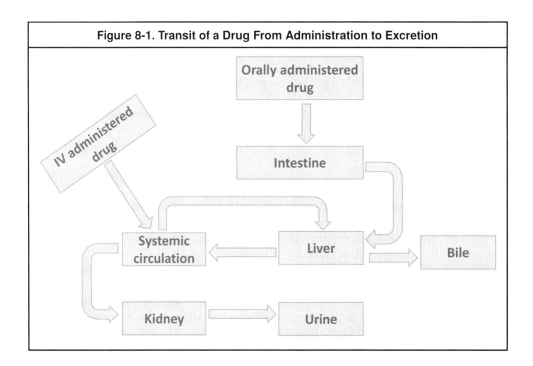

Figure 8-1. Transit of a Drug From Administration to Excretion

    3. A drug that is given parenterally bypasses absorption through the gastrointestinal tract but also undergoes distribution, metabolism, and excretion much like an orally administered drug.

  J. The efficiency of metabolism and excretion is critical to ensuring that the optimal dose of the drug is given, adverse side effects are minimized, and the disease condition is effectively treated.

    1. However, these processes are often altered in disease conditions, which potentially leads to variability in the elimination half-life ($t_{1/2}$) of drugs and the patient's response to drug treatment.

    2. Also, because individuals receiving palliative care often take multiple medications, the risk of both drug–drug and drug–disease interactions is increased as a result of changes in these processes (Koh & Koo, 2002; Kotlinska-Lemieszek, Paulsen, Kaasa, & Klepstad, 2014).

    3. Therefore, it is essential that healthcare workers, especially those who care for patients under palliative care, possess an understanding of drug metabolism and excretion pathways (see Figure 8-1), mechanisms of the alterations of these processes, and how these alterations affect drug therapy.

III. Relevance to practice

  A. Hepatic diseases

    1. The liver has the highest expression of metabolic enzymes in the human body and is the principal site of biotransformation for most endogenous and exogenous substances.

    2. Hepatic enzymes catalyze the conversion of drugs into metabolites that are usually, but not always, more hydrophilic, thereby reducing reabsorption and facilitating the excretion of these drugs via the kidneys.

    3. Drugs and their metabolites can likewise be excreted into bile, which is a digestive fluid produced by the liver that is needed for fat emulsification.

    4. The liver also synthesizes plasma proteins such as albumin.

    5. Albumin binds a plethora of drugs, and the albumin–drug complex serves as a depot from which the drug can be released.

    6. Pathologic changes in the metabolic, biosynthetic, and excretory functions of the liver will affect the concentration of drugs in the systemic circulation, the ratio of free and bound drug, and the levels of extrahepatic metabolism of drugs.

    7. This makes the liver a critical organ in controlling the fate of drugs in the body.

    8. The liver has remarkable functional reserve capacity.

      a) An estimated 75% of a normal liver can be resected without any fatality because the liver can regenerate itself (Schindl, Redhead, Fearon, Garden, & Wigmore, 2005; Shoup et al., 2003).

      b) Therefore, the effect of liver diseases on drug metabolism and excretion may not always be clinically observed unless there is significant liver damage such as that seen in liver failure and cirrhosis.

    9. The clearance of a drug by the liver depends on the blood supply to the liver, the expression and activity of metabolic enzymes, and the extent of drug binding with albumin and other protein components of plasma. Disruption of the blood supply to the liver has the potential to reduce drug metabolism and increase the duration of action and the incidence of adverse reactions related to the drug, with the exception being a prodrug.

    10. The liver is unique in that it has two primary sources of blood supply: the hepatic artery and the hepatic portal vein.

11. The hepatic artery carries oxygenated blood from the heart to the liver, whereas the portal vein collects blood rich in nutrients and other substances from the gastrointestinal tract.

    a) Liver cirrhosis often is associated with a disruption of the blood supply via the portal veins leading to portal hypertension and development of portosystemic shunts in which the blood from the gastrointestinal tract bypasses the liver (Zardi et al., 2009).

    b) Portosystemic shunts limit first-pass metabolism and increase the bioavailability of drugs (see Figure 8-2).

    c) This increases the risk of adverse events, especially with drugs that undergo extensive first-pass metabolism (low oral bioavailability) and have a narrow therapeutic index.

12. The drug-metabolizing potential of the liver progressively decreases with disease severity.

    a) The loss of hepatocytes in liver diseases causes a reduction in both the expression (at both mRNA and protein levels) and activity of the metabolizing enzymes (Villeneuve & Pichette, 2004; Yang et al., 2003).

    b) Orally administered drugs therefore undergo reduced first-pass metabolism and also are not readily metabolized once in the circulation, which often leads to an increase in bioavailability and the elimination of $t_{1/2}$, respectively.

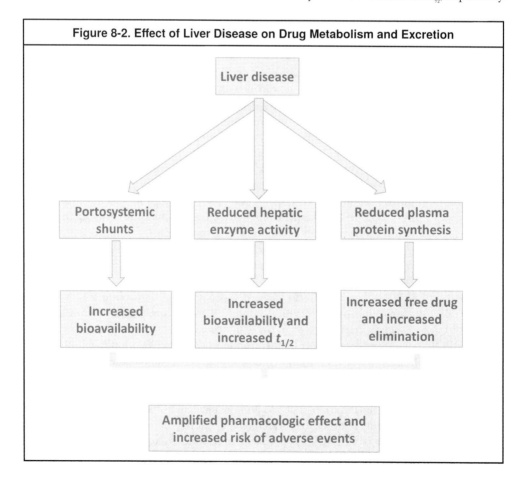

Figure 8-2. Effect of Liver Disease on Drug Metabolism and Excretion

Liver disease

Portosystemic shunts

Reduced hepatic enzyme activity

Reduced plasma protein synthesis

Increased bioavailability

Increased bioavailability and increased $t_{1/2}$

Increased free drug and increased elimination

Amplified pharmacologic effect and increased risk of adverse events

    c) Interestingly, metabolizing enzymes are affected to different extents by liver diseases. This is evident in the observation that the hepatic metabolism of some drugs is significantly or modestly altered in patients with chronic liver diseases while that of other drugs is unaffected in the same patient population—a factor that should inform drug selection for patients with liver diseases (Frye et al., 2006; Rhee & Broadbent, 2007).

13. One area in which this has profound consequences is in sedation for patients with liver disease, as excessive sedation can lead to coma and ultimately death.

    a) The choice of benzodiazepine that is used is based on an understanding of the metabolism of the drugs.

    b) Because of its different metabolic pathways, temazepam is preferred and diazepam is not recommended in patients with liver disease.

14. Diazepam is extensively metabolized by CYP enzymes into several metabolites including temazepam, which is primarily metabolized to the O-glucuronide and subsequently eliminated via the kidneys (Andersson, Miners, Veronese, & Birkett, 1994; Ghabrial et al., 1986; Klotz, Avant, Hoyumpa, Schenker, & Wilkinson, 1975; Locniskar & Greenblatt, 1990).

15. Although both CYP and conjugating enzymes are abundant in the liver, conjugation reactions such as glucuronidation are comparatively less affected in liver disease (Elbekai, Korashy, & El-Kadi, 2004; Schenker, Bergstrom, Wolen, & Lemberger, 1988). As a result, the elimination half-life ($t_{1/2}$) of diazepam is increased more than twofold in patients with cirrhosis, whereas that of temazepam remains relatively unaltered (Ghabrial et al., 1986; Klotz et al., 1975).

16. Most drugs are bound to plasma proteins, usually either albumin or α-1-acid glycoprotein in the systemic circulation. Albumin binds acidic and neutral drugs, whereas α-1-acid glycoprotein binds to basic drugs.

17. The extent and strength of the plasma protein–drug interaction affect the activity and elimination half-life of the drug because only the free drug can traverse biologic membranes to elicit the desired pharmacologic effect, be metabolized by the liver, or be excreted by the kidney.

    a) Because the liver synthesizes these plasma proteins, chronic liver diseases often lead to hypoalbuminemia, a reduction in the levels of other plasma proteins, and consequently an increase in the free–bound drug ratio.

    b) The clinical consequences of a change in the free–bound drug ratio depend on the drug and the functional state of the liver.

    c) In individuals with normal liver function, modest changes in protein binding of a drug usually are not of significant clinical relevance (Benet & Hoener, 2002).

    d) However, depending on the drug, it can be very important in the context of liver disease. In drugs such as warfarin, there is no sustained increase in the plasma concentration of the free drug because the drug clearance is proportional to the amount of free drug available, such that an increase in the free fraction of the drug leads to an increase in hepatic clearance of the drug.

    e) With drugs such as propranolol, the drug clearance rate is unchanged despite an increase in free–bound drug ratio (Arthur et al., 1985; Branch & Shand, 1976).

    f) This may result in a sustained increase in the concentration of the free drug and an increase in toxicity.

18. Dosage adjustment is essential in patients with liver failure more so with drugs that undergo extensive hepatic metabolism or induce or inhibit hepatic enzymes.

    a) However, unlike in renal disease, where creatinine clearance is used to predict a drug's renal clearance, no single in vivo parameter can be used to correct for liver disease.

    b) Therefore, adjustments must be made based on the kinetic profiles of the drugs in patients with hepatic failure.

    c) The existence of genetic polymorphism with metabolizing enzymes should also be considered.

    d) Four categories of metabolizers are recognized: poor, intermediate, extensive, and ultra-rapid (Lea, 2005; Ng, Schweitzer, Norman, & Easteal, 2004).

    e) Poor metabolizers have reduced baseline enzyme activity, whereas ultra-rapid metabolizers have an elevated baseline enzyme activity, with the result being a different kinetic profile for the same drug.

    f) Genotyping of a patient's CYP enzyme profile is a vital tool that will help optimize treatment.

B. Renal diseases

1. The kidney remains the major organ for drug excretion, although the lungs can be important for gaseous compounds and metabolites.

2. Drugs and their metabolites can also be excreted via the feces, sweat, saliva, and breast milk, although taken together, these represent a small fraction of the routes of excretion for most drugs.

    a) Renal clearance of a drug is defined as the volume of plasma from which a drug is completely removed by the kidney in a given amount of time.

    b) It involves the delivery of the drug or its metabolite into the renal tubules either by glomerular filtration (passive diffusion), tubular secretion (active transport), or both.

    c) Diseases of the kidney, such as chronic kidney disease, also called chronic renal failure, often reduce these processes and alter protein and tissue binding of drugs, which modifies the patient's exposure to the drug (Nolin, Naud, Leblond, & Pichette, 2008; Reidenberg & Drayer, 1984).

    d) The need for dose adjustment when giving renally cleared drugs to patients with renal impairment is now well recognized.

3. Reduced glomerular filtration rate and reduced tubular secretion decrease the amount of drug or its metabolite that is removed from the renal vasculature into the nephrons for excretion.

    a) This causes a buildup of compounds in the systemic circulation and the potentiation of the desired or adverse effects of a drug or its metabolite, which can lead to potentially significant toxic events.

    b) It therefore is imperative that other alternative drugs be explored or the dosage be adjusted when individuals with renal diseases are receiving drugs that undergo significant renal clearance.

4. Nowhere is this more relevant than in pain management for patients with renal diseases.

5. Pain is very common in patients with end-stage renal disease (ESRD), with an estimated 50% of patients with this disease experiencing chronic pain (Davison, Chambers, & Ferro, 2010; Kuebler, 2001).

6. Ensuring adequate analgesia while minimizing significant adverse effects is critical in this patient subpopulation.

7. Although opioids are the mainstay of pain management in these patients, the choice of opioid used is dependent on many factors with special consideration given to the role of the kidneys in the excretion of the particular drug from the body.
    a) For example, although morphine is the gold standard in treating severe pain in individuals with normal renal function, it is not recommended for long-term use in individuals with ESRD because of the accumulation of the morphine-3-glucuronide (M3G) and morphine-6-glucuronide (M6G), the latter metabolite having twice the analgesic potency of morphine (Arnold, Verrico, & Davison, 2015; Davison et al., 2010).
    b) Increased systemic levels of M3G and M6G will lengthen the duration of action of morphine and elicit an increased incidence of morphine-related adverse events.
8. Other common opioid analgesics such as meperidine, codeine, dextropropoxyphene, and oxycodone either accumulate or have pharmacologically active or toxic metabolites that accumulate when administered to patients with renal failure, which can lead to significant central nervous system toxicity. Fentanyl, hydromorphone, and methadone are preferred for pain management in renal failure because of a lack of active metabolites or as a result of a favorable excretion profile for both parent drugs and metabolites from the body (Arnold et al., 2015; Davison et al., 2010; Kuebler, 2001).
9. It is important to note that dosage adjustment often is still necessary, even with the preferred drugs, based on the severity of renal failure as measured by the creatinine clearance (Broadbent, Khor, & Heaney, 2003).
10. In addition to the effect on glomerular filtration and tubular secretion of drugs, renal diseases also alter the hepatic clearance of some drugs (Nolin, 2008; Nolin et al., 2008; Sun, Frassetto, & Benet, 2006).
    a) These drugs display changes in total clearance from the body that cannot be explained solely by a change in renal clearance.
    b) The hepatic clearance of drugs including but not limited to captopril, cefotaxime, erythromycin, lovastatin, metoclopramide, raloxifene, repaglinide, verapamil, and warfarin is reduced in renal failure (Czock, Keller, Heringa, & Rasche, 2005; Dreisbach & Lertora, 2003; Kanfer et al., 1987; Marbury et al., 2000; Pichette & Leblond, 2003; Quérin et al., 1991; Sun et al., 2006).
    c) Despite this observation, the need to correct for this observation in patients with renal failure taking these drugs has not been readily recognized and would likely involve the consideration of a complex interplay of factors related to the specific drug.
    d) Nevertheless, it is important to use these drugs with caution and preferably titrate the dose of the drug to optimize the patient's exposure to the drug.
11. The expression levels and the activity of specific hepatic enzymes catalyzing both phase I and phase II reactions are suppressed in renal failure (Dreisbach & Lertora, 2003; Pichette & Leblond, 2003).
    a) The expression and activity of hepatic and intestinal uptake and efflux transporters also are altered in renal failure (Nolin, 2008; Nolin et al., 2008; Sun et al., 2006).
    b) The net effects of these changes is an increased bioavailability as a result of increased absorption from the gastrointestinal tract and decreased first-

pass metabolism, decreased hepatic uptake, and decreased metabolism of the drugs once inside the circulation.

   c) These changes have been shown to be secondary to accumulation of uremic toxins such as urea, indoxyl sulfate, 3-carboxy-4-methyl-5-propyl-2-furan-propanoic acid (known as CMPF) and hippuric acid (Vanholder et al., 2003).

   d) The mechanism by which these toxins alter the expression and activity of hepatic enzymes, transporters, and intestinal transporters is not entirely clear, but it is believed to be due to either direct inhibition or inhibition of the transcription and translation of these macromolecules (Sun et al., 2006).

IV. Interface to palliative care

   A. The elimination profile of most drugs is determined by the activity of the liver and kidneys.

   1. Drugs undergo chemical biotransformation catalyzed by hepatic enzymes to produce metabolites that are usually, although not always, less lipophilic.

   2. The parent drug and the metabolites can then be removed from the systemic circulation and excreted by the kidneys.

   3. Hepatic and renal diseases reduce the clearance of drugs from the systemic circulation, which causes drug accumulation and toxicity.

   B. An understanding of changes to the metabolism and excretion of drugs is critical to drug selection in particular disease settings as well as determination of the optimal dosage for therapy.

   1. In patients with renal failure, dosage adjustment based on the creatinine clearance has long been recognized for drugs with significant renal clearance.

   2. However, with liver failure, no single in vivo parameter can be used to determine the needed dosage adjustment. Hence, adjustment will need to be made based on the kinetics of that drug in a particular patient or patient population starting with the lowest effective dose.

References

Andersson, T., Miners, J.O., Veronese, M.E., & Birkett, D.J. (1994). Diazepam metabolism by human liver microsomes is mediated by both S-mephenytoin hydroxylase and CYP3A isoforms. *British Journal of Clinical Pharmacology, 38,* 131–137. doi:10.1111/j.1365-2125.1994.tb04336.x

Arnold, R., Verrico, P., & Davison, S.N. (2015). Fast Facts and Concepts #161: Opioid use in renal failure. Retrieved from http://www.mypcnow.org/blank-x9494

Arthur, M.J., Tanner, A.R., Patel, C., Wright, R., Renwick, A.G., & George, C.F. (1985). Pharmacology of propranolol in patients with cirrhosis and portal hypertension. *Gut, 26,* 14–19. doi:10.1136/gut.26.1.14

Benet, L.Z., & Hoener, B.-A. (2002). Changes in plasma protein binding have little clinical relevance. *Clinical Pharmacology and Therapeutics, 71,* 115–121. doi:10.1067/mcp.2002.121829

Branch, R.A., & Shand, D.G. (1976). Propranolol disposition in chronic liver disease: A physiological approach. *Clinical Pharmacokinetics, 1,* 264–279. doi:10.2165/00003088-197601040-00002

Broadbent, A., Khor, K., & Heaney, A. (2003). Palliation and chronic renal failure: Opioid and other palliative medications—Dosage guidelines. *Progress in Palliative Care, 11,* 183–190. doi:10.1179/096992603225002627

Czock, D., Keller, F., Heringa, M., & Rasche, F.M. (2005). Raloxifene pharmacokinetics in males with normal and impaired renal function. *British Journal of Clinical Pharmacology, 59,* 479–482. doi:10.1111/j.1365-2125.2004.02326.x

Davison, S.N., Chambers, E.J., & Ferro, C.J. (2010). Management of pain in renal failure. In E.J. Chambers, E.A. Brown, & M. Germain (Eds.), *Supportive care for the renal patient* (2nd ed., pp. 140–188). New York, NY: Oxford University Press.

Dreisbach, A.W., & Lertora, J.J.L. (2003). The effect of chronic renal failure on hepatic drug metabolism and drug disposition. *Seminars in Dialysis, 16,* 45–50. doi:10.1046/j.1525-139X.2003.03011.x

Elbckai, R.H., Korashy, H.M., & El-Kadi, A.O.S. (2004). The effect of liver cirrhosis on the regulation and expression of drug metabolizing enzymes. *Current Drug Metabolism, 5,* 157–167. doi:10.2174/1389200043489054

Frye, R.F., Zgheib, N.K., Matzke, G.R., Chaves-Gnecco, D., Rabinovitz, M., Shaikh, O.S., & Branch, R.A. (2006). Liver disease selectively modulates cytochrome P450–mediated metabolism. *Clinical Pharmacology and Therapeutics, 80,* 235–245. doi:10.1016/j.clpt.2006.05.006

Ghabrial, H., Desmond, P.V., Watson, K.J.R., Gijsbers, A.J., Harman, P.J., Breen, K.J., & Mashford, M.L. (1986). The effects of age and chronic liver disease on the elimination of temazepam. *European Journal of Clinical Pharmacology, 30,* 93–97. doi:10.1007/BF00614203

Kanfer, A., Stamatakis, G., Torlotin, J.C., Fredj, G., Kenouch, S., & Méry, J.P. (1987). Changes in erythromycin pharmacokinetics induced by renal failure. *Clinical Nephrology, 27,* 147–150.

Klotz, U., Avant, G.R., Hoyumpa, A., Schenker, S., & Wilkinson, G.R. (1975). The effects of age and liver disease on the disposition and elimination of diazepam in adult man. *Journal of Clinical Investigation, 55,* 347–359. doi:10.1172/JCI107938

Koh, N.Y., & Koo, W.H. (2002). Polypharmacy in palliative care: Can it be reduced? *Singapore Medical Journal, 43,* 279–283.

Kotlinska-Lemieszek, A., Paulsen, O., Kaasa, S., & Klepstad, P. (2014). Polypharmacy in patients with advanced cancer and pain: A European cross-sectional study of 2282 patients. *Journal of Pain and Symptom Management, 48,* 1145–1159. doi:10.1016/j.jpainsymman.2014.03.008

Kuebler, K.K. (2001). Palliative nursing care for the patient experiencing end-stage renal failure. *Urologic Nursing, 21,* 167–168, 171–178.

Lea, D.H. (2005). Tailoring drug therapy with pharmacogenetics. *Nursing, 35*(4), 22–23. doi:10.1097/00152193-200504000-00013

Locniskar, A., & Greenblatt, D.J. (1990). Oxidative versus conjugative biotransformation of temazepam. *Biopharmaceutics and Drug Disposition, 11,* 499–506. doi:10.1002/bdd.2510110604

Marbury, T.C., Ruckle, J.L., Hatorp, V., Andersen, M.P., Nielsen, K.K., Huang, W.C., & Strange, P. (2000). Pharmacokinetics of repaglinide in subjects with renal impairment. *Clinical Pharmacology and Therapeutics, 67,* 7–15. doi:10.1067/mcp.2000.103973

Ng, C.H., Schweitzer, I., Norman, T., & Easteal, S. (2004). The emerging role of pharmacogenetics: Implications for clinical psychiatry. *Australian and New Zealand Journal of Psychiatry, 38,* 483–489. doi:10.1111/j.1440-1614.2004.01400.x

Nolin, T.D. (2008). Altered nonrenal drug clearance in ESRD. *Current Opinion in Nephrology and Hypertension, 17,* 555–559. doi:10.1097/MNH.0b013e3283136732

Nolin, T.D., Naud, J., Leblond, F.A., & Pichette, V. (2008). Emerging evidence of the impact of kidney disease on drug metabolism and transport. *Clinical Pharmacology and Therapeutics, 83,* 898–903. doi:10.1038/clpt.2008.59

Pichette, V., & Leblond, F.A. (2003). Drug metabolism in chronic renal failure. *Current Drug Metabolism, 4,* 91–103. doi:10.2174/1389200033489532

Quérin, S., Lambert, R., Cusson, J.R., Grégoire, S., Vickers, S., Stubbs, R.J., … Larochelle, P. (1991). Single-dose pharmacokinetics of ^{14}C-lovastatin in chronic renal failure. *Clinical Pharmacology and Therapeutics, 50,* 437–441. doi:10.1038/clpt.1991.161

Reidenberg, M.M., & Drayer, D.E. (1984). Alteration of drug-protein binding in renal disease. *Clinical Pharmacokinetics, 9*(Suppl. 1), 18–26.

Rhee, C., & Broadbent, A.M. (2007). Palliation and liver failure: Palliative medications dosage guidelines. *Journal of Palliative Medicine, 10,* 677–685. doi:10.1089/jpm.2006.0246

Schenker, S., Bergstrom, R.F., Wolen, R.L., & Lemberger, L. (1988). Fluoxetine disposition and elimination in cirrhosis. *Clinical Pharmacology and Therapeutics, 44,* 353–359. doi:10.1038/clpt.1988.161

Schindl, M.J., Redhead, D.N., Fearon, K.C.H., Garden, O.J., & Wigmore, S.J. (2005). The value of residual liver volume as a predictor of hepatic dysfunction and infection after major liver resection. *Gut, 54,* 289–296. doi:10.1136/gut.2004.046524

Shoup, M., Gonen, M., D'Angelica, M., Jarnagin, W.R., DeMatteo, R.P., Schwartz, L.H., … Fong, Y. (2003). Volumetric analysis predicts hepatic dysfunction in patients undergoing major liver resection. *Journal of Gastrointestinal Surgery, 7,* 325–330. doi:10.1016/S1091-255X(02)00370-0

Sun, H., Frassetto, L., & Benet, L.Z. (2006). Effects of renal failure on drug transport and metabolism. *Pharmacology and Therapeutics, 109,* 1–11. doi:10.1016/j.pharmthera.2005.05.010

Vanholder, R., De Smet, R., Glorieux, G., Argilés, A., Baurmeister, U., Brunet, P., … Zidek, W. (2003). Review on uremic toxins: Classification, concentration, and interindividual variability. *Kidney International, 63,* 1934–1943. doi:10.1046/j.1523-1755.2003.00924.x

Villeneuve, J.-P., & Pichette, V. (2004). Cytochrome P450 and liver diseases. *Current Drug Metabolism, 5,* 273–282. doi:10.2174/1389200043335531

Yang, L.-Q., Li, S.-J., Cao, Y.-F., Man, X.-B., Yu, W.-F., Wang, H.-Y., & Wu, M.-C. (2003). Different alterations of cytochrome P450 3A4 isoform and its gene expression in livers of patients with chronic liver diseases. *World Journal of Gastroenterology, 9,* 359–363. doi:10.3748/wjg.v9.i2.359

Zardi, E.M., Uwechie, V., Caccavo, D., Pellegrino, N.M., Cacciapaglia, F., Di Matteo, F., ... Afeltra, A. (2009). Portosystemic shunts in a large cohort of patients with liver cirrhosis: Detection rate and clinical relevance. *Journal of Gastroenterology, 44,* 76–83. doi:10.1007/s00535-008-2279-1

CHAPTER 9

Cytochrome P450 in Palliative Care

Vicky V. Mody, PhD, Adegoke O. Adeniji, RPh, PhD, and Launa M.J. Lynch, PhD

I. Definitions
   A. A *substrate* is a compound that binds to an enzyme and undergoes chemical biotransformation to a structural analog.
   B. An enzyme *inhibitor* is a compound that interacts with the enzyme to prevent it from metabolizing other substrates.
   C. An enzyme *inducer* is a compound that can stimulate the activity of an enzyme.

II. Key aspects
   A. The cytochrome P450 (CYP) superfamily is a large family of heme proteins that catalyze the monooxygenation of large variety of structurally diverse compounds such as exogenous xenobiotics or endogenously synthesized cholesterol, steroid hormones, and fatty acids.
      1. A drug or chemical can inhibit the enzyme even if it is not a substrate for the enzyme. An inhibitor will increase the concentration of concomitantly administered drug if the simultaneously administered drug is a substrate for the enzyme that has been inhibited.
      2. A drug or chemical can induce the enzyme even if it is not a substrate for the enzyme. An inducer will decrease the concentration of concomitantly administered drug if the simultaneously administered drug is a substrate for the enzyme that has been induced.
   B. Substrates for CYP include exogenous xenobiotics or endogenously synthesized cholesterol, steroid hormones, and fatty acids that are ingested, inhaled, or absorbed through the skin.
      1. CYP isoenzymes are involved in various reactions such as synthesis of steroid hormones, metabolism of fatty acids, prostaglandins, leukotrienes, retinoids, and inactivation and activation of various xenobiotics.
      2. Structurally, the CYP isoenzymes are heme-containing, membrane-bound proteins. When the iron of heme (prosthetic group) of the enzyme is bound to carbon monoxide (CO), they attain a unique absorption spectrum that peaks at approximately 450 nm, hence the name *P450* (Lynch & Price, 2007).
      3. The general monooxygenation reaction catalyzed by CYP enzymes is $NADPH + H^+ + O_2 + SH \rightarrow NADP^+ + H_2O + SOH$ (Roman & Masters, 2011).
      4. Here, "S" can be any molecule that serves as the site for oxygenation.

5. The catalytic metabolism of substrates (SH) using CYP involves a two-electron reduction of molecular oxygen to form a reactive oxygen species (SOH in the reaction previously shown) and water.

6. The drug metabolism via CYP is one of the most common metabolic pathways to detoxify a xenobiotic. There are 57 known human CYP enzymes; these have been classified into various families and subfamilies based on their nomenclature as determined by the CYP nomenclature committee (Nelson et al., 1996).

C. "CYP" denotes a human enzyme as compared to "Cyp" for mouse or drosophila (Nelson et al., 1996).

1. An Arabic numeral following CYP indicates the family (e.g., CYP1, CYP2, CYP3).

2. Letters A, B, and C following the family indicate the subfamily (e.g., CYP1A, CYP2C, CYP3A).

3. Another numeral added after the subfamily indicates the gene/isoenzyme/isoform (e.g., CYP3A4, CYP2C9).

D. Isoenzymes in the same family have more than 40% homology in their protein structure, whereas the members of the same subfamily have more than 55% homology. The difference in the protein structure make them more substrate specific (Nelson et al., 1996).

E. Many members of the CYP family are known to metabolize active agents in humans. Among the various isoenzymes, those belonging to the CYP 1, 2, and 3 families (CYP1A2, CYP2C9, CYP2C19, CYP2D6, CYP3A4, and CYP3A5) carry out phase I metabolism of more than 90% of the clinical drugs (Slaughter & Edwards, 1995; Wilkinson, 2005).

F. The human CYP3A family has the highest abundance in the liver and intestine, with CYP3A4 involved in the metabolism of more than 50% of clinically used drugs (Slaughter & Edwards, 1995).

1. These metabolic reactions involving CYP3A4 predominantly take place in the liver, although some of them also take place in the kidney, skin, lungs, and gastrointestinal tract (Slaughter & Edwards, 1995).

2. However, significant differences have been observed in the expression and activity of the individual CYP enzymes among different races.

3. Genetics, environment, and physiologic factors play an important role for these noted variations.

4. Apart from being a substrate, some of the compounds also can act as inhibitors or inducers of certain CYP enzymes.

5. For example, omeprazole is both a substrate and an inhibitor of CYP2C19.

6. Affinity of the drug to the substrate and the inhibitor binding site of the enzyme might be due to a small change in conformation of the CYP enzyme when it is bound by either a substrate or an inhibitor (Williams et al., 2004)

7. Similarly, a compound might be a substrate of one specific genotype and an inducer or inhibitor of another genotype.

8. For example, phenytoin is a substrate of both CYP2C9 and CYP2C19 and an inducer of CYP3A4.

9. This difference in activity of a drug (substrate, inhibitor, or inducer) toward different genotypes accounts for a large amount of the drug–drug interactions that can occur in a patient on multiple medications.

G. These interactions remain a major concern for the entire healthcare industry (Badyal & Dadhich, 2001).

H. In fact, it is one of the top 10 major causes of death (Badyal & Dadhich, 2001). Hence, it is imperative to understand the molecular biology of the CYP enzymes and several patient-specific factors that can influence the activity of CYP enzymes.

III. Relevance to practice

A. Patient-specific factors such as age, health, diet, smoking, and alcohol use play an important role in CYP-catalyzed metabolism and are of significance to healthcare professionals.

B. In addition to these factors, ethnicity plays a prominent role and has been extensively studied over the past two decades.

C. This is important because several CYP enzymes (CYP2C subfamily, namely CYP2C8, CYP2C9, CYP2C18, and CYP2C19, and CYP2D6) are known to be genetically polymorphic, which can lead to interindividual variation in substrate metabolism (Martínez et al., 2005).

D. Thus, individuals with variants of specific CYP (e.g., CYP2C9 and its variants) enzymes may have reduced or no catalytic activity.

1. This can lead to poor metabolizers (PMs) of substrate or extensive metabolizers (EMs) of substrate.

2. These genetic polymorphisms vary by ethnicity. Thus, the Caucasian populations are PMs of CYP2D6 substrates, whereas Asians are EMs of CYP2D6 substrates.

3. Conversely, Asians are PMs of CYP2C19 substrates, whereas Caucasians are EMs of CYP2C19 substrates.

4. Therefore, care must be taken when dispensing therapeutic substrates of these enzymes.

E. By understanding these unique characteristics of CYP enzymes, medical professionals can anticipate or explain an individual's response to a particular therapeutic regimen.

F. This is especially important in palliative care, as polypharmacy often is the course of action to maintain patients' quality of life.

1. Figure 9-1 lists drugs used in palliative care as recommended by the World Health Organization (WHO) based on their therapeutic potential (International Association for Hospice and Palliative Care, n.d.; WHO, 2015).

2. However, the use of additional drugs not included in this list is warranted if the patient cannot use one of those listed in this table.

G. Enzyme substrates

1. Currently, the isoenzymes in the CYP 1, 2, and 3 families—such as CYP1A2, CYP2C9, CYP2C19, CYP2D6, CYP3A4, and CYP3A5—carry out most of the metabolism of the drugs in the market.

2. Among them, CYP3A4 is the most abundant in the liver and is responsible for metabolizing compounds into metabolites that are usually more hydrophilic.

3. Others, such as CYP2C9, CYP2C19, and CYP2D6, also play an important role in metabolism (see Figure 9-2).

4. Figure 9-2 lists various drugs used in palliative care and the corresponding CYP enzymes used to metabolize them. Thus, a particular drug such as warfarin, haloperidol, or phenytoin might be a substrate for multiple enzymes.

5. The CYP3A4 enzyme covers a very broad range of substrates where the molecules often are metabolized based on their functional groups and stereochemistry (Zhou, 2008).

Figure 9-1. Drugs Recommended for Use in Palliative Care

Anorexia
- Dexamethasone
- Megestrol acetate

Anticonvulsant
- Carbamazepine

Anxiety
- Diazepam
- Lorazepam[a]
- Midazolam

Constipation
- Bisacodyl[b]
- Docusate sodium[b]
- Senna (children)
- Sodium picosulfate[b]

Delirium
- Haloperidol
- Levomepromazine

Depression
- Amitriptyline
- Citalopram
- Desvenlafaxine[a]
- Duloxetine
- Escitalopram
- Fluoxetine
- Levomilnacipran[a]
- Milnacipran[a]
- Mirtazapine
- Sertraline
- Sibutramine[b]

Diarrhea
- Loperamide
- Octreotide

Dyspnea
- Morphine[a]

Insomnia
- Lorazepam
- Trazodone
- Zolpidem

Nausea and Vomiting
- Dexamethasone
- Diphenhydramine
- Haloperidol
- Hyoscine butylbromide
- Metoclopramide
- Octreotide

Pain
- Amitriptyline (neuropathic)
- Carbamazepine (neuropathic)
- Codeine
- Dexamethasone (neuropathic)
- Diclofenac
- Fentanyl
- Gabapentin[a] (neuropathic)
- Hyoscine butylbromide (visceral)
- Ibuprofen
- Methadone
- Morphine[a]
- Oxycodone
- Paracetamol
- Tramadol

Respiratory Tract Secretions
- Hyoscine butylbromide

[a] No CYP metabolism involved

[b] Metabolized by CYP2B6; enzyme not included in Figures 9-2, 9-3, and 9-4.

Note. Based on information from International Association for Hospice and Palliative Care, n.d.; World Health Organization, 2015.

---

6. The substrates of CYP3A4 are structurally diverse and exhibit a wide range of sizes and affinities because of its relatively large and flexible substrate-binding cavity (Zhou, 2008).

7. Most common phase I metabolic pathways for these substrates involving CYP3A4 enzymes include common oxidation reactions such as hydroxylation of aromatic rings or aliphatic chains, *N*-oxidation, *N*-dealkylation, and *O*-dealkylation.

   a) Studies also suggest that there are two different substrate-binding domains and an allosteric effector binding domain on the CYP3A4 enzyme (Guengerich, 1999).

   b) Three binding sites influence the metabolism of CYP3A4 substrates. These binding sites can act to increase the metabolism of one compound in the presence of another (similar to catalysis) or can competitively inhibit the metabolism of another by blocking the catalytic site (e.g., metoclopramide and diphenhydramine) (Akutsu et al., 2007; Desta, Wu, Morocho, & Flockhart, 2002).

   c) Thus, these multiple binding sites provide an opportunity to metabolize many drugs so that a more hydrophilic moiety is synthesized to ensure faster excretion from the body.

d) Figure 9-2 lists CYP3A4 substrates that are often used in palliative care. This table indicates whether a drug is partly or completely metabolized by that particular isoform. However, this in no way indicates that the isoform has the primary role in metabolism. This table is intended to help practicing healthcare specialists determine potential drug–drug interactions.

Figure 9-2. Drugs Catalyzed by Cytochrome P450 Used in Palliative Care

CYP1A2	CYP2C9	CYP2C19	CYP2D6	CYP2E1	CYP3A4
• Acetaminophen	• Carbamazepine	• Amitriptyline	• Citalopram	• Acetaminophen	• Alprazolam
• Carbamazepine	• Diclofenac	• Citalopram	• Codeine		• Amlodipine
• Duloxetine	• Ibuprofen	• Diazepam	• Diphenhydramine		• Carbamazepine
• Haloperidol	• Methadone	• Diclofenac	• Duloxetine		• Citalopram
• *R*-Warfarin	• Phenytoin	• Diltiazem	• Escitalopram		• Clarithromycin
	• *S*-Warfarin	• Escitalopram	• Fluoxetine		• Dexamethasone
		• Methadone	• Metoclopramide		• Diazepam
		• Omeprazole	• Methadone		• Diltiazem
		• Phenytoin	• Mirtazapine		• Erythromycin
		• Sertraline	• Ondansetron		• Escitalopram
			• Oxycodone		• Felodipine
			• Promethazine		• Fentanyl
			• Sertraline		• Haloperidol
			• Tramadol		• Hyoscine
					• Levomepromazine
					• Megestrol acetate
					• Methadone
					• Midazolam
					• Mirtazapine
					• Nifedipine
					• Nisoldipine
					• Omeprazole
					• Ondansetron
					• Oxycodone
					• *R*-Warfarin
					• Sertraline
					• Telithromycin
					• Tramadol
					• Trazodone
					• Triazolam
					• Verapamil
					• Zolpidem

Note. Based on information from Abelö et al., 2000; Akutsu et al., 2007; Bajpai et al., 1996; Bessems & Vermeulen, 2001; Bort et al., 1999; Cuttle et al., 2000; Davis, 2012; Desta et al., 2002; Kamei et al., 2015; Kaminsky & Zhang, 1997; Kosuge et al., 2001; Kudo & Ishizaki, 1999; Labroo et al., 1997; Lynch & Price, 2007; Mandrioli et al., 2006; Martínez et al., 2005; Nakamura et al., 1996; Nelson et al., 1996; Obach et al., 2005; Olesen & Linnet, 1997; Olkkola & Ahonen, 2008; Pai et al., 2002; Patki et al., 2003; Pearce et al., 2008; Renner et al., 2005; Rotzinger et al., 1998; Shi et al., 2005; Skinner et al., 2003; Slaughter & Edwards, 1995; Smith, 2009; Stamer et al., 2011; Sun et al., 2015; Suzuki et al., 2003; Timmer et al., 2000; Tomlinson et al., 1997; Tracy et al., 1999; von Moltke et al., 2001; Watkins et al., 1989; Wójcikowski et al., 2014; World Health Organization, 2015; Zhu et al., 2014.

8. CYP2C9, CYP2C19, and CYP2D6 are other isoforms of CYP enzymes primarily expressed in the liver and are responsible for the phase I metabolic clearance of active agents and psychotherapeutic agents, mainly by CYP2D6 (Van Booven et al., 2010).
    a) Structurally, CYP2C9 can use multiple binding ligands during its drug interaction or an allosteric binding site, which is also used in the metabolism of substrates such as warfarin (Wester et al., 2004).
    b) The gene encoding CYP2C9 is highly polymorphic, and changes in metabolism due to genetic variation in *CYP2C9* play an important role in drug–drug interactions (Pirmohamed & Park, 2003).
    c) Hence, a healthcare professional should be cautious in patients with low enzyme activity of CYP2C9, especially with substrates such as phenytoin and warfarin. On the other hand, CYP2C19 is encoded by the *CYP2C19* gene.
    d) Patients can be classified as EMs or PMs of CYP2C19 substrates based on their ability to metabolize *S*-mephenytoin or other CYP2C19 substrates.
9. As discussed earlier, ethnicity is one of the most important factors for the interindividual variation of EM and PM genotypes.
10. Patients who are EMs clear most of the doses (approximately 80%) of the proton pump inhibitors (PPIs) omeprazole, lansoprazole, and pantoprazole by CYP2C19, whereas those who are PMs use their CYP3A enzymes to metabolize PPIs (Desta et al., 2002).
    a) Thus, a patient who is a PM of CYP2C19 substrate will have more effective control of gastroesophageal reflux disease and ulcer compared to those who are EMs.
    b) This is because an increase in plasma concentration of a PPI allows for a longer duration of the drug.
    c) However, the difference in CYP2C19 activity does not seem to increase the risk for adverse drug reactions or interactions of PPIs.
11. Among all the enzymes, CYP2D6 is the second most abundant enzyme (after CYP3A4) that extensively metabolizes many drugs used in palliative care (see Figure 9-2). Like CYP2C9 and CYP2C19, it is highly polymorphic in nature, and the ethnicity of the patient plays an important role in its expression and activity.
12. Drugs such as warfarin, haloperidol, and phenytoin might be a substrate for multiple enzymes (see Figure 9-2), and care must be taken in the use of these drugs in a polypharmacy situation in palliative care.

H. Enzyme inhibitors
1. Enzyme inhibitors are compounds that interact with an enzyme and prevent it from metabolizing other substrates. In other words, they modulate the structure of the enzyme so that its function is inhibited.
2. Enzyme inhibition often involves competition between two active agents for the substrate-binding site of the enzyme, although other mechanisms for inhibition exist.
3. Based on the type of inhibition, a compound can be classified as a nonspecific, irreversible, reversible competitive, or reversible noncompetitive inhibitor.
    a) A compound can inhibit the enzyme even if it is not a substrate for the enzyme.
    b) Likewise, if two drugs are substrates for the same CYP enzyme, then the metabolism of one can delay the metabolism of another.

    c) This may be due to competition for the substrate-binding site on the enzyme, which might be occupied by the other.

    d) For example, when a patient takes erythromycin and midazolam, both of which are substrates for CYP3A4 isoenzymes, there is competition for enzyme sites by the two drugs, leading to the delay in the metabolism of the other.

    e) In this specific case, the metabolism of midazolam is inhibited, leading to an increase in plasma concentration of the drug (Olkkola et al., 1993).

4. Enzyme inhibition also can be due to drugs that are not substrates of the specific CYP enzyme.

    a) For example, the fluoroquinolone and macrolide antibiotics cause reversible inhibition of CYP3A4 isoenzyme.

    b) Hence, a patient on fluoroquinolones or macrolides should be very careful when also taking a CYP3A4 substrate (see Figure 9-2).

    c) This becomes more important when a patient is taking a drug such as haloperidol that also is a CYP3A4 substrate, as concentrations in plasma can change substantially because of the presence of macrolide or fluoroquinolone antibiotics.

5. Some selective CYP inhibitors are synthesized in situ by the CYP isoforms; these compounds are substrates of those CYP isoforms that catalyze their synthesis.

6. However, once converted to reactive species in vivo, they can lead to enzyme inactivation.

7. This type of inhibition, called *suicide inhibition*, is irreversible.

    a) Aspirin is the best example of a suicide inhibitor and can be used in palliative care even though it is not included in the list by WHO.

    b) The irreversible inhibitor will decrease the metabolism of other concomitantly administered substrates, which will lead to increased drug effect or toxicity of the substrate.

8. Figure 9-3 lists some of the most important CYP inhibitors commonly used in palliative care (Indiana University Clinical Pharmacology Research Institute, n.d.). Hence, healthcare professionals need to evaluate the CYP reactivity of all concomitantly administered drugs.

I. Enzyme inducers

1. Enzyme inducers are drugs or other chemical substances that can instigate the activity of the CYP enzymes.

2. Enzyme induction occurs when an active agent activates an enzyme or stimulates the synthesis of more enzymes, enhancing the enzyme's metabolizing capacity.

3. The most common enzyme-inducing drugs used in palliative care are barbiturates and phenytoin.

    a) Apart from induction of CYP enzymes by active agents, drug metabolism also can be induced by other factors such as diet, exposure to environmental pollutants, alcohol use, and smoking.

    b) Notably, smoking induces the activity of CYP1A2 and CYP2B6. Therefore, in a patient who smokes and is taking psychoactive drugs such as haloperidol or an anticoagulant such as warfarin, a clinician might have trouble adjusting the therapeutic dose of these drugs.

    c) Thus, if a drug is taken concomitantly with the inducer, drug efficacy is usually reduced.

Figure 9-3. Cytochrome P450 Inhibitors Used in Palliative Care

CYP1A2	CYP2C8	CYP2C9	CYP2C19	CYP2D6	CYP3A4
• Amiodarone • Chlorpromazine • Cimetidine • Ciprofloxacin • Omeprazole • Ranitidine	• Trimethoprim	• Cimetidine • Fluconazole • Lansoprazole • Pantoprazole • *R*-Omeprazole • Sulfamethoxazole • Voriconazole	• Carbamazepine • Cimetidine • Fluoxetine • Lansoprazole • Oxcarbazepine • Pantoprazole • Rabeprazole • *R*-Omeprazole • Topiramate • Voriconazole	• Amiodarone • Bupropion • Chlorpromazine • Cimetidine • Citalopram • Clomipramine • Diphenhydramine • Doxepin • Duloxetine • Escitalopram • Fluoxetine • Haloperidol • Metoclopramide • Paroxetine • Ranitidine • Sertraline	• Amiodarone • Cimetidine • Ciprofloxacin • Diltiazem • Fluconazole • Ketoconazole • Omeprazole • Verapamil • Voriconazole

Note. Based on information from Akutsu et al., 2007; Alfaro et al., 2000; Badyal & Dadhich, 2001; Benedetti, 2000; Brüggemann et al., 2009; Desta et al., 2002; Furuta et al., 2001; Gervasini et al., 2013; Granfors et al., 2004; Harvey & Preskorn, 2001; Indiana University Clinical Pharmacology Research Institute, n.d.; Kosuge et al., 2001; Kotlyar et al., 2005; Kudo & Ishizaki, 1999; Lakehal et al., 2002; Li et al., 2004; Malhotra et al., 2011; Martínez et al., 1999, 2005; Shahzadi et al., 2011; Shirasaka et al., 2013; Skinner et al., 2003; von Moltke et al., 2001; Wang et al., 2005; Wen et al., 2002; Williams et al., 2004; World Health Organization, 2015.

---

    d) However, in certain cases, such as with a prodrug or the formation of a toxic metabolite, enzyme induction can result in increased toxicity of the drug.

4. A drug also can induce its own metabolism by a process called *autoinduction*, which occurs with carbamazepine.

5. Fortunately, drug interactions involving enzyme induction are not as commonly observed as interactions with enzyme inhibitors, especially in palliative care, but they are as clinically important.

6. It is somewhat difficult to predict the time course of enzyme induction because several factors, including the half-life of the drug and the enzyme turnover, determine induction.

7. Understanding these mechanisms of enzyme induction and inhibition is extremely important in order to give appropriate multiple drug therapy.

8. Figure 9-4 lists various drugs that act as an inducer and are of major concern in palliative care. Clinicians should research the induction properties of new drugs before administering them to patients.

  J. Significant interactions by drug class

    1. Antiepileptic drugs

      a) Interactions from most of the clinically important antiepileptic drugs such as carbamazepine, phenytoin, and phenobarbital result from induction or inhibition (valproic acid) of drug-metabolizing enzymes (Perucca, 2006).

b) These enzyme inducers (carbamazepine, phenytoin, and phenobarbital) intensify the activity of several CYP enzymes, such CYP1A2, CYP2C9, CYP2C19, and CYP3A4 (Anderson, 1998; Benedetti & Bani, 1999; Perucca et al., 1984).

c) Thus, patients taking antiepileptic drugs will trigger the induction of these specific CYP isoforms and consequently stimulate the metabolism of concomitantly administered substrates of these specific isoforms.

d) Hence, clinicians may need to increase the dose of these concomitantly administered drugs.

e) For example, when primidone is concomitantly administered with phenytoin, the enzyme induction by phenytoin increases the serum concentrations of the active metabolite of primidone, phenobarbital, which increases the risk of phenobarbital-related adverse effects.

f) Under these circumstances, it would be prudent to change primidone, or, if that is not possible, to reduce the doses.

g) Newer antiepileptic drugs such as oxcarbazepine, lamotrigine, felbamate, and topiramate are relatively safer than the older generations; however, they display a concentration-dependent induction of CYP enzymes, especially CYP3A4, at dosages of 200 mg/day or greater (Perucca, 2006).

h) This is seen in the observation that the simultaneous use of either oxcarbazepine, lamotrigine, felbamate, or topiramate can decrease the concentration of steroids such as megestrol (Wilbur & Ensom, 2000).

i) Hence, care must be taken to monitor the concentration of simultaneously administered drugs if the concentration of antiepileptic drugs is greater than 200 mg/day.

2. Antidepressants

a) Selective serotonin reuptake inhibitors (SSRIs) have become the drug of choice for the treatment of depressive disorders, mainly because of their tolerability and better pharmacokinetic profile (Spina, Santoro, & D'Arrigo, 2008).

b) Among the second-generation SSRIs, fluoxetine and paroxetine are potent inhibitors of CYP2D6 (Hemeryck & Belpaire, 2002; Hiemke & Härtter, 2000).

c) Thus, if a patient is taking fluoxetine or paroxetine and is given codeine, then the codeine will lose its analgesic activity because it cannot be converted to morphine in the absence of CYP2D6. Duloxetine and

---

Figure 9-4. Cytochrome P450 Inducers Used in Palliative Care

CYP2B6	CYP2C19	CYP2D6	CYP3A4
• Phenobarbital	• Carbamazepine • Prednisone	• Reduced haloperidol	• Carbamazepine • Glucocorticoids • Oxcarbazepine • Phenobarbital • Phenytoin • Topiramate

Note. Based on information from Benedetti, 2000; DrugBank, n.d.; Indiana University Clinical Pharmacology Research Institute, n.d.; Kudo & Ishizaki, 1999; Martínez et al., 2005; Waxman & Azaroff, 1992.

bupropion, both moderate inhibitors of CYP2D6, will have a similar effect on codeine (Hemeryck & Belpaire, 2002; Hiemke & Härtter, 2000).

d) Similarly, fluvoxamine and nefazodone are inhibitors of CYP2C19 and CYP3A4, respectively (Hemeryck & Belpaire, 2002; Hiemke & Härtter, 2000).

e) Several other interactions can happen with the use of SSRIs; thus, knowing these potential interactions from antidepressants, clinicians may foresee and prevent certain drug combinations that can be potentially harmful to patients.

3. Cardiovascular drugs

a) Cardiovascular disease is one of the most prevalent diseases in the United States and is the leading cause of death (Centers for Disease Control and Prevention, 2015).

b) Patients taking cardiovascular drugs can experience potential drug interactions due to CYP inhibition or induction.

c) For example, verapamil is metabolized by CYP3A4 enzymes, whereas ciprofloxacin, a fluoroquinolone, has an inhibitory effect on those CYP isoforms (Zhou et al., 2014).

d) Thus, concomitant use of verapamil and ciprofloxacin can lead to an increase in the systemic levels of verapamil and an increased risk of potential side effects such as hypotension and constipation. This also can be seen in the use of verapamil with other CYP3A4 inhibitors, such as macrolide antibiotics (Martin & Fay, 2001).

e) Similarly, a patient taking cisapride (a CYP3A4 substrate) along with CYP3A4 inhibitors, such as diltiazem or macrolides, will see QT prolongation because of the increase in the concentration of cisapride (Martin & Fay, 2001).

f) Warfarin is one of the most common anticoagulants prescribed and is subject to many potential drug–drug interactions. This is mainly due to its complex metabolic pathway, which involves multiple CYP isoforms. Changes in the activity of CYP isoforms due to any additional medication in patients on warfarin can have a tremendous impact on warfarin's international normalized ratio (INR) value. Hence, close monitoring of patients' warfarin INR is required if additional medications are warranted (Martin & Fay, 2001).

IV. Interface to palliative care

A. This chapter gives a snapshot of common drug interactions in patients involved in polypharmacy in a palliative care setting.

B. Drug interactions can be due to the different types of interactions of the drug with CYP enzymes, leading to either activation or inactivation of the enzyme.

C. Activation and inactivation of enzymes can have potentially fatal consequences. Healthcare professionals should ensure that such interactions between two medications are avoided.

D. The presence and absence of the CYP isoforms also can be influenced by a variety of factors such as physical health, age, genetic polymorphism, and ethnicity.

E. Pharmacogenomics also plays an important role in the current healthcare system; hence, it might be helpful to have some genetic screening for the most common CYP isoforms to have a better idea about patients' metabolic profile.

F. The age and health of the patient play an important role in the metabolism of drugs via CYP enzymes, as both of these factors influence CYP enzymes.

G. Also, as patients become older or their disease progresses, the effectiveness of their medication should be evaluated regularly to ensure optimal therapeutic outcome.

References

Abelö, A.A., Andersson, T.B., Antonsson, M., Naudot, A.K., Skånberg, I., & Weidolf, L. (2000). Stereoselective metabolism of omeprazole by human cytochrome P450 enzymes. *Drug Metabolism and Disposition, 28,* 966–972.

Akutsu, T., Kobayashi, K., Sakurada, K., Ikegaya, H., Furihata, T., & Chiba, K. (2007). Identification of human cytochrome P450 isozymes involved in diphenhydramine *N*-demethylation. *Drug Metabolism and Disposition, 35,* 72–78. doi:10.1124/dmd.106.012088

Alfaro, C.L., Lam, Y.W.F., Simpson, J., & Ereshefsky, L. (2000). CYP2D6 inhibition by fluoxetine, paroxetine, sertraline, and venlafaxine in a crossover study: Intraindividual variability and plasma concentration correlations. *Journal of Clinical Pharmacology, 40,* 58–66. doi/10.1177/009127000004000108

Anderson, G.D. (1998). A mechanistic approach to antiepileptic drug interactions. *Annals of Pharmacotherapy, 32,* 554–563. doi:10.1345/aph.17332

Badyal, D.K., & Dadhich, A.P. (2001). Cytochrome P450 and drug interactions. *Indian Journal of Pharmacology, 33,* 248–259.

Bajpai, M., Roskos, L.K., Shen, D.D., & Levy, R.H. (1996). Roles of cytochrome P4502C9 and cytochrome P4502C19 in the stereoselective metabolism of phenytoin to its major metabolite. *Drug Metabolism and Disposition, 24,* 1401–1403.

Benedetti, M.S. (2000). Enzyme induction and inhibition by new antiepileptic drugs: A review of human studies. *Fundamental and Clinical Pharmacology, 14,* 301–319. doi:10.1111/j.1472-8206.2000.tb00411.x

Benedetti, M.S., & Bani, M. (1999). Metabolism-based drug interactions involving oral azole antifungals in humans. *Drug Metabolism Reviews, 31,* 665–717. doi:10.1081/DMR-100101941

Bessems, J.G.M., & Vermeulen, N.P.E. (2001). Paracetamol (acetaminophen)-induced toxicity: Molecular and biochemical mechanisms, analogues and protective approaches. *Critical Reviews in Toxicology, 31,* 55–138. doi:10.1080/20014091111677

Bort, R., Macé, K., Boobis, A., Gómez-Lechón, M.-J., Pfeifer, A., & Castell, J. (1999). Hepatic metabolism of diclofenac: Role of human *CYP* in the minor oxidative pathways. *Biochemical Pharmacology, 58,* 787–796. doi:10.1016/S0006-2952(99)00167-7

Brüggemann, R.J.M., Alffenaar, J.-W.C., Blijlevens, N.M.A., Billaud, E.M., Kosterink, J.G.W., Verweij, P.E., … Saravolatz, L.D. (2009). Clinical relevance of the pharmacokinetic interactions of azole antifungal drugs with other coadministered agents. *Clinical Infectious Diseases, 48,* 1441–1458. doi:10.1086/598327

Centers for Disease Control and Prevention. (2015, August 10). Heart disease facts. Retrieved from http://www.cdc.gov/heartdisease/facts.htm

Cuttle, L., Munns, A.J., Hogg, N.A., Scott, J.R., Hooper, W.D., Dickinson, R.G., & Gillam, E.M. (2000). Phenytoin metabolism by human cytochrome P450: Involvement of P450 3A and 2C forms in secondary metabolism and drug-protein adduct formation. *Drug Metabolism and Disposition, 28,* 945–950.

Davis, M.W. (2012). *U.S. Patent No. 8,231,915.* Washington, DC: U.S. Patent and Trademark Office.

Desta, Z., Wu, G.M., Morocho, A.M., & Flockhart, D.A. (2002). The gastroprokinetic and antiemetic drug metoclopramide is a substrate and inhibitor of cytochrome P450 2D6. *Drug Metabolism and Disposition, 30,* 336–343. doi:10.1124/dmd.30.3.336

DrugBank. (n.d.). Biointeractions for DB00564 (carbamazepine): Enzyme mediated interactions [DrugBank version 4.3]. Retrieved from http://www.drugbank.ca/drugs/DB00564/biointeractions#enzyme-tab

Furuta, S., Kamada, E., Suzuki, T., Sugimoto, T., Kawabata, Y., Shinozaki, Y., & Sano, H. (2001). Inhibition of drug metabolism in human liver microsomes by nizatidine, cimetidine and omeprazole. *Xenobiotica, 31,* 1–10. doi:10.1080/00498250110035615

Gervasini, G., Caballero, M.J., Carrillo, J.A., & Benitez, J. (2013). Comparative cytochrome P450 *in vitro* inhibition by atypical antipsychotic drugs. *ISRN Pharmacology, 2013,* Article 792456. doi:10.1155/2013/792456

Granfors, M.T., Backman, J.T., Neuvonen, M., & Neuvonen, P.J. (2004). Ciprofloxacin greatly increases concentrations and hypotensive effect of tizanidine by inhibiting its cytochrome P450 1A2–mediated presystemic metabolism. *Clinical Pharmacology and Therapeutics, 76,* 598–606. doi:10.1016/j.clpt.2004.08.018

Guengerich, F.P. (1999). Cytochrome P-450 3A4: Regulation and role in drug metabolism. *Annual Review of Pharmacology and Toxicology, 39,* 1–17. doi:10.1146/annurev.pharmtox.39.1.1

Harvey, A.T., & Preskorn, S.H. (2001). Fluoxetine pharmacokinetics and effect on CYP2C19 in young and elderly volunteers. *Journal of Clinical Psychopharmacology, 21,* 161–166. doi:10.1097/00004714-200104000-00007

Hemeryck, A., & Belpaire, F.M. (2002). Selective serotonin reuptake inhibitors and cytochrome P-450 mediated drug-drug interactions: An update. *Current Drug Metabolism, 3,* 13–37. doi:10.2174/1389200023338017

Hiemke, C., & Härtter, S. (2000). Pharmacokinetics of selective serotonin reuptake inhibitors. *Pharmacology and Therapeutics, 85,* 11–28. doi:10.1016/S0163-7258(99)00048-0

Indiana University Clinical Pharmacology Research Institute. (n.d.). P450 drug interaction table. Retrieved from http://medicine.iupui.edu/clinpharm/ddis/main-table

International Association for Hospice and Palliative Care. (n.d.). IAHPC list of essential medicines for palliative care. Retrieved from http://hospicecare.com/resources/palliative-care-essentials/iahpc-essential-medicines-for-palliative-care

Kamei, S., Kaneto, H., Tanabe, A., Irie, S., Hirata, Y., Shimoda, M., … Kaku, K. (2015). Rapid onset of syndrome of inappropriate antidiuretic hormone secretion induced by duloxetine in an elderly type 2 diabetic patient with painful diabetic neuropathy. *Journal of Diabetes Investigation, 6,* 343–345. doi:10.1111/jdi.12301

Kaminsky, L.S., & Zhang, Z.-Y. (1997). Human P450 metabolism of warfarin. *Pharmacology and Therapeutics, 73,* 67–74. doi:10.1016/S0163-7258(96)00140-4

Kosuge, K., Jun, Y., Watanabe, H., Kimura, M., Nishimoto, M., Ishizaki, T., & Ohashi, K. (2001). Effects of CYP3A4 inhibition by diltiazem on pharmacokinetics and dynamics of diazepam in relation to CYP2C19 genotype status. *Drug Metabolism and Disposition, 29,* 1284–1289.

Kotlyar, M., Brauer, L.H., Tracy, T.S., Hatsukami, D.K., Harris, J., Bronars, C.A., & Adson, D.E. (2005). Inhibition of CYP2D6 activity by bupropion. *Journal of Clinical Psychopharmacology, 25,* 226–229. doi:10.1097/01.jcp.0000162805.46453.e3

Kudo, S., & Ishizaki, T. (1999). Pharmacokinetics of haloperidol. *Clinical Pharmacokinetics, 37,* 435–456. doi:10.2165/00003088-199937060-00001

Labroo, R.B., Paine, M.F., Thummel, K.E., & Kharasch, E.D. (1997). Fentanyl metabolism by human hepatic and intestinal cytochrome P450 3A4: Implications for interindividual variability in disposition, efficacy, and drug interactions. *Drug Metabolism and Disposition, 25,* 1072–1080.

Lakehal, F., Wurden, C.J., Kalhorn, T.F., & Levy, R.H. (2002). Carbamazepine and oxcarbazepine decrease phenytoin metabolism through inhibition of CYP2C19. *Epilepsy Research, 52,* 79–83. doi:10.1016/S0920-1211(02)00188-2

Li, X.-Q., Andersson, T.B., Ahlström, M., & Weidolf, L. (2004). Comparison of inhibitory effects of the proton pump-inhibiting drugs omeprazole, esomeprazole, lansoprazole, pantoprazole, and rabeprazole on human cytochrome P450 activities. *Drug Metabolism and Disposition, 32,* 821–827. doi:10.1124/dmd.32.8.821

Lynch, T., & Price, A. (2007). The effect of cytochrome P450 metabolism on drug response, interactions, and adverse effects. *American Family Physician, 76,* 391–396.

Malhotra, B., Dickins, M., Alvey, C., Jumadilova, Z., Li, X., Duczynski, G., & Gandelman, K. (2011). Effects of the moderate CYP3A4 inhibitor, fluconazole, on the pharmacokinetics of fesoterodine in healthy subjects. *British Journal of Clinical Pharmacology, 72,* 263–269. doi:10.1111/j.1365-2125.2011.04007.x

Mandrioli, R., Forti, G.C., & Raggi, M.A. (2006). Fluoxetine metabolism and pharmacological interactions: The role of cytochrome P450. *Current Drug Metabolism, 7,* 127–133. doi:10.2174/138920006775541561

Martin, J., & Fay, M. (2001). Cytochrome P450 drug interactions: Are they clinically relevant? *Australian Prescriber, 24,* 10–12. doi:10.18773/austprescr.2001.007

Martínez, C., Albet, C., Agúndez, J.A.G., Herrero, E., Carrillo, J.A., Márquez, M., … Ortiz, J.A. (1999). Comparative in vitro and in vivo inhibition of cytochrome P450 CYP1A2, CYP2D6, and CYP3A by H_2-receptor antagonists. *Clinical Pharmacology and Therapeutics, 65,* 369–376. doi:10.1016/S0009-9236(99)70129-3

Martínez, C., García-Martín, E., Blanco, G., Gamito, F.J.G., Ladero, J.M., & Agúndez, J.A.G. (2005). The effect of the cytochrome P450 CYP2C8 polymorphism on the disposition of (R)-ibuprofen enantiomer in healthy subjects. *British Journal of Clinical Pharmacology, 59,* 62–68. doi:10.1111/j.1365-2125.2004.02183.x

Nakamura, K., Yokoi, T., Inoue, K., Shimada, N., Ohashi, N., Kume, T., & Kamataki, T. (1996). CYP2D6 is the principal cytochrome P450 responsible for metabolism of the histamine 111 antagonist promethazine in human liver microsomes. *Pharmacogenetics and Genomics, 6,* 449–457.

Nelson, D.R., Koymans, L., Kamataki, T., Stegeman, J.J., Feyereisen, R., Waxman, D.J., … Nebert, D.W. (1996). P450 superfamily: Update on new sequences, gene mapping, accession numbers and nomenclature. *Pharmacogenetics and Genomics, 6,* 1–42.

Obach, R.S., Cox, L.M., & Tremaine, L.M. (2005). Sertraline is metabolized by multiple cytochrome P450 enzymes, monoamine oxidases, and glucuronyl transferases in human: An in vitro study. *Drug Metabolism and Disposition, 33,* 262–270. doi:10.1124/dmd.104.002428

Olesen, O.V., & Linnet, K. (1997). Metabolism of the tricyclic antidepressant amitriptyline by cDNA-expressed human cytochrome P450 enzymes. *Pharmacology, 55,* 235–243. doi:10.1159/000139533

Olkkola, K.T., & Ahonen, J. (2008). Midazolam and other benzodiazepines. In J. Schüttler & H. Schwilden (Eds.), *Handbook of Experimental Pharmacology: Vol. 182. Modern anesthetics* (pp. 335–360). doi:10.1007/978 -3-540-74806-9_16

Olkkola, K.T., Aranko, K., Luurila, H., Hiller, A., Saarnivaara, L., Himberg, J.-J., & Neuvonen, P.J. (1993). A potentially hazardous interaction between erythromycin and midazolam. *Clinical Pharmacology and Therapeutics, 53,* 298–305. doi:10.1038/clpt.1993.25

Pai, H.V., Upadhya, S.C., Chinta, S.J., Hegde, S.N., & Ravindranath, V. (2002). Differential metabolism of alprazolam by liver and brain cytochrome (P4503A) to pharmacologically active metabolite. *Pharmacogenomics Journal, 2,* 243–258. doi:10.1038/sj.tpj.6500115

Patki, K.C., von Moltke, L.L., & Greenblatt, D.J. (2003). In vitro metabolism of midazolam, triazolam, nifedipine, and testosterone by human liver microsomes and recombinant cytochromes P450: Role of CYP3A4 and CYP3A5. *Drug Metabolism and Disposition, 31,* 938–944. doi:10.1124/dmd.31.7.938

Pearce, R.E., Lu, W., Wang, Y., Uetrecht, J.P., Correia, M.A., & Leeder, J.S. (2008). Pathways of carbamazepine bioactivation in vitro. III. The role of human cytochrome P450 enzymes in the formation of 2,3-dihydroxy-carbamazepine. *Drug Metabolism and Disposition, 36,* 1637–1649. doi:10.1124/dmd.107.019562

Perucca, E. (2006). Clinically relevant drug interactions with antiepileptic drugs. *British Journal of Clinical Pharmacology, 61,* 246–255. doi:10.1111/j.1365-2125.2005.02529.x

Perucca, E., Hedges, A., Makki, K.A., Ruprah, M., Wilson, J.F., & Richens, A. (1984). A comparative study of the relative enzyme inducing properties of anticonvulsant drugs in epileptic patients. *British Journal of Clinical Pharmacology, 18,* 401–410. doi:10.1111/j.1365-2125.1984.tb02482.x

Pirmohamed, M., & Park, B.K. (2003). Cytochrome P450 enzyme polymorphisms and adverse drug reactions. *Toxicology, 192,* 23–32. doi:10.1016/S0300-483X(03)00247-6

Renner, U.D., Oertel, R., & Kirch, W. (2005). Pharmacokinetics and pharmacodynamics in clinical use of scopolamine. *Therapeutic Drug Monitoring, 27,* 655–665. doi:10.1097/01.ftd.0000168293.48226.57

Roman, L.J., & Masters, B.S.S. (2011). The cytochromes P450 and nitric oxide synthases. In T.M. Devlin (Ed.), *Textbook of biochemistry with clinical correlations* (7th ed., pp. 435–456). Hoboken, NJ: John Wiley & Sons.

Rotzinger, S., Fang, J., & Baker, G.B. (1998). Trazodone is metabolized to m-chlorophenylpiperazine by CYP3A4 from human sources. *Drug Metabolism and Disposition, 26,* 572–575.

Shahzadi, A., Javed, I., Aslam, B., Muhammad, F., Asi, M.R., Ashraf, M.Y., & Rahman, Z.U. (2011). Therapeutic effects of ciprofloxacin on the pharmacokinetics of carbamazepine in healthy adult male volunteers. *Pakistan Journal of Pharmaceutical Sciences, 24,* 63–68.

Shi, J., Montay, G., & Bhargava, V.O. (2005). Clinical pharmacokinetics of telithromycin, the first ketolide antibacterial. *Clinical Pharmacokinetics, 44,* 915–934. doi:10.2165/00003088-200544090-00003

Shirasaka, Y., Sager, J.E., Lutz, J.D., Davis, C., & Isoherranen, N. (2013). Inhibition of CYP2C19 and CYP3A4 by omeprazole metabolites and their contribution to drug-drug interactions. *Drug Metabolism and Disposition, 41,* 1414–1424. doi:10.1124/dmd.113.051722

Skinner, M.H., Kuan, H.-Y., Pan, A., Sathirakul, K., Knadler, M.P., Gonzales, C.R., ... Wise, S.D. (2003). Duloxetine is both an inhibitor and a substrate of cytochrome P4502D6 in healthy volunteers. *Clinical Pharmacology and Therapeutics, 73,* 170–177. doi:10.1067/mcp.2003.28

Slaughter, R.L., & Edwards, D.J. (1995). Recent advances: The cytochrome P450 enzymes. *Annals of Pharmacotherapy, 29,* 619–624.

Smith, H.S. (2009). Opioid metabolism. *Mayo Clinic Proceedings, 84,* 613–624. doi:10.1016/S0025 -6196(11)60750-7

Spina, E., Santoro, V., & D'Arrigo, C. (2008). Clinically relevant pharmacokinetic drug interactions with second-generation antidepressants: An update. *Clinical Therapeutics, 30,* 1206–1227. doi:10.1016/S0149 -2918(08)80047-1

Stamer, U.M., Lee, E.H., Kleine-Brueggeney, M., Zhang, L., Musshoff, F., & Stuber, F. (2011). CYP2D6 and CYP3A genotypes influence metabolism of *R*- and *S*-ondansetron: BAPCPC1-3 (Abstract). *European Journal of Anaesthesiology, 28,* 1. doi:10.1097/00003643-201106001-00003

Sun, Y., Jia, P., Yuan, L., Liu, Y., Zhang, Z., Du, Y., & Zhang, L. (2015). Investigating the *in vitro* stereoselective metabolism of *m*-nisoldipine enantiomers: Characterization of metabolites and cytochrome P450 isoforms involved. *Biomedical Chromatography, 29,* 1893–1900. doi:10.1002/bmc.3512

Suzuki, A., Iida, I., Hirota, M., Akimoto, M., Higuchi, S., Suwa, T., … Chiba, K. (2003). CYP isoforms involved in the metabolism of clarithromycin in vitro: Comparison between the identification from disappearance rate and that from formation rate of metabolites. *Drug Metabolism and Pharmacokinetics, 18,* 104–113. doi:10.2133/dmpk.18.104

Timmer, C.J., Sitsen, J.M.A., & Delbressine, L.P. (2000). Clinical pharmacokinetics of mirtazapine. *Clinical Pharmacokinetics, 38,* 461–474. doi:10.2165/00003088-200038060-00001

Tomlinson, E.S., Lewis, D.F.V., Maggs, J.L., Kroemer, H.K., Park, B.K., & Back, D.J. (1997). *In vitro* metabolism of dexamethasone (DEX) in human liver and kidney: The involvement of CYP3a4 and CYP17 (17,20 LYASE) and molecular modelling studies. *Biochemical Pharmacology, 54,* 605–611. doi:10.1016/S0006-2952(97)00166-4

Tracy, T.S., Korzekwa, K.R., Gonzalez, F.J., & Wainer, I.W. (1999). Cytochrome P450 isoforms involved in metabolism of the enantiomers of verapamil and norverapamil. *British Journal of Clinical Pharmacology, 47,* 545–552. doi:10.1046/j.1365-2125.1999.00923.x

Van Booven, D., Marsh, S., McLeod, H., Carrillo, M.W., Sangkuhl, K., Klein, T.E., & Altman, R.B. (2010). Cytochrome P450 2C9-CYP2C9. *Pharmacogenetics and Genomics, 20,* 277–281. doi:10.1097/FPC.0b013e3283349e84

von Moltke, L.L., Greenblatt, D.J., Giancarlo, G.M., Granda, B.W., Harmatz, J.S., & Shader, R.I. (2001). Escitalopram (*S*-citalopram) and its metabolites in vitro: Cytochromes mediating biotransformation, inhibitory effects, and comparison to *R*-citalopram. *Drug Metabolism and Disposition, 29,* 1102–1109.

Wang, Y.-H., Jones, D.R., & Hall, S.D. (2005). Differential mechanism-based inhibition of CYP3A4 and CYP3A5 by verapamil. *Drug Metabolism and Disposition, 33,* 664–671. doi:10.1124/dmd.104.001834

Watkins, P.B., Murray, S.A., Winkelman, L.G., Heuman, D.M., Wrighton, S.A., & Guzelian, P.S. (1989). Erythromycin breath test as an assay of glucocorticoid-inducible liver cytochromes P-450: Studies in rats and patients. *Journal of Clinical Investigation, 83,* 688–697. doi:10.1172/JCI113933

Waxman, D.J., & Azaroff, L. (1992). Phenobarbital induction of cytochrome *P*-450 gene expression. *Biochemical Journal, 281,* 577–592. doi:10.1042/bj2810577

Wen, X., Wang, J.-S., Backman, J.T., Laitila, J., & Neuvonen, P.J. (2002). Trimethoprim and sulfamethoxazole are selective inhibitors of CYP2C8 and CYP2C9, respectively. *Drug Metabolism and Disposition, 30,* 631–615. doi:10.1124/dmd.30.6.631

Wester, M.R., Yano, J.K., Schoch, G.A., Yang, C., Griffin, K.J., Stout, C.D., & Johnson, E.F. (2004). The structure of human cytochrome P450 2C9 complexed with flurbiprofen at 2.0-Å resolution. *Journal of Biological Chemistry, 279,* 35630–35637. doi:10.1074/jbc.M405427200

Wilbur, K., & Ensom, M.H.H. (2000). Pharmacokinetic drug interactions between oral contraceptives and second-generation anticonvulsants. *Clinical Pharmacokinetics, 38,* 355–365. doi:10.2165/00003088-200038040-00004

Wilkinson, G.R. (2005). Drug metabolism and variability among patients in drug response. *New England Journal of Medicine, 352,* 2211–2221. doi:10.1056/NEJMra032424

Williams, P.A., Cosme, J., Vinković, D.M., Ward, A., Angove, H.C., Day, P.J., … Jhoti, H. (2004). Crystal structures of human cytochrome P450 3A4 bound to metyrapone and progesterone. *Science, 305,* 683–686. doi:10.1126/science.1099736

Wójcikowski, J., Basińska, A., & Daniel, W.A. (2014). The cytochrome P450-catalyzed metabolism of levomepromazine: A phenothiazine neuroleptic with a wide spectrum of clinical application. *Biochemical Pharmacology, 90,* 188–195. doi:10.1016/j.bcp.2014.05.005

World Health Organization. (2015). WHO model list of essential medicines (19th ed.). Retrieved from http://www.who.int/medicines/publications/essentialmedicines/en

Zhou, S.-F. (2008). Drugs behave as substrates, inhibitors and inducers of human cytochrome P450 3A4. *Current Drug Metabolism, 9,* 310–322. doi:10.2174/138920008784220664

Zhou, Y.-T., Yu, L.-S., Zeng, S., Huang, Y.-W., Xu, H.-M., & Zhou, Q. (2014). Pharmacokinetic drug–drug interactions between 1,4-dihydropyridine calcium channel blockers and statins: Factors determining interaction strength and relevant clinical risk management. *Therapeutics and Clinical Risk Management, 10,* 17–26. doi:10.2147/TCRM.S55512

Zhu, Y., Wang, F., Li, Q., Zhu, M., Du, A., Tang, W., & Chen, W. (2014). Amlodipine metabolism in human liver microsomes and roles of CYP3A4/5 in the dihydropyridine dehydrogenation. *Drug Metabolism and Disposition, 42,* 245–249. doi:10.1124/dmd.113.055400

CHAPTER 10

Drug–Drug Interactions in Palliative Care

Launa M.J. Lynch, PhD, Vicky V. Mody, PhD, and Adegoke O. Adeniji, RPh, PhD

I. Definitions
  A. *Drug–drug interactions* refers to the ability of a drug to modify the pharmacologic effects of another drug when drugs are administered concurrently.
  B. A drug with the ability to increase the metabolism of another drug is called an *inducer*.
  C. A drug that acts to decrease the metabolism of another drug is called an *inhibitor*.
  D. The number of drug–drug interactions is higher in palliative care because of the use of polypharmacy.
  E. *Polypharmacy* is when a patient is taking multiple drugs for the treatment of a number of symptoms related to one or more disease states.
  F. Cytochrome P450 (CYP) enzymes are membrane-bound, heme-containing oxidases that are responsible for the metabolic inactivation of most drugs and toxins.
  G. These enzymes are also able to metabolize prodrugs into active drugs (Hunter, Cruz, Cheyne, McManus, & Granville, 2004).
  H. Drugs metabolized by CYP enzymes are *substrates*.
      1. Genetic variations in the patient population can change the metabolism rates of CYP enzymes.
      2. Patients with the *poor metabolizer* phenotype with respect to a specific CYP enzyme usually do not have functional CYP enzymes or have remarkably reduced expression of the enzyme. This slows the elimination of the drug from the body, which can result in drug toxicity.
      3. A person with the *intermediate metabolizer* phenotype can have CYP enzymes that are partially active, causing the drug to be cleared at a slower than normal rate from the body, although the drug is still cleared at a faster rate relative to a poor metabolizer.
      4. Individuals with the *extensive metabolizer* phenotype have more active CYP enzymes present, and the drug is eliminated faster than normal from the body.
      5. Patients with the *ultra-rapid metabolizer* phenotype have the most CYP enzymes present, and the drug is eliminated very fast from the body.
  I. The clinical implications for both extensive and ultra-rapid metabolizers are increased risk of therapeutic failure (Weston, 2010).
II. Key aspects
  A. The most common drug–drug interactions involve the metabolism of drugs through the CYP enzyme system.

1. The CYP enzyme system is a superfamily of monooxygenases located predominantly in the liver.
2. These enzymes also are located at lower levels in other tissues such as the lungs, kidneys, and intestines.
3. The CYP enzymes are involved in the conversion of a lipid-soluble drug into a water-soluble metabolite for elimination from the body.
4. The CYP enzyme system metabolizes more than 30 classes of drugs (Kudzma & Carey, 2009).

B. The CYP enzyme system has been classified into 74 families are numerically designated as CYP1, CYP2, and CYP3.
   1. These families can be further divided into subfamilies by adding an alphabetical letter—examples include CYP1A, CYP2B, and CYP3A (Haddad, Davis, & Lagman, 2007).
   2. The subfamilies CYP1A2, CYP3A4, CYP2B6, CYP2C9, and CYP2D6 are the CYP enzymes involved in the majority of drug metabolism (Kudzma & Carey, 2009).
   3. Approximately 53% of drugs are metabolized by CYP3A4 and 25% are metabolized by CYP2D6 (Davis & Homsi, 2001).

C. Drugs can be classified as a CYP enzyme substrate, inhibitor, or inducer.

D. Patients can be classified as an ultra-rapid, extensive, intermediate, or poor metabolizer. Each of these genetic variations in a patient can have an effect on drug clearance.
   1. Patients with the ultra-rapid metabolizer phenotype may require a higher dose to achieve therapeutic level, whereas patients with the extensive metabolizer phenotype may not require a dose adjustment.
   2. Patients with the intermediate or poor metabolizer phenotype may require a reduced drug dose to avoid symptoms of an overdose (Kudzma & Carey, 2009; Kuebler, Varga, & Mihelic, 2003).
   3. The variability in the patient population and the interaction of drugs in the CYP enzyme system have the potential to affect drug metabolism and cause drug–drug interactions (Kuebler et al., 2003).

III. Current findings
   A. Polypharmacy is the main risk factor for drug–drug interactions in patients. The drugs most commonly involved in drug–drug interactions in palliative care are antipsychotics, antiemetics, antidepressants, glucocorticoids, and nonsteroidal anti-inflammatory drugs (Frechen, Zoeller, Ruberg, Voltz, & Gaertner, 2012).
   B. The principal CYP enzymes involved in the metabolism of drugs are CYP1A2, CYP3A4, CYP2B6, CYP2C9, and CYP2D6 (Kudzma & Carey, 2009). Of these, CYP3A4 and CYP2D6 are the main enzymes involved in drug metabolism (Davis & Homsi, 2001).
   C. Current lists for drug–drug interactions involving the CYP enzyme system include multiple drugs (Ogu & Maxa, 2000). These lists can make it difficult to determine which medications would be important to focus on in a clinical setting (Lynch & Price, 2007; Malone et al., 2004).
   D. Clinically relevant medications used in palliative care settings can be found in Figures 10-1 and 10-2.
   E. Substrates, inhibitors, and inducers of the CYP3A4 enzyme are in Figure 10-1 (Haddad et al., 2007).

Figure 10-1. CYP3A4 Substrates, Inhibitors, and Inducers Used in Palliative Care

CYP3A4 Substrates

Analgesics
- Alfentanil
- Buprenorphine
- Codeine
- Fentanyl
- Methadone

Anticonvulsant
- Carbamazepine

Antidepressant
- Trazodone

Antiemetics
- Granisetron
- Ondansetron

Antipsychotic
- Haloperidol

Anxiolytic
- Buspirone

Benzodiazepines
- Alprazolam
- Diazepam
- Midazolam
- Triazolam

Corticosteroids
- Dexamethasone
- Prednisone

Psychostimulant
- Modafinil

CYP3A4 Inhibitors

Anti-Infective Agents
- Ciprofloxacin
- Fluconazole

Selective Serotonin Reuptake Inhibitor
- Fluoxetine

CYP3A4 Inducers

Anticonvulsant
- Carbamazepine

Corticosteroid
- Dexamethasone

Note. Based on information from Haddad et al., 2007.

F. Figure 10-2 contains information for the CYP2D6 enzyme. These drugs can only be substrates and inhibitors because this enzyme is not inducible (Davis & Homsi, 2001; Haertter, 2013).

G. The most commonly prescribed drugs in the palliative care setting are dexamethasone, diazepam, fentanyl, haloperidol, lorazepam, metoclopramide, and morphine (Frechen et al., 2012).

H. Analgesics
   1. Codeine and tramadol are prodrugs, which need to be metabolized by the CYP2D6 enzyme to their active metabolite to be able to exert analgesic effects.
   2. A patient who has the poor metabolizer phenotype in CYP2D6 will be unable to convert codeine or tramadol to the active compound to relieve pain.

Figure 10-2. CYP2D6 Substrates and Inhibitors Used in Palliative Care

CYP2D6 Substrates

Analgesics
- Codeine
- Dextromethorphan
- Dihydrocodeine
- Ethylmorphine
- Hydrocodone
- Oxycodone
- Tramadol

Antiemetics
- Dolasetron
- Metoclopramide
- Ondansetron
- Palonosetron
- Promethazine

Antihistamine
- Diphenhydramine

Antipsychotics
- Chlorpromazine
- Haloperidol
- Olanzapine
- Risperidone
- Thioridazine

Other Antidepressants
- Duloxetine
- Mirtazapine
- Venlafaxine

Selective Serotonin Reuptake Inhibitors
- Fluoxetine
- Mirtazapine
- Paroxetine
- Sertraline
- Venlafaxine

Tricyclic Antidepressants
- Amitriptyline
- Doxepin
- Nortriptyline

CYP2D6 Inhibitors

Antihistamines
- Chlorpheniramine
- Diphenhydramine

Antiemetics
- Metoclopramide
- Promethazine

Antipsychotics
- Chlorpromazine
- Haloperidol
- Thioridazine

Selective Serotonin Reuptake Inhibitors
- Fluoxetine
- Fluvoxamine
- Paroxetine
- Sertraline

Note. Based on information from Davis & Homsi, 2001; Haertter, 2013.

---

3. Overdose symptoms would be observed in a patient who has the ultra-rapid CYP2D6 metabolizer phenotype because the prodrug would be rapidly converted to the active metabolite (Kudzma & Carey, 2009).

4. Dextromethorphan and hydrocodone are substrates of the CYP2D6 enzyme, and when administered with a CYP2D6 inhibitor, the drug levels in plasma will increase.

5. When dextromethorphan is combined with fluoxetine, a CYP2D6 substrate and inhibitor, an increase in the plasma concentration of both drugs will occur,

as well as associated side effects and the potential for serotonin syndrome (Davis & Homsi, 2001).

6. Alfentanil, buprenorphine, fentanyl, and methadone are metabolized by the CYP3A4 enzyme.
7. Caution should be exercised when using these drugs with a CYP3A4 enzyme inhibitor or inducer (Haddad et al., 2007).

I. Antidepressants
1. Fluoxetine, a selective serotonin reuptake inhibitor (SSRI), is a strong CYP2D6 enzyme inhibitor and a moderate CYP3A4 enzyme inhibitor.
   a) Fluoxetine causes an increase in the plasma levels of haloperidol when these drugs are taken together.
   b) Fluoxetine will slow the clearance of alprazolam, diazepam, and methadone.
   c) An alternative to fluoxetine may be venlafaxine.
2. Venlafaxine is a weak inhibitor of both the CYP2D6 and CYP3A4 enzymes and is associated with a lower incidence of drug–drug interactions (Haddad et al., 2007).
3. Tricyclic antidepressants are substrates for the CYP2D6 enzyme. The clearance of tricyclic antidepressants from the body can be slowed by CYP2D6 inhibitors such as SSRIs (Davis & Homsi, 2001).

J. Antipsychotics
1. Haloperidol is a substrate for CYP3A4 and CYP2D6, but it is mainly cleared by CYP3A4.
2. Interactions occur when haloperidol is combined with alprazolam, fluoxetine, or carbamazepine.
   a) Alprazolam is a competitive inhibitor of CYP3A4 metabolism and will slow the metabolism of haloperidol, resulting in increased plasma levels and potentially increased adverse side effects.
   b) Fluoxetine is a CYP3A4 enzyme inhibitor and increases the plasma levels of haloperidol when these two drugs are administered together.
   c) Carbamazepine is an inducer of CYP3A4 metabolism and will decrease plasma levels of haloperidol when coadministration occurs and may result in haloperidol not being therapeutically effective (Frechen et al., 2012).
3. The CYP2D6 enzyme is responsible for the metabolism of chlorpromazine, olanzapine, risperidone, and thioridazine (Davis & Homsi, 2001).
4. CYP2D6 inhibitors will decrease the enzyme activity and cause these drugs to be slowly cleared from the body.
5. Slow clearance of a drug from the body increases the plasma levels and the toxic effects of the drug.
6. The clinical effectiveness of chlorpromazine, haloperidol, and thioridazine is not altered even though these drugs are both substrates and inhibitors of the CYP2D6 enzyme (Davis & Homsi, 2001).

K. Benzodiazepines
1. Alprazolam, diazepam, midazolam, and triazolam are all substrates for the CYP3A4 enzyme.
2. CYP3A4 inhibitors such as fluconazole and fluoxetine will cause an increase in the plasma levels of the substrate drugs when taken together.
3. When a combination of a CYP3A4 enzyme substrate and inhibitor is administered, the patient should be monitored for adverse side effects of the substrate (Haddad et al., 2007).

    L. Corticosteroids
       1. When dexamethasone is used in high doses, the drug becomes a CYP3A4 inducer.
       2. When a CYP3A4 substrate is taken by a patient who is on high doses of dexamethasone, the substrate will be cleared from the body faster than normal and may have lower clinical efficacy (Haddad et al., 2007).

IV. Relevance to practice
    A. Polypharmacy is a reality for patients in the palliative care setting.
    B. In these settings, clinicians need to periodically monitor and evaluate the combination of drugs being taken by a patient.
    C. In general, a CYP enzyme–inhibiting drug will decrease the clearance and raise the plasma levels of a substrate drug for the same CYP enzyme.
       1. For example, the combination of methadone (a CYP3A4 substrate) and ciprofloxacin (a CYP3A4 inhibitor) may result in methadone causing fatal respiratory depression.
       2. A patient on this combination will need to be monitored closely, and a dose adjustment of methadone may be needed to avoid this life-threatening adverse side effect (*Nursing2015 Drug Handbook*, 2015).
    D. A CYP enzyme–inducing drug will increase the clearance and lower the plasma levels of a substrate drug for the same CYP enzyme.
       1. In this situation, the substrate drug may not be effective.
       2. For example, carbamazepine is a CYP3A4 inducer and will increase the clearance of CYP3A4 substrates such as buprenorphine, fentanyl, and methadone.
       3. Patients taking this combination will need to be monitored for pain because buprenorphine, fentanyl, or methadone may not be as effective.
       4. Patients will still be in pain because of the reduced analgesic effects (*Nursing2015 Drug Handbook*, 2015).
    E. Observations will be key in patients in the palliative care setting.
       1. When combinations of substrates and inhibitors are being taken together, clinicians need to monitor patients for adverse side effects.
       2. The clinician may need to administer a lower dose of the substrate drug or use an alternative drug.
       3. When a patient is taking a combination of a substrate and an inducer, clinicians need to monitor for therapeutic effectiveness of the substrate.
       4. Clinicians may need to increase the dose of the substrate drug or use another therapeutic agent.

References

Davis, M.P., & Homsi, J. (2001). The importance of cytochrome P450 monooxygenase CYP2D6 in palliative medicine. *Supportive Care in Cancer, 9*, 442–451. doi:10.1007/s005200000222

Frechen, S., Zoeller, A., Ruberg, K., Voltz, R., & Gaertner, J. (2012). Drug interactions in dying patients: A retrospective analysis of hospice inpatients in Germany. *Drug Safety, 35*, 745–758. doi:10.1007/bf03261971

Haddad, A., Davis, M., & Lagman, R. (2007). The pharmacological importance of cytochrome CYP3A4 in the palliation of symptoms: Review and recommendations for avoiding adverse drug interactions. *Supportive Care in Cancer, 15*, 251–257. doi:10.1007/s00520-006-0127-5

Haertter, S. (2013). Recent examples on the clinical relevance of the CYP2D6 polymorphism and endogenous functionality of CYP2D6. *Drug Metabolism and Drug Interactions, 28*, 209–216. doi:10.1515/dmdi-2013-0032

Hunter, A.L., Cruz, R.P., Cheyne, B.M., McManus, B.M., & Granville, D.J. (2004). Cytochrome p450 enzymes and cardiovascular disease. *Canadian Journal of Physiology and Pharmacology, 82,* 1053–1060. doi:10.1139/y04-118

Kudzma, E.C., & Carey, E.T. (2009). Pharmacogenomics: Personalizing drug therapy. *American Journal of Nursing, 109*(10), 50–57. doi:10.1097/01.NAJ.0000361493.75589.06

Kuebler, K.K., Varga, J., & Mihelic, R.A. (2003). Why there is no cookbook approach to palliative care: Implications of the P450 enzyme system. *Clinical Journal of Oncology Nursing, 7,* 569–572. doi:10.1188/03.CJON.569-572

Lynch, T., & Price, A. (2007). The effect of cytochrome P450 metabolism on drug response, interactions, and adverse effects. *American Family Physician, 76,* 391–396. Retrieved from http://www.aafp.org/afp/2007/0801/p391.html

Malone, D.C., Abarca, J., Hansten, P.D., Grizzle, A.J., Armstrong, E.P., Van Bergen, R.C., … Lipton, R.B. (2004). Identification of serious drug–drug interactions: Results of the partnership to prevent drug–drug interactions. *Journal of the American Pharmacists Association, 44,* 142–151.

Nursing2015 drug handbook (35th ed.). (2015). Philadelphia, PA: Wolters Kluwer.

Ogu, C.C., & Maxa, J.L. (2000). Drug interactions due to cytochrome P450. *Baylor University Medical Center Proceedings, 13,* 421–423. Retrieved from http://www.ncbi.nlm.nih.gov/pmc/articles/PMC1312247

Weston, G.S. (2010). The pharmacogenetics of drug metabolism. In M.M. Zdanowicz (Ed.), *Concepts in pharmacogenomics* (pp. 85–127). Bethesda, MD: American Society of Health-System Pharmacists.

CHAPTER 11

Palliative Care and Concomitant Medications

Kimberly L. Barefield, PharmD, BCPS, CDE

I. Definitions
   A. The goal of palliative care is to achieve optimal quality of life, reduce symptom burden and healthcare resource use, and potentially increase survival.
   B. Patients with advanced disease experience many physical and emotional symptoms during the disease trajectory as a result of progressing illness, disease-related therapy, or comorbidities (Berger, Yennu, & Million, 2013).
   C. Symptoms can occur in *clusters*, which are defined as two or more concurrent and interrelated symptoms that occur with a high degree of predictability (Miaskowski, Dodd, & Lee, 2004).
      1. Evidence shows that symptom clusters have a more complicated and synergistic negative association with treatment outcomes, functional status, prognosis, and overall quality of life compared to individual symptoms (Aktas, Walsh, & Rybicki, 2012; Fan, Filipczak, & Chow, 2007).
      2. Symptoms within a cluster do not require a common etiology but may be grouped together based on presentation.
      3. Symptom clusters have a "core" or "defining" symptom, which represents the presence of a symptom cluster (Dong, Butow, Costa, Lovell, & Agar, 2014). Consider, for example, the influence that poorly managed depression has on increased patient-reported pain intensity from chronic pain.
      4. All symptoms within the cluster may not be present throughout the entire disease course; therefore, it is critical to continuously monitor patients for symptoms and adverse effects related to treatment.
II. Key aspects
   A. Palliative care interventions include anticancer therapy and treatment of comorbidities and symptoms (World Health Organization, 2002).
   B. The most common comorbidities and symptoms are listed in Figure 11-1 (de Lima, 2006).
   C. Over time, palliative care treatment progresses from treatment of comorbidities to management of symptoms.
   D. Patients with chronic illnesses experience complex symptoms from both disease and disease treatment (Rangachari & Smith, 2013).
   E. A key aspect of management is the assessment of symptoms and therapy for drug interactions and adverse effects.

F. Donnelly, Walsh, and Rybicki characterized symptoms that occur in patients with cancer (Donnelly & Walsh, 1995; Walsh, Donnelly, & Rybicki, 2000).
  1. The median number of symptoms identified was 11, with the most frequently reported being pain, fatigue, weakness, anorexia, weight loss, lack of energy, dry mouth, constipation, and dyspnea.
  2. The prevalence differed with gender, age, and type of cancer.
  3. Gastrointestinal symptoms were related to female gender, and overall survival favored females.
  4. Younger patients exhibited more symptoms of anxiety, depression, and insomnia, likely related to psychosocial stress.

Figure 11-1. Common Comorbidities and Symptoms in Palliative Care

- Pain
  - Bone
  - Neuropathic
  - Inflammation
  - Visceral
- Dyspnea
- Xerostomia
- Hiccups
- Increased secretions
- Anorexia or cachexia
- Gastrointestinal disorders
  - Nausea
  - Vomiting
  - Constipation
  - Diarrhea
  - Heartburn
- Psychological disorders
- Fatigue
- Sweating
- Terminal agitation

Note. Based on information from de Lima, 2006.

G. Therapy based on symptom clusters can decrease the medication burden and adverse effects related to treatment.
H. A review article by Dong et al. (2014) identified the most common symptom cluster groupings as anxiety and depression; nausea and appetite loss; nausea and vomiting; and fatigue, dyspnea, drowsiness, and pain.
  1. The symptom cluster of anxiety and depression appears to be consistent across age and gender.
  2. It may represent psychological stress more than clinical anxiety or depression, with the possibility of other psychological components.
  3. The symptom cluster of fatigue, dyspnea, drowsiness, and pain has been associated with the symptom cluster of anorexia and cachexia, suggesting that a treatment approach for fatigue, dyspnea, drowsiness, and pain may positively affect the other symptom cluster.

III. Current findings and relevance to practice
  A. Recognition of these symptoms along with safe and effective treatment is critical in the management of palliative care patients.
  B. The International Association for Hospice and Palliative Care was appointed by the World Health Organization to develop a list of essential medications for use in palliative care (de Lima, 2006).
    1. Medications were evaluated based on safety and efficacy in the treatment of identified common comorbidities and symptoms (see Figure 11-1).
    2. The final list contained 33 medications, but consensus could not be reached on safe and effective treatment of bone pain, dry mouth, fatigue, hiccups, and sweating.
    3. Table 11-1 lists the essential medications based on symptom management.

Table 11-1. Essential Medications	
Class	**Medications**
Analgesics—opioids	Codeine, fentanyl transdermal, methadone, morphine, oxycodone, tramadol
Analgesics—nonopioids	Acetaminophen, diclofenac, ibuprofen
Antidepressants	Amitriptyline, citalopram, mirtazapine, trazodone
Benzodiazepines	Diazepam, lorazepam, midazolam
Laxatives	Bisacodyl, mineral oil enema, senna
Gastrointestinal agents	Hyoscine butylbromide, loperamide
Steroids	Dexamethasone, prednisone
Other	Diphenhydramine, gabapentin, haloperidol, megestrol, metoclopramide, octreotide, zolpidem

Note. Based on information from de Lima, 2006.

4. Many of the agents on the list may be used to treat more than one symptom in a patient or symptoms clusters (Miaskowski et al., 2004).
C. Prevention of drug interactions and adverse effects is a priority when designing a treatment plan for palliative care patients. Designing therapeutic plans that address symptom clusters rather than individual symptoms will reduce the drug burden, as well as minimize drug interactions and adverse effects.
D. Patients who transition from curative treatment to palliative care require a thorough review of their therapy for medications that may no longer be appropriate (Lindsay et al., 2014).
   1. Medications for treatment of current disease states or those without short-term benefit may not be suitable and may be potentially harmful because of the greater pill burden for the patient and possible adverse effects.
   2. Riechelmann, Krzyzanowska, and Zimmermann (2009) performed a retrospective chart review of patients with advanced cancer receiving supportive care and found that 22% were using at least one unnecessary or duplicate medication.
E. The identification of symptom clusters in practice reduces medication burden and adverse effects related to disease treatment.
F. Practitioners should reassess patients' symptoms routinely to make adjustments in therapy.
IV. Role of the advanced practice registered nurse (APRN)
   A. APRNs are an essential part of the interdisciplinary team to meet the complex care needs of patients with symptomatic advanced disease.
   B. APRNs provide ongoing physical and diagnostic assessment of symptoms and effective disease and symptom management.
   C. APRNs should remain current and relevant in the pharmacologic and physiologic changes that can occur by patient ethnicity and whenever introducing new medications.
   D. APRNs need to consider cytochrome P450 system metabolism with all drug combinations and the inhibitory or accelerated mechanisms of combined medication classes.

Case Study

C.K. is a 57-year-old man with advanced (stage IV) lung cancer and is complaining of poorly managed neuropathic pain, dyspnea, and depression. The patient also complains of abdominal pain and fullness. He describes his pain as shooting-like and radiating from the cervical neck down into his bilateral shoulders and into the right elbow, medially. He describes his pain as intermittent and rates it as a 7 out of 10. Because of the widely metastatic disease, he is prescribed morphine extended release 90 mg every 12 hours, and for breakthrough pain, he uses morphine sulfate immediate release 10–20 mg every 4 hours. C.K. continues to complain of pain and now has constipation accompanied with intermittent nausea and vomiting. He has tried increasing his breakthrough opioid dose, but it only makes him sleepy. He has lost eight pounds in the past month because of his gastrointestinal complaints.

Physical examination of vital signs shows a blood pressure of 135/69 mm Hg, respiratory rate of 26 breaths per minute, heart rate of 80 beats per minute, and temperature of 99°F (37.2°C). Cardiovascular findings show regular rate and rhythm, and pulmonary findings show diminished lung sounds in bilateral lobes, tight wheezing in upper lobes bilaterally, and increased anteroposterior diameter.

On assessment, the APRN notes neuropathic pain, depression, anorexia-cachexia, nausea and vomiting, constipation, and sedation. The APRN prescribes duloxetine 20 mg daily for depression and radiculopathy. The APRN also infuses 1,000 ml of normal saline to relieve constipation, improve nausea and vomiting, and aid in reducing the systemic circulation of medication metabolites. Following a thorough discussion with the patient about the short-term benefit of a steroid, the patient consent to receive dexamethasone 10 mg intramuscular injection to improve appetite and reduce pain, dyspnea, and nausea and vomiting. The APRN prescribes oxygen per nasal cannula at 2 L/min. The APRN also makes a referral for physical therapy and a registered dietitian, and orders a complete metabolic panel, complete blood count diagnostics, and follow-up in one week.

References

Aktas, A., Walsh, D., & Rybicki, L. (2012). Symptom clusters and prognosis in advanced cancer. *Supportive Care in Cancer, 20,* 2837–2843. doi:10.1007/s00520-012-1408-9

Berger, A.M., Yennu, S., & Million, R. (2013). Update on interventions focused on symptom clusters: What has been tried and what have we learned? *Current Opinion in Supportive and Palliative Care, 7,* 60–66. doi:10.1097/SPC.0b013e32835c7d88

de Lima, L. (2006). The International Association for Hospice and Palliative Care list of essential medicines for palliative care. *Palliative Medicine, 20,* 647–651. doi:10.1177/0269216306072058

Dong, S.T., Butow, P.N., Costa, D.S.J., Lovell, M.R., & Agar, M. (2014). Symptom clusters in patients with advanced cancer: A systematic review of observational studies. *Journal of Pain and Symptom Management, 48,* 411–450. doi:10.1016/j.jpainsymman.2013.10.027

Donnelly, S., & Walsh, D. (1995). The symptoms of advanced cancer. *Seminars in Oncology, 22*(2, Suppl. 3), 67–72.

Fan, G., Filipczak, L., & Chow, E. (2007). Symptom clusters in cancer patients: A review of the literature. *Current Oncology, 14,* 173–179. doi:10.3747/co.2007.145

Lindsay, J., Dooley, M., Martin, J., Fay, M., Kearney, A., & Barras, M. (2014). Reducing potentially inappropriate medications in palliative cancer patients: Evidence to support deprescribing approaches. *Supportive Care in Cancer, 22,* 1113–1119. doi:10.1007/s00520-013-2098-7

Miaskowski, C., Dodd, M., & Lee, K. (2004). Symptom clusters: The new frontier in symptom management research. *Journal of the National Cancer Institute Monographs, 2004*(32), 17–21. doi:10.1093/jncimonographs/lgh023

Rangachari, D., & Smith, T.J. (2013). Integrating palliative care in oncology: The oncologist as a primary palliative care provider. *Cancer Journal, 19,* 373–378. doi:10.1097/PPO.0b013e3182a76b9c

Riechelmann, R.P., Krzyzanowska, M.K., & Zimmermann, C. (2009). Futile medication use in terminally ill cancer patients. *Supportive Care in Cancer, 17,* 745–748. doi:10.1007/s00520-008-0541-y

Walsh, D., Donnelly, S., & Rybicki, L. (2000). The symptoms of advanced cancer: Relationship to age, gender, and performance status in 1,000 patients. *Supportive Care in Cancer, 8,* 175–179. doi:10.1007/s005200050281

World Health Organization. (2002). *Cancer pain relief and palliative care: Report of a WHO expert committee.* Geneva, Switzerland: Author.

Section III.

Chronic Conditions and Malignancy

CHAPTER 12

Cardiovascular Disease

Myrshia L. Woods, MHS, PA-C, and Kim Kuebler, DNP, APRN, ANP-BC

I. Definition
   A. Heart failure (HF) is "a complex clinical syndrome that results from any structural or functional impairment of ventricular filling or ejection of blood" (Yancy et al., 2013, p. e246). The term *heart failure* is preferred over *congestive heart failure* because signs or symptoms of volume overload may not be present (Yancy et al., 2013).
   B. The term *heart failure* is used to signify that the heart is failing to adequately meet the metabolic demands and basic physiologic functions of the body.
   C. The clinical understanding of HF is directly correlated to disorders of the pericardium, myocardium, endocardium, heart valves, or major vessels or from certain metabolic abnormalities. The majority of patients with HF have symptoms resulting from impaired left ventricular myocardial function (Yancy et al., 2013).
      1. The particular impairment of the left ventricle may be related to the diastolic phase (relaxation or filling phase) or systolic phase (contraction or ejection phase) of the cardiac cycle.
      2. HF is associated with a wide spectrum of left ventricular functional abnormalities that can range from patients with normal left ventricular size and a preserved or normal ejection fraction (EF) to those with severe vascular dilatation and markedly reduced EF. Most patients present with abnormalities of coexisting systolic and diastolic dysfunction regardless of EF findings (Yancy et al., 2013).
         a) Evaluation of EF is a diagnostic tool and a requirement when discerning the specific type of HF for an individualized patient. It also is important to note that diastolic and systolic impairment can coexist in the same ventricle at once.
         b) HF with a reduced EF of 40% or less is recognized as *systolic HF*. U.S. Food and Drug Administration–approved medications for systolic HF have been mainly studied in the population of patients specifically with low ejection fractions, less than 40%. These medications have been approved because they each showed a mortality benefit (Yancy et al., 2013).
         c) HF with a preserved EF of 50 or greater is referred to as *diastolic HF*.
         d) The diagnosis of diastolic HF is challenging because it is largely one of excluding other potential noncardiac causes of symptoms suggestive of HF.
         e) Limited evidence currently exists in providing efficacious therapies in diastolic HF (Yancy et al., 2013).

125

3. A common cause of diastolic HF is uncontrolled hypertension. Effective management of diastolic HF will likely entail aggressive use of antihypertensive medications to meet blood pressure goals designated in the Eighth Joint National Committee (JNC 8) guidelines (James et al., 2014).
4. Patients with borderline or intermediate HF with preserved EF of 40–49 present similarly as patients with diastolic HF (Yancy et al., 2013).
5. The classifications and stages of HF are directed by the American College of Cardiology Foundation and the American Heart Association.
    a) These criteria can help to identify the development and progression of HF and are often used to describe individuals and populations at risk. These criteria, together with the New York Heart Association (NYHA) functional classification system, provide useful information for determining the severity of HF (see Table 12-1).

Table 12-1. Comparison of ACCF/AHA Stages of Heart Failure and NYHA Functional Classifications

ACCF/AHA Stages of Heart Failure		NYHA Functional Classifications	
A	At high risk for heart failure (HF) but without structural heart disease or symptoms of HF	None	–
B	Structural heart disease but without signs or symptoms of HF	I	No limitation of physical activity. Ordinary physical activity does not cause symptoms of HF.
C	Structural heart disease with prior or current symptoms of HF	I	No limitation of physical activity. Ordinary physical activity does not cause symptoms of HF.
	–	II	Slight limitation of physical activity. Comfortable at rest, but ordinary physical activity results in symptoms of HF.
	–	III	Marked limitation of physical activity. Comfortable at rest, but less than ordinary activity causes symptoms of HF.
	–	IV	Unable to carry on any physical activity without symptoms of HF, or symptoms of HF at rest.
D	Refractory HF requiring specialized interventions	IV	Unable to carry on any physical activity without symptoms of HF, or symptoms of HF at rest.

ACCF/AHA—American College of Cardiology Foundation/American Heart Association; NYHA—New York Heart Association

Note. Based on information from Criteria Committee of the New York Heart Association, 1994; Hunt et al., 2009.

From "2013 ACCF/AHA Guideline for the Management of Heart Failure: A Report of the American College of Cardiology Foundation/American Heart Association Task Force on Practice Guidelines," by C.W. Yancy, M. Jessup, B. Bozkurt, J. Butler, D.E. Casey, Jr., M.H. Drazner, … B.L. Wilkoff, 2013, *Circulation, 128,* p. e248. Copyright 2013 by American College of Cardiology Foundation and American Heart Association, Inc. Reprinted with permission.

  b) With both of these tools, providers will have a better understanding on the prognosis, treatment options, and care required for individual patients (Yancy et al., 2013).

 6. As of 2010, 5.1 million people in the United States were clinically diagnosed with HF (Go et al., 2013), and the prevalence has continued to rise.

 7. Medicare beneficiaries diagnosed with HF from 1994 to 2003 rose from 90 to 121 per 1,000 beneficiaries. By 2050, 1 out of 5 Americans will be aged 65 and older. HF is the highest in this age group, and the prevalence of HF will significantly worsen in the future (U.S. Department of Health and Human Services, 2005).

 8. The lifetime risk for developing HF is 20% for Americans older than 40 years (Djoussé, Driver, & Gaziano, 2009).

D. Long-term effective management of systolic and diastolic hypertension can reduce the risk of HF by approximately 50%. Lifetime risk for developing HF is greater than 75% in the United States (Izzo & Gradman, 2004).

E. Additional risk factors

 1. Obesity and insulin resistance are risk factors that can markedly lend to the development of HF and metabolic syndrome (Izzo & Gradman, 2004).

 2. Metabolic syndrome includes three of the following conditions: abdominal adiposity, hypertriglyceridemia, decreased high-density lipoprotein, hypertension, and fasting hyperglycemia. Nearly 35% of all U.S. adults and 50% of those aged 60 years or older were estimated to have the metabolic syndrome in 2011–2012 (JAMA, 2015).

 3. Cigarette smoking, excessive alcohol use, excessive intake of sodium, and sedentary lifestyle can all contribute over time to HF (Izzo & Gradman, 2004).

F. In 2009, 1 in 9 deaths in the United States included HF as a contributing cause (Go et al., 2013).

G. Half of Americans who are diagnosed with HF are expected to die within five years of diagnosis (Go et al., 2013).

H. The annual financial burden of HF on the nation's health system was estimated at $32 billion in 2013. This total included the cost of healthcare services, medications, and missed days of productivity (Go et al., 2013).

I. HF is the primary diagnosis in more than one million hospitalizations annually in the United States. Patients who are hospitalized with HF are at high risk for all-cause rehospitalizations, with a one-month readmission rate of 25% (Go et al., 2013).

J. In 2010, there were 1.8 million office visits with a primary diagnosis of HF (Go et al., 2013).

K. Centers for Medicare and Medicaid Services (CMS) Hospital Readmissions Reduction Program

 1. Because of the excessive financial burden in the United States related to the care and management of HF, section 3025 of the Patient Protection and Affordable Care Act (ACA) of 2010 added section 1886(q) to the Social Security Act establishing the Hospital Readmissions Reduction Program, mandating CMS to reduce payments to Medicare-participating hospitals with excess readmissions for disease-specific conditions following hospital discharge beginning on October 1, 2012 (CMS, 2016).

 2. These conditions have been updated and are reviewed annually. Currently, HF is the number-one diagnosis for readmission penalty because of the excessive

cost management of HF and from the exacerbations that occur from poorly managed symptoms (CMS, 2016).

3. In 2012, CMS finalized the policy rule for short-term acute care hospitals that receive Medicare reimbursement under the inpatient prospective payment system (IPPS) to collect and report readmission measures under the Hospital Readmissions Reduction Program (CMS, 2016).

    a) CMS defines readmission as an admission to an IPPS participating hospital within 30 days of a discharge from the same or another IPPS participating hospital.

    b) The policy rule adopted the initial readmission measures in 2012 for acute myocardial infarction, HF, and pneumonia (CMS, 2016).

    c) From 2014 to 2016, the addition of readmission measures includes patients admitted with acute exacerbation of chronic obstructive pulmonary disease (COPD) and patients admitted for elective total hip arthroplasty and total knee replacement (CMS, 2016).

    d) In 2015, these measures were expanded to patients admitted for coronary artery bypass graft (beginning with the 2017 program) and, in 2016, CMS expanded the pneumonia readmission measures to include diagnoses of aspiration pneumonia and sepsis (CMS, 2016).

II. Pathophysiology

A. Several compensatory mechanisms occur within the body as the failing heart attempts to maintain adequate function. These include increasing cardiac output via the Frank-Starling mechanism, increasing ventricular volume and myocardial wall thickness through ventricular remodeling, and maintaining tissue perfusion by increasing the mean arterial pressure through activation of the neurohormonal systems (Kemp & Conte, 2012).

B. The body attempts to maintain normal cardiac output to provide adequate tissue perfusion. Cardiac output is equal to heart rate times the stroke volume.

C. Stroke volume is the amount of blood ejected out of the left ventricle with each heartbeat. When the heart is failing, the stroke volume decreases, and the heart rate increases to compensate for the reduced stroke volume to maintain a normal cardiac output.

D. These compensatory efforts by the body cause deleterious effects of increasing myocardial strain, lending to ischemia, hemodynamic compromise, apoptosis, fibrosis, arrhythmias, and cellular alterations, all of which can be catastrophic to the failing heart.

1. The prolonged activation of the compensatory mechanisms eventually leads to a vicious circle of worsening heart failure and enlargement and thickening of the myocardium (Kemp & Conte, 2012).

2. This process is called *remodeling*.

    a) Remodeling is the undesirable end result of the culmination of all the compensatory neurohormonal processes triggered in the body.

    b) The myocardium changes morphologically over time and changes from an oval-shaped, small-chamber ventricle into a larger, dilated, spherical-shaped ventricle that is less compliant and less efficient in its contractility (James et al., 2014).

3. Neurohormonal adaptations that include the activation of the renin-angiotensin-aldosterone and the sympathetic nervous systems by the low-output state help to maintain perfusion maintenance to the vital organs in the following two ways:

a) Maintenance of systemic pressure through vascular vasoconstriction results in redistribution of blood flow to vital organs. As blood flow is redirected or shunted toward the vital organs, the extremities become cold and pale because of decreased tissue perfusion. The skin and extremities are ischemic as a result of low cardiac output (James et al., 2014).

b) Cardiac output is restored by an increase in myocardial contractility and heart rate and by expansion of the extracellular fluid volume (Sarraf, Masoumi, & Schrier, 2009). Increasing myocardial contractility increases the myocardial oxygen consumption requirement by the myocardium itself, and the heart is unable to meet this requirement adequately because of low perfusion, thus resulting in ischemia.

4. In HF, these adaptations tend to overwhelm the vasodilatory and natriuretic effects of the compensatory pathways including natriuretic peptides, nitric oxide, prostaglandins, and bradykinin (Logeart et al., 2008). On laboratory investigation, these respective levels are markedly abnormal. In the worst cases of decompensated HF, B-type natriuretic peptide (BNP, also termed *brain natriuretic peptide*) levels can reach to a level greater than 5,000 pg/ml (James et al., 2014).

5. Volume expansion is often effective because the heart can respond to an increase in venous return with an elevation in end-diastolic volume that results in a rise in stroke volume (via the Frank-Starling mechanism) (Logeart et al., 2008). Over time, this process can overwhelm the heart as a whole, and each chamber can begin to dilate because of the increased volume, which potentiates further remodeling of the myocardium.

E. Neurohormonal influence
   1. Sympathetic nervous system (SNS)
      a) The SNS is one of the main branches of the autonomic nervous system and commonly is referred to as the fight-or-flight response.
      b) In HF, the SNS becomes activated and releases norepinephrine in response to decreased cardiac output of the failing heart, reflected by an increased heart rate and inotropy (contractility) of the left ventricle (Kemp & Conte, 2012).
      c) Although activation of the SNS initially is compensatory for the failing heart, over time it causes further damage to the myocardium by increasing peripheral vasoconstriction and triggering the remodeling process.
      d) Remodeling ends in increased ventricular hypertrophy, arrhythmias, and alterations in molecular and biochemical processes (Kemp & Conte, 2012).
   2. Role of myocardial adrenergic receptors
      a) The beta-1 adrenoreceptors of the myocardium are stimulated by the release of norepinephrine.
      b) In the failing ventricle with systolic dysfunction, this stimulation is insufficient to restore normal inotropy (Kemp & Conte, 2012).
      c) Significant downregulation of the beta-1 adrenoreceptors occurs, leading to a blunting of the inotropic response.
      d) Prolonged sympathetic activation worsens HF over time.
   3. Renin–angiotensin–aldosterone system (RAAS)
      a) Similarly, the RAAS is upregulated by increased sympathetic outflow to the kidneys, causing the release of renin.
      b) Renin is an important hormone that regulates blood pressure and fluid balance.

  c) Renin production is mediated by the beta-1 adrenoreceptors in the kidneys.

  d) With persistent increased sympathetic activation, there is production of angiotensin II, a potent vasoconstrictor peripherally, and later aldosterone, which leads to alterations in sodium and fluid retention.

  e) Activation of all these hormones contributes to the development of peripheral edema and eventual volume overload (Sarraf et al., 2009).

4. Aldosterone

  a) Aldosterone is an important mineralocorticoid released by the adrenal glands that aids in blood pressure regulation, sodium conservation, potassium excretion, and water retention.

  b) As plasma levels of angiotensin II increase, aldosterone is produced. Increasing aldosterone production worsens HF by increasing overall blood volume (Sarraf et al., 2009).

5. Angiotensin-converting enzyme (ACE) gene polymorphism

  a) Genetic studies have been performed on individuals expressing different genotypic variations of the ACE polymorphism.

  b) A strong association exists between the ACE polymorphism and the plasma level of ACE, which can directly affect a patient's disease progression of HF.

  c) This has been found to be most prevalent in African Americans and generated the changes in the JNC 8 guidelines discouraging the use of ACE inhibitor medications in this patient population (James et al., 2014).

6. Antidiuretic hormone (ADH)

  a) ADH, also known as vasopressin, plays a key role in homeostasis and aids in the regulation of salt and water in the body.

  b) It also causes peripheral vasoconstriction and plays a role in regulating arterial blood pressure.

  c) It plays an important compensatory role in extreme conditions such as hypovolemic shock.

  d) In HF, impaired water excretion and an inappropriate response to plasma ADH occur (Sarraf et al., 2009).

7. Atrial natriuretic peptide (ANP) and BNP

  a) ANP and BNP are peptide hormones of cardiac origin released both from the atria and the ventricles in response to pressure or volume overload in the failing myocardium (James et al., 2014).

  b) The release of ANP or BNP promotes natriuresis by the kidneys.

   (1) ANP serves to maintain sodium homeostasis and inhibits the activation of the RAAS.

   (2) ANP is released by the atria in response to atrial distension from volume or pressure overload (Sarraf et al., 2009).

   (3) BNP is an important biomarker in the diagnosis of HF, and many studies demonstrate a direct correlation with the BNP level and NYHA classification (Logeart et al., 2008).

   (4) BNP is released from the myocardial ventricles. The release decreases systemic vascular resistance and central venous pressure while promoting natriuresis.

   (5) Both of these peptide hormones are compensatory mechanisms of the body to decrease volume overload in patients with congestive HF (Kemp & Conte, 2012).

8. Endothelin is a peptide that constricts blood vessels and raises blood pressure.
   a) The release of endothelin is a mechanism of the body to compensate for hemodynamic collapse by the failing heart (James et al., 2014).
   b) Overexpression of endothelin levels can occur in HF, which leads to hypertension.
   c) Hypertension further exacerbates the progression of HF with subsequent development of pulmonary hypertension (James et al., 2014).
9. Differentiation between right-sided and left-sided HF (see Figure 12-1)
   a) Right-sided HF results from increased pulmonary arterial pressures causing increased pulmonary resistance.
   b) The forward flow of blood from the right ventricle is decreased because of the increased pulmonary resistance, and the right ventricle is overwhelmed with increased volume and pressure overload (Kemp & Conte, 2012).
   c) Right ventricular failure is dominated by venous congestion. The manifestations of right-sided HF are systemic, leading to jugular venous distension, hepatic congestion with hepatomegaly, ascites, intestinal edema, lower-extremity edema, and anasarca (Kemp & Conte, 2012).
   d) Left-sided HF is dominated mainly by pulmonary congestion. Left ventricular failure results in backward circulatory congestion causing left atrial dilatation, which builds up pressure within the pulmonary circulation, leading to crackles, rales, and pulmonary edema (Kemp & Conte, 2012).
   e) This process causes decreased oxygenation and ultimately a decreased cardiac output caused by increased sympathetic stimulation. There is persistent atrial contraction against a noncompliant ventricle, leading to increased intracardiac pressures. Peripheral vasoconstriction is enhanced, which potentiates the progression of HF (Logeart et al., 2008).

III. Presenting symptoms
   A. Patients with HF sometimes do not suspect they have a problem with their heart or have unrelated cardiac symptoms. Early symptoms can include dyspnea, cough, or a sensation of not being able to take a deep breath, especially when lying down (O'Brien, 2016).
   B. Patients with a pulmonary history of asthma or COPD may link their symptoms as an exacerbation of their underlying disease. Patients without a pulmonary his-

---

Figure 12-1. Characteristics of Left- and Right-Sided Heart Failure

Left-sided heart failure	Right-sided heart failure
• Ineffective ventricular contractibility	• Ineffective right ventricular contractibility
• Reduced left ventricular pumping ability	• Reduced right ventricular pumping ability
• Decreased cardiac output to body	• Decreased cardiac output to lungs
• Blood backup into left atrium and lungs	• Blood backup into right atrium and peripheral circulation
• Pulmonary congestion, dyspnea, activity intolerance	• Weight gain, peripheral edema, engorgement of kidneys and other organs
• Pulmonary edema and right-sided heart failure	

Note. From *Pathophysiology: An Incredibly Visual!™ Pocket Guide* (p. 29), by Lippincott Williams & Wilkins, 2010, Ambler, PA: Author. Copyright 2010 by Lippincott Williams & Wilkins. Reprinted with permission.

tory may consider having a common cold, flu, or bronchitis rather than a condition related to their heart (O'Brien, 2016).

C. Primary symptoms of HF
   1. Exercise intolerance
      a) Patients begin to notice they are no longer able to perform simple activities they were able to do before, such as walking to the mailbox. The inability to exercise or walk at a normal pace can develop into symptoms of tiredness, fatigue, or dyspnea (O'Brien, 2016).
      b) Patients with HF have difficulty breathing or become dyspneic with activity. Simple activities like walking around the house can precipitate dyspnea that usually resolves with rest (O'Brien, 2016).
   2. Nocturnal dyspnea occurs as HF progresses and excessive fluid backs into the lungs and interferes with systemic oxygen saturation, causing dyspnea at rest or orthopnea (O'Brien, 2016).
   3. Peripheral edema and fluid retention occur in patients with prolonged sitting. Pitting edema of the lower ankles or lower leg also can be a symptom of other conditions, including hepatic and renal failure. Nonpitting edema is generally not caused by HF (O'Brien, 2016).
   4. Edema can extend beyond the lower extremities to include the hips, scrotum, abdominal wall, or abdominal cavity (ascites).

IV. Physical examination
   A. Perform a full history with the patient to determine the specific etiology of HF. A careful family history can identify the presence of familial cardiomyopathy (Hershberger & Siegfried, 2011).
   B. Identify the duration of illness—a patient who presents with a recent-onset systolic HF has a better prognosis over time (Hershberger & Siegfried, 2011; McNamara et al., 2011).
   C. Evaluate the severity and precipitating triggers of dyspnea or fatigue. If angina is elicited, or there is a cited diminished exercise tolerance or limited sexual activity, then evidence exists to support that HF is negatively affecting the patient's quality of life (Yancy et al., 2013).
   D. Assess for the presence of anorexia, early satiety, or weight loss. Gastrointestinal symptoms are common in patients with HF. Cardiac cachexia and significant weight loss are associated with a poor prognosis (de Lemos et al., 2009). Obesity can be a contributing cause of HF.
   E. Assess for weight gain, especially rapid weight gain in days or one week, which suggests volume overload (Sarraf et al., 2009).
   F. Ask the patient about palpitations to rule out paroxysmal atrial fibrillation or ventricular tachycardia (Kociol et al., 2011).
   G. Assess for development of peripheral edema or abdominal ascites to determine fluid overload.
   H. Ascertain whether the patient has difficulty breathing, the inability to lie flat to sleep, history of sleep apnea, or a smoking history.
   I. Assess for excessive use of nonsteroidal anti-inflammatory drugs for pain or any medications that can exacerbate HF.
   J. Evaluate the patient's awareness of diet, salt intake, fluid intake, and adherence to medication use.
   K. Physical examination of the patient with HF
      1. Assess the patient's body mass index for evidence of weight loss.

2. Blood pressure taken supine and upright allows the clinician to evaluate for hypertension or hypotension. The width of pulse pressure can reflect the adequacy of cardiac output.
3. Evaluate the strength, quality, and regularity of the patient's pulses.
4. Identify any orthostatic changes in blood pressure and heart rate.
5. Palpate and evaluate jugular venous pressure at rest and when performing abdominal compression (Kasai & Bradley, 2011).
6. Auscultate for presence of extra heart sounds and murmurs. The presence of S_3 is associated with a poor prognosis (Hershberger & Siegfried, 2011). Murmurs can suggest valvular heart disease.
7. Palpate and assess the size and location of the point of maximal impulse. An enlarged and displaced point of maximal impulse can suggest ventricular enlargement (Yancy et al., 2013).
8. Assess for the presence of right ventricular heave. This finding suggests significant right ventricular dysfunction or is a positive finding for pulmonary hypertension (Yancy et al., 2013).
9. Auscultate for the presence of pulmonary rales, pleural effusion, and rate of respirations. In advanced HF, rales may be absent because of major pulmonary congestion (Yancy et al., 2013).
10. Perform an abdominal examination to evaluate for hepatomegaly or the presence of abdominal ascites, which indicates evidence of volume overload.
11. Identify the presence of peripheral edema. Younger patients may not have positive findings for peripheral edema despite intravascular overload. Obese and older adult patients can have pedal edema that may or may not be associated with HF (Yancy et al., 2013).
12. Evaluate the warmth and perfusion of the lower extremities; cool, pale, or cyanotic lower extremities can reflect inadequate cardiac output (Yancy et al., 2013).

V. Diagnostics
   A. Echocardiogram
      1. An echocardiogram is an ultrasound test that uses sound waves to measure the size of the heart chambers and the condition of the valves and analyzes how well they are performing.
      2. An echocardiogram provides various ways to produce an ejection fraction and identifies the type of HF.
      3. It also provides information about pulmonary pressures, diastology, and hemodynamics (King, Kingery, & Casey, 2012).
   B. Electrocardiogram (ECG)
      1. An ECG provides a quick electrical assessment of the heart that records the heart rhythm and rate. It also can reflect heart wall damage or active ischemia occurring in the myocardium.
      2. An ECG can detect other medical conditions as well, such as COPD, cerebral vascular accident, pulmonary embolism, or pericardial effusion (King et al., 2012).
   C. Right heart catheterization, or Swan-Ganz catheter
      1. This is an invasive procedure performed to directly measure the pressures within the heart chambers.
      2. This important procedure can identify the amount of fluid overload a patient is experiencing, and the data obtained can influence the choice in medical therapies given, as well as medication titration (Kasai & Bradley, 2011).

D. Left heart catheterization, or coronary angiography
   1. This is an invasive procedure that enables the cardiology interventionist to visualize the coronary arteries to determine the degree of atherosclerosis.
   2. This procedure aids in the evaluation of valvular heart disease and the assessment for ventricular aneurysms or rupture (King et al., 2012).
E. Chest radiograph
   1. A radiograph helps to detect pleural effusions, cardiomegaly, pulmonary edema, and pericardial effusion.
   2. These conditions can be the result of or can coexist with congestive heart failure (Yancy et al., 2013).
F. Cardiac magnetic resonance imaging (MRI)
   1. A cardiac MRI is a noninvasive study incorporating MRI to assess the structure and function of the myocardium.
   2. A cardiac MRI is useful for studying coronary artery disease, in addition to analyzing for infiltrative processes affecting the myocardium and contributing to HF.
   3. The use of a contrast agent, such as gadolinium, can enhance the imaging of the myocardium to highlight the coronary vessels and assess for abnormalities (King et al., 2012).
G. Cardiac positron-emission tomography
   1. Cardiac positron-emission tomography is a form of myocardial perfusion imaging that uses radiotracers and allows for assessment of coronary artery disease.
   2. This tool is useful in determining the cause of HF with an ischemic etiology (King et al., 2012).
H. Holter and event monitors
   1. These rhythm monitors can be worn on the thorax or implanted subcutaneously in the thorax to offer constant heart rhythm monitoring.
   2. As HF progresses, heart rhythm disturbances are common, and these monitors offer a tracking method to determine if patients are experiencing arrhythmias.
   3. These devices aid in determining whether patients with HF qualify for pacemakers or cardiac defibrillators (King et al., 2012).
I. Nuclear stress testing or dobutamine stress echocardiogram
   1. Nuclear stress testing is a noninvasive study used to determine if ischemia is present within the myocardium, essentially evaluating the blood flow to the myocardium.
   2. This type of testing is useful to identify if ischemic heart disease is the etiology of left ventricular diastolic or systolic impairment.
   3. A nuclear exercise or pharmacologic stress test is a diagnostic test that uses a small amount of radioactive tracer injected into a vein.
   4. A gamma camera detects the radiation released by the tracer to produce computer images of the heart.
   5. A dobutamine stress echocardiogram uses dobutamine to accelerate the heart rate, which is followed by ultrasound imaging to evaluate for any wall motion abnormalities occurring during "stress" within the myocardium (King et al., 2012; Yancy et al., 2013).
VI. Differential diagnosis
   A. Congestive airway disease

 B. Pulmonary hypertension
 C. Portal hypertension
 D. Medication-induced side effects (dihydropyridines: amlodipine)
 E. Hypoalbuminemia
 F. Cellulitis and fasciitis
 G. Scleroderma
 H. Lymphedema
 I. Myxedema
 J. Venous insufficiency
 K. Thromboembolic disease: Deep vein thrombosis
 L. Hypothyroidism
VII. Interventions
 A. Treatment strategies have been developed based on the understanding of the physiologic compensatory mechanisms.
 1. Medical therapy includes diuresis, suppression of the overactive neurohormonal systems, and augmentation of contractility (Yancy et al., 2013) (see Table 12-2).

Table 12-2. Recommended Medications for Stage C Heart Failure With Reduced Ejection Fraction

Medications	Initial Daily Dose(s)	Maximum Dose(s)	Mean Doses Achieved in Clinical Trials
Angiotensin-Converting Enzyme Inhibitors			
Captopril	6.25 mg 3 times	50 mg 3 times	122.7 mg/d
Enalapril	2.5 mg twice	10–20 mg twice	16.6 mg/d
Fosinopril	5–10 mg once	40 mg once	N/A
Lisinopril	2.5–5 mg once	20–40 mg once	32.5–35 mg/d
Perindopril	2 mg once	8–16 mg once	N/A
Quinapril	5 mg twice	20 mg twice	N/A
Ramipril	1.25–2.5 mg once	10 mg once	N/A
Trandolapril	1 mg once	4 mg once	N/A
Angiotensin Receptor Blockers			
Candesartan	4 to 8 mg once	32 mg once	24 mg/d
Losartan	25–50 mg once	50–150 mg once	129 mg/d
Valsartan	20–40 mg twice	160 mg twice	254 mg/d
Aldosterone Antagonists			
Spironolactone	12.5–25 mg once	25 mg once or twice	26 mg/d
Eplerenone	25 mg once	50 mg once	42.6 mg/d

(Continued on next page)

Table 12-2. Recommended Medications for Stage C Heart Failure With Reduced Ejection Fraction *(Continued)*

Medications	Initial Daily Dose(s)	Maximum Dose(s)	Mean Doses Achieved in Clinical Trials
Beta-Blockers			
Bisoprolol	1.25 mg once	10 mg once	8.6 mg/d
Carvedilol	3.125 mg twice	50 mg twice	37 mg/d
Carvedilol CR	10 mg once	80 mg once	N/A
Metoprolol succinate extended release (metoprolol CR/XL)	12.5–25 mg once	200 mg once	159 mg/d
Hydralazine and Isosorbide Dinitrate			
Fixed-dose combination	37.5 mg hydralazine/20 mg isosorbide dinitrate 3 times daily	75 mg hydralazine/40 mg isosorbide dinitrate 3 times daily	~175 mg hydralazine/90 mg isosorbide dinitrate daily
Hydralazine and isosorbide dinitrate	Hydralazine: 25–50 mg, 3 or 4 times daily and isosorbide dinitrate: 20–30 mg 3 or 4 times daily	Hydralazine: 300 mg daily in divided doses and isosorbide dinitrate: 120 mg daily in divided doses	N/A

CR—controlled release; CR/XL—controlled release/extended release; N/A—not applicable

Note. From "2013 ACCF/AHA Guideline for the Management of Heart Failure: A Report of the American College of Cardiology Foundation/American Heart Association Task Force on Practice Guidelines," by C.W. Yancy, M. Jessup, B. Bozkurt, J. Butler, D.E. Casey, Jr., M.H. Drazner, … B.L. Wilkoff, 2013, *Circulation, 128,* p. e266. Copyright 2013 by American College of Cardiology Foundation and American Heart Association, Inc. Reprinted with permission.

2. Close adherence to lifestyle modifications and strict compliance with medications can lead to a relatively symptom-free existence for patients, decreased hospitalizations, and ultimately lengthened survival rates.
3. Surgical options include ventricular resynchronization therapy, surgical ventricular remodeling, ventricular assist device implantation, and heart transplantation.
4. Pharmacologic management should be reviewed and evaluated based on the patient's diagnostic stage of HF and include the use of guidelines and the consideration of concomitant conditions.
5. Pharmacologic interventions based on guideline recommendations (Yancy et al., 2013)
    a) ACE inhibitor
    b) Angiotensin receptor blockade
    c) Beta-blockers
    d) Added diuretics (e.g., loop diuretics, hydralazine nitrates, aldosterone antagonists) (see Table 12-3)
6. Nonpharmacologic interventions

Table 12-3. Oral Diuretics Guideline Recommendations in Treatment of Chronic Heart Failure

Drug	Initial Daily Dose(s)	Maximum Total Daily Dose	Duration of Action
Loop Diuretics			
Bumetanide	0.5–1 mg once or twice	10 mg	4–6 hr
Furosemide	20–40 mg once or twice	600 mg	6–8 hr
Torsemide	10–20 mg once	200 mg	12–16 hr
Thiazide Diuretics			
Chlorothiazide	250–500 mg once or twice	1,000 mg	6–12 hr
Chlorthalidone	12.5–25 mg once	100 mg	24–72 hr
Hydrochlorothiazide	25 mg once or twice	200 mg	6 to 12 hr
Indapamide	2.5 mg once	5 mg	36 hr
Metolazone	2.5 mg once	20 mg	12–24 hr
Potassium-Sparing Diuretics[a]			
Amiloride	5 mg once	20 mg	24 hr
Spironolactone	12.5–25 mg once	50 mg[b]	1–3 hr
Triamterene	50–75 mg twice	200 mg	7–9 hr
Sequential Nephron Blockade			
Metolazone	2.5–10 mg once plus loop diuretic	N/A	N/A
Hydrochlorothiazide	25–100 mg once or twice plus loop diuretic	N/A	N/A
Chlorothiazide (IV)	500–1,000 mg once plus loop diuretic	N/A	N/A

[a] Eplerenone, although also a diuretic, is primarily used in chronic heart failure.

[b] Higher doses may occasionally be used with close monitoring.

N/A—not applicable

Note. From "2013 ACCF/AHA Guideline for the Management of Heart Failure: A Report of the American College of Cardiology Foundation/American Heart Association Task Force on Practice Guidelines," by C.W. Yancy, M. Jessup, B. Bozkurt, J. Butler, D.E. Casey, Jr., M.H. Drazner, … B.L. Wilkoff, 2013, *Circulation, 128,* p. e265. Copyright 2013 by American College of Cardiology Foundation and American Heart Association, Inc. Reprinted with permission.

a) Integration of the interdisciplinary team to assess and evaluate specific patient and family needs

b) Referral to a self-management program to empower patients and families to become educated and informed on symptoms and preventive practices to reduce disease exacerbation

c) Referral to a registered dietitian to provide information on a low-sodium diet *d)* Referral to a physical therapy to educate patients on realistic physical activity that can be incorporated into daily fitness planning

  B. Referrals and follow-up

    1. After the initial diagnosis of HF is made, close follow-up is prudent to closely monitor patients' symptoms so that proper medication adjustments are made. Titration of standard-of-care HF medications is essential to slow disease progression and reduce the incidence of exacerbation and hospitalizations.

    2. Engaging patients in self-management practices is necessary in helping them to recognize physical signs and to report their symptoms early for prevention of exacerbations.

    3. Cardiac rehabilitation is beneficial following an acute care admission for an exacerbation.

    4. Patients with HF may be considered candidates for pacemakers or automated implantable cardiac defibrillators to reduce the risk for sudden death.

        a) As HF progresses, referral to an advanced HF program becomes necessary.

        b) HF specialists will evaluate patients with end-stage heart failure for device interventions such as left ventricular assist devices versus heart transplantation.

        c) Patients with concomitant pulmonary conditions (e.g., COPD, pulmonary hypertension, cor pulmonale, prior pulmonary embolism, obstructive sleep apnea) should be followed and monitored by pulmonary medicine.

Case Study

    S.M. is a 61-year-old woman who presents in the emergency department after suddenly awakening around midnight with breathlessness. She has been requiring two or three pillows to sleep comfortably. Sitting upright with her legs dangling from the side of the bed helped some, but she still remained dyspneic. She has a history of coronary artery disease and a large anterior myocardial infarction six months prior. Her left ventricular EF following her myocardial infarction was 30%. She has not been following her diet or taking her medications regularly. She reports weight gain of "several pounds" over the past two months, increasing dyspnea while doing her housework, and increasing fatigue.

    She appears tired and in moderate distress. She has cool, moist skin; dusky nail beds; slow capillary refill; and weak peripheral pulses. She exhibits jugular vein distension, crackles in bilateral lower lungs, an irregular pulse, and a systolic heart murmur loudest at the cardiac apex. She has hepatomegaly and moderate lower-leg pitting edema. Vital signs include blood pressure of 100/70 mm Hg, heart rate of 120 beats per minute and irregular, and respirations of 24 breaths per minute and shallow.

    By the afternoon of the day of admission, S.M.'s condition had deteriorated despite treatment with furosemide 20 mg by mouth daily, a potassium supplement, lisinopril 20 mg by mouth daily, and oxygen 2 L per nasal cannula. She exhibited increased fatigue, crackles throughout all lung fields, pulsus alternans, and a cough occasionally productive of frothy sputum. Her blood gases at this time are pH of 7.24, partial pressure of carbon dioxide of 60 mm Hg, partial pressure of oxygen of 60 mm Hg, oxygen saturation of 88%, and bicarbonate level of 24 mEq/L. She was changed to a 40% ventimask and a nitroglycerin IV drip.

    Two days later, her condition had improved and her IV fluids were tapered off. She was discharged home with skilled nursing care with the expectation that the nurse would help S.M. to recognize early symptoms of an exacerbation and reduce her symptoms that warranted hospitalization. The nurse taught S.M. about dietary changes and weight management. S.M. was followed by her primary care provider through the chronic care management Medicare benefit.

References

Centers for Medicare and Medicaid Services. (2016). Readmissions Reduction Program (HRRP). Retrieved from https://www.cms.gov/medicare/medicare-fee-for-service-payment/acuteinpatientpps/readmissions -reduction-program.html

Criteria Committee of the New York Heart Association. (1994). *Nomenclature and criteria for diagnosis of diseases of the heart and great vessels* (9th ed.). Boston, MA: Little, Brown.

de Lemos, J.A., McGuire, D.K., Khera, A., Das, S.R., Murphy, S.A., Omland, T., & Drazner, M.H. (2009). Screening the population for left ventricular hypertrophy and left ventricular systolic dysfunction using natriuretic peptides: Results from the Dallas Heart Study. *American Heart Journal, 157,* 746–753. doi:10.1016/ j.ahj.2008.12.017

Djoussé, L., Driver, J.A., & Gaziano, J.M. (2009). Relation between modifiable lifestyle factors and lifetime risk of heart failure. *JAMA, 302,* 394–400. doi:10.1001/jama.2009.1062

Go, A.S., Mozaffarian, D., Roger, V.L., Benjamin, E.J., Berry, J.D., Borden, W.B., … Turner, M.B. (2013). Heart disease and stroke statistics—2013 update: A report from the American Heart Association. *Circulation, 127,* e6–e245. doi:10.1161/CIR.0b013e31828124ad

Hershberger, R.E., & Siegfried, J.D. (2011). Update 2011: Clinical and genetic issues in familial dilated cardiomyopathy. *Journal of the American College of Cardiology, 57,* 1641–1649. doi:10.1016/j.jacc.2011.01.015

Hunt, S.A., Abraham, W.T., Chin, M.H., Feldman, A.M., Francis, G.S., Ganiats, T.G., … Yancy, C.W. (2009). 2009 focused update incorporated into the ACC/AHA 2005 guidelines for the diagnosis and management of heart failure in adults: A report of the American College of Cardiology Foundation/American Heart Association Task Force on Practice Guidelines. *Circulation, 119,* e391–e479. doi:10.1161/CIRCULA TIONAHA.109.192065

Izzo, J.L., Jr., & Gradman, A.H. (2004). Mechanisms and management of hypertensive heart disease: From left ventricular hypertrophy to heart failure. *Medical Clinics of North America, 88,* 1257–1271. doi:10.1016/ j.mcna.2004.06.002

JAMA. (2015, May 19). High prevalence of metabolic syndrome found in U.S. *ScienceDaily.* Retrieved from http://www.sciencedaily.com/releases/2015/05/150519121529.htm

James, P.A., Oparil, S., Carter, B.L., Cushman, W.C., Dennison-Himmelfarb, C., Handler, J., … Ortiz, E. (2014). 2014 evidence-based guideline for the management of high blood pressure in adults: Report from the panel members appointed to the Eighth Joint National Committee (JNC 8). *JAMA, 311,* 507–520. doi:10.1001/ jama.2013.284427

Kasai, T., & Bradley, T.D. (2011). Obstructive sleep apnea and heart failure: Pathophysiologic and therapeutic implications. *Journal of the American College of Cardiology, 57,* 119–127. doi:10.1016/j.jacc.2010.08.627

Kemp, C.D., & Conte, J.V. (2012). The pathophysiology of heart failure. *Cardiovascular Pathology, 21,* 365–371. doi:10.1016/j.carpath.2011.11.007

King, M., Kingery, J., & Casey, B. (2012). Diagnosis and evaluation of heart failure. *American Family Physician, 85,* 1161–1168.

Kociol, R.D., Horton, J.R., Fonarow, G.C., Reyes, E.M., Shaw, L.K., O'Connor, C.M., … Hernandez, A.F. (2011). Admission, discharge, or change in B-type natriuretic peptide and long-term outcomes: Data from Organized Program to Initiate Lifesaving Treatment in Hospitalized Patients with Heart Failure (OPTIMIZE-HF) linked to Medicare claims. *Circulation: Heart Failure, 4,* 628–636. doi:10.1161/ CIRCHEARTFAILURE.111.962290

Logeart, D., Tabet, J.-Y., Hittinger, L., Thabut, G., Jourdain, P., Maison, P., … Solal, A.C. (2008). Transient worsening of renal function during hospitalization for acute heart failure alters outcome. *International Journal of Cardiology, 127,* 228–232. doi:10.1016/j.ijcard.2007.06.007

McNamara, D.M., Starling, R.C., Cooper, L.T., Boehmer, J.P., Mather, P.J., Janosko, K.M., … Dec, W. (2011). Clinical and demographic predictors of outcomes in recent onset dilated cardiomyopathy: Results of the IMAC (Intervention in Myocarditis and Acute Cardiomyopathy)-2 study. *Journal of the American College of Cardiology, 58,* 1112–1118. doi:10.1016/j.jacc.2011.05.033

O'Brien, T.X. (2016, February 10). Congestive heart failure. Retrieved from http://www.emedicinehealth.com/ congestive_heart_failure/article_em.htm

Patient Protection and Affordable Care Act, 42 U.S.C. § 18001 et seq. (2010). Retrieved from http://www.hhs
.gov/healthcare/about-the-law/read-the-law/index.html

Sarraf, M., Masoumi, A., & Schrier, R.W. (2009). Cardiorenal syndrome in acute decompensated heart failure. *Clinical Journal of the American Society of Nephrology, 4,* 2013–2026. doi:10.2215/CJN.03150509

U.S. Department of Health and Human Services. (2005, December). *The booming dynamics of aging: From awareness to action.* White House Conference on Aging. Washington, DC: Author.

Yancy, C.W., Jessup, M., Bozkurt, B., Butler, J., Casey, D.E., Jr., Drazner, M.H., … Wilkoff, B.L. (2013). 2013 ACCF/AHA guideline for the management of heart failure: A report of the American College of Cardiology Foundation/American Heart Association Task Force on practice guidelines. *Circulation, 128,* e240–e327. doi:10.1161/CIR.0b013e31829e8776

CHAPTER 13

Chronic Kidney Disease

Stephanie Banasik, MSN, RN, ANP-BC

I. Definition
   A. Chronic kidney disease (CKD) is a worldwide public health problem with an increasing incidence and prevalence, poor outcomes, and high cost (Levey & Coresh, 2012).
      1. Incidence and prevalence of CKD are difficult to assess accurately because early stages are usually asymptomatic (Haynes & Winearls, 2010).
      2. The Centers for Disease Control and Prevention (2014) estimates that more than 10% of adults in the United States may have CKD, and the National Health and Nutrition Examination Survey estimates the prevalence in the United States to be about 16% (Haynes & Winearls, 2010).
   B. CKD is defined as kidney damage with a glomerular filtration rate (GFR) of less than 60 ml/min/1.73 m^2 on two separate occasions separated by at least 90 days (Krol, 2011).
   C. CKD encompasses the continuum of kidney dysfunction—from mild kidney damage to kidney failure—and also includes the term *end-stage renal disease* (Krol, 2011).
   D. An informed interpretation of the GFR is required because GFR is still considered the best overall index of kidney function in stable, nonhospitalized patients.
   E. The five stages of CKD based on GFR (Krol, 2011)
      1. Stage 1: GFR ≥ 90 ml/min/1.73 m^2
      2. Stage 2: GFR 60–89 ml/min/1.73 m^2
      3. Stage 3: GFR 30–59 ml/min/1.73 m^2
      4. Stage 4: GFR 15–29 ml/min/1.73 m^2
      5. Stage 5: < 15 ml/min/1.73 m^2
II. Pathophysiology
   A. CKD usually progresses from two mechanisms: those of primary kidney disease and those of nonspecific injury, with the former being disease specific (e.g., hypertension [HTN] or diabetes) and the latter representing a common pathophysiologic course once the initial injury has occurred.
   B. All chronic renal diseases cause a loss of functioning nephrons (Haynes & Winearls, 2010).
   C. The remaining healthy nephrons maintain GFR by compensatory hypertrophy and increasing intraglomerular pressure, causing hyperfiltration.
   D. Increased glomerular pressure is harmful and causes progressive endothelial injury, glomerular sclerosis, and eventually nephron loss (Haynes & Winearls, 2010).
   E. Plasma levels of substances, such as urea and creatinine, start to show measurable increases only after total GFR has decreased to 50% (Arora, 2015).

F. Proteinuria, caused by hyperfiltration and glomerular injury, overwhelms the proximal tubule's ability to reabsorb and protein overflows into the distal tubule, causing inflammation, interstitial fibrosis, and systemic loss of albumin.

G. The progression of CKD is largely independent of the initial injury, and renal function declines linearly (Haynes & Winearls, 2010).

H. Factors other than the underlying disease process and glomerular hypertension that may cause progressive renal injury include the following (Arora, 2015):
   1. Systemic hypertension
   2. Nephrotoxins (e.g., nonsteroidal anti-inflammatory drugs, IV contrast media)
   3. Decreased perfusion (e.g., from severe dehydration or episodes of shock)
   4. Proteinuria (in addition to being a marker of CKD)
   5. Hyperlipidemia
   6. Hyperphosphatemia with calcium phosphate deposition
   7. Smoking
   8. Uncontrolled diabetes

III. Presenting symptoms
   A. Stage 1 and 2 CKD usually have no presenting symptoms; however, HTN often is present.
      1. Symptoms develop in the later stages of CKD and only when end-stage renal disease is imminent.
      2. Symptoms of uremia include pruritus, muscle cramps, anorexia, nausea, and cognitive impairment or confusion.
   B. The presence of these symptoms, if attributable to CKD, is a good indication that renal replacement therapy (RRT) should be initiated (Haynes & Winearls, 2010).
   C. The early symptoms of CKD are also symptoms of other illnesses.
      1. These symptoms may be the only signs of kidney disease until the condition is more advanced.
      2. Symptoms include anorexia, malaise and fatigue, headaches, pruritus and dry skin, nausea, and cachexia (National Institutes of Health, 2012).
      3. Other symptoms that may develop, especially when kidney function has gotten worse, include the following (National Institutes of Health, 2012):
         a) Abnormally dark or light skin
         b) Bone pain
         c) Central nervous system
            (1) Drowsiness and confusion
            (2) Problems concentrating or thinking
            (3) Numbness in hands, feet, or other areas
            (4) Muscle twitching or cramps
         d) Breath odor
         e) Easy bruising, bleeding, or blood in the stool
         f) Excessive thirst
         g) Frequent hiccups
         h) Low level of sexual interest and impotence
         i) Amenorrhea
         j) Dyspnea
         k) Sleep problems, such as insomnia, restless legs syndrome, and obstructive sleep apnea
         l) Edema in hands or feet
         m) Vomiting, typically in the mornings

IV. Physical examination
  A. A careful physical examination may reveal findings characteristic of the condition that is underlying CKD or its complications. However, the lack of findings on physical examination does not exclude kidney disease.
  B. In fact, CKD is frequently clinically silent, so screening of patients without signs or symptoms at routine health visits is important (Arora, 2015).
  C. General examination
    1. Patients with moderate or severe CKD often appear pale, cachectic, or ill.
    2. Kussmaul breathing, or labored respiration, suggests hyperventilation in response to metabolic acidosis with acidemia.
  D. Chest examination
    1. Auscultate the lungs for rales.
    2. Auscultate the heart for gallops or rubs.
  E. Abdominal examination
    1. Inspect for distension of the upper abdomen, which may indicate polycystic kidney disease, a kidney or abdominal mass, or hydronephrosis.
    2. Auscultate to evaluate for a soft, lateralizing bruit, which may be audible in the epigastrium or the flank in renal artery stenosis.
    3. Palpate the kidneys; normal kidneys usually are not palpable. However, in some women, the lower pole of the right kidney can occasionally be felt with palpation during deep inspiration, and large kidneys or masses can sometimes be felt without special maneuvers.
    4. Pain elicited by mild striking of the back or flanks and costovertebral tenderness may indicate pyelonephritis or urinary tract obstruction.
  F. Skin examination
    1. Xerosis
    2. Pallor
    3. Hyperpigmentation
    4. Sallow or yellow-brown skin
    5. Petechiae or ecchymoses
    6. Excoriation due to itching
    7. Uremic frost, the deposition of white-to-tan urea crystals on the skin after sweat evaporation (rare)
  G. Neurologic examination
    1. Patients with acute renal failure may be drowsy or confused, and speech may be slurred.
    2. Asterixis can be detected in handwriting or by observation of outstretched hands maximally extended at the wrists; after several seconds in this position, a hand flap in the flexor direction is asterixis.
    3. Asterixis suggests one of the following:
      a) CKD
      b) Chronic liver failure
      c) Carbon dioxide narcosis
      d) Toxic encephalopathy
V. Diagnostics
  A. Diagnostic evaluation is critical in ascertaining the stage, course, chronicity, and complications of CKD.
  B. Appropriate laboratory testing includes the following (National Institutes of Health, 2012):

    1. Comprehensive metabolic panel
    2. Lipid profile and triglycerides
    3. Complete blood count
    4. Electrolytes
       a) Magnesium
       b) Phosphorus
       c) Potassium
       d) Sodium
    5. Urinalysis or urine protein to creatinine ratio for protein
    6. Creatinine clearance
    7. Serum creatinine
    8. Blood urea nitrogen
    9. GFR
VI. Differential diagnosis
  A. Acute kidney injury
  B. Alport syndrome
  C. Autosomal dominant polycystic kidney disease
  D. Chronic glomerulonephritis
  E. Diabetic nephropathy
  F. Goodpasture syndrome
  G. Multiple myeloma
  H. Nephrolithiasis
  I. Nephrosclerosis
  J. Rapidly progressive glomerulonephritis
VII. Interventions
  A. General interventions
    1. Provide support to patients, including patient education and social and financial support.
    2. Refer patients to a nephrologist.
    3. For stages 4 and 5 CKD, access devices for RRT such as arteriovenous fistula, requiring several months to fully mature and heal
  B. Patient teaching
    1. Educate patients about how the kidneys work and how their body is affected by CKD.
    2. Emphasize the importance of following instructions to prevent further kidney damage.
    3. Instruct patients when to notify the provider with urgent signs or symptoms or changes in kidney function.
  C. Pharmacologic therapy: The intended use of medications is to prevent the progression of CKD and associated complications.
  D. Evaluation and follow-up: Regular follow-up appointments to monitor progression of CKD, management of complications, and management of comorbidities (e.g., diabetes mellitus, HTN) are recommended.
  E. Referrals
    1. Consult with the physician for patients with chronic renal insufficiency who have abnormal laboratory tests beyond baseline and when indicated by symptoms and physical examination.
    2. For increases in proteinuria, follow with 24-hour urine for protein; refer and consult if abnormal.

3. Early referral to a nephrologist is recommended for anyone with CKD.
4. Patients with stage 4 and 5 CKD need specialized interventions provided by a nephrologist and should be immediately referred.
5. Consult with an endocrinologist or HTN specialist in cases of escalating HTN.
6. Refer patients for counseling on renal transplantation by a nephrologist.
7. Refer patients to a dietitian for nutritional counseling and education.
8. Referral to a renal social worker for patients with stage 4 or 5 CKD is recommended for counseling regarding the psychosocial and financial effect of progressive renal disease.
9. Patients should be referred to educational and support organizations for further education regarding CKD.
10. Refer patients to useful websites.
    a) National Kidney Foundation: www.kidney.org
    b) National Kidney Disease Education Program: www.nkdep.nih.gov

Case Study

C.C. is a 56-year-old Caucasian woman presenting to the dialysis clinic and reports, "I'm really itchy and have chills." The advanced practice registered nurse (APRN) notes pruritus all over the patient's body, worsened over the past two weeks. C.C. also has developed weakness, dyspnea on exertion, and fatigue. She has been receiving treatment for recurrent furuncle methicillin-resistant *Staphylococcus aureus* infection for several months with sulfamethoxazole and trimethoprim, clindamycin, and nonsteroidal anti-inflammatory drugs with some relief. She sees her primary care provider sporadically. The patient does not have a fever but has chills. She has had hypertension for 12 years, proteinuria, pneumonia, hematuria, and oral candidiasis. She had a renal biopsy in 2004 that indicated chronic renal failure.

The patient is currently taking lisinopril 10 mg PO once a day, hydrocodone/acetaminophen 5/300 mg 1–2 tablets PO every four to six hours, clindamycin 450 mg PO every six hours, sulfamethoxazole and trimethoprim 500 mg PO twice a day, and fluconazole 200 mg PO on the first day as a loading dose, followed with 100 mg PO once a day for 14 days. The patient has no known drug allergies.

The patient has been divorced twice and has two daughters. The oldest daughter lives in another state, and the youngest lives in town. C.C. is a high school graduate with some college. She is a 60-pack-year smoker with significant alcohol consumption of 8–12 beers nearly every day until a few months ago. The patient states she is now a social drinker having two to four drinks every four to five days. She admits to marijuana use but denies use of all other illicit drugs. Her mother died at age 60 of lung cancer. Her father died at age 88 from complications of diabetes mellitus.

On examination, the patient denies having a fever, weight loss, or lymphadenopathy. She denies visual disturbances, eye discharge, diminished hearing, tinnitus, epistaxis, sore throat, or dysphagia. Her neck shows no lumps, goiters, or masses. She denies angina at rest, angina with exertion, palpitations, and orthopnea. She also denies hemoptysis, cough, and wheezing. She has no nausea, vomiting, diarrhea, constipation, or abdominal pain. She has no dysuria, frequency, nocturia, or urgency. She reports no joint or muscle pain or limited range of motion. The patient has no dizziness, syncope, seizures, paresthesia, numbness, or loss of balance. She has four lesions on her upper back. She is not suicidal and has no homicidal thoughts or mania. The nurse notices no bruising, bleeding, or endocrine problems.

During examination, the nurse notes C.C.'s height is 6 ft and weight is 90 kg (198 lbs), with a body mass index of 27.1 kg/m². Her blood pressure is 133/65 mm Hg, pulse is 85 beats per minute, respiration is 18 breaths per minute, and temperature is 98.6°F (37°C). The patient is well-appearing; alert; oriented to person, place, and time; demonstrates normal mood and affect; and ambulates without difficulty. Her skin is pale gray, dusky, dry, and scaly, with no tenting. There are four furuncle-type lesions on her upper back, one of which is draining purulent discharge. There are no abnormalities of her head and neck. Pupils are equal, reactive, and accommodate to light bilaterally. Her extraocular movements are intact and she has no sinus pain bilaterally. Her tympanic membranes are pearly and intact, bilaterally. No oropharynx erythema is present, and her uvula rises and falls. Her neck is supple; there is no jugular vein distension, thyromegaly, lymphadenopathy, or carotid bruits audible bilaterally. Respiration is regular and nonlabored, and lungs are clear to auscultation bilaterally throughout all lobes. Cardiovascular evaluation reveals regular rate and rhythm, with S_1 and S_2 audible, no S_3 or S_4, and no murmur or rub. The abdomen is soft, nontender, nondistended, with positive bowel sounds in all four quadrants and no hepatosplenomegaly. Genitalia show no lesions, rash, or discharge. The patient shows full range of motion without limitations in all extremities, normal strength in upper extremities, and no deformities. Spine is midline and straight. Gait is normal. There is no clubbing, cyanosis, or edema in extremities. The patient has normal motor and sensation responses, normal balance and negative Romberg, and patellar reflexes 2+ bilaterally. She is cooperative and coherent, with appropriate mood and affect.

Diagnostic testing included electrocardiogram, complete blood count with differential, urinalysis, microalbumin test, comprehensive metabolic profile, hepatitis studies, C-reactive protein, hepatic panel, sedimentation rate, iron panel, vitamin B_{12}, and folate.

C.C. was diagnosed with acute kidney injury, acute or chronic renal failure, with hypertension. She was referred for renal ultrasound, 24-hour urine, computed tomography scan of the abdomen and pelvis without contrast, and echocardiogram for baseline ejection fraction. She was scheduled for temporary central line venous access into the intrajugular vasculature while awaiting abdominal peritoneal dialysis catheter placement. The APRN made a referral for behavioral health.

References

Arora, P. (2015, April). Chronic kidney disease: Practice essentials. Retrieved from http://emedicine.medscape.com/article/238798-overview

Centers for Disease Control and Prevention. (2014). National chronic kidney disease fact sheet, 2014. Retrieved from http://www.cdc.gov/diabetes/pubs/pdf/kidney_Factsheet.pdf

Haynes, R.J., & Winearls, C.G. (2010). Chronic kidney disease. *Surgery, 28,* 525–529. doi:10.1016/j.mpsur.2010.08.003

Krol, G.D. (2011). Chronic kidney disease staging and progression. In J. Yee & G.D. Krol (Eds.), *Chronic kidney disease (CKD): Clinical practice recommendations for primary care physicians and healthcare providers—A collaborative approach* (6th ed., pp. 4–10). Detroit, MI: Henry Ford Health System.

Levey, A.S., & Coresh, J. (2012). Chronic kidney disease. *Lancet, 379,* 165–180. doi:10.1016/S0140-6736(11)60178-5

National Institutes of Health. (2012). Kidney disease statistics for the United States. Retrieved from http://www.niddk.nih.gov/health-information/health-statistics/Pages/kidney-disease-statistics-united-states.aspx

CHAPTER 14

Chronic Obstructive Pulmonary Disease

Kim Kuebler, DNP, APRN, ANP-BC

I. Definition
   A. The World Health Organization (WHO, n.d.) defines chronic obstructive pulmonary disease (COPD) as a lung disease characterized by chronic obstruction of lung airflow that interferes with normal or eupneic breathing and is not fully reversible.
   B. The terms *chronic bronchitis* and *emphysema* are no longer used and are included in the diagnosis of COPD (WHO, n.d.).
   C. COPD is not a "smoker's cough" but rather an underdiagnosed and life-threatening lung disease (WHO, n.d.).
   D. Global Strategy for the Diagnosis, Management, and Prevention of Chronic Obstructive Pulmonary Disease (Global Initiative for Chronic Obstructive Lung Disease [GOLD], 2016)
      1. Sets the standard of care in annual updated guidelines to guide the clinical management of COPD, which is the third most common chronic condition in the United States (Centers for Disease Control and Prevention, 2012)
      2. Defines COPD as a common preventable and treatable condition characterized by persistent airflow limitation that is usually progressive and associated with an inflammatory response of the airways and the lung to noxious particles or gases (GOLD, 2016)
   E. COPD is a chronic inflammatory lung disease that causes obstructed airflow in the bronchial airways, preventing air from entering and exiting the lungs. It includes cough, sputum production, and dyspnea. It is caused by long-term exposure to oxidative stress associated with prolonged use of smoking cigarettes (National Heart, Lung, and Blood Institute, 2011).
   F. *COPD* refers to a group of diseases that cause airflow blockage and breathing-related problems. It includes emphysema, chronic bronchitis, and in some cases asthma (Centers for Disease Control and Prevention, 2015).
   G. COPD is a leading cause of morbidity and mortality worldwide and creates a global economic and social burden that is on the rise (WHO, n.d.).
II. Pathophysiology
   A. Oxidative stress from ongoing exposure to noxious particles that come from cigarette smoke, biomass fuels, and air pollution eventually leads to inflammation of the airways and lung tissue (GOLD, 2016).

1. COPD reflects the sum of pathologic changes that occur in the airway epithelium, which can occur in large central airways, small peripheral airways, and in the lung parenchyma (Fischer, Pavlisko, & Voynow, 2011).
2. Chronic inflammation causes parenchymal tissue destruction, which reduces the body's ability to perform normal repair and provide a defense mechanism within the airways.
3. Pathologic conditions occur within the airways, lung parenchyma, and pulmonary vasculature (Chen, Chen, Hanaoka, Droma, & Kubo, 2008).
4. Oxidative stress may serve as an amplifying agent in the progression of COPD. Oxidants are released from inflamed macrophages and neutrophil cells (Kirkham & Barnes, 2013).

B. Data suggest an imbalance between proteases (which break down connective tissue) and antiproteases (which protect against tissue breakdown) within the lungs. Patients with COPD have an increase in inflammatory and epithelial cells that release several proteases.

1. Different biologic or molecular markers have been found that help to describe the mechanistic or pathogenic triad of inflammation, proteases, and oxidants that occur in patients with COPD.
2. These markers correspond to the different aspects of COPD histopathology (Fischer et al., 2011).
3. Genetic variations or polymorphisms have been linked to COPD-associated inflammation, protease–antiprotease imbalance, and oxidative stress (Fischer et al., 2011).
4. Recent data suggest that aging-associated mechanistic markers develop as progressive consequences of the pathogenic triad and imbalance of the protease and antiprotease effects on the lungs of patients with COPD (Fischer et al., 2011).

C. Inflammatory cells and mediators are characteristic of COPD.

1. The number of CD8+ cytotoxic cells and Tc1 lymphocytes increases.
2. These cells, together with increased neutrophils and macrophages, release inflammatory mediators and enzymes that affect the structural cells in the airways, lung parenchyma, and pulmonary vascular (van den Berge, ten Hacken, Cohen, Douma, & Postma, 2011).
   a) The increase in inflammatory mediators attracts inflammatory cells from the systemic circulation, a result of chemotactic factors.
   b) This amplifies the systemic inflammatory processes known as proinflammatory cytokines, which promotes growth factors that induce pulmonary and systemic structural changes (Sin, Anthonisen, Soriano, & Agusti, 2006).
   c) Inflammation and obstruction from narrowing of peripheral airways contribute to a decrease in pulmonary function or the patient's ability to forcefully exhale air in one second—known as forced expiratory volume in one second, or FEV_1 (GOLD, 2016).

D. Air trapping occurs within the lungs as a result of progressive inflammation, which leads to fibrosis and ischemic changes within the airway epithelium. This creates narrowing of the bronchial lumen, thus obstructing airflow exchange within the lungs (GOLD, 2016).

1. The lungs become hyperinflated with progressive air trapping on expiration. This becomes more pronounced as the alveoli lose their structural walls and the elastin in the lung parenchyma is destroyed by repetitive oxidative stress (National Heart, Lung, and Blood Institute, 2011).

2. Hyperinflation reduces inspiratory capacity and, in turn, increases the functional residual capacity of the lung; this is more pronounced with physical exercise or what is termed *hyperinflation* (GOLD, 2016).

3. Hyperinflation occurs early in the disease process and is considered one of the main contributors to the symptoms of dyspnea or exercise intolerance (Waschki et al., 2011).

4. Changes in lung capacities eventually create intrinsic changes to the contractile properties of the respiratory muscles; the hyperinflation causes the diaphragm to become thin and flattened (GOLD, 2016).

E. Hypoxemia and hypercapnia occur as a result of impaired gas exchange between the lungs and systemic circulation.

1. As the disease trajectory progresses, the oxygen and carbon dioxide exchange worsens (Rodríguez-Roisin et al., 2009).

2. The impaired gas exchange causes the systemic retention of carbon dioxide due to reduced ventilator drive. This is further worsened with obstruction, hyperinflation, and reduced ventilator muscle strength (GOLD, 2016).

F. Patients with COPD have an overproduction of mucus secretion, or hypersecretion.

1. This is a direct result of oxidative stress on the airway epithelium, which stimulates an increase of goblet cells and enlarges submucosal glands when irritated by noxious gas particles (Turner & Jones, 2009).

2. Inflammatory mediators and abnormal proteases contribute to the stimulation of mucus hypersecretion by exerting effects through the activation of epidermal growth factor receptor (Turner & Jones, 2009).

III. Presenting symptoms

A. The classic symptoms of COPD include chronic cough, sputum production, and chronic and progressive dyspnea with a history of exposure to tobacco smoke, biomass fuels, home cooking smoke, and occupational irritants and chemicals (GOLD, 2016).

B. Chronic cough and sputum production can occur long before the presence of airflow limitation and vary from one day to another (Miravitlles, 2011).

C. Dyspnea is the cardinal symptom of COPD (WHO, n.d.). Additional terms for this symptom include breathlessness, difficulty breathing, chest heaviness, air hunger, gasping, or an increased effort to breathe (GOLD, 2016). (See Chapter 27.)

D. Chronic cough usually is the first symptom associated with COPD. Cough may initially present as intermittent in nature and often is underreported by patients who assume it is a consequence of smoking (GOLD, 2016). (See Chapter 23.)

E. Sputum production often occurs following a course of coughing.

1. The classic definition of bronchitis is the regular production of sputum for three or more months in two consecutive years. This definition, however, does not provide a specific measurement for COPD (GOLD, 2016).

2. Excessive amounts of sputum production should warrant an investigation for bronchiectasis, and purulent sputum suggests an increase in inflammatory mediators that develop into an exacerbation (Hill, Pasteur, Cornford, Welham, & Bilton, 2011).

F. Systemic consequences of progressive COPD should always be assessed; these include fatigue, osteoporosis, anxiety, depression, cachexia, and poor appetite (Nussbaumer-Ochsnre & Rabe, 2011).

IV. Physical examination
  A. Prior to the physical examination, the provider should review the patient's past medical history and the presence of any risk factors that can exacerbate the symptoms of COPD, including the following (Mosenifar & Kamangar, 2016):
    1. Pack-year smoking history, which is calculated by multiplying the number of years smoked by the number of cigarette packs per day (e.g., a patient who has smoked 1 pack of cigarettes a day for 22 years is a 22-pack-year smoker).
    2. History of bronchitis or hospitalization for COPD exacerbation in the past year
    3. Asthma history, allergies, or prior respiratory infections such as tuberculosis
    4. Familial history of COPD or other respiratory conditions
    5. Concomitant chronic conditions such as cardiac disease, peripheral vascular insufficiency, depression, anxiety, sinus problems, or headache
    6. Weight loss, which needs emergent attention because this can indicate a poor prognosis
  B. Physical examination is relatively poor in detecting mild to moderate COPD.
    1. More pronounced physical findings exist in patients with severe COPD.
    2. Patients with severe COPD can be observed for tachypnea, pursed-lip breathing, and distress with simple activities (Mosenifar & Kamangar, 2016).
      a) Increased respiratory rate occurs in direct proportion to disease severity.
      b) Obvious accessory muscle use and what is considered paradoxical indrawing of the lower intercostal spaces reflect a positive Hoover sign (Mosenifar & Kamangar, 2016).
      c) As COPD worsens, cyanosis, elevated jugular venous pulse more pronounced on expiration, and peripheral edema can be expected (Mosenifar & Kamangar, 2016).
      d) Additional findings from a thoracic physical examination in a patient with severe COPD will include the following (Mosenifar & Kamangar, 2016; National Center for Biotechnology Information, 2016):
        (1) Barrel chest from compensation for hyperinflated lungs
        (2) Diffusely decreased lung sounds throughout all lobes
        (3) Hyperresonance on percussion
        (4) Pursed-lip breathing
        (5) Prolonged expiration
        (6) Inspiratory coarse crackles
        (7) Muscle wasting or cachexia
        (8) Positioning of self in the tripod position
        (9) Asterixis due to severe hypercapnia
        (10) Hepatomegaly if concomitant right-sided heart failure
        (11) Smell of cigarette smoke and yellow stains on the fingers from the tar and nicotine created from burning tobacco
V. Diagnostics
  A. The only way to confirm a diagnosis of COPD is with spirometry (GOLD, 2016; WHO, n.d.).
  B. A positive history of cough, dyspnea, sputum production, and prolonged exposure to tobacco smoke, industrial gas and particles, or home heating and cooking smoke should be considered when combined with spirometry to confirm a COPD diagnosis (GOLD, 2016).
    1. Spirometry measurements are evaluated by reference and include additional values: patient age, height, sex, and ethnicity.

2. Spirometry measures the volume of air forcibly exhaled from the point of maximal inspiration, or what is termed *forced vital capacity* (FVC), the volume of air exhaled during the first second of this maneuver, or *forced expiratory volume in one second* (FEV$_1$), and the ratio of these two measurements (GOLD, 2016).

C. Spirometric criterion for airflow limitation remains a post-bronchodilator fixed ratio of FEV$_1$/FVC less than 0.7 (GOLD, 2016).

1. FEV$_1$ and FVC predict all-cause mortality independent of tobacco smoking.
2. Abnormal lung function can be used to help identify a subgroup of smokers at increased risk of lung cancer.
3. Weak correlation exists between FEV$_1$, patient symptoms, and impairment in patients' health-related quality of life (GOLD, 2016).
4. Fixed FEV$_1$/FVC ratio is used to define and determine airflow limitation and validates the diagnosis of COPD in patients aged 45 years and older (GOLD, 2016).
5. FVC and FEV$_1$ should be the largest volume obtained from any three spirometry readings and not vary by more than 5% or 150 ml, whichever is greater (GOLD, 2016).
6. According to the GOLD (2015) guidelines, bronchodilator protocols are 400 mcg short-acting beta-2 agonist (albuterol), 160 mcg short-acting anticholinergic (ipratropium), or the two combined.
7. FEV$_1$ should be measured 10–15 minutes following a short-acting beta-2 agonist or 30–45 minutes following inhaled short-acting anticholinergic.
8. FEV$_1$/FVC ratios are used to determine the classification of COPD, which assists in determining the prognosis and severity of COPD. These ratios can assist in determining which patients are at risk for exacerbation (see Table 14-1).

D. A chest radiograph is not used to diagnosis COPD but can be used to rule out other comorbidities. A radiograph of a flat plate can confirm hyperinflation and a flattened diaphragm in patients with COPD (GOLD, 2016).

E. A computed tomography (CT) scan is rarely used to diagnose COPD. However, it is helpful when ruling out differential diagnoses (GOLD, 2016).

F. Exercise testing is helpful in determining exercise capacity. The shuttle walk test and six-minute walk test can be used to determine exercise capacity for specific patients with COPD (Holland, Hill, Conron, Munro, & McDonald, 2008).

G. Oximetry is used to determine oxygen saturation.

Table 14-1. Spirometry Classification for Chronic Obstructive Pulmonary Disease	
Intensity	**FEV$_1$**
Mild	FEV$_1$ ≥ 80% predicted
Moderate	50% ≤ FEV$_1$ < 80% predicted
Severe	30% ≤ FEV$_1$ < 50% predicted
Very severe	FEV$_1$ < 30% predicted

FEV$_1$—forced expiratory volume in one second

Note. Based on information from Global Initiative for Chronic Obstructive Lung Disease, 2016.

1. Pulse oximetry should routinely be evaluated in stable patients with COPD with an FEV_1 less than 35% predicted or in those who demonstrate respiratory failure or right-sided heart failure.
2. If peripheral saturation is less than 92%, arterial blood gases should be considered (García-Talavera & Aguirre-Jaime, 2009).

H. Alpha-1 antitrypsin deficiency screening should be performed in patients who are younger than age 45, have a familial history, and are symptomatic with cough, dyspnea, and sputum production. A serum concentration of alpha-1 antitrypsin of less than 15%–20% below normal value is indicative of this genetic disorder (GOLD, 2016).

VI. Differential diagnosis
A. Other diagnoses to confirm a diagnosis of COPD include the following (GOLD, 2016):
1. Asthma—should never be a differential in a patient older than age 45 without a past medical history of childhood or early adult-onset asthma. Asthmatic patients who smoke can develop COPD, and the management of these patients will differ (see Table 14-2).
2. Congestive heart failure—confirmed on chest radiograph showing enlarged heart and pulmonary edema
3. Bronchiectasis—present with a large volume of purulent sputum. Chest radiograph or CT scan confirms bronchodilation and bronchial wall thickening.
4. Tuberculosis—affects people of all ages in areas with a high prevalence of this disorder. A chest radiograph shows lung infiltrates.
5. Obliterative bronchiolitis—occurs in younger ages and nonsmokers. Associated with past medical history of autoimmune disorders. CT on expiration reveals hypodense areas throughout the lung fields.
6. Diffuse panbronchiolitis—occurs in men of Asian ethnicity, nonsmokers, and those with chronic sinusitis. A chest radiograph or CT shows diffuse small centrilobular nodular opacities on hyperinflation.

	Table 14-2. Differentiating Chronic Obstructive Pulmonary Disease From Asthma	
Characteristic	**Chronic Obstructive Pulmonary Disease**	**Asthma**
Wheezing	Can occur in patients with chronic obstructive pulmonary disease, particularly with a past medical history of asthma	Is considered the hallmark symptom of asthma
Breathing	Prolonged expiratory effort and pursed-lip breathing, with accessory muscle use and nasal flaring during an acute exacerbation	During an exacerbation, pursed-lip breathing, accessory muscle use, and nasal flaring
Cyanosis	In severe exacerbation	During an acute attack
Percussion hyperresonance (air trapping)	Chronic	During an acute episode
Note. Based on information from Global Initiative for Asthma, 2016; Global Initiative for Chronic Obstructive Lung Disease, 2016; Kuebler et al., 2008.		

B. COPD exacerbation is an acute onset of changes and variations in symptoms to include increased dyspnea, increased production of sputum or purulence, productive or nonproductive cough that has increased from baseline, febrile state, chest tightness or pressure, and fatigue and other systemic consequences (Mackay et al., 2012).

C. Exacerbation diagnosis relies exclusively on the patient's clinical presentation and chief complaint.

D. The most common trigger is viral and bacterial infection in the airways.

E. In patients with concomitant asthma, seasonal allergies can precipitate exacerbations. Exacerbations negatively affect patients' health-related quality of life and reduce and impair pulmonary function.

F. Increased mortality occurs with exacerbation and hospitalization (Mackay et al., 2012). Long-term prognosis following hospitalization for a COPD exacerbation is poor, with a five-year mortality rate of 50% (Mackay et al., 2012).

VII. Interventions

A. Goals for treatment of COPD include the following (GOLD, 2016):
   1. Reduce morbidity through optimal symptom management.
   2. Improve exercise tolerance.
   3. Improve health status.
   4. Prevent disease progression.
   5. Prevent and proactively manage exacerbations.
   6. Reduce mortality.

B. Nonpharmacologic interventions
   1. Smoking cessation with nicotine replacement
   2. Increased physical activity
   3. Annual influenza vaccine
   4. Pneumococcal vaccine
   5. Pulmonary rehabilitation (Dodd et al., 2011)

C. Pharmacologic interventions are primarily based on the GOLD classification of COPD and associated symptomatology. GOLD (2015) recommends the following interventions to support the care needs of patients based on the criteria found in Table 14-3.

D. Maintenance and rescue dosing of long-acting and short-acting bronchodilators is required to reduce symptoms and prevent exacerbations. Maximizing bronchodilator therapy in advanced COPD is required (GOLD, 2016).

E. No evidence exists to suggest the routine use of inhaled corticosteroids or use of monotherapy inhaled corticosteroids in patients with mild or moderate COPD.
   1. It should be used in patients with severe or very severe COPD or in those with frequent exacerbations who are not adequately managed with a combined long-acting bronchodilator (GOLD, 2016).
   2. Long-term use is not recommended because of the increased propensity for pneumonia and fractures related to progressive osteoporosis (GOLD, 2016).

F. Phosphodiesterase-4 inhibitors (e.g., roflumilast) can be used in patients with severe or very severe disease (GOLD classification 3–4) to reduce exacerbations (GOLD, 2016).

G. The use of theophylline should only be considered if the patient is unable to tolerate beta-2 agonists or anticholinergics, or if it is the only available bronchodilator. Theophylline has limited bronchodilator effect and, given its narrow therapeutic window, carries more disadvantages than advantages (GOLD, 2016).

Table 14-3. Pharmacologic Intervention Based on GOLD Classification Criteria			
GOLD Classification	**Symptom Burden**	**Exacerbations**	**First-Line Recommendations**
GOLD 1–2	Low risk, less symptoms	≤ 1	Short-acting anticholinergic (ipratropium) OR short-acting beta-2 agonist (albuterol) as needed
GOLD 1–2	Low risk, more symptoms	≤ 1	Long-acting anticholinergic (tiotropium) or long-acting beta-2 agonist (e.g., salmeterol) daily
GOLD 3–4	High risk, less symptoms	≥ 2	Long-acting anticholinergic (tiotropium) or long-acting beta-2 agonist with combined inhaled corticosteroid (e.g., salmeterol, fluticasone propionate)
GOLD 3–4	High risk, more symptoms	≥ 2	Long-acting anticholinergic (tiotropium) plus long-acting beta-2 agonist with combined inhaled corticosteroid (e.g., salmeterol, fluticasone propionate)

GOLD—Global Initiative for Chronic Obstructive Lung Disease

Note. Based on information from Global Initiative for Chronic Obstructive Lung Disease, 2016.

H. Pharmacologic management of COPD exacerbations requires emergent attention, as these patients can progress to respiratory failure if not properly evaluated and managed.

I. Pharmacologic interventions for a COPD exacerbation include the following (GOLD, 2016):
1. Combined long-acting bronchodilators (anticholinergic plus beta-2 agonist combined with inhaled corticosteroid) as maintenance therapy
2. Short-acting beta-2 agonist bronchodilator as rescue
3. Systemic prednisone 40 mg for five days
4. Empiric anti-infectives in patients with severe or very severe COPD before receiving culture and sensitivity data from sputum culture. Macrolides are preferred if affordable.
5. Anti-infectives should only be considered in patients with an increase in dyspnea, purulent sputum, and fever.

J. Never underestimate the patient's fragile condition in the face of an exacerbation that may require emergent IV anti-infectives and corticosteroid use.

Case Study

O.G. is a 54-year-old African American man who presents to the clinic with complaints of a progressive cough that is productive with copious amounts of thick, purulent mucus; a fever with chills; and worsening dyspnea preventing him from walking upstairs to his bedroom. From his social history, the advanced practice registered nurse (APRN) notes that O.G. is a 54-pack-year smoker. His past FEV_1 from spirometry was 48% predicted. The APRN also notes that he has decreased O_2 saturation per oximetry of 89%. He has a blood pressure of 148/96 mm Hg, pulse of 94 beats per minute, respiration rate of 22 breaths per minute, and a temperature of 101.5°F (38.6°C).

On physical examination, O.G. appears cachectic, frail, and dyspneic with obvious accessory muscle use. He is bent forward and using pursed-lip breathing, his lips are cyanotic, and his skin is pale and dry. Auscultation of his lung fields reveals diminished bilateral lower and mid-lobe lung sounds. He has rhonchi in his bilateral upper lobes that clear with cough. He has an increased anterior and posterior diameter and is unable to speak a full sentence without stopping to catch his breath. The index finger and thumb on his right hand have yellowed fingernails.

The APRN codes the clinic visit with the following diagnosis and differentials: COPD exacerbation, dyspnea, cough, increased sputum, dehydration, cachexia, and fever. Based on these findings, the nurse encourages O.G. to continue with his once-daily tiotropium, one inhalation every day, and adds an inhalation powder of fluticasone propionate 250 mcg and salmeterol 50 mcg, 2 puffs BID; albuterol HFA 2 puffs every four hours; and 40 mg of prednisone for five days. The APRN instructs the patient to increase fluids and to use acetaminophen over-the-counter 500 mg PO TID as needed for fever and chills. An azithromycin dose pack was prescribed. O.G. is encouraged to be adherent to these recommendations and, if his condition worsens, to call 911 or go immediately to the local emergency department. The nurse will follow up in one week.

References

Centers for Disease Control and Prevention. (2012). Chronic obstructive pulmonary disease among adults—United States, 2011. *Morbidity and Mortality Weekly Report, 61,* 938–943. Retrieved from http://www.cdc.gov/mmwr/preview/mmwrhtml/mm6146a2.htm

Centers for Disease Control and Prevention. (2015). Indicator definitions—Chronic obstructive pulmonary disease. Retrieved from http://www.cdc.gov/cdi/definitions/chronic-obstructive.html

Chen, Y., Chen, P., Hanaoka, M., Droma, Y., & Kubo, K. (2008). Enhanced levels of prostaglandin E_2 and matrix metalloproteinase-2 correlate with the severity of airflow limitation in stable COPD. *Respirology, 13,* 1014–1021. doi:10.1111/j.1440-1843.2008.01365.x

Dodd, J.W., Hogg, L., Nolan, J., Jefford, H., Grant, A., Lord, V.M., … Hopkinson, N.S. (2011). The COPD assessment test (CAT): Response to pulmonary rehabilitation. A multicentre, prospective study. *Thorax, 66,* 425–429. doi:10.1136/thx.2010.156372

Fischer, B.M., Pavlisko, E., & Voynow, J.A. (2011). Pathogenic triad in COPD: Oxidative stress, protease–antiprotease imbalance, and inflammation. *International Journal of Chronic Obstructive Pulmonary Disease, 6,* 413–421. doi:10.2147/COPD.S10770

García-Talavera, I., & Aguirre-Jaime, A. (2009). COPD, normoxia, and early desaturation [Letter to the editor]. *Chest, 135,* 885–886. doi:10.1378/chest.08-2286

Global Initiative for Asthma. (2016). *Global strategy for asthma management and prevention.* Retrieved from http://ginasthma.org/2016-gina-report-global-strategy-for-asthma-management-and-prevention

Global Initiative for Chronic Obstructive Lung Disease. (2016). *Global strategy for the diagnosis, management, and prevention of chronic obstructive pulmonary disease.* Retrieved from http://goldcopd.org

Hill, A.T., Pasteur, M., Cornford, C., Welham, S., & Bilton, D. (2011). Primary care summary of the British Thoracic Society Guideline on the management of non-cystic fibrosis bronchiectasis. *Primary Care Respiratory Journal, 20,* 135–140. doi:10.4104/pcrj.2011.00007

Holland, A.E., Hill, C.J., Conron, M., Munro, P., & McDonald, C.F. (2008). Short term improvement in exercise capacity and symptoms following exercise training in interstitial lung disease. *Thorax, 63,* 549–554. doi:10.1136/thx.2007.088070

Kirkham, P.A., & Barnes, P.J. (2013). Oxidative stress in COPD. *Chest, 144,* 266–273. doi:10.1378/chest.12-2664

Kuebler, K.K., Buchsel, P.C., & Balkstra, C.R. (2008). Differentiating chronic obstructive pulmonary disease from asthma. *Journal of the American Academy of Nurse Practitioners, 20,* 445–454. doi:10.1111/j.1745-7599.2008.00332.x

Mackay, A.J., Donaldson, G.C., Patel, A.R.C., Jones, P.W., Hurst, J.R., & Wedzicha, J.A. (2012). Usefulness of the chronic obstructive pulmonary disease assessment test to evaluate severity of COPD exacerbations. *American Journal of Respiratory and Critical Care Medicine, 185,* 1218–1224. doi:10.1164/rccm.201110-1843OC

Miravitlles, M. (2011). Cough and sputum production as risk factors for poor outcomes in patients with COPD. *Respiratory Medicine, 105,* 1118–1128. doi:10.1016/j.rmed.2011.02.003

Mosenifar, Z., & Kamangar, N. (2016). Chronic obstructive pulmonary disease (COPD) clinical presentation. Retrieved from http://emedicine.medscape.com/article/297664-clinical

National Center for Biotechnology Information. (2016). Nicotine. Retrieved from http://pubchem.ncbi.nlm .nih.gov/compound/nicotine#section=Top

National Heart, Lung, and Blood Institute. (2011, June). Oxidative stress/inflammation and heart, lung, blood, and sleep disorders (Meeting summary). Retrieved from http://www.nhlbi.nih.gov/research/reports/2004 -oxidative-stress

Nussbaumer-Ochsnre, Y., & Rabe, K. (2011). Systemic manifestations of COPD. *Chest, 139,* 165–173. doi:10.1378/chest.10-1252

Rodríguez-Roisin, R., Drakulovic, M., Rodríguez, D.A., Roca, J., Barberà, J.A., & Wagner, P.D. (2009). Ventilation-perfusion imbalance and chronic obstructive pulmonary disease staging severity. *Journal of Applied Physiology, 106,* 1902–1908. doi:10.1152/japplphysiol.00085.2009

Sin, D.D., Anthonisen, N.R., Soriano, J.B., & Agusti, A.G. (2006). Mortality in COPD: Role of comorbidities. *European Respiratory Journal, 28,* 1245–1257. doi:10.1183/09031936.00133805

Turner, J., & Jones, C.E. (2009). Regulation of mucin expression in respiratory diseases. *Biochemical Society Transactions, 37,* 877–881. doi:10.1042/bst0370877

van den Berge, M., ten Hacken, N.H.T., Cohen, J., Douma, R., & Postma, D.S. (2011). Small airway disease in asthma and COPD: Clinical implications. *Chest, 139,* 412–423. doi:10.1378/chest.10-1210

Waschki, B., Kirsten, A., Holz, O., Müller, K.-C., Meyer, T., Watz, H., & Magnussen, H. (2011). Physical activity is the strongest predictor of all-cause mortality in patients with COPD: A prospective cohort study. *Chest, 140,* 331–342. doi:10.1378/chest.10-2521

World Health Organization. (n.d.). Chronic respiratory diseases: COPD: Definition. Retrieved from http:// www.who.int/respiratory/copd/definition/en

CHAPTER 15

Endocrine Disorders

Denise Soltow Hershey, PhD, FNP-BC

I. Type 2 diabetes mellitus (T2DM)
   A. Definition: A progressive metabolic disorder characterized by alterations in glucose metabolism caused by islet beta cells not being able to secrete adequate insulin (American Diabetes Association [ADA], 2015a; Kahn, Cooper, & Del Prato, 2014; Nolan, Damm, & Prentki, 2011)
   B. Physiology and pathophysiology
      1. Physiology
         a) Carbohydrates that are unneeded at the time of consumption are stored as glycogen in liver and muscle cells.
         b) Insulin, which is produced in the beta cells of the islets of Langerhans of the pancreas, is necessary for the transportation of glucose into the cells for use or storage.
         c) Insulin stimulates enzymes that make glycogen as well as those that break down glycogen for use.
         d) Glucose is also produced by the liver from protein and the glycerol production from the breakdown of fats.
         e) When insulin is absent, the process of breaking down carbohydrates into storage substances is too rapid, causing the liver to overproduce glucose and resulting in hyperglycemia. This hyperglycemia is a result of either insulin deficiency or insulin resistance (Guthrie & Guthrie, 2004).
      2. Pathophysiology: T2DM results from both inadequate insulin secretion (insulin deficiency) and peripheral insulin resistance.
         a) Insulin resistance
            (1) Can begin several years before the onset of symptoms or the development of hyperglycemia
            (2) Caused by both genetic and environmental (e.g., aging, sedentary lifestyle, obesity) factors
            (3) Develops as a result of increased insulin production in the beta cells as a way to compensate and maintain blood glucose levels for normal body function
         b) Insulin deficiency: Develops as a result of one or more of the following (Guthrie & Guthrie, 2004; Kahn et al., 2014; Nolan et al., 2011):
            (1) Beta cell exhaustion due to hypersecretion of insulin
            (2) Glucose and lipid toxicity to the beta cells
            (3) Genetic factors
   C. Presenting symptoms
      1. T2DM is a global health problem.

a) T2DM is no longer a problem associated only with older adults and those of affluence.

b) T2DM affects more than 28.9 million individuals in the United States and more than 285 million individuals worldwide (Chen, Magliano, & Zimmet, 2012).

c) Currently, it is estimated that 1 in 3 adults in the United States will develop T2DM in their lifetime (Chen et al., 2012).

d) The increase in T2DM is attributed to excessive caloric diets and reduced physical activity.

e) The increase in obesity is one of the main factors driving this worldwide increase (Chen et al., 2012; Hu, 2011; Miller, Nguyen, Hu, Lin, & Nguyen, 2014; Nolan et al., 2011).

2. Some patients with T2DM will present with classic symptoms of polyuria, polydipsia, polyphagia, and unexplained changes in weight.

   a) More commonly, patients will present with gradually increasing fatigue, recurrent infections, prolonged wound healing, and vision changes.

   b) Patients also may present with macro- and microvascular complications associated with diabetes at the time of diagnosis, including the following (Spears & Schub, 2014):

   (1) Renal dysfunction

   (2) Eye disease

   (3) Atherosclerotic cardiovascular and peripheral vascular disease

   (4) Peripheral neuropathy

   (5) Bowel and bladder dysfunction

   (6) Dry pruritic skin

   (7) Infection or gangrene of the extremities

3. Risk factors and determinants

   a) Demographics

   (1) Family history: First-degree relative with diabetes

   (2) Age older than 45 years

   b) Culture and race and ethnicity

   (1) African

   (2) Asian

   (3) Native American

   (4) Latino

   (5) Pacific Islander

   c) Lifestyle and behavioral

   (1) Sedentary lifestyle and physical inactivity

   (2) Diet—excessive caloric intake

   (3) Smoking

   d) Medical (ADA, 2015a; Chen et al., 2012; Spears & Schub, 2014)

   (1) Previous gestational diabetes

   (2) Women who delivered a baby weighing more than nine pounds

   (3) Abnormal fasting blood glucose or glucose tolerance tests

   (4) Overweight or obese

   (5) Hypertension

   (6) Polycystic ovary syndrome

   (7) Prediabetes

   (8) Metabolic syndrome

(9) Dyslipidemia
(10) Acanthosis nigricans
D. Physical examination
  1. History
    a) Age at onset and characteristics of onset
    b) Comorbidities
    c) Eating patterns
    d) Nutritional status
    e) Physical activity habits
    f) Weight history
    g) Psychosocial problems
    h) Dental disease
    i) Diabetes education history
    j) Previous treatment regimens and response to them
    k) Hemoglobin A1c history
    l) Hypoglycemic or hyperglycemic episodes
    m) History of diabetes-related complications
      (1) Retinopathy
      (2) Nephropathy
      (3) Neuropathy
      (4) Sexual dysfunction
      (5) Coronary heart disease
      (6) Cerebrovascular disease
      (7) Peripheral artery disease
  2. Physical
    a) Height, weight, and body mass index (BMI)
    b) Blood pressure
    c) Funduscopic examination
    d) Thyroid examination
    e) Skin examination
    f) Comprehensive foot examination
      (1) Inspection
      (2) Palpation of dorsalis pedis and tibial pulses
      (3) Assessment of patellar and Achilles reflexes
      (4) Assessment of proprioception, vibration, and monofilament sensation
E. Diagnostics (ADA, 2015b; Redmon et al., 2014)
  1. Hemoglobin A1c
    a) A value of 5.7%–6.4% is considered prediabetes.
    b) A value of 6.5% or greater is considered diabetes.
    c) The test is usually performed every three months.
  2. Glucose
    a) Fasting plasma glucose level of 126 mg/dl or greater is diagnostic of diabetes.
    b) Random plasma glucose level of 200 mg/dl or greater is diagnostic of diabetes. A two-hour oral glucose tolerance test (OGTT) can be done to diagnose diabetes; 200 mg/dl or greater on a 75 g OGTT is diagnostic of diabetes.
  3. Fasting lipid profile
  4. Liver function tests
  5. Urine albumin

      6. Creatinine and glomerular filtration rate

      7. Thyroid-stimulating hormone (TSH) in women older than age 50 or in those with dyslipidemia

F. Differential diagnosis (ADA, 2015a)

      1. Type 1 diabetes

      2. Prediabetes

      3. Maturity-onset diabetes of the young

      4. Gestational diabetes

G. Interventions

      1. Treatment goals (ADA, 2015d; Nolan et al., 2011; Redmon et al., 2014)

         a) Maintain good glycemic control as indicated by hemoglobin A1c levels of 7% or lower, or 8% or lower in individuals with a history of severe hypoglycemia, limited life expectancy, advanced micro- or macrovascular complications, and extensive comorbid conditions.

         b) A hemoglobin A1c goal of 6.5% or lower may be appropriate for individuals if they do not incur significant hypoglycemia or other adverse effects associated with the treatment regimen; are newly diagnosed and have had a short duration of T2DM; are treated with lifestyle modifications or metformin only; have a long life expectancy; or have no significant cardiovascular disease.

         c) Reduce diabetes-related micro- and macrovascular complications.

         d) Reduce diabetes-related and all-cause mortality.

         e) Improve quality of life.

      2. Therapies

         a) Lifestyle modifications

            (1) Diet and nutrition

               (a) Set goals.

               (b) Promote and support healthy eating patterns.

               (c) Achieve and maintain body weight goals.

               (d) Address individual nutritional needs incorporating personal and cultural beliefs, health literacy, access to healthy food choices, and willingness to make changes.

               (e) Maintain pleasure of eating.

               (f) Provide practical tools for day-to-day meal planning (ADA, 2015c).

               (g) Nutrition recommendations include the following (ADA, 2015c):

                  i. Nutrition therapy is recommended for all individuals with T2DM.

                  ii. All patients should have an individualized nutrition plan developed in consultation with a registered dietitian.

                  iii. Individuals who are overweight or obese should be encouraged to follow a reduced-calorie diet while maintaining a healthy eating pattern to promote weight loss.

                  iv. Substituting low-glycemic foods for high-glycemic foods may modestly improve glycemic levels.

                  v. Evidence does not identify an ideal percentage of calories from carbohydrates, proteins, or fats for individuals with T2DM.

- Distribution of percentages should be based on individualized assessment, current eating patterns, preferences, and metabolic goals.
- For recommendations specific to carbohydrates, protein, and fat, see Table 15-1.

    vi. Individuals should be encouraged to consume 14 g/100 kcals of dietary fiber daily.

    vii. No clear evidence exists to support the use of vitamin or mineral supplements in individuals with diabetes who do not have identified deficiencies.

    viii. Routine supplementation of antioxidants is not advised.

    ix. Insufficient evidence exists to support the use of cinnamon or other herbal supplements in the treatment of diabetes.

    x. Alcohol should be consumed in moderation (no more than one drink per day for women and no more than two per day for men). If individuals choose to consume alcohol, they should be made aware of the potential delayed hypoglycemic effects, especially if they take insulin.

    xi. Sodium consumption should be limited to the recommendation of 2,300 mg/day.

(2) Exercise (ADA, 2015c; Redmon et al., 2014)

    (a) Individuals with T2DM should follow the same exercise recommendations as those identified for the general population.

Table 15-1. American Diabetes Association Nutrition Recommendations

Macronutrient	Recommendations
Carbohydrates	Monitoring carbohydrate intake either by carbohydrate counting or experience-based estimation is critical in achieving glycemic control. Carbohydrates from vegetables, fruits, whole grains, legumes, and dairy products are preferred over those from other sources. Intake of sugar-sweetened beverages should be avoided. Consumption of sucrose-containing foods should be minimized. Carbohydrate food sources high in protein should not be used to treat or prevent hypoglycemia.
Protein	The amount of daily protein should be individualized. Protein tends to increase insulin response without increasing plasma glucose levels.
Fat	Increased consumption of foods with long-chain omega-3 fatty acids (eicosapentaenoic acid and docosahexaenoic acid) is encouraged. At least 2 servings of fish (particularly fatty fish) per week is recommended. The amount of dietary saturated fat, cholesterol, and trans fats for individuals with diabetes is the same as that recommended for the general population. Evidence does not support the use of omega-3 supplements for prevention or treatment of cardiovascular events. Evidence supports that the use of a Mediterranean-style diet rich in monounsaturated fatty acids can benefit the level of glycemic control and can be used as an alternative to a low-fat, high-carbohydrate diet.

Note. Based on information from American Diabetes Association, 2015c.

       (b) Adults should be advised to perform at least 150 minutes per week of moderate-intensity aerobic physical activity.

       (c) See the Obesity section later in this chapter for further information on exercise recommendations.

  (3) Smoking (Redmon et al., 2014)

       (a) All individuals with diabetes should be advised not to use tobacco products.

       (b) Smoking cessation counseling should be a component of regular diabetes care.

  (4) Weight management (Redmon et al., 2014)

       (a) Weight and BMI should be obtained at every visit.

       (b) Overweight and obese individuals should be counseled regarding weight loss.

       (c) Bariatric surgery should be considered for obese patients unable to lose weight through nutrition and exercise programs.

b) Pharmacologic treatment (Handelsman et al., 2015; Inzucchi et al., 2015; Qaseem, Humphrey, Sweet, Starkey, & Shekelle, 2012; Redmon et al., 2014)

  (1) Use of medications is recommended for adults with T2DM who do not have adequate glycemic control with lifestyle modifications of diet, exercise, and weight loss.

  (2) Monotherapy with metformin is recommended for first-line therapy in most patients with T2DM.

  (3) Second agents should be added in cases of persistent hyperglycemia in patients where lifestyle modifications and metformin alone have failed.

  (4) See Table 15-2 for a description of glucose-lowering agents available in the United States.

  (5) Glucose self-monitoring (Handelsman et al., 2015; Hill et al., 2014; International Diabetes Federation, 2009)

       (a) Self-monitoring of blood glucose in patients with T2DM is only recommended in certain situations (see Table 15-3).

       (b) All patients in whom self-monitoring is recommended should receive education, as well as assessment of their self-monitoring skills and ability to perform the test.

  (6) Diabetes self-management education (DSME) (ADA, 2015c; Powers et al., 2015)

       (a) DSME is an ongoing process that facilitates a patient's knowledge, skill, and ability to perform the necessary self-care for their diabetes and maintain effective self-management.

       (b) It assists patients in optimizing metabolic control and preventing and managing complications.

       (c) It has been shown to increase use of primary care services and decrease use of inpatient hospital services for patients with diabetes.

       (d) ADA recommends that all patients diagnosed with diabetes receive DSME and support at four critical points in time including the following:

         i. At diagnosis

         ii. Annually to assess education, nutrition, and emotional needs

Table 15-2. Available Glucose-Lowering Agents for the Treatment of Type 2 Diabetes Mellitus

Class	Drug	Mechanism	Benefits	Side Effects/Disadvantages
Amylin mimetics	Pramlintide	Activates amylin receptors Decreases glucagon secretion Slows gastric emptying Increases satiety	Decreased postprandial glucose excursions Weight loss	Generally modest hemoglobin A1c decrease GI side effects Hypoglycemia unless insulin dose is simultaneously reduced Injectable Frequent dosing schedule Training requirements
Biguanides	Metformin	Activates AMP-kinase Decreases hepatic glucose production	Extensively used No hypoglycemia Decreased CVD events	GI side effects: diarrhea, abdominal cramping Lactic acidosis Vitamin B_{12} deficiency Multiple contraindications: CKD, acidosis, hypoxia, dehydration
Bile acid sequestrants	Colesevelam	Binds bile acids in the intestinal tract, increasing hepatic bile acid production Decreases hepatic glucose production Possibly increases incretin levels	No hypoglycemia Decreased LDL-C	Generally modest hemoglobin A1c reduction Constipation Increased triglycerides May decrease absorption of other medications
Dopamine-2 agonists	Bromocriptine	Activates dopaminergic receptors Modulates hypothalamic regulation of metabolism Increases insulin sensitivity	No hypoglycemia Possibly CVD events	Generally modest hemoglobin A1c reduction Dizziness, syncope Nausea Fatigue Rhinitis

(Continued on next page)

Table 15-2. Available Glucose-Lowering Agents for the Treatment of Type 2 Diabetes Mellitus (Continued)

Class	Drug	Mechanism	Benefits	Side Effects/Disadvantages
DPP-4 inhibitors	Alogliptin Linagliptin Saxagliptin Sitagliptin	Inhibits DPP-4 activity, increasing postprandial active incretin (GLP-1, GIP) concentrations Increases insulin secretion Decreases glucagon secretion	No hypoglycemia Well tolerated	Angioedema/urticaria and other immune-mediated dermatologic effects Possibly acute pancreatitis Possibly increased heart failure hospitalizations
GLP-1 receptor agonists	Albiglutide Dulaglutide Exenatide Exenatide ER Liraglutide	Activates GLP-1 receptors Increases insulin secretion Decreases glucagon secretion Slows gastric emptying Increases satiety	No hypoglycemia Weight loss Decreased postprandial glucose excursions Decrease in some cardiovascular risk factors	GI side effects Increased heart rate Possibly acute pancreatitis C-cell hyperplasia, medullary thyroid tumors in animals Injectable Training requirements
Glucosidase inhibitors	Acarbose Miglitol	Inhibits intestinal alpha-glycosidase Slows intestinal carbohydrate digestion/absorption	No hypoglycemia Decreased postprandial glucose excursions Possibly decreased CVD events Nonsystemic	Generally modest hemoglobin A1c reduction GI side effects Frequent dosing schedule
Insulins	Rapid-acting • Aspart • Glulisine • Lispro Short-acting • Human regular Intermediate-acting • NPH Basal insulin analogs • Detemir • Glargine Premixed	Activates insulin receptors Increases glucose disposal Decreases hepatic glucose production	Nearly universal response Theoretically unlimited efficacy Decreased microvascular risk	Hypoglycemia Weight gain Possibly mitogenic effects Injectable Patient reluctance Training requirements

(Continued on next page)

Table 15-2. Available Glucose-Lowering Agents for the Treatment of Type 2 Diabetes Mellitus (Continued)

Class	Drug	Mechanism	Benefits	Side Effects/Disadvantages
Meglitinides	Nateglinide Repaglinide	Closes KATP channels on β-cell plasma membranes Increases insulin secretion	Decreased postprandial glucose excursions Dosing flexibility	Hypoglycemia Weight gain Possibly blunts myocardial ischemic pre-conditioning Frequent dosing schedule
SGLT2 inhibitors	Canagliflozin Dapagliflozin Empagliflozin Ipragliflozin Tofogliflozin	Inhibits SGLT2 in the proximal nephron Blocks glucose reabsorption by the kidney, increasing glycosuria	No hypoglycemia Weight loss Decreased blood pressure Effective at all stages of T2DM	Genitourinary infections Polyuria Volume depletion, hypotension, dizziness Increased LDL-C Increased creatinine
Sulfonylureas	Glimepiride Glipizide Glyburide/gliben-clamide	Closes K_{ATP} channels on beta-cell plasma membranes Increases insulin secretion	Extensive experience Decreased microvascular risk	Hypoglycemia Weight gain Possibly blunts myocardial ischemic pre-conditioning Low durability
TZDs	Pioglitazone Rosiglitazone	Activates the nuclear transcription factor PPAR-γ Increases insulin secretion	No hypoglycemia Durability Increased HDL-C Decreased triglycerides Possibly decreased CVD events	Weight gain Edema/heart failure Bone fractures Increased LDL-C (rosiglitazone) Possibly increased MI risk (rosiglitazone)

CKD—chronic kidney disease; CVD—cardiovascular disease; DPP-4—dipeptidyl peptidase-4; ER—extended release; GI—gastrointestinal; GIP—gastric inhibitory polypeptide; GLP-1—glucagon-like peptide-1; HDL-C—high-density lipoprotein cholesterol; K_{ATP}—ATP-sensitive potassium channel; LDL-C—low-density lipoprotein cholesterol; MI—myocardial infarction; NPH—neutral protamine Hagedorn; PPAR-γ—peroxisome proliferator-activated receptor gamma; SGLT2—sodium-glucose cotransporter 2; T2DM—type 2 diabetes mellitus; TZDs—thiazolidinediones

Note. Based on information from Inzucchi et al., 2015; Miller et al., 2014.

Table 15-3. Blood Glucose Self-Monitoring Recommendations for Patients With Type 2 Diabetes Mellitus

Patient Population	Recommendation
Patients on monotherapy or in combination with diet and lifestyle	Self-monitoring of blood glucose (SMBG) should not be routinely ordered. May be useful in certain situations, including the following: • At time of diagnosis to assist patients in understanding their disease and to provide feedback on lifestyle changes • During periods of acute illness • When changing therapy to assess effectiveness • Preconception and duration of pregnancy
Patients using sulfonylureas or glinides as monotherapy or in combination with other agents	SMBG should not be routinely ordered, except in the following situations: • To identify hypoglycemia in the first 3 months of starting a sulfonylurea • In patients who experience episodes of hypoglycemia who are drivers or who have reduced awareness of hypoglycemia • Patients who fast
Patients using insulin as monotherapy or in combination with other agents	Frequency of SMBG should be: • Individualized • Dependent on number of insulin injections • Dependent on the patient's degree of awareness regarding hypoglycemia Increased testing will be needed during periods of acute illness, with change of routine and activity levels, and when dose adjustment is required.

Note. Based on information from Hill et al., 2014; International Diabetes Federation, 2009.

---

       iii. When a new complicating factor occurs that can influence self-management
       iv. When a transition in care occurs
   (e) The American Association of Diabetes Educators (AADE) has included the following seven topics in its AADE7 Self-Care Behaviors™, which provides a framework for DSME (AADE, n.d.).
       i. Healthy eating
       ii. Being active
       iii. Monitoring
       iv. Taking medication
       v. Problem solving
       vi. Reducing risks
       vii. Health coping
  c) Psychosocial care (ADA, 2015c)
    (1) All patients should be screened regularly for psychosocial problems, including depression, diabetes-related distress, eating disorders, and cognitive impairment.
    (2) Assessment of psychosocial issues should also include patients' attitude about having diabetes, expectations for management and outcomes, and resources to assist with managing their diabetes (financial, social, and emotional).
    (3) Patients with diabetes and depression should receive a coordinated collaborative approach for the management of both their diabetes and depression.

      d) Immunizations
         (1) Routine vaccinations recommended for adults in the general population should be continued for patients with diabetes.
         (2) Patients should receive the influenza vaccine annually.
         (3) Pneumococcal vaccine recommendations include the following
            (a) Adults aged 65 years or older with diabetes who have not previously received a pneumococcal vaccine or whose history is unknown should receive a dose of PCV13, followed by a dose of PPSV23 6–12 months later.
            (b) Adults aged 65 years or older with diabetes who have received a previous PPSV23 vaccine should receive a PCV13. This should not be given sooner than 12 months after receipt of the most recent PPSV23.
         (4) The hepatitis B vaccine should be given to all unvaccinated adults with diabetes aged 19–59 years and should be considered for those older than age 60.
    3. Evaluation and follow-up (Handelsman et al., 2015; Redmon et al., 2014)
      a) Assess blood pressure, weight, and BMI at every visit.
      b) Obtain hemoglobin A1c every three months for patients on insulin or those on oral agents who are not well controlled and every six months for patients on oral agents or diet only who are well controlled.
      c) Review and reinforce diet and physical activity recommendations.
      d) Perform visual inspection of the feet at every visit and a neuropathy evaluation that includes pulse check and monofilament examination annually.
      e) Assess smoking status at least annually; if the patient is a smoker, encourage smoking cessation.
      f) An eye care specialist should perform a dilated eye examination annually.
      g) Screen for albuminuria annually. Levels greater than 30 mg/g creatinine indicate kidney damage.
      h) Assess glomerular filtration rate annually to evaluate kidney function.
      i) See Table 15-4 for comprehensive diabetes treatment goals.
II. Obesity
  A. Definition: A chronic condition due to an excess of body fat created from an imbalance of energy intake and expenditure; BMI of 30 kg/m^2 or greater (Fitch et al., 2013; Maggi, Busetto, Noale, Limongi, & Crepaldi, 2015)
  B. Physiology and pathophysiology
    1. Body weight is determined by energy intake and energy expenditure.
    2. Body weight regulation and energy homeostasis is controlled by myriad metabolic pathways.
      a) Food intake is controlled or regulated by the central nervous system.
      b) Energy expenditure is regulated by the autonomic nervous system, particularly the hypothalamus and various endocrine hormones: thyroid, insulin, leptin, and ghrelin (Jéquier & Tappy, 1999).
    3. The hypothalamus is the central processing unit for soluble factors from the bloodstream, particularly the release of leptin from the adipocytes, and plays an essential role in appetite regulation by affecting the stimulation or suppression of hunger (Jéquier & Tappy, 1999; Klok, Jakobsdottir, & Drent, 2007; Sainsbury & Zhang, 2012).

Table 15-4. Treatment Goals for Adults With Type 2 Diabetes Mellitus	
Consideration	**Treatment Goal**
Hemoglobin A1c	A1c levels should be personalized based on individual patient factors to achieve a hemoglobin A1c < 7%. Goal of hemoglobin A1c < 8% may be appropriate if patient has the following: • Known cardiovascular disease or high risk for cardiovascular disease (i.e., has 2 or more cardiovascular risk factors, such as body mass index > 30 kg/m², hypertension, dyslipidemia, smoking, or microalbuminuria) • Inability to recognize and treat hypoglycemia • Inability to comply with standard goals • Limited life expectancy or survival of less than 10 years • Cognitive impairment • Extensive comorbid conditions
Fasting plasma glucose	Based on patient's established hemoglobin A1c goal: • < 100 mg/dl for A1c goal of < 6% • 90–130 mg/dl for A1c goal of 7% • 120–160 mg/dl for A1c goal of 8% • 160–190 mg/dl for A1c goal of 9%
Blood pressure	Individualized based on patient's medical history. Treatment should be initiated for patients with a blood pressure ≥140/90 mm Hg with a treatment goal of < 140/90 mm Hg.
Lipids	Moderate- to high-intensity statin therapy should be recommended for all patients aged 40–75 with a low-density lipoprotein cholesterol ≥ 70 mg/dl.
Weight loss	Clinicians should work with individuals who are overweight or obese to develop a healthful eating plan that promotes weight loss. Weight reduction of 6% has been shown to be beneficial if done early in the treatment process.
Anticoagulant therapy: Aspirin	Aspirin therapy should be initiated in patients with established atherosclerotic cardiovascular disease and considered for others when the benefits outweigh the risk.

Note. Based on information from Redmon et al., 2014.

4. The role of thyroid function in the development of obesity is unclear (Reinehr, 2010).
   a) TSH (thyrotropin levels) tends to be slightly above or at the upper levels of normal in obese individuals.
   b) Thyroid hormones play a role in resting energy expenditure.
   c) Individuals with thyroid disease will demonstrate changes in body weight, thermogenesis, and lipolysis in adipose tissue.
   d) Weight gain and decreased thermogenesis and metabolic rates occur with hypothyroidism.
   e) Weight loss and elevated metabolic rates occur with hyperthyroidism.
5. Insulin assists in the regulation of energy homeostasis and body weight through its effects in the central nervous system and its effect on lipid and glucose metabolism. Insulin promotes the storage of glucose and fat.
   a) The role of insulin in regard to appetite is unclear.
   b) Insulin is known to work as an appetite suppressant in regard to inhibiting food intake. It also has been noted that insulin levels in the post-

prandial period are correlated with an increase in appetite (Dokken & Tsao, 2007).

6. Leptin is a hormone that acts as a satiety signal to decrease or inhibit appetite and is secreted by adipose tissue as a substrate. Obese individuals are usually in a state of leptin resistance and are unable to respond adequately to increased leptin levels (Klok et al., 2007).

7. Ghrelin is a hormone secreted by the stomach and functions as an appetite stimulant. Ghrelin is thought to send signals to the hypothalamus when there is a need to increase metabolic efficiency and serves as a meal-initiation signal (Klok et al., 2007).

8. Metabolic efficiency also plays a role in body weight regulation.
   a) Metabolic efficiency is the amount of energy an organism must exert to perform a given amount of work.
   b) Metabolic efficiency varies among individuals. Individuals with high metabolic efficiency, compared to those with low efficiency, are better able to preserve body weight during negative daily imbalances (when expenditure exceeds intake) and are more likely to gain weight during positive daily imbalances (when intake exceeds expenditure) (Dokken & Tsao, 2007).
   c) Factors that influence metabolic efficiency include the following (Dokken & Tsao, 2007):
      (1) Lifestyle—active versus sedentary
      (2) Genetics is thought to play a partial role.

C. Presenting symptoms
   1. Obesity is at epidemic levels with 78 million adults in the United States having a BMI that is 30 kg/m² or higher (Fitch et al., 2013).
   2. The prevalence of either being overweight or obese continues to increase worldwide (Fitch et al., 2013).
   3. In 2009–2010, an estimated 35.5% of men, 35.8% of women, and 16.9% of children were considered obese (Fitch et al., 2013).
   4. Obesity is the second leading cause of preventable death in the United States and is associated with several comorbidities (T2DM, heart disease, hypertension, dyslipidemia, and certain cancers) (Fitch et al., 2013).
   5. Risk factors and determinants of obesity (Affenito, Franko, Striegel-Morre, & Thompson, 2012; Brook, Lee, Finch, Balka, & Brook, 2013; Siddarth, 2013)
      a) Demographic factors
         (1) Age older than 40
         (2) Lower education level
         (3) Male sex
         (4) Being married
         (5) Lower income level
      b) Cultural factors, race, and ethnicity: Minorities such as African Americans and Hispanic Americans have higher risk for obesity.
      c) Lifestyle and behavioral factors
         (1) Sedentary lifestyle (lower physical activity levels)
         (2) Lack of meal planning
         (3) Eating habits (i.e., skipping breakfast and being a fast eater increases risk for obesity)
         (4) Frequent fast food consumption
         (5) Eating out frequently

        (6) Alcohol use

        (7) Tobacco use

        (8) Television watching of more than two to three hours per day

        (9) Diet high in sugar and cholesterol

    d) Medical factors

        (1) Eating disorders (i.e., binge eating or night eating syndrome)

        (2) Leptin deficiency

        (3) Hypothyroidism

        (4) Hypercortisolism

        (5) Psychiatric disorders

        (6) Peri- and postmenopausal status

        (7) Sleep deprivation

    e) Medication classes that may affect weight

        (1) Antipsychotics

        (2) Beta-blockers

        (3) Antidepressants

        (4) Corticosteroids

        (5) Adjuvant breast cancer therapy

  6. Classification: According to the World Health Organization (n.d.), individuals fit into one of six categories based on their BMI. See Table 15-5 for these categories and their associated comorbidity risk.

D. Physical examination (Fitch et al., 2013)

  1. History

    a) Age at onset

    b) Recent weight changes

    c) Family history of obesity

    d) Occupational history

    e) Eating and exercise behavior

    f) Cigarette and alcohol use

    g) Previous weight loss experience

    h) Psychosocial factors, including assessment of depression and eating disorders

    i) Current medications, including the use of laxatives, diuretics, hormones, nutritional supplements, and over-the-counter medications

Table 15-5. Adult Body Mass Index Categories and Comorbidity Risk Level		
Body Mass Index (kg/m²)	**Category**	**Associated Comorbidity Risk**
< 18.5	Underweight	—
18.5–24.9	Normal weight	Normal
25–29.9	Overweight	Increased
30–34.9	Obese—class I	Moderate
35–39.9	Obese—class II	High
≥ 40	Extreme obesity—class III	Very high

Note. Based on information from Busetto & De Stefano, 2015.

      j) Symptoms suggestive of cardiorespiratory complications, including obstructive sleep apnea

2. Assessment for history or presence of obesity-associated comorbidities
   a) Diabetes
   b) Hypertension
   c) Cardiovascular disease
   d) Hyperlipidemia
3. Physical examination
   a) Vital signs: Blood pressure, pulse
   b) BMI: Calculate for all patients at least once a year and as needed for management (Fitch et al., 2013).
   c) Calculating BMI
       (1) English: Weight in pounds divided by height in inches squared multiplied by 703
       (2) Metric: Weight in kilograms divided by height in meters squared
       (3) Limitation of BMI
           (a) BMI does not convey information on fat distribution. Visceral fat or fatty infiltration around organs is considered an important determinant of metabolic and cardiovascular risk.
           (b) It is recommended that clinicians use their judgment in interpreting BMI, particularly in athletes or others who may have higher levels of lean muscle mass.
   d) Waist circumference yearly and as needed
       (1) Waist circumference along with BMI is considered clinically to be a reliable indicator of visceral fat accumulation.
       (2) Procedure: Hold measuring tape firmly and wrap around a level midway between the lower rib margin and iliac crest (usually at level of umbilicus). The tape should be loose enough to allow the measurer to place one finger between the tape and the person's body. Record measurement taken on an exhalation.
       (3) Risk for obesity-associated diseases increases with a waist circumference greater than 40 inches in men and greater than 35 inches in women (see Table 15-6).
   e) Other screening tools
       (1) Dual-energy x-ray absorptiometry
           (a) Good reproducibility of total body fat mass and total body mass or lean tissue
           (b) Not feasible in routine practice because of cost
       (2) Body adiposity index
           (a) Indirect measurement of body composition from electrical data
           (b) Debatable reliability in accuracy of determining fat mass from fat-free mass
           (c) Some units are able to measure percent of visceral fat mass as well as total body fat.

E. Diagnostics
   1. Diagnosis is based on history and physical examination findings, including BMI and waist circumference.

Table 15-6. Disease Risk Based on Waist Circumference and Body Mass Index Category

Category	BMI (kg/m²)	Obesity Class	Disease Risk[a] Relative to Normal Weight and Waist Circumference	
			Men: ≤ 102 cm (40 in.) Women: ≤ 88 cm (35 in.)	Men: > 102 cm (40 in.) Women: > 88 cm (35 in.)
Underweight	< 18.5	–	–	–
Normal	18.5–24.9	–	–	–
Overweight	25–29.9	–	Increased	High
Obesity	30–34.9	I	High	Very high
	35–39.9	II	Very high	Very high
Extreme obesity	40+[b]	III	Extremely high	Extremely high

[a] Disease risk for type 2 diabetes, hypertension, and cardiovascular disease.

[b] Increased waist circumference also can be a marker for increased risk, even in persons of normal weight.

Note. From "Classification of Overweight and Obesity by BMI, Waist Circumference, and Associated Disease Risks," by National Institutes of Health, n.d. Retrieved from https://www.nhlbi.nih.gov/health/educational/lose_wt/BMI/bmi_dis.htm.

    2. Consider hemoglobin A1c or fasting blood glucose, fasting lipid panel, and hepatic panel to screen for obesity-related comorbidities.

    3. Consider sleep apnea study to screen for obesity-related sleep disorders.

F. Differential diagnosis

    1. Mesomorphic body states: Seen in body builders and people in related occupations (e.g., professional wrestling) and may be associated with elevated BMIs as a result of increased muscle mass rather than excess adiposity

    2. Hypothyroidism

    3. Cushing syndrome

    4. Anasarca

    5. Ascites

    6. Acromegaly

G. Interventions

    1. Treatment goals

      a) Patients should undertake healthy weight loss to obtain a normal-range BMI and prevent the onset of obesity-related comorbidities.

      b) Patients should be encouraged to set small achievable goals. A 10% weight loss has been shown to decrease the risk for development of obesity-related comorbidities (Fitch et al., 2013).

    2. Therapies

      a) Lifestyle modification

        (1) Dietary changes

          (a) For weight reduction, the National Institutes of Health recommends a 1,000–1,200 kcal diet for women and a 1,200–1,600 kcal diet for men (Fitch et al., 2013).

    (b) A low-carbohydrate, high-protein diet has been shown to produce greater weight loss than a low-fat diet.

  (2) Physical activity

    (a) American College of Sports Medicine recommendations (Donnelly et al., 2009)

      i. Moderate-intensity activity for 150–250 minutes per week for prevention of weight gain and facilitation of weight loss (see Table 15-7)

      ii. At least 30 minutes of moderate-intensity cardiorespiratory exercise training on five or more days per week, vigorous-intensity cardiorespiratory exercise training for at least 20 minutes on three or more days per week, or a combination of moderate and vigorous exercise (see Figure 15-1)

    (b) Resistance training also should be performed two to three days per week.

    (c) Exercise intensity is defined as light, moderate, or vigorous (see Table 15-7).

    (d) Weight loss is greater in diet-plus-exercise regimens than in diet-only regimens.

    (e) Exercise-only regimens without reduced-calorie diets are not effective for weight loss.

 b) Psychological therapy and counseling

  (1) Psychotherapy is an effective adjunct to diet and exercise and is recommended in all receptive patients. It is most effective in the form of behavioral or cognitive behavioral therapy.

  (2) The 5 A's approach is useful in primary care (Fitch et al., 2013).

    (a) Ask every patient on an annual basis about weight management.

    (b) Advise patients to be physically active and eat a healthy diet, and, for patients who are overweight, communicate recommendations for weight loss in a direct but sensitive manner.

    (c) Assess readiness to change and motivation for weight loss.

    (d) Assist in weight loss attempts.

    (e) Arrange for follow-up or referral.

Table 15-7. American College of Sports Medicine Physical Activity Recommendations

Goal	Intensity	Minutes/Week
Prevention of weight gain	Moderate	150
Modest weight loss	Moderate	150–250
Clinically significant weight loss	Moderate	≥ 250
Weight maintenance after weight loss	Moderate	≥ 250

Note. Based on information from Garber et al., 2011.

Figure 15-1. Physical Activity Intensity Levels With Examples

Light Intensity
- Equivalent to < 3.0 METs
- Requires little effort
- Does not elevate heart rate

Examples:
- Walking, slowly
- Sitting, using a computer
- Standing, light work (cooking, washing dishes)
- Fishing, sitting

Moderate Intensity
- Equivalent to 3.0–6.0 METs
- Requires moderate effort
- Noticeably elevates heart rate

Examples:
- Walking, very briskly (4 mph)
- Cleaning, heavy (washing windows, vacuuming, mopping)
- Mowing lawn (walking with power mower)
- Bicycling, light effort (5–9 mph)
- Tennis, doubles
- Swimming, recreational

Vigorous Intensity
- Equivalent to > 6.0 METs
- Requires large amount of effort
- Causes heavy breathing and a substantial increase in heart rate

Examples:
- Jogging (6 mph)
- Shoveling
- Bicycling, fast (> 10 mph)
- Tennis, singles
- Backpacking
- Playing basketball
- Swimming, steady paced laps
- Mowing lawn (nonmotorized mower)

METs—metabolic equivalents

Note. Based on information from Centers for Disease Control and Prevention, 1999; Harvard School of Public Health Obesity Prevention Source, n.d.

---

    c) Pharmacologic treatment
        (1) Medication is indicated as an adjunct to diet and exercise in people whose BMI is 30 kg/m² or higher or 27 kg/m² if associated with obesity-related comorbidity.
        (2) Currently, four medications are approved by the U.S. Food and Drug Administration to assist with weight loss (see Table 15-8).
    d) Surgical treatment
        (1) Recommended for individuals with a BMI of 40 or greater or those with a BMI of 35 or greater with significant comorbidities and in whom dietary attempts at weight control have been ineffective.
        (2) Currently, four bariatric procedures to assist with weight loss are available (see Table 15-9).
  3. Evaluation and follow-up
    a) Obesity is a lifelong problem in the majority of cases; therefore, regular follow-up is strongly recommended.
    b) Follow-up should include weekly contact for the first three months, then continued support for up to four years.
    c) Patients on pharmacotherapy need to have regular evaluation of blood pressure, assessment of nutrition adequacy, and surveillance for specific nutrient deficiencies.
    d) Patients who have had bariatric surgery require procedure-specific follow-up.
    e) Ongoing reinforcement of important behavioral strategies that includes provision of new information; strategies to cope with restaurant eating, snacking, and high-calorie beverage intake; and strategies for achieving regular physical activity is essential.

Table 15-8. U.S. Food and Drug Administration–Approved Medications for Weight Loss

Medication	Description	Indications	Contraindications	Dosing	Monitoring
Naltrexone hydrochloride and bupropion (Contrave®) ("Contrave," 2015)	Combination of naltrexone, an opioid antagonist, and bupropion, an inhibitor of neuronal reuptake of dopamine and norepinephrine	An adjunct to a reduced-calorie diet and increased physical activity for chronic weight management in adults with BMI ≥ 30 kg/m² or ≥ 27 kg/m² and at least one weight-related comorbidity	• **Black box warning:** Suicidality—not indicated for major depressive or other psychiatric disorders • Hypersensitivity to drug, class, or component • Pregnancy • MAOI use within 14 days • End-stage renal disease • Uncontrolled HTN • Seizure disorder or history • Bulimia • Opioid use or dependence • Alcohol use	8 mg/90 mg—2 tablets BID, according to schedule: • Week 1: 1 tablet in morning; no evening dose • Week 2: 1 tablet in morning; 1 tablet in evening • Week 3: 2 tablets in morning; 1 tablet in evening • Week 4 and onward: 2 tablets morning and evening Do not cut, crush, or chew tablet. Avoid administration with a high-fat meal.	Creatine at baseline; BP and HR at baseline then periodically. Monitor for suicidality, clinical worsening, or unusual behavior changes, especially during initial treatment or after dose changes.

(Continued on next page)

Table 15-8. U.S. Food and Drug Administration–Approved Medications for Weight Loss (Continued)

Medication	Description	Indications	Contraindications	Dosing	Monitoring
Liraglutide (rDNA origin) injection (Saxenda®) ("Saxenda," 2015)	Glucagon-like peptide-1 (GLP-1) receptor agonist. GLP-1 is a regulator of appetite and calorie intake.	An adjunct to a reduced-calorie diet and increased physical activity for chronic weight management in adults with BMI ≥ 30 kg/m² or ≥ 27 kg/m² and at least one weight-related comorbidity	• **Black box warning:** Thyroid C-cell tumor risk in patients with a personal or family history of medullary thyroid carcinoma and patients with multiple endocrine neoplasia syndrome type 2 • Type 1 diabetes mellitus • Diabetic ketoacidosis • Gastroparesis, severe • History of pancreatitis • Hypersensitivity to drug, class, or component • Intramuscular or IV administration	3 mg daily via subcutaneous injection in the abdomen, thigh, or upper arm. Injection site and timing can be changed without dose adjustment. Start at 0.6 mg per day for one week, then increase the dose in weekly intervals until a dose of 3 mg is reached.	No routine tests are recommended.
Lorcaserin hydrochloride (Belviq®) ("Belviq," 2015)	A serotonin 2C receptor agonist; has been shown to decrease food consumption and promote satiety by selectively activating serotonin 2C receptors in the brain	An adjunct to a reduced-calorie diet and increased physical activity for chronic weight management in adults with BMI ≥ 30 kg/m² or ≥ 27 kg/m² and at least one weight-related comorbidity	• Hypersensitivity to drug, class, or component • Pregnancy • Creatinine clearance < 30 ml/min	10 mg PO BID; discontinue if weight loss is < 5% of total body weight after 12 weeks.	Monitor for signs and symptoms of depression, behavior changes, and suicidality. Measure glucose at baseline, then periodically if patient has diabetes. Consider complete blood count.

(Continued on next page)

Table 15-8. U.S. Food and Drug Administration–Approved Medications for Weight Loss (*Continued*)

Medication	Description	Indications	Contraindications	Dosing	Monitoring
Phentermine and topiramate extended-release (Qsymia®) ("Qsymia," 2015)	Combination of phentermine, a sympathomimetic amine anorectic, and topiramate extended-release, an antiepileptic drug The effect of phentermine on weight management is most likely due to the release of catecholamines in the hypothalamus, resulting in reduced appetite and decreased food consumption. Topiramate's effect on weight management is most likely due to its effects on both appetite suppression and satiety enhancement.	An adjunct to a reduced-calorie diet and increased physical activity for chronic weight management in adults with BMI ≥ 30 kg/m^2 or ≥ 27 kg/m^2 and at least one weight-related comorbidity	• Hypersensitivity to drug, class, or component • MAOI use within 14 days • Pregnancy • Breast-feeding • Cardiovascular disease or history of • Hyperthyroidism • Glaucoma • Agitation • Drug abuse history	7.5 mg/46 mg or 15 mg/92 mg PO every morning. Start 3.75 mg/23 mg PO every morning × 14 days, then increase to 7.5 mg/46 mg PO every morning. Max dose: 15 mg/92 mg/day If weight loss < 3% of body weight after 12 weeks, consider discontinuing or increase dose to 11.25 mg/69 mg PO every morning × 14 days, then 15 mg/92 mg PO every morning. Discontinue if weight loss is < 5% after 12 weeks on max dose. Taper max dose to every other day for at least 1 week to discontinue.	Pregnancy test at baseline, then monthly; chemistry profile and HR at baseline, then periodically; BP at baseline then periodically if patient has HTN. Monitor for signs and symptoms of depression, behavior changes, and suicidality. Avoid abrupt withdrawal.

BMI—body mass index; BP—blood pressure; HR—heart rate; HTN—hypertension; MAOI—monoamine oxidase inhibitor

Table 15-9. Bariatric Surgical Procedures

Procedure	Estimated Weight Loss	Contraindications	Complications/Side Effects	Preoperative Workup	Medical Follow-Up
All procedures	–	Unstable psychological conditions, endocrine disorders, and pregnancy	Hair loss Excess skin Nausea Vomiting Dehydration	Three months to document compliance	Follow-up laboratory tests 3 months after surgery and then annually
Adjustable band	45.1% at 1 year	Esophageal dysmotility Inflammatory bowel disease	Slippage Erosion Concentric dilation Port-related problems	Upper gastrointestinal series including motility	Clinic visit to assess wound 1–4 weeks after surgery 2 months after surgery for first band adjustment 3 months after surgery for second band adjustment Then every 1–2 months until the end of the first year Then every 6 months for rest of life with annual laboratory data Upper gastrointestinal series every year and as needed
Sleeve gastrectomy	45% at 1 year	–	Leak Stenosis Bowel obstruction	–	1, 3, 6, and 12 months after surgery, then annually

(Continued on next page)

Table 15-9. Bariatric Surgical Procedures *(Continued)*

Procedure	Estimated Weight Loss	Contraindications	Complications/Side Effects	Preoperative Workup	Medical Follow-Up
Gastric bypass	49% at 14 years	History of gastric cancer Need for nonsteroidal inflammatory drug Bile duct pathology Inflammatory bowel disease	Nutritional issues Leak Stricture Marginal ulcer Bowel obstruction Internal hernia	Psychological evaluation Nutritional assessment Mandatory weight loss program Sleep study Esophagogastroduodenoscopy if history of ulcer Testing for *Helicobacter pylori*	1, 3, 6, and 12 months after surgery, then annually
Duodenal switch	75% at 12 years	Vegetarianism Inflammatory bowel disease	Malnutrition Leak Stricture Bowel obstruction	—	1, 3, 6, and 12 months after surgery, then annually

Note. Based on information from Fitch et al., 2013.

Case Study

M.J., a 53-year-old African American woman, presents to the clinic with complaints of fatigue, no motivation, and dry, itchy skin for the past six months. Her medical history includes hypertension and hypercholesterolemia. She has not seen a provider in more than two years. In the past, she was on triamterene and hydrochlorothiazide for her hypertension and simvastatin for her elevated cholesterol. She is also concerned that she has gained a significant amount of weight over the past three years. She lives with her daughter and three grandchildren. She does not follow any specific diet, and her current diet consists of fried and prepackaged foods and fast food. She works as a cashier at a local department store. Other than work, she denies any type of exercise or physical activity.

Her physical examination findings include height of 5 ft, 6 in., weight of 265 lbs, BMI of 42.8 (obese class III), blood pressure of 150/88 mm Hg, and pulse of 80 beats per minute. The remainder of her physical examination was unremarkable. The advanced practice registered nurse (APRN) orders a fasting complete metabolic panel, hemoglobin A1c, fasting lipid, and TSH. Her laboratory results were all unremarkable except for fasting glucose of 175 mg/dl and hemoglobin A1c of 7.2%.

The APRN meets with M.J. and discusses the findings from her examination. The nurse shares with her that she has T2DM and that her weight places her in an obesity category that puts her at high risk for the diabetes and other chronic conditions. The nurse discusses with her the importance of weight loss to help with managing her diabetes, as well as her other chronic conditions. She is willing to lose weight but is concerned she will not be able to follow a strict diet. The nurse provides her with a healthy eating plan based on the ADA guidelines and gives her the AADE7 nutrition printout. Through this discussion, M.J. feels she can make changes in her diet that would decrease the amount of fast food and fried food she is eating. The APRN also discusses the importance of regular exercise. The nurse and patient together develop a plan for M.J. to start a regular walking program with the goal of increasing to a total of 150 minutes of moderate-intensity activity per week. She understands that this is something that she will need to work up to but feels she can do it and plans on recruiting her grandchildren to walk with her. At this time, with the agreed-upon changes in her diet and exercise regimens, the nurse decides not to start M.J. on medications for the diabetes. The nurse also refers her to a local diabetes educator to assist her with learning more about her diabetes and how to manage it.

The APRN sees M.J. three months later for routine follow-up for her diabetes and obesity. Her weight is down 10 lbs, putting her BMI at 41.2. Her hemoglobin A1c is now 6.8%. She has been walking on a regular basis and has achieved the goal of 150 minutes of moderate-intensity activity per week. She is still struggling with her diet but is not eating as much fast food and is incorporating more fruits and vegetables now. She shares that she is very frustrated about her weight and that most of her family is overweight or obese, and she has struggled with her weight for most of her life. She knows if she loses weight, she would feel better and that this would help her diabetes. After a long discussion, the APRN decides to start M.J. on metformin to help with the diabetes and refers her to a weight management center for evaluation and treatment of the obesity.

At M.J.'s next follow-up visit, her hemoglobin A1c is down to 6.2%, and her weight is down another 10 lbs. She says that the weight loss continues to be a struggle but she continues to exercise regularly and is now up to 200 minutes per week of moderate-intensity activity. The weight loss center is working with her on ways to continually improve her diet, which she feels is helping. The APRN decides to continue the metformin, congratulates her on her successes to date, and encourages her to continue working on her diet and exercise regimens.

References

Affenito, S.G., Franko, D.L., Striegel-Morre, R.H., & Thompson, D. (2012). Behavioral determinants of obesity: Research findings and policy implications. *Journal of Obesity, 2012,* Article 150732. doi:10.1155/2012/150732

American Association of Diabetes Educators. (n.d.). AADE7 Self-Care Behaviors™. Retrieved from https://www.diabeteseducator.org/patient-resources/aade7-self-care-behaviors

American Diabetes Association. (2015a). 2. Classification and diagnosis of diabetes. *Diabetes Care, 38*(Suppl. 1), S8–S16. doi:10.2337/dc15-S005

American Diabetes Association. (2015b). 3. Initial evaluation and diabetes management planning. *Diabetes Care, 38*(Suppl. 1), S17–S19. doi:10.2337/dc15-S006

American Diabetes Association. (2015c). 4. Foundations of care: Education, nutrition, physical activity, smoking cessation, psychosocial care, and immunization. *Diabetes Care, 38*(Suppl. 1), S20–S30. doi:10.2337/dc15-S007

American Diabetes Association. (2015d). 6. Glycemic targets. *Diabetes Care, 38*(Suppl. 1), S33–S40. doi:10.2337/dc15-S009

Belviq. (2015). Retrieved from Epocrates Online: https://online.epocrates.com/drugs/662410/Belviq/Monograph

Brook, J.S., Lee, J.Y., Finch, S.J., Balka, E.B., & Brook, D.W. (2013). Physical factors, personal characteristics, and substance use: Associations with obesity. *Substance Abuse, 34,* 273–276. doi:10.1080/08897077.2013.770425

Busetto, L., & De Stefano, F. (2015). Clinical evaluation. In A. Lenzi, S. Migliaccio, & L.M. Donini (Eds.), *Multidisciplinary approach to obesity: From assessment to treatment* (pp. 157–169). New York, NY: Springer. doi:10.1007/978-3-319-09045-0_15

Centers for Disease Control and Prevention. (1999). General physical activities defined by level of intensity. Retrieved from http://www.cdc.gov/nccdphp/dnpa/physical/pdf/PA_Intensity_table_2_1.pdf

Chen, L., Magliano, D.J., & Zimmet, P.Z. (2012). The worldwide epidemiology of type 2 diabetes mellitus—Present and future perspectives. *Nature Reviews Endocrinology, 8,* 228–236.

Contrave. (2015). Retrieved from Epocrates Online: https://online.epocrates.com/noFrame/showPage?method=drugs&MonographId=6957

Dokken, B.B., & Tsao, T.-S. (2007). The physiology of body weight regulation: Are we too efficient for our own good? *Diabetes Spectrum, 20,* 166–170. doi:10.2337/diaspect.20.3.166

Donnelly, J.E., Blair, S.N., Jakicic, J.M., Manore, M.M., Rankin, J.W., & Smith, B.K. (2009). Appropriate physical activity intervention strategies for weight loss and prevention of weight regain for adults [Position stand]. *Medicine and Science in Sports and Exercise, 41,* 459–471. doi:10.1249/MSS.0b013e3181949333

Fitch, A., Everling, L., Fox, C., Goldberg, J., Heim, C., Johnson, K., ... Webb, B. (2013, May). *Institute for Clinical Systems Improvement health care: Prevention and management of obesity for adults.* Retrieved from https://www.icsi.org/_asset/s935hy/Obesity-Interactive0411.pdf

Garber, C.E., Blissmer, B., Deschenes, M.R., Franklin, B.A., Lamonte, M.J., Lee, I.-M., ... Swain, D.P. (2011). Quantity and quality of exercise for developing and maintaining cardiorespiratory, musculoskeletal, and neuromotor fitness in apparently healthy adults: Guidance for prescribing exercise. *Medicine and Science in Sports and Exercise, 43,* 1334–1359. doi:10.1249/MSS.0b013e318213fefb

Guthrie, R.A., & Guthrie, D.W. (2004). Pathophysiology of diabetes mellitus. *Critical Care Nursing Quarterly, 27,* 113–125. doi:10.1097/00002727-200404000-00003

Handelsman, Y., Bloomgarden, Z.T., Grunberger, G., Umpierrez, G., Zimmerman, R.S., Bailey, T.S., ... Zangeneh, F. (2015). American Association of Clinical Endocrinologists and American College of Endocrinology—Clinical practice guidelines for developing a diabetes mellitus comprehensive care plan—2015. *Endocrine Practice, 21*(Suppl. 1), 1–87. doi:10.4158/EP15672.GLSUPPL

Harvard School of Public Health Obesity Prevention Source. (n.d.). Examples of moderate and vigorous physical activity. Retrieved from http://www.hsph.harvard.edu/obesity-prevention-source/moderate-and-vigorous-physical-activity

Hill, J., Hicks, D., James, J., Vanterpool, G., Brown, P., Diggle, J., & Hardman, H. (2014, May). *Blood glucose monitoring guidelines: Consensus document* [Version 1.0]. Retrieved from http://www.trend-uk.org/documents/TREND_BG_Consensus_May_Final_HIGHRES.pdf

Hu, F.B. (2011). Globalization of diabetes: The role of diet, lifestyle, and genes. *Diabetes Care, 34,* 1249–1257. doi:10.2337/dc11-0442

International Diabetes Federation. (2009). *Guideline on self-monitoring of blood glucose in non-insulin treated type 2 diabetes.* Retrieved from http://www.idf.org/webdata/docs/SMBG_EN2.pdf

Inzucchi, S.E., Bergenstal, R.M., Buse, J.B., Diamant, M., Ferrannini, E., Nauck, M., ... Matthews, D.R. (2015). Management of hyperglycemia in type 2 diabetes, 2015: A patient-centered approach: Update to a position statement of the American Diabetes Association and the European Association for the Study of Diabetes. *Diabetes Care, 38,* 140–149. doi:10.2337/dc14-2441

Jéquier, E., & Tappy, L. (1999). Regulation of body weight in humans. *Physiological Reviews, 79,* 451–480. Retrieved from http://physrev.physiology.org/content/79/2/451.long

Kahn, S.E., Cooper, M.E., & Del Prato, S. (2014). Pathophysiology and treatment of type 2 diabetes: Perspectives on the past, present, and future. *Lancet, 383,* 1068–1083. doi:10.1016/S0140-6736(13)62154-6

Klok, M.D., Jakobsdottir, S., & Drent, M.L. (2007). The role of leptin and ghrelin in the regulation of food intake and body weight in humans: A review. *Obesity Reviews, 8,* 21–34. doi:10.1111/j.1467-789X.2006.00270.x

Maggi, S., Busetto, L., Noale, M., Limongi, F., & Crepaldi, G. (2015). Obesity: Definition and epidemiology. In A. Lenzi, S. Migliaccio, & L.M. Donini (Eds.), *Multidisciplinary approach to obesity: From assessment to treatment* (pp. 31–39). New York, NY: Springer.

Miller, B.R., Nguyen, H., Hu, C.J.-H., Lin, C., & Nguyen, Q.T. (2014). New and emerging drugs and targets for type 2 diabetes: Reviewing the evidence. *American Health and Drug Benefits, 7,* 452–463. Retrieved from http://www.ncbi.nlm.nih.gov/pmc/articles/PMC4280522/pdf/ahdb-07-452.pdf

Nolan, C.J., Damm, P., & Prentki, M. (2011). Type 2 diabetes across generations: From pathophysiology to prevention and management. *Lancet, 378,* 169–181. doi:10.1016/S0140-6736(11)60614-4

Powers, M., Bardsley, J., Cypress, M., Duker, P., Funnell, M., Fischl, A., … Vivian, E. (2015). Diabetes self-management education and support in type 2 diabetes: A joint positon statement of the American Diabetes Association, the American Association of Diabetes Educators, and the Academy of Nutrition and Dietetics. *Diabetes Educator, 41,* 417–430. doi:10.1177/0145721715588904

Qaseem, A., Humphrey, L.L., Sweet, D.E., Starkey, M., & Shekelle, P. (2012). Oral pharmacologic treatment of type 2 diabetes mellitus: A clinical practice guideline from the American College of Physicians. *Annals of Internal Medicine, 156,* 218–231. doi:10.7326/0003-4819-156-3-201202070-00011

Qsymia. (2015). Retrieved from Epocrates Online: https://online.epocrates.com/noFrame/showPage?method= drugs&MonographId=6442

Redmon, B., Caccamo, D., Flavin, P., Michels, R., O'Connor, P., Roberts, J., … Sperl-Hillen, J. (2014, July). *Institute for Clinical Systems Improvement health care guideline: Diagnosis and management of type 2 diabetes mellitus in adults.* Retrieved from https://www.icsi.org/_asset/3rrm36/Diabetes.pdf

Reinehr, T. (2010). Obesity and thyroid function. *Molecular and Cellular Endocrinology, 316,* 165–171. doi:10.1016/j.mce.2009.06.005

Sainsbury, A., & Zhang, L. (2012). Role of the hypothalamus in the neuroendocrine regulation of body weight and composition during energy deficit. *Obesity Reviews, 13,* 234–257. doi:10.1111/j.1467-789X.2011.00948.x

Saxenda. (2015). Retrieved from Epocrates Online: https://online.epocrates.com/noFrame/showPage?metho d=drugs&MonographId=7106

Siddarth, D. (2013). Risk factors for obesity in children and adults. *Journal of Investigative Medicine, 61,* 1039–1042. doi:10.2310/JIM.0b013e31829c39d0

Spears, T.-L., & Schub, T. (2014). Diabetes mellitus, type 2. Glendale, CA: CINAHL Information Systems.

World Health Organization. (n.d.). Global database on body mass index. Retrieved from http://apps.who.int/ bmi/index.jsp

CHAPTER 16

General Oncology

Peg Esper, DNP, MSN, MSA, ANP-BC, AOCN®

I. Definition
   A. *Cancer* is a generic term to describe diseases that can occur virtually anywhere in the body. It is characterized by dysregulated cell growth and the potential to invade or spread to other areas of the body (American Cancer Society [ACS], 2016; Hanahan & Weinberg, 2011; Holland et al., 2010; National Cancer Institute [NCI], 2015b).
   B. *Metastasis* or *metastatic disease* is the spread of cancer to other parts of the body from the site of origin and is the major cause of death from cancer (World Health Organization [WHO], 2015).
   C. The most common causes of cancer death in the United States are lung and bronchus, prostate, and colorectal cancers in men, and lung and bronchus, breast, and colorectal cancers in women (ACS, 2016).
   D. In the United States, the lifetime risk of developing an invasive cancer is 38% for women and 42% for men (ACS, 2016).
II. Pathophysiology
   A. A multistep process by which an accumulation of inherited or acquired genetic mutations leads to cellular proliferation and tumor development (Biological Sciences Curriculum Study, 2007).
   B. Normal cells are affected by a variety of assaults that can lead to DNA damage.
      1. Behavioral risks—obesity, alcohol abuse
      2. Dietary risks—diets low in fruits and vegetables
      3. Environmental risks
         a) Physical (e.g., ultraviolet radiation)
         b) Chemical (e.g., smoke, asbestos)—Smoking accounts for the cause of approximately 20% of global cancer-related deaths (WHO, 2015), and mesothelioma is related to asbestos exposure.
         c) Biologic—viruses and parasites (e.g., human papillomavirus, HIV, hepatitis, Epstein-Barr virus)
   C. Damaged DNA (unrepaired) can lead to abnormal cell proliferation and tumor development.
   D. Most cancer is considered sporadic, with hereditary (nonsporadic) accounting for approximately 3%–10% of all cancers (i.e., *VHL* mutations in kidney cancer; *BRCA1* and *BRCA2* mutations in breast and ovarian cancers; *MLH1* mutations in colon cancer; *CDKN2A* mutations in skin cancer).
   E. In metastatic disease, malignant cells invade blood vessels or lymphatics to travel to other sites of the body (Bevers, Brown, Maresso, & Hawk, 2014; Eggert, 2011;

Fidler, 2011; Hanahan & Weinberg, 2011; Holland et al., 2010; MacDonald, 2011; NCI, 2015b; WHO, 2015).

III. Presenting symptoms
  A. Persistent cough, hemoptysis
  B. Abnormal growths, enlarged lymph nodes
  C. Mole changes
  D. Abnormal bleeding
  E. Difficulty swallowing
  F. Headaches, seizures
  G. New-onset pain
  H. Unexplained weight loss

IV. Physical examination
  A. All body systems require evaluation.
  B. Observation of skin for abnormal moles or growths
  C. Oral examination for abnormal lesions
  D. Examination of cervical, supraclavicular, infraclavicular, axillary, and inguinal lymph nodes for adenopathy
  E. Evaluation of lungs for adventitious breath sounds, effusions, anterior and posterior diameter, clubbing of fingers, and cyanosis
  F. Abdominal examination for positive Murphy sign for tenderness, organomegaly, and ascites
  G. Genitourinary examination for cervical changes, rectal masses, testicular masses, guaiac-positive stool, enlarged or nodular prostate, and hematuria
  H. Neurologic examination for pupillary changes, cranial nerve deficits, changes in proprioception, brisk or flaccid reflexes, and bowel or bladder incontinence
  I. Musculoskeletal examination for motor weakness, peripheral edema, changes in ambulation, and bone pain

V. Diagnostics
  A. Laboratory findings
    1. Complete blood count: Changes in hemoglobin and hematocrit can be the result of blood loss and commonly are due to involved bone marrow or paraneoplastic syndromes. Changes in white blood cell counts can be seen in hematologic cancers such as leukemia. Neutropenia and thrombocytopenia often are associated with cancer therapies. Leukocytosis must be differentiated to rule out infection.
    2. Hypercalcemia: Increased serum calcium may be associated with paraneoplastic syndromes or bone metastasis.
    3. Tumor markers (NCI, 2015a): These are substances produced by the body in response to cancer or by the cancer cells themselves, such as the following:
      a) Prostate-specific antigen in prostate cancer
      b) Alpha-fetoprotein and beta-human chorionic gonadotropin in testicular cancer
      c) Carcinoembryonic antigen in colorectal cancer
      d) CA-125 in ovarian cancer
  B. Imaging (Jaffray, 2013)
    1. Radiographic films can show pathologic fractures or sites of bone metastasis.
    2. Computed tomography scans can show initial identification of tumors as well as the extent of disease and sites of metastasis; good for soft tissue discrimination, tumor measurement and reproducibility.

3. Magnetic resonance imaging scans show excellent soft tissue discrimination and are the gold standard for the staging and evaluation of central nervous system tumors.

4. Nuclear medicine scans are useful in skeletal evaluation and for showing uptake of radioactive substances (e.g., thyroid cancer).

5. Ultrasound is useful in characterizing lesions as well as localization of lesions for some treatment modalities (i.e., seed placement in prostate cancer treatment).

6. Positron-emission tomography scans show metabolism and may increase the accuracy of staging in some tumors.

C. Pathology
   1. Pathologic evaluation is fundamental and the only way an actual diagnosis of cancer can be made (Jazieh, 2009; Tannock, Hill, Bristow, & Harrington, 2013).
   2. Immunohistochemistry staining assists pathologists in identification of the specific histology of the tumor (e.g., S100 and HMB-45 in melanoma).
   3. Identification of genetic mutations: Certain genetic mutations may cause a growth of or confer a survival advantage to cancer cells (chromosome translocations such as *BCR-ABL*; mutations such as *BRAF*, *KRAS*, and *EGFR*) (Beamer, Linder, Wu, & Eggert, 2013; MacDonald, 2011).
   4. Prognostic indicators: The presence or absence of markers can have prognostic significance, such as estrogen and progesterone receptor and HER2/neu status in breast cancer.

D. Staging
   1. Staging is used for both establishing prognosis and determining disease management (Jazieh, 2009).
   2. Standard staging systems are used, such as the American Joint Committee on Cancer's tumor-node-metastasis, or TNM, system (Jazieh, 2009).

VI. Differential diagnosis
   A. Evaluation for nonmalignant symptom etiology
      1. Infections
      2. Trauma
      3. Neurologic disorders
      4. Benign skin lesions or growths
      5. Nutritional deficits
      6. Psychological disorders
      7. Chronic comorbid conditions
      8. Symptom burden
   B. Biopsy for pathologic confirmation, including fine needle aspirate, bronchial washings, incisional or excisional biopsies, or surgical excisions

VII. Interventions
   A. All interventions have unique toxicity profiles.
   B. Surgery
      1. With curative intent
      2. With palliative intent (to control symptoms)
      3. Primary site of disease or resection of metastatic sites of disease
   C. Radiation
      1. With curative intent
      2. With palliative intent
      3. Multiple methods of delivery
         a) External beam (i.e., intensity-modulated radiation therapy)

    b) Radioactive implants (e.g., seed implants for prostate cancer)

    c) Infusion of radioactive substances (e.g., radium-223)

    d) High-intensity focused radiation such as stereotactic radiosurgery used in central nervous system malignancies

D. Chemotherapy (Brown, 2014)

   1. Curative intent—few cancers are cured with chemotherapy

   2. Palliative intent—most common use of chemotherapy

   3. Agents and regimens are selected using evidence-based data from clinical trials.

E. Targeted therapy

   1. Newer therapies that interfere with signal transduction pathways believed to be essential for tumor survival

   2. Used as single agents or in combination with other targeted therapies, radiation therapy, immunologic therapies, or chemotherapies (Esper, 2014; Lemoine, 2014)

F. Immunotherapy

   1. Biologic agents designed to modulate or alter the body's own immune system to mount a defense against the cancer

   2. May have unique toxicity profiles based on immune-related adverse events, referred to as irAEs (Curiel, 2013)

G. Clinical trials (Heckman-Stoddard & Smith, 2014)

   1. Critical in advancing the science of oncology

   2. Separated into phase I, II, III, and IV trials based on the extent of human testing, available safety data, and level of established efficacy (Tannock et al., 2013)

H. Evaluation and follow-up (Brennan, Gormally, Butow, Boyle, & Spillane, 2014; Esper, 2011; Esper & Kuebler, 2008; Johnson et al., 2013)

   1. Palliative care—care that starts from the time of diagnosis with a serious illness focusing on the patient, not the disease, with the goal of optimizing quality of life

   2. Survivorship—focuses on the life of the individual following treatment until the end of life

   3. Hospice—care provided during the last phases of life and includes palliative care

   4. Risk for secondary malignancies—typically seen as a late effect of cancer therapies, including chemotherapy and radiation therapy

I. Referrals

   1. Specialists

    a) Surgical oncologists

    b) Oncologists

    c) Hematologists

    d) Radiation oncologists

   2. Psychosocial

    a) Social workers

    b) Chaplains

    c) Sexual counselors

    d) Grief counselors

   3. Symptoms from disease and treatment

    a) Pain specialists

    b) Symptom management clinics

    c) Interventional radiology (Glynos & Malagari, 2014)

    d) Physical and occupational therapists

    e) Rehabilitation

References

American Cancer Society. (2016). *Cancer facts and figures 2016.* Retrieved from http://www.cancer.org/research/cancerfactsstatistics/cancerfactsfigures2016/index

Beamer, L.C., Linder, L., Wu, B., & Eggert, J. (2013). The impact of genomics on oncology nursing. *Nursing Clinics of North America, 48,* 585–626. doi:10.1016/j.cnur.2013.09.007

Bevers, T.B., Brown, P.H., Maresso, K.C., & Hawk, E.T. (2014). Cancer prevention, screening, and early detection. In J.E. Niederhuber, J.O. Armitage, J.H. Doroshow, M.B. Kastan, & J.E. Tepper (Eds.), *Abeloff's clinical oncology* (5th ed., pp. 322–359). Philadelphia, PA: Elsevier Saunders.

Biological Sciences Curriculum Study. (2007). Understanding cancer. *NIH Curriculum Supplement Series.* Retrieved from http://www.ncbi.nlm.nih.gov/books/NBK20362

Brennan, M.E., Gormally, J.F., Butow, P., Boyle, F.M., & Spillane, A.J. (2014). Survivorship care plans in cancer: A systematic review of care plan outcomes. *British Journal of Cancer, 111,* 1899–1908. doi:10.1038/bjc.2014.505

Brown, D.L. (2014). Cellular mechanisms of chemotherapy. In M.M. Gullatte (Ed.), *Clinical guide to antineoplastic therapy: A chemotherapy handbook* (3rd ed., pp. 1–23). Pittsburgh, PA: Oncology Nursing Society.

Curiel, T.J. (Ed.). (2013). *Cancer immunotherapy: Paradigms, practice and promise.* New York, NY: Springer. doi:10.1007/978-1-4614-4732-0

Eggert, J. (2011). The biology of cancer: What do oncology nurses really need to know? *Seminars in Oncology Nursing, 27,* 3–12. doi:10.1016/j.soncn.2010.11.002

Esper, P. (2011). Principles and issues in palliative care. In C.H. Yarbro, D. Wujcik, & B.H. Gobel (Eds.), *Cancer nursing: Principles and practice* (7th ed., pp. 1815–1828). Burlington, MA: Jones & Bartlett Learning.

Esper, P. (2014). Targeted therapy: Agents and targets. In M.M. Gullatte (Ed.), *Clinical guide to antineoplastic therapy: A chemotherapy handbook* (3rd ed., pp. 73–92). Pittsburgh, PA: Oncology Nursing Society.

Esper, P., & Kuebler, K.K. (Eds.). (2008). *Palliative practices from A–Z for the bedside clinician* (2nd ed.). Pittsburgh, PA: Oncology Nursing Society.

Fidler, I.J. (2011). The biology of cancer metastasis [Editorial]. *Seminars in Cancer Biology, 21,* 71. doi:10.1016/j.semcancer.2010.12.004

Glynos, M.K., & Malagari, K.S. (2014). Interventional radiology in oncology. In A.D. Gouliamos, J.A. Andreou, & P.A. Kosmidis (Eds.), *Imaging in clinical oncology* (5th ed., pp. 43–64). Milan, Italy: Springer.

Hanahan, D., & Weinberg, R.A. (2011). Hallmarks of cancer: The next generation. *Cell, 144,* 646–674. doi:10.1016/j.cell.2011.02.013

Heckman-Stoddard, B.M., & Smith, J.J. (2014). Precision medicine clinical trials: Defining new treatment strategies. *Seminars in Oncology Nursing, 30,* 109–116. doi:10.1016/j.soncn.2014.03.004

Holland, J.F., Frei, E., Hong, W.K., Kufe, D.W., Bast, R.C., Jr., Hait, W.N., … Weichselbaum, R.R. (2010). Cardinal manifestations of cancer. In W.K. Hong, R.C. Bast Jr., W.N. Hait, D.W. Kufe, R.E. Pollock, R.R. Weichselbaum, … E. Frei III (Eds.), *Holland-Frei cancer medicine* (8th ed., pp. 1–3). Shelton, CT: People's Medical Publishing House.

Jaffray, D.A. (2013). Imaging in oncology. In I.F. Tannock, R. Hill, R. Bristow, & L. Harrington (Eds.), *The basic science of oncology* (5th ed., pp. 317–332). New York, NY: McGraw-Hill.

Jazieh, A.-R. (2009). The principles of oncology care: Back to basics. *American Journal of Clinical Oncology, 32,* 330–331. doi:10.1097/COC.0b013e318184b326

Johnson, F.E., Maehara, Y., Browman, G.P., Margenthaler, J.A., Audisio, R.A., Thompson, J.F., … Virgo, K.S. (Eds.). (2013). *Patient surveillance after cancer treatment.* New York, NY: Springer.

Lemoine, C. (2014). Precision medicine for nurses: 101. *Seminars in Oncology Nursing, 30,* 84–99. doi:10.1016/j.soncn.2014.03.002

MacDonald, D.J. (2011). Germline mutations in cancer susceptibility genes: An overview for nurses. *Seminars in Oncology Nursing, 27,* 21–33. doi:10.1016/j.soncn.2010.11.004

National Cancer Institute. (2015a, November 4). Tumor markers. Retrieved from http://www.cancer.gov/about-cancer/diagnosis-staging/diagnosis/tumor-markers-fact-sheet

National Cancer Institute. (2015b, February 9). What is cancer? Retrieved from http://www.cancer.gov/about-cancer/what-is-cancer

Tannock, I.F., Hill, R.P., Bristow, R., & Harrington, L. (2013). *The basic science of oncology* (5th ed.). New York, NY: McGraw-Hill.

World Health Organization. (2015). Cancer (Fact sheet No. 297). Retrieved from http://www.who.int/mediacentre/factsheets/fs297/en

CHAPTER 17

Musculoskeletal Disorders: Osteoarthritis

Catherine Fowler, DHSc, RN

I. Definition
   A. Osteoarthritis (OA) is defined as a painful, chronic joint condition which is characterized by structural joint changes and focal loss of articular hyaline cartilage (Bennell, Hunter, & Hinman, 2012).
      1. OA commonly affects the knees, hips, and hands. Loss of bone is progressive, and muscle wasting can occur (Courtney & Doherty, 2014; Negoescu & Ostör, 2014).
      2. OA is a significant cause of chronic musculoskeletal pain in older adults (Voorn et al., 2013).
      3. Arthritis is the most common cause of disability in the United States; 52.5 million U.S. adults have arthritis (Centers for Disease Control and Prevention, 2013).
      4. Arthritis accounts for approximately $128 billion in lost earnings and costs of medical care annually (Centers for Disease Control and Prevention, 2013).
   B. Issues associated with OA include decreased quality of life, fatigue, depression, falls, obesity, and cardiovascular disease (Courtney & Doherty, 2013; Voorn et al., 2013).
      1. Patients with OA may have an increased rate of falls, possibly due to gait changes or loss of balance (Ng & Tan, 2013).
      2. In addition, depression is associated with increased fall rates in patients (Ng & Tan, 2013).

II. Pathophysiology
   A. Characteristics of OA (Bennell et al., 2012)
      1. Hyaline cartilage loss
      2. Subchondral trabecular condensation, characterized by altered cell integrin expression
         a) This process modifies chondrocyte synthesis with an imbalance of destructive cytokines over regulatory factors.
         b) Procatabolic cytokines activate the degradation of cartilage matrix and are not counterbalanced by adequate synthesis of inhibitors.
         c) The chronic inflammatory response is caused by upregulation of sodium ion channels, production of nitric oxide, and degeneration of joint cartilage (Girbés, Nijs, Torres-Cueco, & Cubas, 2013).

      3. Marginal new bone and osteophytes

      4. Subchondral cysts, synovial hypertrophy

      5. Capsular thickening

      6. Osteochondral bodies embedded in the synovium

      7. Damage to the menisci

      8. Ligamentous laxity

      9. Pain, which is related to deformation of periarticular tissues and synovial inflammation

III. Presenting symptoms

  A. Pain

      1. Pain may be acute and chronic.

      2. The somatic pain may be described as sharp, dull, aching, constant, or intermittent.

      3. Neuropathic pain is described as burning, stabbing, or pins and needles and is not associated with OA.

      4. Pain can cause limited mobility.

      5. The hands, hips, and knees are commonly affected. Chronic back pain may be due to OA.

  B. Joint deformity

  C. Morning stiffness that lasts no longer than 30 minutes

  D. Limited range of motion of the affected joint, which can be unilateral

  E. Muscle weakness

  F. Fatigue; mood and sleep disturbance

IV. Physical examination

  A. Patient history

      1. Type of pain (acute versus chronic)

      2. Pain assessment

         a) Onset of pain

         b) Type of pain: Morning stiffness—should last no longer than 30 minutes

         c) Impact on quality of life and daily activities

      3. Family history of OA

      4. History of trauma, injury to joints

      5. Mood, sleep disturbance

      6. Activity level—exercise, activities of daily living

      7. Medications—prescribed and over the counter

      8. Risk factors for OA include age, obesity, genetics, female gender, low muscle strength, vitamin D deficiency, occupational hazards, and menopause (Girbés et al., 2013).

  B. Physical examination and findings

      1. Musculoskeletal limited movement, swelling, limited range of motion, especially of the hands, knees, and hips

      2. Range of motion: Patient may have limited range of motion. Assess adduction and abduction of hips and flexion and extension of legs, knees, shoulders, and hands.

      3. Joint laxity, joint instability

      4. Abnormal joint shape, structural joint changes, bony enlargement and deformity

      5. Periarticular tenderness, crepitus

      6. Effusion, which, if present, is usually mild and felt on light palpation (Girbés et al., 2013).

V. Diagnostics
   A. The clinician should diagnose OA without further investigation when the following two conditions are met:
      1. Patient has activity-related joint pain with either no morning joint-related stiffness or morning stiffness that lasts no longer than 30 minutes (National Clinical Guideline Centre, 2014; Negoescu & Ostör, 2014).
      2. Patient is age 45 years or older.
   B. Radiography is the only diagnostic to confirm the diagnosis. Findings may include the following (Negoescu & Ostör, 2014):
      1. Joint space narrowing
      2. Osteophytes
      3. Subchondral cysts
      4. Subchondral bony sclerosis
   C. Aspirate joint fluid for culture to rule out infection in the presence of an acutely swollen and painful joint, with or without fever (Negoescu & Ostör, 2014).
VI. Differential diagnosis
   A. Gout
   B. Rheumatoid arthritis
   C. Septic arthritis
   D. Malignancy, characterized by bone pain; bone metastasis from solid tumor malignancies or multiple myeloma
   E. Degenerative bone disease
   F. Osteoporosis
   G. Rule out an alternative condition or diagnosis in addition to OA with the following (National Clinical Guideline Centre, 2014):
      1. Prolonged morning joint-related stiffness
      2. Rapid worsening of symptoms or the presence of a hot, swollen joint
      3. History of trauma
VII. Interventions
   A. Management of OA should use a holistic approach. Assess OA effect on function, quality of life, occupation, relationships, and leisure activities.
   B. Consider any concomitant conditions, patient preference, and risk-benefit ratio of treatments (National Clinical Guideline Centre, 2014) (see Figure 17-1).
   C. Nonpharmacologic interventions
      1. Footwear and durable medical equipment
         a) Offer advice on appropriate footwear that includes shock-absorbing properties.

Figure 17-1. Treatments and Management

Core Treatments	**Self-Management and Patient Education**
Access to information Interventions for weight management for overweight and obese patients Instruction for land- and water-based exercise Strength training	Assess feasibility of self-management techniques. Individualize treatment goals. Provide written information in addition to discussion. Ensure patient understanding of the disease, disease progression, and lack of a cure.

Note. Based on information from McAlindon et al., 2014; National Clinical Guideline Centre, 2014.

        b) If the patient has biomechanical joint pain or instability, consider joint brace support.

        c) Use of a cane is appropriate for patients with knee-only OA.

        d) Consider consultation with occupational therapy and assistive devices for patients who have trouble with activities of daily living.

           (1) Transcutaneous electrical nerve stimulation can be used as adjunctive therapy for knee OA (McAlindon et al., 2014).

           (2) Balneotherapy and spa therapy may be appropriate for patients with multiple joint OA and relevant comorbidities (McAlindon et al.,2014).

           (3) Thermotherapy, including heat and cold, can be used locally and as adjuncts to core therapy.

D. Pharmacologic interventions (McAlindon et al., 2014)

    1. Acetaminophen (paracetamol) for patients with no relevant concomitant conditions

    2. Duloxetine for patients with multiple joint OA

    3. Oral nonspecific nonsteroidal anti-inflammatory drugs (NS-NSAIDs) can be prescribed without a proton pump inhibitor if no concomitant risk exists. It is not appropriate to prescribe an NS-NSAID in patients with high comorbidity risk (McAlindon et al., 2014).

    4. An oral cyclooxygenase-2 (COX-2) NSAID, such as celecoxib, may have similar pain relief as NS-NSAIDs, but side effect profiles differ.

        a) COX-2 NSAIDs generally have fewer gastrointestinal side effects than NS-NSAIDs.

        b) Use the lowest dose for the shortest amount of time.

        c) COX-2 NSAIDs are appropriate for patients with or without comorbidities with multiple joint OA.

    5. Other

        a) Intra-articular corticosteroid injection may be considered as adjunctive therapy to core treatments in patients with moderate to severe OA pain.

        b) Topical NSAIDs or topical capsaicin should be considered before starting oral NSAID therapy (see Figure 17-2).

E. Guidelines for care of patients with OA were developed by the Osteoarthritis Research Society International based on the RAND/UCLA approach to methodology for reaching decisions for appropriateness of treatments (McAlindon et al., 2014) and by the National Clinical Guideline Centre (2014).

F. Evaluation and follow-up

    1. Monitor symptoms, the course of the disease, and quality-of-life changes (National Clinical Guideline Centre, 2014).

    2. Discuss patient knowledge of the disease, disease progression, and patient concerns.

    3. Evaluate the efficacy of current treatments and the tolerability of treatments (National Clinical Guideline Centre, 2014).

    4. Offer support, evaluate the family support system, and assess the patient's self-management progress.

    5. Cases requiring an annual review (National Clinical Guideline Centre, 2014)

        a) Patients with troublesome joint pain

        b) Patients with more than one symptomatic joint

        c) Patients with more than one comorbidity

        d) Patients who are taking regular medication for OA

Figure 17-2. Interventions for Osteoarthritis			
Pharmacologic	**Nonpharmacologic**	**Other**	**Not Recommended**
• Acetaminophen • Duloxetine • Oral nonspecific nonsteroidal anti-inflammatory drug • Oral cyclooxygenase-2 specific inhibitor	• Durable medical equipment • Footwear • Spa therapy • Transcutaneous electrical nerve stimulation • Thermotherapy	• Intra-articular steroid injection • Topical treatments: capsaicin, diclofenac gel • Diclofenac epolamine patch	• Opioids • Electrotherapy • Intra-articular hyaluronic injection • Crutches • Nutraceuticals

Note. Based on information from McAlindon et al., 2014; National Clinical Guideline Centre, 2014.

    G. Referrals
        1. Prior to referral to an orthopedic surgeon, ensure the patient has been offered the core treatments.
            a) The decision to refer should be based on discussions with the patient, family, clinician, and surgeon (National Clinical Guideline Centre, 2014).
            b) Consider referral when patients have increasing pain, stiffness, and effect on quality of life.
        2. Ensure that discussions with the patient include risk-benefit ratio of procedures, recovery, rehabilitation, and course of care (National Clinical Guideline Centre, 2014).
        3. OA study participants who were referred to a specialist and had follow-up with a nurse practitioner and physical therapist showed improvements in pain, function, and quality of life (Voorn et al., 2014).
        4. The patient's age and sex, smoking behavior, obesity, and comorbidities should not be barriers to referral (National Clinical Guideline Centre, 2014).

Case Study

M.A. is a 70-year-old woman with a long history of pain in both hips, knees, and hands. She has difficulty walking and getting up from sitting or kneeling positions because of discomfort and stiffness. Her joints are more painful in rainy weather; however, she reports loosening up in the morning after activity. Her body mass index is 24 kg/m². She presents today with worsening pain in her hips and knees and limited mobility.

The care objectives for the advanced practice registered nurse (APRN) who manages M.A. are to evaluate her pain management and assess for a potential referral to a joint specialist. The patient has no redness or swelling of joints. She has mild low back pain, rated 2–3 on the visual pain scale. She denies numbness, tingling, weakness, or shooting pain in her legs. She takes aspirin, 81 mg twice a week, for the pain.

M.A.'s medical history includes gravida 3 para 3 adult healthy children. Her mother had complained of achy joints. M.A. does not have osteoporosis. She does not exercise regularly but gardens in the summer months. She has no known drug allergies and denies tobacco use. The physical assessment reveals full range of motion at shoulders and elbows; decreased range of motion of the hands; nodules present on both hands; and decreased flexion of the back. Her hips have decreased range of motion with internal and external rotation, and her knees are enlarged with decreased flexion and extension; crepitus bilaterally. No joint heat is noted. The laboratory and radiographic results show normal complete blood count, comprehensive metabolic panel, and thyroid function. Radiograph of knees shows joint space narrowing and bone cysts bilaterally.

The APRN confirms the diagnosis of OA. She discusses the core management strategies of exercise and pain management with M.A. The patient agrees to begin walking 10 minutes per day and to gradually increase the time. The APRN prescribes celecoxib 200 mg PO daily for pain management. The patient has no known gastrointestinal history or cardiovascular contraindications.

The APRN schedules a follow-up clinic appointment in one month to assess M.A.'s pain and function and the need for referral to an orthopedic specialist.

References

Bennell, K.L., Hunter, D.J., & Hinman, R.S. (2012). Management of osteoarthritis of the knee. *BMJ, 345,* e4934. doi:10.1136/bmj.e4934

Centers for Disease Control and Prevention. (2013). Prevalence of doctor-diagnosed arthritis and arthritis-attributable activity limitation—United States, 2010–2012. *Morbidity and Mortality Weekly Report, 62,* 869–873. Retrieved from http://www.cdc.gov/mmwr/preview/mmwrhtml/mm6244a1.htm?s_cid=mm624a1_w

Courtney, P., & Doherty, M. (2014). Osteoarthritis. *British Journal of Hospital Medicine, 75*(Suppl. 5), C66–C70. doi:10.12968/hmed.2014.75.Sup5.C66

Girbés, E.L., Nijs, J., Torres-Cueco, R., & Cubas, C.L. (2013). Pain treatment for patients with osteoarthritis and central sensitization. *Physical Therapy, 93,* 842–851. doi:10.2522/ptj.20120253

McAlindon, T.E., Bannuru, R.R., Sullivan, M.C., Arden, N.K., Berenbaum, F., Bierma-Zeinstra, S.M., … Underwood, M. (2014). OARSI guidelines for the non-surgical management of knee osteoarthritis. *Osteoarthritis and Cartilage, 22,* 363–388. doi:10.1016/j.joca.2014.01.003

National Clinical Guideline Centre. (2014). *Osteoarthritis: Care and management in adults* (Clinical Guideline No. 177). Retrieved from http://www.guideline.gov/content.aspx?id=47862&search=osteoarthritis

Negoescu, A., & Ostör, A.J. (2014). Self-management pivotal in osteoarthritis. *Practitioner, 258*(1770), 25–28.

Ng, C.T., & Tan, M.P. (2013). Osteoarthritis and falls in the older person. *Age and Ageing, 42,* 561–566. doi:10.1093/ageing/aft070

Voorn, V.M.A., Vermeulen, H.M., Nelissen, R.G.H.H., Kloppenburg, M., Huizinga, T.W.J., Leijerzapf, N.A.C., … van der Linden, H.M.J. (2013). An innovative care model coordinated by a physical therapist and nurse practitioner for osteoarthritis of the hip and knee in specialist care: A prospective study. *Rheumatology International, 33,* 1821–1828. doi:10.1007/s00296-012-2662-3

CHAPTER 18

Neurologic Conditions

Mary Margaret Hillstrand, DNP, ANP

I. Alzheimer disease (AD)
  A. Definition
    1. AD is the most common cause of dementia in the general population but most commonly overlaps with other chronic disorders that contribute to the loss of brain cells (Desai & Grossberg, 2005; Toledo et al., 2013).
    2. AD is one of several neurodegenerative disorders that result in deterioration of cognitive ability.
    3. Patients with dementia, including AD, lose their visuospatial abilities, language functions, reasoning, and the ability to obtain and retain new information.
    4. Patients with AD may develop personality and behavioral changes (McKhann et al., 2011; Talan, 2014).
  B. Pathophysiology
    1. The cellular pathology of AD begins at least a decade before symptoms begin to emerge (Talan, 2014).
       a) At the cellular level, nerve cell degeneration and subsequent synaptic loss occur.
       b) Although specific cellular pathophysiology is associated with AD, any progressive brain cell loss will result in the inability to acquire and process information.
    2. Numerous diseases and disorders can cause acquired dementia.
       a) The three most common causes of dementia are AD, dementia with Lewy bodies, and vascular dementia.
       b) The plaques and tangles frequently described in AD pathophysiology are caused by an accumulation of misfolded proteins causing intracellular neurofibrillary tangles.
       c) These abnormally functioning cells are associated with insoluble extracellular amyloid beta plaques that accumulate along characteristic patterns and densities in specific areas of the brain (Sepulcre, Sabuncu, Becker, Sperling, & Johnson, 2013).
  C. Presenting symptoms
    1. AD generally has a gradual onset over months to years.
       a) AD alone does not have a sudden or episodic onset.
       b) Because cellular disruption starts 10 or more years before patients have obvious symptoms, patients may experience an acute event such as infection, trauma, or stroke, and the dementia may be unmasked, seeming to have a sudden onset (Talan, 2014).

      c) Individuals with unidentified or mild memory problems can compensate for deficiencies.

      d) If the patient has a sudden compromise of brain cells, such as from hypoxia due to pneumonia or complete loss of functioning brain cells due to stroke, the dementia will be more apparent.

2. Usually patients with AD present to the clinic accompanied by a family member or friend who has noticed changes in the individual's activities or behavior as a result of memory failure. Patients with AD will have little insight into their memory problem and will likely deny any problems related to memory (Desai & Grossberg, 2005).

3. Patients often describe memory problems including apathy, problems finding words, difficulty with daily activities, sequencing tasks, indecision, confusion, difficulty sleeping, depression, and anxiety (Knopman, 2012).

4. If individuals live with a spouse or family member, they will gradually rely more on the other individual to prepare meals, do laundry, manage finances, or keep appointments.

      a) If individuals with AD live alone, they decrease activities that require intact short-term memory.

      b) This can manifest as limiting social activities, having problems with finances, missing social engagements, or losing weight because they are unable to sequence the necessary activities.

5. Numerous screening tools to evaluate dementia are available.

      a) Choose a proven tool that fits your practice.

      b) Objective tests include global cognitive functioning such as the Mini-Mental State Examination (Pangman, Sloan, & Guse, 2000), the Clinical Dementia Rating (Morris, 1993), and domain-specific deficits found with neuropsychological testing (Desai & Grossberg, 2005).

      c) Scores from these evaluations are only a minor contribution to the diagnosis and treatment plan for patients with AD, although insurance companies and home health agencies ask for these scores.

      d) Sometimes family members need the evidence of a specific score to realize the level of disability in their family member (Desai & Grossberg, 2005).

D. Physical examination

1. Cardiovascular and circulatory system examination includes evaluation of blood pressure, perfusion, and pulse rhythm and rate. Treat causes for low cardiac output or inadequate perfusion pressures.

2. Pulmonary examination includes evaluation and treatment for any evidence of pulmonary inefficiency such as fibrosis, asthma, chronic obstructive pulmonary disease, pneumonia, or other causes of poor oxygen perfusion.

3. Neurologic examination includes evaluation of patients' general level of functioning.

      a) This is achieved by observing patients' ability to interact with their surroundings, including verbal and nonverbal abilities.

      b) Full neurologic examination consists of general cognitive ability, cranial nerves, and motor and sensory evaluation.

      c) Treat or refer if evidence exists of poor vision, hearing loss, vestibular dysfunction, or focal neurologic deficit.

         (1) Level of motor function is based on manual resistance using a scale of 1–5. Evaluate limbs for flexion and extension against resistance.

(2) Normal motor strength is documented as 5/5 for normal motor strength and 1/5 for flaccid paralysis.

(3) Sensory examination includes light touch, pinprick, vibratory sensation, and proprioception. Examine the face, limbs, and trunk if focal deficits are suspected.

E. Diagnostics

   1. Laboratory

      a) Complete blood count, cyanocobalamin level (more commonly known as vitamin B_{12}), intrinsic factor, and methylmalonic acid may be abnormal in vitamin B_{12} or iron-deficiency anemia, infection, or other systemic illness.

      b) Comprehensive metabolic panel and hemoglobin A1c may be abnormal in diabetes, renal insufficiency, or liver disease, or with aging.

      c) Thyroid-stimulating hormone and free T4 can be measured to evaluate for thyroid abnormalities.

   2. Radiology

      a) Magnetic resonance imaging (MRI) of the brain will show structural abnormalities.

         (1) Contrast should be included if there is a suspicion for recent cell injury or focal changes on the examination.

         (2) MRI of the brain with and without contrast, computed tomography (CT) or magnetic resonance angiography, and carotid artery and cardiac echocardiogram including a "bubble study" can be performed to evaluate for embolic sources that may contribute to stroke.

         (3) Brain cell loss occurs with normal aging and may be accelerated in patients with a history of diabetes, hypertension, stroke, smoking, or trauma.

         (4) More brain cell loss occurs in dementia than would normally be expected in patients based on their medical history.

      b) CT is the most efficient diagnostic tool if hemorrhagic injury is suspected.

      c) Neuropsychology evaluation is recommended, especially if cognitive deterioration will affect employment, resource allocation, or safety.

F. Differential diagnosis

   1. Cardiac dysrhythmias, such as atrial fibrillation, bradycardia, or paroxysmal atrial tachycardia

   2. Cardiovascular disorders, such as hypertension, transient ischemic attack (TIA), stroke, coronary artery disease, and diabetes, which can cause loss of brain cells and require appropriate treatment to reduce further cell loss

   3. Delirium related to polypharmacy

   4. Metabolic causes, such as diabetes, hypertension, vitamin deficiency, or nutritional deficit (Balion et al., 2012)

   5. Sleep disorders, such as obstructive sleep apnea, restless legs syndrome, rapid eye movement sleep disorder, or insomnia

   6. Depression or other underlying psychiatric disorders

G. Interventions

   1. The challenges for caregivers and patients with dementia are similar despite differing cellular pathophysiology (Desai & Grossberg, 2005).

   2. Establish a regular schedule of sleeping, eating, fluid intake, and physical activity patterns.

3. Develop a safety net of community resources for the patient and family, including respite care.
4. Establish a baseline and trajectory of dementia including patient's strengths and deficiencies. Rule out or treat other possible causes of cognitive decline and reevaluate in three to six months.
5. Establish a regular schedule of social activities such as participation in adult daycare programs for socialization.
6. Treat behavioral or sleep disorders while establishing other regularly scheduled activities. Establish social activities including family members.
7. Medications indicated for AD are not intended to reverse or cure this disorder but are useful to slow disease progression.
    a) Cholinesterase inhibitors
        (1) Donepezil—dosage forms are 5, 10, and 23 mg tablets or 5 and 10 mg orally disintegrating tablets. Start with 5 mg PO nightly at bedtime for four to six weeks, then may increase to the standard dose of 10 mg PO nightly at bedtime.
        (2) Rivastigmine—dosage forms are 1.5, 3, 4.5, and 6 mg tablets. Start with 1.5 mg PO BID and increase by 1.5 mg/dose every two weeks as tolerated up to 12 mg/day.
        (3) Galantamine—dosage forms are 4, 8, and 12 mg tablets or 4 mg/ml liquid. Start with 4 mg PO BID and increase by 4 mg BID every four weeks to 12 mg PO BID.
    b) N-methyl-D-aspartate, or NMDA, receptor antagonist: Memantine— dosage forms are 5 and 10 mg tablets or 2 mg/ml oral solution. Start with 5 mg PO once daily and increase by 5 mg per day each week to a maximum of 20 mg per day.
    c) Avoid benzodiazepines because they may cause greater disinhibition.
    d) Consider treatment for agitated dementia and problems with sleep.
8. Evaluation and follow-up: Initially schedule monthly 30-minute office visits with the patient and family or support people, such as patient care attendants, to establish safety and adequacy of the treatment plan.
9. Referrals
    a) Neurology consultation to confirm the diagnosis and expand resources for patients and caregivers
    b) Community and home services for family caregivers, including respite care
    c) Consideration of psychiatric evaluation for treatment for depression or other psychiatric concomitant conditions
    d) Physical and occupational rehabilitation therapy as needed
II. Parkinson disease (PD)
    A. Definition: PD is a progressive neurodegenerative movement disorder.
        1. Dopamine released from the substantia nigra activates motor neuron receptors to produce movement in both smooth and striated muscle.
        2. The loss of dopamine producing cells in the substantia nigra results in slowing of muscle movement and, as a result, patients experience muscle stiffness or rigidity.
        3. This manifests as postural instability, shuffling stooped gait, micrographia, and nonmotor symptoms such as sleep disorders, loss of smell, hallucinations, and dementia (Jankovic, 2008).
    B. Pathophysiology

1. The substantia nigra and the ventral tegmental nuclei overlap in the midbrain. The neurons in these areas project to subcortical and cortical areas and provide electrophysiologic effects that are important for voluntary movement and control.
2. By the time a patient demonstrates motor symptoms consistent with PD, approximately 60% of the dopamine-producing cells are lost (Dragicevic, Schiemann, & Liss, 2015; Rajput & Rajput, 2014).
3. Age is the largest risk factor for development of PD, although some environmental and genetic factors have been indicated in a small number of patients.
4. RNA metabolism and misfolded proteins due to oxidative stress contribute to damage, degeneration, and death of dopaminergic cells (Fu & Fu, 2015).
5. Secondary parkinsonism results from head trauma, medications, infectious encephalitis, toxins, metabolic disorders, other degenerative brain disorders, and vascular events.

C. Presenting symptoms
1. Motor symptoms in PD occur as a result of deterioration of neurotransmitters and circuits that allow and control movement.
    a) Early symptoms include unilateral, progressive stiffness in muscles or joints.
    b) Balance, coordination, and gait changes contribute to decreased overall activity levels that result in generalized deconditioning (Jankovic, 2008; Rajput & Rajput, 2014).
2. Nonmotor symptoms may be subtle, including anosmia, rapid eye movement sleep disorders, depression, apathy, anxiety, depression, hallucinations, and cognitive decline. Patients with PD also can have autonomic dysfunction with complaints of constipation and erectile and urinary abnormalities (Berg & Bandmann, 2013; Schrag, Horsfall, Walters, Noyce, & Petersen, 2015).
3. Patients can have the typical PD symptoms that can be attributed to other physiologic factors in addition to tremor, postural instability, rigidity, and gait abnormalities.
4. Symptoms including poor response to dopaminergic medications, labile blood pressure, and limited ocular movements may represent disorders classified as Parkinson-plus syndromes or multiple system degeneration. These disorders may present with similar symptoms but have differing progression and response to treatments (Moran, 2014).

D. Physical examination
1. The Hoehn and Yahr staging score is used to assess the motor disability based on five stages of PD (Hoehn & Yahr, 1967).
2. The Movement Disorder Society–sponsored revision of the Unified Parkinson's Disease Rating Scale is a four-part evaluation that includes motor and nonmotor experiences of daily living, patient-based items, and physical examination for a total score (Harrison et al., 2009).
3. Neurologic examination: Full neurologic examination includes assessment of general cognitive ability, cranial nerves, and motor and sensory function. Treat or refer if evidence exists of poor vision, hearing loss, vestibular dysfunction, or focal neurologic deficit.
    a) The level of motor function is based on manual resistance using a scale of 1–5. Evaluate limbs for flexion and extension against resistance. Normal motor strength is documented as 5/5 for normal motor strength and 1/5 for flaccid paralysis.

    b) The sensory system includes light touch, pinprick, vibratory sensation, and proprioception of the face, limbs, and trunk if focal deficits are suspected.

    c) Assess cranial nerves and treat if evidence exists of poor vision, hearing loss, or vestibular dysfunction.

4. Mental status and cognitive function may be completely normal but deteriorate over years. Evaluate patients' ability to ambulate safely, orientation, ability to communicate, affect, and general level of function.

5. Cardiovascular and circulatory system examination includes evaluation of blood pressure, perfusion, and pulse rhythm and rate. Treat causes for low cardiac output or inadequate perfusion pressures.

6. Pulmonary examination includes evaluation and treatment for any evidence of pulmonary inefficiency such as fibrosis, asthma, chronic obstructive pulmonary disease, pneumonia, or other causes of poor oxygen perfusion.

7. Evaluate for focal symptoms from prior injury or deficits.

E. Diagnostics

1. Currently, no specific tests exist to confirm the diagnosis of PD, so diagnosis is made by the clinician based on presence and presentation of clinical criteria (Jankovic, 2008).

2. Clinical diagnosis may be made if there is no evidence of other neurologic disorders when two of the following motor features are present: resting tremor, bradykinesia, and rigidity or loss of postural reflexes (Rajput & Rajput, 2014).

F. Differential diagnosis

1. Patients can present with complaints of balance problems, muscle and joint stiffness prior to classic PD manifestation of rigidity, tremor, or cognitive changes.

2. Disorders mistaken for PD may include multisystem atrophy, cortical basal ganglia degeneration, Lewy body disease, and progressive supranuclear palsy (Silver & Ruggieri, 1998).

G. Interventions

1. Treat or refer focal neurologic deficits such as poor vision, hearing loss, or changes in motor or sensory system, then reevaluate.

2. The cornerstone of PD treatment remains dopamine enhancement or replacement.

    a) Currently levodopa-carbidopa is supplied in various combinations and should be used in amounts adequate to support normal motor function.

    b) Dosages and frequency will change as the disease progresses.

    c) Levodopa-carbidopa 25 mg/100 mg tablets. Start with half of a tablet two or three times per day and increase every three days to a dose that allows the patient to move more easily.

    d) Avoid overdosing because this will cause dyskinesia and can cause hallucinations.

3. Catechol-O-methyltransferase in the form of entacapone may be added to extend the half-life of dopamine.

4. Dopamine agonists also can enhance and extend native dopamine or extend the efficiency of levodopa-carbidopa (Moran, 2014; Silver & Ruggieri, 1998).

5. The patient may be started on a dopamine agonist and levodopa-carbidopa may be added later, or the patient may be started on the levodopa-carbidopa and an agonist may be added to achieve the desired level of mobility.

    a) Ropinirole immediate-release can be started at 0.25 mg TID and increased by 0.5 mg TID every week to a maximum of 24 mg/day.

    b) Ropinirole extended-release can be used once the patient is on a stable level of the immediate-release form starting at 2 mg extended-release PO every day for one to two weeks to a maximum of 24 mg/day.

    c) Pramipexole immediate-release is started at 0.124 mg PO TID for a week, then increased by 0.25 mg per dose to a maximum of 4.5 mg/day.

    d) Pramipexole extended-release form is started at 0.375 mg/day for five to seven days then can be increased by 0.75 mg/day to a maximum of 4.5 mg/day. The immediate-release form can be switched to the extended-release form overnight at the same daily dose.

    e) Monoamine oxidase inhibitors, specifically type A, also will extend and enhance the effect of dopamine.

      (1) These medications can improve wakefulness, so they need to be dosed at least 12 hours before bed.

      (2) Use caution when dosed with antidepressants, triptans, and some aged foods.

      (3) Although it is rare, risk of serotonin syndrome exists.

    f) Selegiline is supplied in 5 mg tablets and may be given with breakfast or lunch.

    g) Rasagiline is supplied in 0.5 and 1 mg tablets and can be started at 0.5 mg PO every morning with a maximum of 1 mg PO each day.

6. Evaluation and follow-up

    a) Establish regular evaluations with a neurology practitioner to evaluate disease progression and optimize medication.

    b) Patients with PD should be instructed to adhere to the medication schedule to ensure stable motor function and avoid motor fluctuations (Samson, 2014).

      (1) Adjust doses to optimize functioning.

      (2) Adjust one medication at a time, gradually increasing or decreasing the doses to achieve smooth flexion and extension of limbs and the ability to perform spontaneous movement.

7. Referrals

    a) Refer patients for a physical therapy evaluation and continuing therapy to maintain strength, balance, endurance, and gait training.

    b) Refer patients to a speech-language pathologist for baseline and continuing therapy. Maintaining coordination necessary for speech and swallow is a safety issue, not a convenience (Samson, 2014).

    c) Consider referral to a sleep specialist to evaluate for sleep abnormalities.

    d) Refer patients for a psychiatric evaluation for prolonged depression and other organic or nonorganic factors that do not resolve with adequate dopamine replacement therapy (Martínez-Martín et al., 2015).

III. Stroke

  A. Definition

    1. Stroke is defined as a focal episode of neurologic dysfunction caused by a vascular event that disrupts normal brain function with or without identifiable physical changes in the patient (Sacco et al., 2013).

    2. Stroke is the fourth leading cause of death and disability in the U.S. population (Jauch et al., 2013).

    3. According to the American Stroke Association (2015), 40% of strokes occur in men and 60% in women.

B. Pathophysiology
1. A predominance of strokes occur in patients aged 65 years and older, and 90% of these patients have at least one chronic disease such as diabetes, hypertension, obesity, coronary artery disease, sleep disorders, or cancer, which increased the prevalence of comorbidity (Schmidt, Jacobsen, Johnsen, Bøtker, & Sørensen, 2014).
2. About 80% of strokes are embolic or thrombotic. Ischemic strokes occur as a result of an embolism or thrombosis that lodges in a blood vessel that supplies the brain (American Stroke Association, 2015).
   a) A thrombosis forms at the location of the infarct. An embolic occlusion is a thrombus that arises from another location and breaks off or dislodges then travels to a smaller vessel in the brain where it becomes lodged.
   b) Common origins include the heart or large arteries of the chest or neck. The territory of the brain distal to the blockage is injured or dies, and the resulting symptoms depend on the location and functions of the brain that are damaged.
3. About 20% of strokes are hemorrhagic, resulting from the rupture of an arteriovenous malformation or aneurysm concomitantly with hypertension (American Stroke Association, 2015).
4. TIA, commonly called a "mini stroke," is caused by a partial or temporary blockage in a cerebral blood vessel.
   a) By definition, a TIA is stroke-like symptoms that last less than 24 hours.
   b) No evidence of brain damage will be present on CT or MRI.
   c) The risk of having a stroke after TIA increases with comorbid factors, specifically blood pressure of 140/90 mm Hg or higher, unilateral weakness or speech impairment with duration greater than 60 minutes, and diabetes (Rempe, 2014).
C. Presenting symptoms
1. Carotid disruption presents as contralateral weakness and hemisensory changes in the face and limbs. Patients can have altered consciousness and aphasia.
2. Anterior cerebral artery vascular disruption presents with emotional lability, contralateral weakness, and sensory changes in the face and limbs. Frequently, the leg will be more affected than the face. If the left anterior cerebral artery is blocked, patients will have aphasia, and if the right is blocked, apraxia.
3. Patients with left middle cerebral artery disruption have varying levels of aphasia.
   a) If the right middle cerebral artery is affected, they will have apraxia.
   b) Both left and right middle cerebral artery disruptions result in altered sensation in the contralateral face and limbs.
4. When the cerebellar circulation is disrupted, patients may have ipsilateral weakness and sensory changes in the face or deafness.
   a) They may have diplopia or nystagmus.
   b) They may have decreased sensation, including loss of pain and temperature sensation, on the contralateral side.
   c) They may develop chorea or ballism, visual neglect, agnosia, and dyslexia.
5. Patients with basilar vascular disruption will develop intraocular ophthalmoplegia and contralateral weakness. Bilateral occlusion may result in locked-in syndrome (Jauch et al., 2013; Sacco et al., 2013).

D. Physical examination
    1. Cardiovascular and circulatory system examination: Evaluate blood pressure and pulse rhythm and rate, and treat causes for low cardiac output or abnormal perfusion pressures.
    2. Pulmonary examination: Evaluate and treat if evidence exists of pulmonary inefficiency from chronic lung disease or other causes of poor oxygenation perfusion.
    3. Neurologic examination
        a) Assess cranial nerves and treat if evidence exists of poor vision, hearing loss, or vestibular dysfunction.
        b) Assess motor function by manual resistance using a scale of 1–5 with 5 for normal motor strength and 1 for flaccid paralysis.
        c) Assess the sensory system for light touch, pinprick, vibratory sensation, and proprioception.
        d) Muscle stretch reflexes are graded on a scale of 0–3+, with 0 demonstrating absent reflexes and 3+ demonstrating normal reflexes.
E. Diagnostics
    1. Complete a thorough initial patient history and physical examination to confirm the diagnosis and establish a baseline, including the region and severity of stroke.
    2. Eliminate any other diagnosis contributing to the patient's symptoms. Complete the physical examination, laboratory studies, and imaging with analysis of results within 60 minutes from contact with the patient (Jauch et al., 2013).
    3. Laboratory studies include complete blood count to identify the cause or contributing factors such as anemia, polycythemia, or clotting abnormalities.
        a) Obtain a comprehensive metabolic panel to document comorbid diagnoses, including diabetes, renal insufficiency, hypoglycemia, or hyponatremia.
        b) Complete baseline clotting studies, including prothrombin time, partial thromboplastin time, and international normalized ratio. After the acute phase of stroke, consider evaluation for contributing disorders.
        c) Evaluate for thyroid abnormalities including thyroid-stimulating hormone, triiodothyronine (T3), and thyroxin (T4).
        d) Perform a complete evaluation for anemias, including an iron profile and vitamin B_{12} level.
    4. Either CT or MRI may be used as initial imaging to identify the area of brain injury.
        a) Digital subtraction angiography remains the gold standard for evaluation of cerebrovascular lesions but is an invasive procedure requiring contrast administration and may require more time and resources to complete.
        b) After the patient is stabilized and if more definitive imaging is required, CT angiography or magnetic resonance angiography may be completed (American Stroke Association, 2015; Jauch et al., 2013).
        c) Numerous scoring formats have been designed to describe the severity and deficits in the acute phase of stroke as well as to predict the stroke outcome.
            (1) Most of these scales include the National Institutes of Health Stroke Scale (NIHSS).
            (2) The NIHSS is helpful in evaluating baseline and is a common denominator if multiple providers or agencies are involved in the patient's care (Rabinstein & Rundek, 2013).

F. Differential diagnosis
   1. TIA
   2. Uncontrolled hypertension
   3. Delirium
   4. Hyperglycemia
   5. Electrolyte imbalance such as low sodium
   6. Seizure
   7. Migraine
   8. Hemiplegic migraine can be eliminated based on patient history and CT scan (American Stroke Association, 2015; Jauch et al., 2013).
G. Interventions
   1. The American Stroke Association has detailed guidelines with extensive evidence to support treatment options (Jauch et al., 2013).
      a) Based on current data, the initial intervention is establishing reperfusion.
      b) Rapid reperfusion to rescue threatened brain cells is imperative.
   2. Options include IV recombinant tissue-type plasminogen activator and intra-arterial injection or thrombectomy (American Stroke Association, 2015; Jauch et al., 2013).
   3. If there is no prior history of stroke and no contraindication such as allergy or concomitant anticoagulation therapy, begin aspirin therapy.
      a) In addition to controlling hypertension, diabetes, and cardiac dysrhythmias, initiate preventive measures to reduce future risk.
      b) Depending on the patient's history, consider the use of platelet antiaggregants and statins.
      c) The importance of maintaining a lifestyle including regular cardiovascular exercise, normal range body surface area, and avoidance or cessation of smoking cannot be overstated (American Stroke Association, 2015; Jauch et al., 2013).
   4. Evaluation and follow-up
      a) Once the acute stroke event is stabilized, attention is directed to avoiding or reducing consequences and preventing recurrence.
      b) Schedule monthly office visits with patients and their support providers to evaluate patients as they return to optimal functioning.
         (1) In about 5% of ischemic strokes, an ischemic infarct can evolve into an area of hemorrhage (Rempe, 2014).
         (2) Patients may or may not have extension of their original stroke symptoms.
      c) Patients have a risk of developing seizure disorder after hemorrhagic stroke. Antiepileptic drugs are indicated if evidence exists by history, electroencephalogram, and patient characteristics (American Stroke Association, 2015).
   5. Referrals
      a) Refer patients for evaluation by a speech-language pathologist for competent swallow and speech-language function.
      b) Physical therapy and occupational therapy are essential referrals for acute rehabilitation and to maintain optimum physical function.
      c) Evaluate, treat, or refer patients to mental health specialists as needed to treat depression or other mental health disorders.

Case Study

J.T. is a 57-year-old Caucasian man who scheduled an appointment with the nurse practitioner for follow-up and to establish primary care after being seen in the emergency department. About a week ago, he woke up with weakness in his right arm and word-finding problems. A friend called him that morning to confirm they were meeting for lunch, but J.T. struggled with speech during the phone conversation, so the friend went to the patient's home. The friend observed J.T.'s right extremity weakness and expressive aphasia and promptly drove him to the hospital. J.T.'s symptoms resolved by the time he was seen in the emergency department (ED) about five hours after awakening.

On evaluation in the office, J.T.'s medical history is remarkable for hypertension and use of lisinopril 20 mg PO daily. He informs the advanced practice registered nurse (APRN) that he ran out of medication more than a month ago. J.T.'s family history identifies both parents are living. His mother has hyperlipidemia, and both of her parents died in their 60s of stroke. His father is being treated for hyperlipidemia. J.T. is a prior 22-pack-year smoker who quit smoking two years ago. He drinks two to three cans of beer one to two times per week and does not use recreational substances. He lives alone. His eating, sleeping, water intake, and exercise patterns are erratic. He informs the APRN that since the event, his right hand is weak and uncoordinated when he types on his computer keyboard.

His physical examination is unremarkable with the exception of grasp on the right is 4+/5 and blood pressure is 156/98 mm Hg. His pulse is 88 beats per minute and regular. His body mass index is 32.5 kg/m².

On review of the ED report, the APRN finds the following: blood pressure of 160/86 mm Hg, pulse of 88 beats per minute and regular, respiration rate of 16 breaths per minute, oxygen saturation of 98%, and temperature of 98.9°F (37.2°C). Laboratory results showed complete blood count with differential in the normal range. Comprehensive metabolic panel showed elevated blood glucose of 138 md/dl but was otherwise unremarkable. The hemoglobin A1c is pending at the time of the ED report. His low-density lipoprotein level was 121 mg/dl. CT scan of his brain was done in the ED and did not show any acute changes. He was advised to take aspirin 81 mg daily and follow up with a primary provider.

The APRN codes this office visit as a new patient and uses the diagnosis codes for left cerebral infarct and right upper extremity or hand muscle weakness, in addition to hypertension, elevated blood glucose, and obesity. Because J.T.'s examination is abnormal, the APRN orders an MRI of the brain with and without contrast to confirm the diagnosis of stroke. The nurse will leave him on the daily dose of 81 mg of aspirin, treat his hypertension, and provide lifestyle, diet, and exercise recommendations to address hypertension and increased fasting serum glucose. J.T. will follow-up in one month to review the MRI results, evaluate blood pressure treatment, and repeat laboratory tests, including clotting studies. The APRN decides to treat the hypertension first and then review the results of the MRI before considering treatment with antiplatelet therapy. They will address the blood glucose and body mass index on the next visit. The APRN tasks an assistant to check on J.T. by telephone in two weeks to be sure he is taking his antihypertensive medication and to see if he has any questions.

References

American Stroke Association. (2015). Impact of stroke (stroke statistics). Retrieved from http://www.strokeassociation.org/STROKEORG/AboutStroke/Impact-of-Stroke-Stroke-statistics_UCM_310728_Article.jsp

Balion, C.G., Griffith, L.E., Strifler, L., Henderson, M., Patterson, C., Heckman, G., … Raina, P. (2012). Vitamin D, cognition, and dementia. *Neurology, 79,* 1397–1405. doi:10.1212/WNL.0b013e31826c197f

Berg, D.B., & Bandmann, O. (2013). Biomarkers for PD: How can we approach complexity? *Neurology, 80,* 608–609. doi:10.1212/WNL.0b013e3182825184

Desai, A.K., & Grossberg, G.T. (2005). Diagnosis and treatment of Alzheimer's disease. *Neurology, 64*(Suppl. 3), S34–S39. doi:10.1212/WNL.64.12_suppl_3.S34

Dragicevic, E.S., Schiemann, J., & Liss, B. (2015). Dopamine midbrain neurons in health and Parkinson's disease: Emerging roles of voltage-gated calcium channels and ATP-sensitive potassium channels. *Neuroscience, 284,* 798–814. doi:10.1016/j.neuroscience.2014.10.037

Fu, L.M., & Fu, K.A. (2015). Analysis of Parkinson's disease pathophysiology using an integrated genomics-bioinformatics approach. *Journal of Pathophysiology, 22,* 15–29. doi:10.1016/j.pathophys.2014.10.002

Harrison, M.B., Wylie, S.A., Frysinger, R.C., Patrie, J.T., Huss, D.S., Currie, L.J., & Wooten, G.F. (2009). UPDRS activity of daily living score as a marker of Parkinson's disease progression. *Movement Disorders, 24,* 224–230. doi;10.1002/mds.22335

Hoehn, M.M., & Yahr, M.D. (1967). Parkinsonism: Onset, progression, and mortality. *Neurology, 17,* 427–442. doi:10.1212/WNL.17.5.427

Jankovic, J. (2008). Parkinson's disease: Clinical features and diagnosis. *Journal of Neurology, Neurosurgery and Psychiatry, 79,* 368–376. doi:10.1136/jnnp.2007.131045

Jauch, E.C., Saver, J.L., Adams, H.P., Jr., Bruno, A., Connors, J.J., Demaerschalk, B.M., … Yonas, H. (2013). Guidelines for the early management of patients with acute ischemic stroke: A guideline for healthcare professionals from the American Heart Association/American Stroke Association. *Stroke, 44,* 870–947. doi:10.1161/STR.0b013e318284056a

Knopman, D.S. (2012). Subjective cognitive impairment: Fickle but fateful [Editorial]. *Neurology, 79,* 1308–1309. doi:10.1212/WNL.0b013e31826c1bd1

Martínez-Martín, P., Rodríguez-Blázquez, C., Alvarez, M., Arakaki, T., Arillo, V.C., Chaná, P., … Merello, M. (2015). Parkinson's disease severity levels and MDS-Unified Parkinson's Disease Rating Scale. *Parkinsonism and Related Disorders, 21,* 50–54. doi:10.1016/j.parkreldis.2014.10.026

McKhann, G.M., Knopman, D.S., Chertkow, H., Hyman, B.T., Jack, C.R., Jr., Kawas, C.H., … Phelps, C.H. (2011). The diagnosis of dementia due to Alzheimer's disease: Recommendations from the National Institute on Aging-Alzheimer's Association workgroups on diagnostic guidelines for Alzheimer's disease. *Alzheimer's and Dementia, 7,* 263–269. doi:10.1016/j.jalz.2011.03.005

Moran, M. (2014). Largest clinical trial of three different types of drugs finds levodopa therapy most effective to start for Parkinson's disease. *Neurology Today, 14*(14), 8, 10. doi:10.1097/01.NT.0000452483.06331.9c

Morris, J.C. (1993). The Clinical Dementia Rating (CDR): Current vision and scoring rules. *Neurology, 43,* 2412–2414. doi:10.1212/WNL.43.11.2412-a

Pangman, V.C., Sloan, J., & Guse, L. (2000). An examination of psychometric properties of the Mini-Mental State Examination and the Standardized Mini-Mental State Examination: Implications for clinical practice. *Applied Nursing Research, 13,* 209–2013. doi:10.1053/apnr.2000.9231

Rabinstein, A., & Rundek, T. (2013). Prediction of outcome after ischemic stroke: The value of clinical scores. *Neurology, 80,* 15–16. doi:10.1212/WNL.0b013e31827b1b5c

Rajput, A.H., & Rajput, A. (2014). Accuracy of Parkinson disease diagnosis unchanged in 2 decades. *Neurology, 83,* 386–387. doi:10.1212/WNL.0000000000000653

Rempe, D.A. (2014). Predicting outcomes after transient ischemic attack and stroke. *Continuum, 20,* 412–428. doi:10.1212/01.con.0000446110.97667.58

Sacco, R.L., Kasner, S.E., Broderick, J.P., Caplan, L.R., Connors, J.J., Culebras, A., … Vinters, H.V. (2013). An updated definition of stroke for the 21st century: A statement for healthcare professionals from the American Heart Association/American Stroke Association. *Stroke, 44,* 2064–2089. doi:10.1161/STR.0b013e318296aeca

Samson, K. (2014). How to prevent falls in Parkinson's patients? A new consensus document offers tips. *Neurology Today, 14*(12), 1, 13–16. doi:10.1097/01.NT.0000451829.59576.c3

Schmidt, M., Jacobsen, J.B., Johnsen, S.P., Bøtker, H.E., & Sørensen, H.T. (2014). Eighteen-year trends in stroke mortality and prognostic influence of comorbidity. *Neurology, 82,* 340–350. doi:10.1212/WNL.0000000000000062

Schrag, A., Horsfall, L., Walters, K., Noyce, A., & Petersen, I. (2015). Prediagnostic presentations of Parkinson's disease in primary care: A case-control study. *Lancet Neurology, 14,* 57–64. doi:10.1016/S1474-4422(14)70287-X

Sepulcre, J., Sabuncu, M.R., Becker, A., Sperling, R., & Johnson, K.A. (2013). *In vivo* characterization of the early states of the amyloid-beta network. *Brain, 136,* 2239–2252. doi:10.1093/brain/awt146

Silver, D.E., & Ruggieri, S. (1998). Initiating therapy for Parkinson's disease. *Neurology, 50*(Suppl. 6), S18–S22. doi:10.1212/WNL.50.6_Suppl_6.S18

Talan, J. (2014). The how and why behind the newest AD prevention trial. *Neurology Today, 14*(8), 12–14. doi:10.1097/01.NT.0000446541.49527.34

Toledo, J.B., Arnold, S.E., Raible, K., Brettschneider, J., Xie, S.X., Grossman, M., … Trojanowski, J.Q. (2013). Contribution of cerebrovascular disease in autopsy confirmed neurodegenerative disease cases in the National Alzheimer's Coordinating Centre. *Brain, 136,* 2697–2706. doi:10.1093/brain/awt188

Section IV.

Symptom Management

CHAPTER 19

Anxiety

Kristi A. Acker, DNP, FNP-BC, AOCNP®, ACHPN

I. Definition
   A. The number of Americans suffering from debilitating multiple chronic conditions (MCCs) continues to rise. Despite the plethora of literature concerning the psychological manifestations that accompany MCCs, a deficit remains by healthcare providers in recognizing and managing prevalent psychological symptoms in the primary care setting (Haws, 2015).
   B. Many patients experience worries and fears related to physical and psychological decline that do not escalate to the level of pathologic anxiety. Patients will experience anxious feelings that readily subside once the perceived threat is removed or an adjustment period has taken place (Haws, 2015; Kessler, Chiu, Demler, Merikangas, & Walters, 2005).
      1. Depending on the severity of symptoms and the patient's perceived effect on quality of life, initial healthcare provider response consists of reassurance of provider support and presence, with open dialogue concerning the anticipated disease progression.
      2. Patients and caregivers often minimize or fail to report anxiety symptoms to their healthcare providers, assuming that the symptoms they experience are inevitably a result of normal disease progression.
      3. Because of the complex and often mixed-state anxiety symptoms reported in patients with MCCs, providers have a difficult task of distinguishing symptoms related to psychological distress from those of underlying somatic disease burden.
      4. Disparities in provider education and support and community resources contribute to underrecognition and undertreatment of anxiety disorders in primary care.
      5. Certain societal and cultural populations interpret anxious behaviors favorably and consider the symptoms to be a normal and accepted part of life and, at times, even motivational.
      6. Societal acceptance, in conjunction with the societal stigma of mental health disorders, further complicates timely diagnosis and management of comorbid anxiety in patients with MCCs.
   C. Occasional worry is a normal phenomenon; approximately 18% of the general U.S. population suffers from potentially pathologic anxiety disorders annually (Kessler et al., 2005).
      1. In the United States, anxiety disorders are the most common mental health problem in primary care (Kavan, Elsasser, & Barone, 2009; Tone, 2005; Weisberg, Beard, Moitra, Dyck, & Keller, 2014).

2. Women are twice as likely as men to be diagnosed with anxiety. Men with unmanaged anxiety disorder are more likely than women to have the comorbidity of substance misuse (Cape, Chan, Lovell, Leibowitz, & Kendall, 2011; Davidson, Feltner, & Dugar, 2010; Kavan et al., 2009; Kessler et al., 2005).

   a) If left untreated, anxiety negatively affects patient quality of life, educational or workforce functioning (increased absenteeism), and family or social relationships (Rovira et al., 2012).

   b) Poorly managed or underdiagnosed anxiety disorders result in an increased use of healthcare services and community resources (Kavan et al., 2009).

   c) Patients with untreated anxiety combined with chronic disease have poorer quality of life and outcomes including intensified somatic symptoms, lower use of disease self-management practices, and increased health complications (Haws, 2015).

   d) Anxiety disorders are not always related to somatic conditions and may include psychological, spiritual, or social origins.

   e) A number of patients who suffer from anxiety disorders are clinically managed by primary care providers (Baldwin, 2015; Barry, 2012; Cape et al., 2011). Primary care is usually the first point of contact for patients with anxiety disorders (Weisberg et al., 2014).

   f) According to the Anxiety and Depression Association of America (2014), generalized anxiety disorder (GAD) affects 6.8 million Americans and is characterized by unprovoked excessive worry and tension (usually more intense than the situation warrants) related to a variety of problems for at least six months.

   g) Patients with GAD maintain unrealistic views concerning money, health, and family well-being without any clear indication of underlying problems (Rovira et al., 2012).

D. Clinical management of anxiety disorders is vital for palliation in patients with MCCs, and patient symptoms should routinely be reassessed throughout the disease trajectory.

   1. In addition, primary care providers should be prepared to recognize and offer strategies for GAD management to reduce this health burden.

   2. To develop a proper treatment plan, healthcare providers must be able to delineate like symptoms associated with other anxiety conditions such as panic, post-trauma, stress, adjustment, and social disorders, among others.

E. GAD is the most common mental health disorder in primary care, affecting 1%–12% of the general population (Baldwin, 2015; Barry, 2012; Davidson et al., 2010).

F. Historically, GAD is believed to only occur early in life, but recent findings indicate that GAD is increasingly reported in adults aged 65 years and older. The 12-year incidence rate of developing late-onset GAD is 8.4% (Zhang et al., 2015).

   1. Late-onset GAD usually results in a more favorable prognosis (Kessler et al., 2005; Turk & Mennin, 2011).

   2. In the older adult population, GAD is the most common mental health disorder (Baldwin, 2015).

   3. GAD has been linked to cardiovascular disease in addition to gastrointestinal and chronic pain disorders (Davidson et al., 2010).

   4. Comorbid GAD and depression significantly decreases the odds of recovery and increases the time for pharmacologic response, resulting in a more chronic course of treatment (Kessler et al., 2008).

     5. Patients with GAD overuse healthcare services and negatively affect workforce productivity, generating higher health costs (Rovira et al., 2012).

     6. GAD accounts for 30% of mental health disorders seen in general practice (Kessler et al., 2005), and 66% of patients with GAD have a minimum of one concurrent disorder (Baldwin, 2015).

     7. Predictors of GAD (Baldwin, 2015)
  - *a)* Female gender
  - *b)* Poverty
  - *c)* Low affective support in childhood
  - *d)* Recent adverse life events
  - *e)* Family history of psychiatric disorders
  - *f)* Chronic physical or psychological illness
  - *g)* Parental and familial factors

II. Pathophysiology

  A. Defining a specific pathophysiology of anxiety can be challenging. Anxiety is thought to be multidimensional and include one or a combination of genetic, neurobiologic, and environmental influences or etiologies, which only adds to the complexity of the disorder.

  B. Genetic influences and the impact on rates of occurrence for patients suffering from GAD are inconclusive.

  C. Some commonalities identified that point to a genetic link in patients with GAD include a family history of major depression and personal neuroticism.

     1. Evidence suggests a greater frequency of specific serotonin transporter gene-linked polymorphic region SS genotypes in patients with known GAD.

     2. In addition, patients may be more susceptible to GAD if variations in two subtypes of the glutamic acid decarboxylase gene are evident (Baldwin, 2015).

  D. Neuropsychological factors have been recognized in patients with GAD with hyper-responses to threatening situations, often with misinterpretation of the significance of the situation that can result in emotional distress.

     1. Abnormalities in neurotransmitters or modulators such as norepinephrine, serotonin, adenosine, cholecystokinin, and gamma-aminobutyric acid have been isolated.

     2. In these patients, psychological and pharmacologic interventions, such as selective serotonin reuptake inhibitors (SSRIs), among others, have been successful.

     3. Additional study findings have demonstrated that patients with GAD have consistent cerebral metabolic variation patterns when undergoing positron-emission tomography scans and identified enhanced anticipatory activity on magnetic resonance imaging studies (Baldwin, 2015).

  E. Environmental factors such as high occupational, social, and physical stress have been identified in patients with GAD. In particular, competitive societal demands, early exposure to significant life stress, and overly protective or hypercritical parents have been identified as risk factors (McGrandles & McCaig, 2010).

III. Presenting symptoms

  A. Patients with MCCs do not recognize symptoms of anxiety or depression and can associate distressing physiologic symptoms with the usual disease trajectory.

     1. Family and caregivers are more apt to raise concerns regarding patient distress burden than the patient.

     2. Healthcare providers should include not only the patient but also family members and caregivers (with patient consent) when collecting a medical history.

B. Healthcare providers can interpret distressing anxiety symptoms as somatic conditions, further complicating the identification of GAD.

C. Presenting symptoms of comorbid anxiety can be varied in populations that are vulnerable to multiple underlying chronic conditions.

1. Symptoms most commonly reported by patients with GAD include restlessness, poor concentration, sleep disturbance, irritability, apprehension, difficulty relaxing, muscle tension, fatigue, nausea, and diarrhea. Additionally, headaches and neck pain are commonly reported.

2. Additional symptoms commonly reported by patients and caregivers and observed by healthcare providers in patients with anxiety disorders include diaphoresis, tachycardia, tachypnea, and cognitive disturbances.

3. A thorough review of symptoms must be elicited from the patient (preferably in combination with family and caregivers) to distinguish presenting symptoms related to anxious etiologies from symptoms that may be attributable to lifestyle factors such as steroid use, substance misuse, caffeine consumption, and nicotine dependence.

IV. Physical examination: Much like the need for a thorough patient history, healthcare providers should perform a detailed physical when assessing patients for anxiety disorders.

A. General: Overall appearance is necessary to document at baseline.

1. Specifically, patients with GAD may appear restless, nervous, and shaky and may display anxious behavior such as nail biting and hand wringing.

2. Poor personal hygiene also may be evident.

3. Providers should perform a functional assessment at baseline to evaluate response to treatment and monitor for adverse effects of treatment.

a) Neurologic: In addition to the psychological distress symptoms already mentioned, providers may observe confusion, cognitive impairments, and an exaggerated startle response in patients with GAD (especially in the vulnerable older adult population).

b) Providers should pay special attention to patients' mood, affect, speech patterns, and judgment.

B. Head, ears, eyes, nose, and throat: Neck pain or tenderness, along with muscle tension, is commonly seen in patients with GAD.

C. Cardiovascular: Tachycardia and hypertension can be recorded in patients with GAD along with adrenergic effects such as irregular heartbeat, palpitations, shortness of breath, and diaphoresis.

D. Respiratory: Tachypnea and bronchial airway constriction (asthma) have been observed in patients with GAD.

E. Gastrointestinal and genitourinary: Diarrhea and emesis can be observed in patients with GAD; however, nausea is more commonly reported in the literature (along with diarrhea) than emesis.

F. Musculoskeletal: Limited range of motion could be observed related to chronic pain and muscle tension experienced in patients with GAD.

G. Dermatologic: Hives and urticaria may be present.

V. Diagnostics

A. Laboratory findings: Evaluate for endocrine disorders, electrolyte imbalance, and other abnormalities.

B. Anxiety disorders are frequently seen in patients with comorbid depression.

1. Healthcare providers should screen patients for both conditions periodically.

2. A brief depression screening tool is the Patient Health Questionnaire for Depression and Anxiety (PHQ-4 or PHQ-9) (Kroenke & Spitzer, 2002; see Figure 19-1).

Figure 19-1. Patient Health Questionnaire-9 (PHQ-9)				
Over the last 2 weeks, how often have you been bothered by any of the following problems? (Use "✓" to indicate your answer)	**Not at all**	**Several days**	**More than half the days**	**Nearly every day**
1. Little interest or pleasure in doing things	0	1	2	3
2. Feeling down, depressed, or hopeless	0	1	2	3
3. Trouble falling or staying asleep, or sleeping too much	0	1	2	3
4. Feeling tired or having little energy	0	1	2	3
5. Poor appetite or overeating	0	1	2	3
6. Feeling bad about yourself — or that you are a failure or have let yourself or your family down	0	1	2	3
7. Trouble concentrating on things, such as reading the newspaper or watching television	0	1	2	3
8. Moving or speaking so slowly that other people could have noticed? Or the opposite — being so fidgety or restless that you have been moving around a lot more than usual	0	1	2	3
9. Thoughts that you would be better off dead or of hurting yourself in some way	0	1	2	3
FOR OFFICE CODING	0 +	_____ +	_____ +	_____
				= Total Score: _____
If you checked off <u>any</u> problems, how <u>difficult</u> have these problems made it for you to do your work, take care of things at home, or get along with other people?				
Not difficult at all ☐	**Somewhat difficult** ☐	**Very difficult** ☐	**Extremely difficult** ☐	
PHQ-9 Scores and Proposed Treatment Actions*				
PHQ-9 Score	**Depression Severity**	**Proposed Treatment Actions**		
0–4	None–minimal	None		
5–9	Mild	Watchful waiting; repeat PHQ-9 at follow-up		
10–14	Moderate	Treatment plan, considering counseling, follow-up and/or pharmacotherapy		
15–19	Moderately severe	Active treatment with pharmacotherapy and/or psychotherapy		
20–27	Severe	Immediate initiation of pharmacotherapy and, if severe impairment or poor response to therapy, expedited referral to a mental health specialist for psychotherapy and/or collaborative management		

* From Kroenke & Spitzer, 2002.

Note. Developed by Drs. Robert L. Spitzer, Janet B.W. Williams, Kurt Kroenke and colleagues, with an educational grant from Pfizer Inc. Retrieved from http://www.phqscreeners.com. No permission required to reproduce, translate, display, or distribute.

C. A valid and reliable screening tool for GAD is the seven-question General Anxiety Disorder Scale (GAD-7) (Spitzer, Kroenke, Williams, & Löwe, 2006; see Figure 19-2).

D. The Hamilton Rating Scale for Anxiety, or HAM-A, is considered the gold standard for GAD symptom severity (see Figure 19-3).

1. This rating scale can better assist healthcare providers in discerning between anxiety and depression (Vaccarino, Evans, Sills, & Kalali, 2008).

2. *Diagnostic and Statistical Manual of Mental Disorders* (DSM-5) criteria for GAD (American Psychiatric Association, 2013; Mayo Clinic, 2014)

   a) Excessive anxiety and worry about several events or activities most days of the week for at least six months

   b) Difficulty controlling feelings of worry

   c) At least three of the following symptoms in adults and one of the following in children: Restlessness, fatigue, trouble concentrating, irritability, muscle tension, or sleep disturbance

   d) Anxiety or worry that causes significant distress that interferes with or impairs social, occupational, or other areas of functioning

   e) Disturbances not attributable to other psychological, substance, or somatic conditions

Figure 19-2. GAD-7 Anxiety Scale				
Over the last 2 weeks, how often have you been bothered by the following problems? (Use "✓" to indicate your answer)	**Not at All**	**Several Days**	**More Than Half the Days**	**Nearly Every Day**
1. Feeling nervous, anxious or on edge	0	1	2	3
2. Not being able to stop or control worrying	0	1	2	3
3. Worrying too much about different things	0	1	2	3
4. Trouble relaxing	0	1	2	3
5. Being so restless that it is hard to sit still	0	1	2	3
6. Becoming easily annoyed or irritable	0	1	2	3
7. Feeling afraid as if something awful might happen	0	1	2	3
(For office coding: Total Score T____ = ____ + ____ + ____)				

GAD-7 anxiety severity is calculated by assigning scores of 0, 1, 2, and 3, to the response categories of "not at all," "several days," "more than half the days," and "nearly every day," respectively. GAD-7 total score for the seven items ranges from 0 to 21. Scores of 5, 10, and 15 represent cutpoints for mild, moderate, and severe anxiety, respectively. Though designed primarily as a screening and severity measure for generalized anxiety disorder, the GAD-7 also has moderately good operating characteristics for three other common anxiety disorders—panic disorder, social anxiety disorder, and post-traumatic stress disorder. When screening for anxiety disorders, a recommended cutpoint for further evaluation is a score of 10 or greater.

Note. Developed by Drs. Robert L. Spitzer, Janet B.W. Williams, Kurt Kroenke and colleagues, with an educational grant from Pfizer Inc. Retrieved from http://www.phqscreeners.com. No permission required to reproduce, translate, display, or distribute.

Figure 19-3. Hamilton Anxiety Rating Scale (HAM-A)

Below is a list of phrases that describe certain feeling that people have. Rate the patients by finding the answer which best describes the extent to which he/she has these conditions. Select one of the five responses for each of the fourteen questions.

0 = Not present,   1 = Mild,   2 = Moderate,   3 = Severe,   4 = Very severe.

---

1   Anxious mood   [0] [1] [2] [3] [4]

Worries, anticipation of the worst, fearful anticipation, irritability.

2   Tension   [0] [1] [2] [3] [4]

Feelings of tension, fatigability, startle response, moved to tears easily, trembling, feelings of restlessness, inability to relax.

3   Fears   [0] [1] [2] [3] [4]

Of dark, of strangers, of being left alone, of animals, of traffic, of crowds.

4   Insomnia   [0] [1] [2] [3] [4]

Difficulty in falling asleep, broken sleep, unsatisfying sleep and fatigue on waking, dreams, nightmares, night terrors.

5   Intellectual   [0] [1] [2] [3] [4]

Difficulty in concentration, poor memory.

6   Depressed mood   [0] [1] [2] [3] [4]

Loss of interest, lack of pleasure in hobbies, depression, early waking, diurnal swing.

7   Somatic (muscular)   [0] [1] [2] [3] [4]

Pains and aches, twitching, stiffness, myoclonic jerks, grinding of teeth, unsteady voice, increased muscular tone.

8   Somatic (sensory)   [0] [1] [2] [3] [4]

Tinnitus, blurring of vision, hot and cold flushes, feelings of weakness, pricking sensation.

9   Cardiovascular symptoms   [0] [1] [2] [3] [4]

Tachycardia, palpitations, pain in chest, throbbing of vessels, fainting feelings, missing beat.

10   Respiratory symptoms   [0] [1] [2] [3] [4]

Pressure or constriction in chest, choking feelings, sighing, dyspnea.

11   Gastrointestinal symptoms   [0] [1] [2] [3] [4]

Difficulty in swallowing, wind abdominal pain, burning sensations, abdominal fullness, nausea, vomiting, borborygmi, looseness of bowels, loss of weight, constipation.

12   Genitourinary symptoms   [0] [1] [2] [3] [4]

Frequency of micturition, urgency of micturition, amenorrhea, menorrhagia, development of frigidity, premature ejaculation, loss of libido, impotence.

13   Autonomic symptoms   [0] [1] [2] [3] [4]

Dry mouth, flushing, pallor, tendency to sweat, giddiness, tension headache, raising of hair.

14   Behavior at interview   [0] [1] [2] [3] [4]

Fidgeting, restlessness or pacing, tremor of hands, furrowed brow, strained face, sighing or rapid respiration, facial pallor, swallowing, etc.

Note. From "The Assessment of Anxiety States by Rating," by M. Hamilton, 1959, *British Journal of Medical Psychology, 32,* pp. 50–55. This material is in the public domain.

---

3. Healthcare providers should refer to the DSM-5 for a full listing of diagnostic criteria.

VI. Differential diagnosis
   A. One of the most challenging and complex aspects for healthcare providers in identifying patients with GAD is differentiating it from other disorders.
   B. Differentials
      1. Other somatic disorders
      2. Depression, which is difficult to distinguish from GAD and is often seen as a comorbid condition with GAD. However, the following symptoms are more specific to depressive disorders: early morning awakening, diurnal variation in mood, and suicidal thoughts (Baldwin, 2015).
      3. Delirium
      4. Chronic stress
      5. Other anxiety disorders, such as panic disorder, obsessive compulsive disorder, and adjustment disorder
      6. Nutritional deficiencies, specifically elemental deficiencies
      7. Hypochondriasis, which presents as excessive worry about one's personal medical condition, whereas in GAD, patients are concerned about multiple things in addition to health and are more focused on others than self

8. Endocrine disturbances such as hyperthyroidism, which can clinically present with many of the same nonspecific patient complaints as in GAD, as well as hormonal imbalances
9. Neurologic conditions
10. Cardiac abnormalities
11. Pulmonary diseases
12. Substance use and self-medication, especially in patients who may misuse alcohol, prescription drugs, caffeine, and nicotine

VII. Interventions

A. After a diagnosis of GAD, it is necessary that healthcare providers, when possible, proceed with a collaborative approach when developing a plan for management, with patient-centered care being the primary objective.
   1. If GAD and depression coexist, then healthcare providers must decide which condition would be best addressed initially.
   2. Often, if distressing symptoms from anxiety are well managed, the patient's depressive symptoms are alleviated or much improved.

B. The effectiveness of treatment for GAD is dependent on the healthcare provider's awareness of current guidelines for both psychological and pharmacologic management (Haws, 2015).

C. GAD management can be approached on many fronts.
   1. Cognitive behavioral therapy (CBT) and pharmacologic interventions are considered first-line approaches and offer successful patient outcomes.
   2. The National Institute for Health and Care Excellence (NICE, formerly the National Institute for Health and Clinical Excellence) recommends a stepped care approach that maintains patient choice as a priority in the management decision-making process (Cape et al., 2011; NICE, 2011).
   3. The least intrusive, most effective intervention should be offered initially (Cape et al., 2011; NICE, 2011). Healthcare providers should reference the comprehensive NICE stepped care model for complete guideline recommendations.
   4. Either treatment option can be initiated as monotherapy or in combination.
   5. Combination therapy has been beneficial in patients who have prior pharmacologic responses, severe and debilitating symptoms accompanied by other comorbidities, or a lack of adequate response to monotherapy (Davidson et al., 2010).

D. Treatment interventions, including the benefits, limitations, and duration, need to be communicated.
   1. Collaboration with patients and caregivers will improve the likelihood of treatment adherence and response.
   2. Because both CBT and pharmacologic approaches have proved beneficial in managing CBT, patient preference should be a priority and respected by the healthcare provider in deciding the initial course of action (Bandelow, Lichte, Rudolf, Wiltink, & Beutel, 2014; Hofmann, Wu, Boettcher, & Strum, 2014).

E. Healthcare providers beginning pharmacologic intervention in the older adult population must carefully consider the increased risk for fall and osteoporotic fractures (Davidson et al., 2010).
   1. If pharmacologic intervention is warranted, thoughtful consideration as to potential drug–drug interactions, contraindications, and concurrent medical conditions is needed.

2. In addition, patients should be counseled on initiation and adherence to the medication regimen along with thorough education on the potential side effects and the monitoring requirements that may be indicated.
3. Other patient considerations prior to pharmacologic interventions
    a) Underlying illness and prognosis
    b) Presence of comorbidities
    c) Medical frailty
    d) General psychosocial and physical status
    e) Patient and caregiver wishes and goals
    f) Community resources
    g) Intervention costs
    h) Outcomes of prior therapies
F. Considerations for GAD intervention
    1. Physiologic therapy
        a) CBT has been shown to be both effective and sustainable in managing GAD (Norton et al., 2013). For any patient diagnosed with GAD, psychological interventions should be offered (Bandelow et al., 2012).
        b) CBT is intended to focus on the "here and now" problems rather than past influences (Haws, 2015).
        c) In the older adult population (older than 65 years old), CBT has demonstrated lower efficacy (Bandelow et al., 2012).
        d) CBT can be offered face to face or as computerized programs that can be navigated independently or with support.
        e) CBT is considered a time-limited treatment and generally lasts for three to four months.
        f) Unfortunately, time constraints and limited access to community resources serve as barriers for physiologic therapy recommendations in primary care.
    2. Pharmacotherapy (Healthcare providers should refer to drug package inserts for full prescribing recommendations, U.S. Food and Drug Administration approvals, side effects, and contraindications.)
        a) SSRIs such as citalopram, escitalopram, paroxetine, and sertraline are considered first-line pharmacologic treatment for GAD.
            (1) Side effects of SSRIs are varied and include sexual dysfunction, nausea, diarrhea, insomnia, and discontinuation withdrawal.
            (2) Bystritsky (2016) suggested that SSRIs such as fluoxetine and fluvoxamine are also effective in managing GAD.
            (3) The average onset of action for SSRIs is four weeks. Citalopram has demonstrated to be preferable in older patients (Davidson et al., 2010).
        b) Serotonin–norepinephrine reuptake inhibitors (SNRIs) such as duloxetine and venlafaxine may offer a better overall safety and tolerability profile than older antidepressants and are suitable to use in patients with chronic health conditions such as cardiovascular disease and chronic obstructive pulmonary disease.
            (1) Side effects may include nausea, dizziness, insomnia, sedation, sweating, and constipation.
            (2) SNRIs' efficacy and tolerability are comparable to those of SSRIs. However, elevations in blood pressure have been reported. Venlafaxine may cause elevated blood pressure in higher dosages (greater

than 300 mg/day). Both duloxetine and venlafaxine should be monitored closely in patients with hypertension (Bystritsky, 2016; Davidson et al., 2010).

(3) Both SSRIs and SNRIs are considered first-line pharmacologic options for managing GAD. Initiating the lowest effective dosage should be considered in order to avoid unnecessary adverse effects. With either class, treatment should be continued for 12 months to minimize the risk for relapse (Fricchione, 2004).

c) Benzodiazepines are rapid and highly effective treatment options for GAD but require caution and careful consideration, as well as a thorough risk-benefit analysis, prior to use in older adult patient populations (Barry, 2012).

(1) Benzodiazepines should not be considered for long-term use.

(2) Sorsdahl et al. (2013) reported that providers used benzodiazepines more frequently than SSRIs and SNRIs in the management of GAD.

(3) However, concomitant treatment can be beneficial in acutely managing distressing anxious symptoms while awaiting the onset of SSRIs or SNRIs.

(4) Side effects of benzodiazepines may include sedation, memory complications, and risk for addiction.

(5) Oxazepam, lorazepam, and temazepam are better choices for patients on multiple medications or methadone or have liver dysfunction (Bystritsky, 2016).

(6) Benzodiazepines are approved for use as monotherapy in the absence of comorbid mood disorders.

d) Although not a first-line option, buspirone has been shown to be helpful for managing GAD in the absence of comorbid major depression and is nonaddictive (Bystritsky, 2016).

e) Likewise, calcium modulators, such as pregabalin, have shown effectiveness in managing GAD symptoms as second-line treatment (Bandelow et al., 2012).

f) Tricyclic antidepressants (TCAs) are less tolerable than other acceptable pharmacologic interventions for managing GAD and have been shown to be cardiotoxic and carry an increased risk for drug–drug interactions.

(1) Additionally, TCAs should be avoided in patients at risk for suicide (Bandelow et al., 2012).

(2) TCAs are considered second-line therapy and are not recommended for use in primary care settings.

g) Some antihistamines, such as hydroxyzine, have been reported to be effective treatment in patients with GAD, although they are not a first-line recommendation (Davidson et al., 2010).

3. Although their safety is not proven, complementary therapies may be beneficial in managing GAD.

a) Many complementary therapies exist, including music and art therapy, relaxation or massage therapy, aromatherapy, acupuncture, and hypnosis.

b) Herbal supplements also have been used in patients with GAD, including kava extract (which may cause hepatotoxicity), valerian, St. John's wort, and passion flower.

c) Insufficient evidence exists as to their effectiveness in managing the distressing symptoms of GAD.

      d) Providers should be cautious when considering these interventions without supportive data to ensure safety and efficacy (Zoberi & Pollard, 2010).

    4. Exercise (sometimes referred to as endurance training) is considered a natural mood enhancer. When it is slowly incorporated, patients may find an increase in functional capacity, leading to improved well-being and less anxious symptomology. Exercise should be given as an adjunct treatment recommendation to other standard interventions for managing GAD (Bandelow et al., 2012).

G. Evaluation and follow-up

    1. Effective communication is the mainstay when evaluating patient response to interventions in managing GAD. Reassessment on a routine basis also is necessary for proper and sustainable management of anxiety.

    2. If patients have demonstrated little to no response to first-line treatment with monotherapy CBT, combining treatment with an SSRI or SRNI is recommended.

        a) Once pharmacotherapy has been implemented, and no response occurs within four weeks of initiation, the healthcare provider should slowly escalate the starting dose.

        b) If the patient still shows little to no improvement in symptoms, a different SSRI or augment to the current treatment plan is warranted.

H. Referrals

    1. Refractory anxiety or worsening anxiety complaints by patients despite provider interventions should result in referral to a mental health specialist.

    2. Likewise, patients with severe anxiety with comorbid major depressive disorders or patients with a high risk for suicide or who exhibit negativity and hopelessness should be considered for urgent referral.

    3. Other indications for mental health specialist referral include patients with significant disease burden; current or prior substance misuse, including alcohol or prescription drugs; prior history of suicidal ideation; patients who have complex anxiety symptoms with increasing personal stress; and patients who have not responded to treatment interventions in the past.

    4. Both patients and caregivers need to be made aware to report any acute mood changes and expressions of hopelessness or suicidal ideations emergently. This is especially important with any recent pharmacologic changes (NICE, 2011).

Case Study

A.F. is a 62-year-old woman with a history of an early-stage right breast cancer diagnosed in 2001. She successfully completed adjuvant endocrine therapy; however, in 2012, she was diagnosed with multiple myeloma. Although treatment (including systemic therapy and bone marrow transplant) was lengthy and challenging, A.F. experienced a complete remission and continues to follow routinely with her oncologist without any evidence of disease. A.F.'s medical history includes hypertension, hypercholesterolemia, breast cancer, multiple myeloma, and peripheral neuropathy. Current medications include lisinopril and hydrochlorothiazide 20 mg/12.5 mg/day, aspirin 81 mg/day, simvastatin 20 mg/day, and a multivitamin daily. She does not report drug allergies and denies a history of depression, drug abuse (including self-medication), or suicidal ideation.

A.F. comes to the primary care clinic to discuss with the advanced practice registered nurse (APRN) her concerns about not sleeping well and always feeling tired. A.F. tells the APRN that she has been overly worried that her cancer will return and she will cause "too much stress" on her family, especially her husband. A.F. reports that she shared these concerns with her visit to oncology approximately six months ago. She stated, "I know this scenario sounds unreasonable, but I can't stop worrying." A.F. is concerned that if her cancer returns, she will cause her family to have financial problems and that she has already caused her family enough stress from her prior illnesses. A.F. states that she is not sleeping because of her continuous thoughts of her cancer returning, and she does not know how she would tell her family she has cancer "again."

The APRN reviews the medical records, and the oncologist will plan a six-month follow-up. Laboratory findings for myeloma surveillance remain negative. The laboratory work obtained today from the APRN (including a complete blood count, comprehensive metabolic panel, thyroid-stimulating hormone, and free T4 levels) were normal. The APRN considers a diagnosis of GAD and discusses this with A.F. The APRN reviews the symptoms of GAD and depression with A.F. After the discussion, A.F. agrees to complete GAD-7 and PHQ-9 screening and scores 13 and 5, respectively. This places A.F. in the parameters for moderate anxiety and minimal depression. The APRN discusses treatment options with A.F., including CBT (facilitated or self-guided) and treatment with an SSRI. The potential adverse effects (including the expected treatment duration before symptoms would be expected to improve) are explored. The APRN recommends investigating a cancer support group in addition to CBT and SSRI treatment. A.F. is also reassured that the APRN, along with the oncologist, would keep close surveillance and would be available to her when needed or if problems were to arise.

After careful consideration, A.F. elects to proceed with counseling and agrees to participate in guided CBT sessions. A.F. voices concerns about the potential cost associated with beginning another medication. Based on the PHQ score in addition to A.F.'s denial of having suicidal ideations or a medical history of depression, the APRN and A.F. elect a conservative approach to management. The APRN encourages A.F. to be consistent with her CBT sessions and shares that depressive symptoms often resolve for many patients who show response to treatment for GAD. Follow-up is then scheduled for six weeks after the start of CBT sessions. The APRN details a plan to discuss the addition of an SSRI if needed (with drug assistance exploration if necessary). In addition, the APRN contacts the oncology social worker to help educate A.F. on cancer survivor support group resources in her area.

References

American Psychiatric Association. (2013). *Diagnostic and statistical manual of mental disorders* (5th ed.). Washington, DC: Author.

Anxiety and Depression Association of America. (2014). Facts and statistics. Retrieved from http://www.adaa .org/about-adaa/Press-room/facts-statistics

Baldwin, D. (2015, July 23). Generalized anxiety disorder in adults: Epidemiology, pathogenesis, clinical manifestations, course, assessment, and diagnosis [Literature review current through March 2016]. Retrieved from http://www.uptodate.com/contents/generalized-anxiety-disorder-in-adults-epidemiology-pathogenesis -clinical-manifestations-course-assessment-and-diagnosis

Bandelow, B., Lichte, T., Rudolf, S., Wiltink, J., & Beutel, M.E. (2014). The diagnosis of and treatment recommendations for anxiety disorders. *Deutsches Ärzteblatt International, 111,* 473–480. doi:10.3238/arztebl.2014.0473

Bandelow, B., Sher, L., Bunevicius, R., Hollander, E., Kasper, S., Zohar, J., & Möller, H.-J. (2012). Guidelines for the pharmacological treatment of anxiety disorders, obsessive-compulsive disorders and posttraumatic stress disorder in primary care. *International Journal of Psychiatry in Clinical Practice, 16,* 77–84. doi:10.3109/ 13651501.2012.667114

Barry, M.J. (2012). Generalized anxiety disorder: Helping patients overcome worry. *Current Psychiatry, 11*(5), 40–44.

Bystritsky, A. (2016, March 18). Pharmacotherapy for generalized anxiety disorder in adults [Literature review current through March 2016]. Retrieved from http://www.uptodate.com/contents/pharmacotherapy-for-generalized-anxiety-disorder-in-adults

Cape, J., Chan, M., Lovell, K., Leibowitz, J., & Kendall, T. (2011). Management of generalized anxiety disorder: The updated NICE guideline. *Healthcare Counselling and Psychotherapy Journal, 11*(2), 12–16.

Davidson, J.R.T., Feltner, D.E., & Dugar, A. (2010). Management of generalized anxiety disorder in primary care: Identifying the challenges and unmet needs. *Primary Care Companion to the Journal of Clinical Psychiatry, 12*(2), e1–e13. doi:10.4088/PCC.09r00772blu

Fricchione, G. (2004). Generalized anxiety disorder. *New England Journal of Medicine, 351,* 675–682. doi:10.1056/NEJMcp022342

Haws, J.M. (2015). Anxiety and depression: The hidden cost of long-term conditions. *Practice Nurse, 45*(4), 41–45.

Hofmann, S.G., Wu, J.Q., Boettcher, H., & Strum, J. (2014). Effect of pharmacotherapy for anxiety disorders on quality of life: A meta-analysis. *Quality of Life, 23,* 1141–1153. doi:10.1007/s11136-013-0573-8

Kavan, M.G., Elsasser, G., & Barone, E.J. (2009). Generalized anxiety disorder: Practical assessment and management. *American Family Physician, 79,* 785–791.

Kessler, R.C., Chiu, W.T., Demler, O., Merikangas, K.R., & Walters, E.E. (2005). Prevalence, severity, and comorbidity of 12-month DSM-IV disorders in the National Comorbidity Survey Replication. *Archives of General Psychiatry, 62,* 617–627. doi:10.1001/archpsyc.62.6.617

Kessler, R.C., Gruber, M., Hettema, J., Hwang, I., Sampson, N., & Yonkers, K.A. (2008). Co-morbid major depression and generalized anxiety disorders in the National Comorbidity Survey follow-up. *Psychological Medicine, 38,* 365–374. doi:10.1017/S0033291707002012

Kroenke, K., & Spitzer, R.L. (2002). The PHQ-9: A new depression and diagnostic severity measure. *Psychiatric Annals, 32,* 509–521. doi:10.3928/0048-5713-20020901-06

Mayo Clinic. (2014, September). Generalized anxiety disorder: Tests and diagnosis. Retrieved from http://www.mayoclinic.org/diseases-conditions/generalized-anxiety-disorder/basics/tests-diagnosis/con-20024562

McGrandles, A., & McCaig, M. (2010). Diagnosis and management of anxiety in primary care. *Nurse Prescribing, 8,* 311–318. doi:10.12968/npre.2010.8.7.48935

National Institute for Health and Care Excellence. (2011). *Generalised anxiety disorder and panic disorder in adults: Management.* Retrieved from https://www.nice.org.uk/guidance/cg113/resources/generalised-anxiety-disorder-and-panic-disorder-in-adults-management-35109387756997

Norton, P.J., Barrera, T.L., Mathew, A.R., Chamberlain, L.D., Szafranski, D.D., Reddy, R., & Smith, A.H. (2013). Effect of transdiagnostic CBT for anxiety disorders on comorbid diagnoses. *Depression and Anxiety, 30,* 168–173. doi:10.1002/da.22018

Rovira, J., Albarracin, G., Salvador, L., Rejas, J., Sánchez-Iriso, E., & Cabasés, J.M. (2012). The cost of generalized anxiety disorder in primary care settings: Results of the ANCORA study. *Community Mental Health Journal, 48,* 372–383. doi:10.1007/s10597-012-9503-4

Sorsdahl, K., Blanco, C., Rae, D.S., Pincus, H., Narrow, W.S., Suliman, S., & Stein, D.J. (2013). Treatment of anxiety disorders by psychiatrists from the American Psychiatric Practice Research Network. *Revista Brasileira de Psiquiatria, 35,* 136–141. doi:10.1590/1516-4446-2012-0978

Spitzer, R.L., Kroenke, K., Williams, J.B.W., & Löwe, B. (2006). A brief measure for assessing generalized anxiety disorder: The GAD-7. *Archives of Internal Medicine, 166,* 1092–1097. doi:10.1001/archinte.166.10.1092

Tone, A. (2005). Listening to the past: History, psychiatry, and anxiety. *Canadian Journal of Psychiatry, 50,* 373–380.

Turk, C.L., & Mennin, D.S. (2011). Phenomenology of generalized anxiety disorder. *Psychiatric Annals, 41,* 72–78. doi:10.3928/00485713-20110203-05

Vaccarino, A.L., Evans, K.R., Sills, T.L., & Kalali, A.H. (2008). Symptoms of anxiety in depression: Assessment of item performance of the Hamilton Anxiety Rating Scale in patients with depression. *Depression and Anxiety, 25,* 1006–1013. doi:10.1002/da.20435

Weisberg, R.B., Beard, C., Moitra, E., Dyck, I., & Keller, M.B. (2014). Adequacy of treatment received by primary care patients with anxiety disorders. *Depression and Anxiety, 31,* 443–450. doi:10.1002/da.22209

Zhang, X., Norton, J., Carrière, I., Ritchie, K., Chaudieu, I., & Ancelin, M.L. (2015). Risk factors for late-onset generalized anxiety disorder: Results from a 12-year prospective cohort (the ESPRIT study). *Translational Psychiatry, 5,* e536. doi:10.1038/tp.2015.31

Zoberi, K., & Pollard, C.A. (2010). Treating anxiety without SSRIs. *Journal of Family Practice, 59,* 148–154.

CHAPTER 20

Chronic Nonmalignant Pain

Kim Kuebler, DNP, APRN, ANP-BC,
Mary Atkinson Smith, DNP, FNP-BC, ONP-C, RNFA, CNOR,
Francois Prizinski, DPT, OCS, COMT, FAAOMPT, and Christopher Schuetz, DPT

I. Definition
   A. Chronic pain affects approximately 117 million American adults—more than the total affected by heart disease, cancer, and diabetes combined—according to a report by the Institute of Medicine (IOM, 2011).
      1. The economic burden of chronic pain costs the nation up to $635 billion each year in medical treatment and lost productivity (IOM, 2011).
      2. The 2010 Patient Protection and Affordable Care Act required the U.S. Department of Health and Human Services (DHHS) to examine chronic pain as a public health problem (IOM, 2011).
   B. In the United States, opioids are frequently prescribed for chronic noncancer pain. The Centers for Disease Control and Prevention estimate that 20% of patients who present to their primary care provider with a chief complaint of chronic pain or any pain-related diagnoses (including acute and chronic pain) receive an opioid prescription (Dowell, Haegerich, & Chou, 2016).
   C. In 2012, healthcare providers ordered more than 259 million individual prescriptions for opioid analgesics. This is enough for every adult in the United States to have a bottle of opioid analgesic medication (Dowell et al., 2016).
   D. Opioid prescriptions per capita in the United States increased 7.3% from 2007 to 2012. This escalation in opioid analgesic prescribing rates rose in primary care settings, including family practice, general practice, and internal medicine, compared to other medical specialties (Dowell et al., 2016).
   E. The lack of consensus by healthcare providers on the use of opioid analgesic prescribing is evident by the extensive variations across states and regions that cannot be explained by the underlying health status of the population (Dowell et al., 2016).
   F. The United States is experiencing an epidemic of opioid drug overdose deaths. Since 2000, the rate of drug-induced deaths increased 137%, with a 200% increase in the rate of opioid analgesic–related deaths, including heroin (Dowell et al., 2016).
   G. Pain is an unpleasant sensory or emotional experience associated with actual or potential tissue damage or described in terms of such damage (World Health Organization [WHO], 2008).

H. Chronic pain persists beyond three months following an injury and extends beyond the usual course of an acute disease or a reasonable time for a comparable injury to heal (International Association for the Study of Pain [IASP], 2009).

   1. Chronic pain is associated with chronic pathologic processes that cause continuous or intermittent pain for more than three months (IASP, 2009).
   2. IASP (2009) defines chronic pain as pain that persists beyond normal tissue healing time, extending past three months.
   3. Chronic pain may occur in the context of numerous diseases and syndromes (IASP, 2009).
   4. Chronic pain is described as persistent pain—a condition that can be continuous or recurrent and of sufficient duration and intensity to adversely affect a person's well-being, level of function, and quality of life (American Chronic Pain Association, 2012).
   5. Chronic pain has been defined as a complex condition with physical, psychological, emotional, and social components (WHO, 2008).

I. Pain that arises from actual or threatened damage to non-neural tissue and activation of nociceptors, a result of actual or potential damage to non-neural tissue, is categorized as visceral or somatic (Cohen & Mao, 2014).

J. Nociceptive pain is caused by damage to body tissue, and patients can subjectively describe their pain as sharp, aching, or throbbing. This kind of pain involves the bones, muscles, or joints or is created from blockage of an organ or blood vessels (American Chronic Pain Association, 2012).

K. Neuropathic pain occurs with nerve damage.

   1. Nerves connect the spinal cord to the rest of the body and allow the brain to communicate with the skin, muscles, and internal organs.
   2. Chronic conditions can precipitate neuropathic pain, such as diabetic neuropathies and other conditions that include autoimmune disease, spinal trauma, failed back surgery, and others. Patients describe this pain as a burning or heavy sensation, numbness, tingling, hot, and shooting along the path of the affected nerve (American Chronic Pain Association, 2012).

L. Chronic back or leg pain can arise from spinal diseases such as spondylosis, degenerative disc disease, epidural fibrosis, failed back surgery syndrome, lumbar disc herniation, osteoporosis, and spinal stenosis, among others (American Chronic Pain Association, 2012).

M. Complex regional pain syndrome (CRPS) is a chronic pain condition affecting one of the limbs (arms, legs, hands, or feet), usually after an injury or trauma to that limb (National Institute of Neurological Disorders and Stroke [NINDS], 2015).

   1. CRPS is believed to be caused by damage to or malfunction of the peripheral and central nervous systems.
   2. CRPS is characterized by prolonged or excessive pain and mild or significant changes in skin color, temperature, and edema in the affected area (NINDS, 2015).
   3. Two forms exist, called CRPS-I and CRPS-II, with common symptoms and treatments.
   4. CRPS-II (causalgia) is the term used to confirm nerve injuries. Patients without confirmed nerve injury are classified as having CRPS-I (reflex sympathetic dystrophy syndrome) (NINDS, 2015).
   5. Symptoms of CRPS (NINDS, 2015)

   a) Changes in skin texture on the affected area; may appear shiny and thin

   b) Abnormal sweating pattern in the affected area or surrounding areas

   c) Changes in nail and hair growth patterns

   d) Stiffness in affected joints

   e) Problems coordinating muscle movement, with decreased ability to move the affected body part

   f) Abnormal movement most often fixed abnormal posture (called *dystonia*), tremors, or jerking, can occur in the affected limb.

II. Pathophysiology

 A. Nociceptive pain can result from either nociceptive input from somatic tissues such as muscles, joints, and ligaments, or from visceral structures such as organs.

  1. Nociceptive pain requires transduction to convert a nonelectrical signal to an electrochemical one (National Research Council Committee on Recognition and Alleviation of Pain in Laboratory Animals, 2009).

  2. Nociceptive pain is attributable to pathophysiologic processes associated with the activation of the peripheral receptive terminals of primary afferent neurons (A delta and C fibers) in response to noxious chemical (inflammatory), mechanical, or thermal stimuli (National Research Council Committee on Recognition and Alleviation of Pain in Laboratory Animals, 2009).

  3. Chemically mediated nociception arises from the activation of nociceptors by proinflammatory mediators released in response to injury or pathology or by a lowering of tissue pH in response to tissue ischemia (Smart, Blake, Staines, Thacker, & Doody, 2012a).

 B. An injury to the peripheral or central nervous system results in maladaptive changes in neurons along the nociceptive pathway that can cause neuropathic pain (Cohen & Mao, 2014).

  1. Neuropathic pain is triggered by lesions to the somatosensory nervous system that alter the structure and function so that pain occurs spontaneously and responds to noxious and innocuous stimuli and are pathologically amplified (Costigan, Scholz, & Woolf, 2009).

  2. *Peripheral neuropathic pain* refers to pain attributable to a lesion or dysfunction in a peripheral nerve, dorsal root ganglion, or dorsal root arising from trauma, compression, inflammation, or ischemia (Smart, Blake, Staines, Thacker, & Doody, 2012b).

  3. Likely causes of peripheral neuropathic pain include entrapment neuropathies of spinal roots, dorsal root ganglia, or peripheral nerve branches.

  4. This type of pain is not a single mechanism but the product of a number of complex pathophysiologic processes that alter the structure and function of peripheral nerves and their central terminals in response to injury (Smart et al., 2012b).

  5. These pathophysiologic processes include sensitization of neural connective tissue nociceptors, ectopic excitability, cross excitation, structural changes, and neuroimmune interactions (Smart et al., 2012b).

 C. An increased sensitization of nociceptors, impaired intraneural circulation, and hypoxia in response to nerve injury can elicit an inflammatory response with neural connective tissues, causing sensitization of nociceptors in nervi nervorum and sinuvertebral nerves (Smart et al., 2012b).

 D. Amplifying nociceptive input following peripheral nerve injury by ectopic excitability and cross excitation produces an exacerbation of neuropathic pain.

1. Ectopic excitability is upregulation of ion channels at sites of nerve injury, leading to formation of abnormal impulse-generating sites, which fire spontaneously and independently of a peripheral stimulus.
2. These sites become thermo-, mechano-, or chemosensitive, causing injured nerves to become abnormally reactive to thermal, mechanical, or chemical stimuli (Smart et al., 2012b; Smart, Blake, Staines, Thacker, & Doody, 2012c).
3. After nerve injury, loss of inhibitory currents occurs as a result of dysfunctional gamma-aminobutyric acid production and release mechanisms, which results in apoptosis of spinal inhibitory interneurons (Janssen, Truin, Van Kleef, & Joosten, 2011).
4. These spinal interneurons synapse with central terminals of primary afferent neurons, thereby reducing their activity, and also regulate activity to ascending secondary order neurons (Cohen & Mao, 2014).

III. Presenting symptoms

    A. Depression and chronic pain often present as concomitant conditions and require prompt assessment to warrant optimal outcomes. Patients who are depressed can somatize (i.e., manifest psychological and emotional pain as physical pain).

    B. Body aches and pains are a common symptom of depression. Studies show that people with more severe depression have an increase in their pain intensity (National Institute of Mental Health [NIMH], 2015).

        1. According to recent evidence, people with depression have higher than normal levels of proteins called *cytokines*.

        2. Cytokines send messages to cells that affect how the immune system responds to infection and disease, including the strength and length of the response (NIMH, 2015).

            a) Cytokines can trigger pain by promoting inflammation, which is the body's response to infection or injury.

            b) Inflammation helps protect the body by destroying, removing, or isolating the infected or injured area (NIMH, 2015).

                (1) In addition to pain, signs of inflammation include swelling, redness, heat, and sometimes loss of function.

                (2) Many studies suggest that inflammation is a link between depression and chronic conditions (NIMH, 2015).

        3. Fibromyalgia has been shown to occur with depression.

            a) Fibromyalgia causes chronic generalized muscle and nerve pain that responds to light touch.

            b) Patients with this condition are more likely than the general population to have depression and other mental disorders (NIMH, 2015).

    C. The 2015 Sleep in America poll found that chronic pain, stress, and poor health were key correlates of shorter sleep durations and worse sleep quality (National Sleep Foundation [NSF], 2015).

        1. This survey indicated that almost one in four people with chronic pain (23%) said they had been diagnosed with a sleep disorder by a doctor, compared with just 6% of all others (NSF, 2015).

        2. Chronic pain triggers poor sleep. A patient who is experiencing low back pain can encounter several intense microarousals (a change in the sleep state to a lighter stage of sleep) per each hour of sleep, which lead to awakenings.

        3. Pain is a serious intrusion to sleep.

  a) Pain is frequently associated with insomnia, and these coexisting problems can be difficult to treat.

  b) One problem can exacerbate the other (NSF, 2015).

4. Quality of sleep in patients with chronic pain is often light and unrefreshing. This nonrestorative sleep pattern can then cause diminished energy, depressed mood, fatigue, and worsening pain during the day (NSF, 2015).

5. Patients with an anxiety disorder concomitant with chronic pain can be difficult to treat. Those who have chronic pain and an anxiety disorder may have a lower tolerance for pain (Anxiety and Depression Association of America, 2015).

6. People with an anxiety disorder may be more sensitive and fearful about medication side effects and more fearful of being in pain than someone who experiences pain without anxiety (Anxiety and Depression Association of America, 2015).

7. Concomitant anxiety, depression, and pain are particularly evident in chronic and sometimes disabling pain syndromes such as fibromyalgia, irritable bowel syndrome, low back pain, headaches, and neuropathic pain (Harvard Men's Health Watch, 2015).

8. Researchers evaluated 250 primary care patients who were being treated at a veterans' medical center in the Midwest. All patients had moderate to severe chronic joint or back pain that had lasted at least three months despite using pain medications (Kroenke et al., 2013).

  a) The participants were screened for five common anxiety disorders, including the following:

  (1) Generalized anxiety, characterized by persistent worry

  (2) Panic, or sudden, repeated attacks of fear

  (3) Social anxiety, characterized by overwhelming anxiety in everyday social interactions

  (4) Post-traumatic stress, or a concurrent feeling of danger or impending doom after a stressful event

  (5) Obsessive-compulsive disorder, characterized by repeated thoughts or rituals that interfere with daily life

  b) Participants were screened for health-related quality-of-life issues, such as fatigue, sleep habits, and work productivity.

  c) The study found that 45% of the patients with pain screened positive for at least one or more of the common anxiety disorders. Those who had an anxiety disorder also reported significantly worse pain and health-related quality of life than patients without a disorder (Kroenke et al., 2013).

D. Social isolation and diminished productivity often occur in patients with chronic pain.

1. Patients may lose their friends, strain their family relationships, and wear down social support systems.

2. This loss of community leads to a loss of interaction and engagement with people or activities that previously helped them in coping with their pain (Canadian Institute for the Relief of Pain and Disability, 2016).

3. Patients living with poorly managed chronic pain often struggle to keep their jobs.

  a) The challenge is convincing employers to modify the patients' job or workload to better manage pain while continuing to work.

  b) Research data have shown that people who return to work earlier have better health outcomes (Canadian Institute for the Relief of Pain and Disability, 2016).

      c) Engaging in work reduces focus on the pain and provides a distraction to the pain experience (Canadian Institute for the Relief of Pain and Disability, 2016).

  E. Lack of intimacy in relationships often occurs with prolonged chronic pain. The combination of limited range of motion, emotional distress, and the possibility of a reduced libido from pain medications can provoke stress and anxiety (Theobald, 2013).

    1. Patients with chronic pain may experience disruptions and inhibitions in sexual expression (Roddie, 2013).

    2. Patients with chronic pain often are fearful of aggravating or exacerbating their pain and reluctant to engage in sexual activity, often resorting to abstinence (Roddie, 2013).

    3. Surprisingly, limited evidence exists on intimacy and chronic pain, yet it is estimated that 75% of people with chronic pain experience some form of sexual dysfunction (Roddie, 2013).

    4. Unfortunately, healthcare practitioners often are reluctant to talk with patients about their sexual problems, and patients may be embarrassed to bring up the subject. This leads to further anxiety, depression, and diminished sexual function (Roddie, 2013).

    5. Medications used for analgesia can decrease libido and induce impotency. Opioid analgesics, tranquillizers, sedatives, and antidepressants can all decrease sexual desire.

    6. Corticosteroids can decrease sensation in the genital area in both men and women (Roddie, 2013).

IV. Physical examination

  A. History and physical examination remain the basis for a medical diagnosis of chronic pain (Dansie & Turk, 2013).

  B. Information gained from the history and physical examination, in combination with a clinical interview, and data obtained from standardized pain assessment tools aid providers in determining the type of pain and specific interventions (Turk & Robinson, 2011).

  C. Healthcare providers should seek any causes of pain through physical examination and diagnostic tests while concomitantly assessing the patient's mood, fears, expectations, coping efforts, resources, responses of significant others, and the effect of pain on the patients' lives (Turk & Robinson, 2011).

  D. Healthcare providers should evaluate the multidimensional aspects of the patient and not just the pain.

  E. Healthcare providers should complete a comprehensive pain assessment on all patients that includes documentation of the pain location, intensity (numeric rating score), quality, onset, duration, variations, rhythms, verbal expression of pain, alleviating and aggravating factors, effects of pain, and response to previous treatments.

  F. Psychological assessment should be included to evaluate for the presence of depression or other factors that increase the pain intensity (Hooten et al., 2013).

  G. Biopsychosocial approach to pain assessment and management requires an evaluation of patients in all of their complexity, including physical and biologic factors and psychological state and beliefs, as well as the family, social, and work environment (Hooten et al., 2013).

  H. Chronic pain usually involves the spine and nervous system and the musculoskeletal system. These body systems require a more detailed assessment and examination with attention to the elicitation of pain found in the patient's history (Hooten et al., 2013).

1. Neurologic and musculoskeletal examination of the upper extremities

   a) Spine alignment, range of motion (lateral side to side, hyperextension and flexion of the cervical spine)

   b) Atrophy, skin changes, hair growth and distribution, nail growth, edema and tenderness on palpation of the cervical facets (unilateral, bilateral)

   c) Speed test for biceps tendinitis, Tinel sign and Phalen maneuver for carpal tunnel syndrome

   d) Bilateral Spurling test and motor reflexes, brachial reflexes to include symmetry, non-brisk and negative Hoffmann sign, intact proprioception of medial aspects of the upper bilateral extremities

2. Shoulder examination: Bilateral assessment of Apley scratch test, Neer sign, Hawkins sign, empty can test, lift-off test, evaluation for pain with external rotation of bilateral wrists

3. Lower extremity examination

   a) Lumbar spine alignment, range of motion (extension, flexion, lateral rotation and lateral bending)

   b) Atrophy, skin changes, edema, hair and nail growth and distribution of hair

   c) Lumbar facet edema and tenderness on palpation, bilateral posterior superior iliac spine tenderness, Patrick test, femoral stretch, Yeoman and Gaenslen tests, bilateral straight leg rise

   d) Intact proprioception, Babinski sign, clonus

   e) Knee examination: Anterior drawer examination, valgus stress test, varus stress test, McMurray test

   f) Hip examination: Log roll, full range of motion (abduction, adduction)

   g) Additionally, cyanosis, pallor, hydration, symmetry of extremities, temperature of painful area

   h) Patient posture, gait, joint effusions, instability of joint (Hooten et al., 2013)

V. Diagnostics

A. No specific diagnostic examination exists for chronic pain. Diagnostics can help determine the pathology or identify the specific etiology generating the pain experience and direct the plan of care (Hooten et al., 2013).

1. Plain radiography is recommended in patients with musculoskeletal pain and generally is used to identify pain related to a bone fracture or mass lesion (Hooten et al., 2013).

2. Magnetic resonance imaging (MRI) is the diagnostic of choice in evaluating spinal abnormalities (e.g., disc bulging, spinal stenosis, disc degeneration) or soft tissue abnormalities in musculoskeletal circumstances (e.g., torn rotator cuff, meniscus tear).

3. Computed tomography with or without contrast is used when patients are unable to undergo MRI or are being considered for surgery or malignancy (Hooten et al., 2013).

4. Electromyography and nerve conduction studies are of use in patients suspected of having motor neuron dysfunction, nerve or nerve root pathology, or myopathy (Hooten et al., 2013).

B. Laboratory diagnostics should rule out systemic physiologic conditions such as anemia, hyperglycemia, hyperlipidemia, high blood pressure, embolism, abnormal thyroid, and dehydration, to name a few.

    1. A complete blood count with differential, comprehensive metabolic profile, lipid panel, and thyroid-stimulating hormone will help when ruling out additional chronic conditions.

    2. These conditions can intensify existing chronic pain.

C. Pain assessment tools: The most important and reliable indicator of the impact of chronic pain is the patient's self-report of the pain experience. This is a key component of chronic pain assessment, effective intervention, and evaluation (WHO, 2008).

D. Tools to assess chronic pain should be appropriate to the person, place, age, ethnicity, education, literacy, socioeconomic status, and psychological or emotional background (Hooten et al., 2013).

    1. Various pain assessment tools exist that determine either multiple dimensions or a single dimension.

    2. A multidimensional tool such as the Brief Pain Inventory should be used at the initial visit to provide a comprehensive overview of the patient's specific pain experience. The Brief Pain Inventory Long Form is available at www.npcrc.org/files/news/briefpain_long.pdf, and the Short Form is available at www.npcrc.org/files/news/briefpain_short.pdf.

    3. Additional multidimensional pain assessment tools include the Neuropathic Pain Scale and the Chronic Pain Grade.

    4. Single-dimension pain assessment tools evaluate the intensity of the pain experience and should be avoided in routine practice except to rate the intensity of the patient's pain (Hooten et al., 2013).

    5. Examples of single-dimension pain assessment tools include the numeric rating scale, visual analog scale, verbal descriptor scale, and Faces Pain Scale (Hooten et al., 2013).

    6. Additional tools that should be considered to effectively manage chronic pain include those that determine the patient's physical functioning, depression, insomnia, and other conditions.

    7. Effective pain management cannot be obtained in the presence of concomitant conditions that add to the intensity of the pain experience.

VI. Differential diagnosis

A. Failed back surgery (e.g., fusion, laminectomy)

B. Osteoarthritis or degenerative disease (e.g., joints, spinal facets)

C. Opioid-induced hyperalgesia is a result of nociceptive sensitization caused by prolonged exposure to opioids (Lee, Silverman, Hansen, Patel, & Manchikanti, 2011).

    1. Opioid-induced hyperalgesia is characterized by a paradoxical response when the patient receiving opioids becomes more sensitive to certain painful stimuli (allodynia) (Lee et al., 2011).

    2. The type of pain experienced might be the same as the underlying pain or different from the original underlying pain (Lee et al., 2011). Allodynia is pain that comes from a stimulus that does not usually provoke pain. Hyperalgesia and allodynia are prominent symptoms in patients with neuropathic pain (Jensen & Finnerup, 2014).

        a) Allodynia and hyperalgesia affect 15%–50% of patients with neuropathic pain (Jensen & Finnerup, 2014).

        b) Allodynia and hyperalgesia are classified according to the sensory modality on physical examination (e.g., touch, pressure, pinprick, cold, and heat) used to elicit the sensation (Jensen & Finnerup, 2014).

        c) Peripheral sensitization and maladaptive central changes contribute to the generation and maintenance of these reactions (Jensen & Finnerup, 2014).

D. Acute trauma from motor vehicle accident or work-related accident

E. Autoimmune disorders (e.g., rheumatoid arthritis, fibromyalgia, chronic fatigue syndrome, lupus)

F. Peripheral neuropathies from poorly managed diabetes mellitus, poor peripheral vascular perfusion, chemotherapy, anemia, dehydration, or other etiologies

G. Malignancy

H. Hormonal (menopause, low testosterone)

I. Depression and anxiety

J. Insomnia

K. Constipation from prolonged opioid exposure

VII. Interventions

A. Pharmacologic and nonpharmacologic interventions should always be considered in promoting optimal analgesia. The pharmacologic management of pain includes prescribing nonopioid analgesics, opioid analgesics, and adjuvant analgesics.

B. The use of appropriate evidence-based prescribing practices is essential in promoting safety and improved quality of life among patients experiencing chronic pain.

    1. Nonopioid analgesics are nonopiates that do not stimulate the central nervous system.

        a) This group of analgesics includes over-the-counter (OTC) acetaminophen, aspirin, and nonsteroidal anti-inflammatory drugs (NSAIDs).

        b) These OTC medications are commonly prescribed and are effective for mild to moderate pain such as headache or pain that originates from the musculoskeletal system (nociceptive or somatic pain).

    2. It is important to understand the black box warning from the U.S. Food and Drug Administration (FDA) for both NSAIDs and acetaminophen and to always quantify the amount of OTC medication that patients are using and whether it is combined with prescribed medications of the same class (polypharmacy).

        a) Opioid analgesics directly adhere to specific receptor sites within the central nervous system, creating a "gate-like" interpretation of pain—from the periphery to the brain's memory.

        b) Opioid prescribing for pain management has increased substantially since the late 1990s.

        c) There is a current paradigm shift in the United States regarding the long-term use of opioids for the management of chronic pain.

        d) The ill effects of prolonged opioid dependency and addiction in the United States has promoted new legislation and federal recommendations suggesting successful chronic pain management without the use of opioids.

    3. This is a controversial public health issue because of the inherent risk for opioid abuse, addiction, diversion, and fatal overdose (Bruehl et al., 2013; Rosenblum, Marsch, Joseph, & Portenoy, 2008). These risks were the impetus for the reclassification of hydrocodone from a schedule III to a schedule II controlled medication in 2014 (Throckmorton, 2014).

    4. Opioids are available in short- and long-acting formulations.

        a) Examples of opioid analgesics include hydrocodone, codeine, morphine, oxycodone, hydromorphone, fentanyl, and methadone.

        (1) Caution should always be taken to reduce the systemic consequences of prolonged opioid use.

        (2) All efforts should be taken to break the memory of pain. This can be accomplished through alternative and healthier interventions.

b) The practice paradigm since the 1990s is changing, and evidence now suggests that alternatives to opioids can successfully manage chronic pain and promote long-term healthier outcomes.

c) Opioid screening tools used in practice have been criticized by medical experts for their inability to provide a valid and reliable prediction of the benefit or harm associated with the initiation of opioids (American Chronic Pain Association, 2012).

d) Other medical experts suggest that screening tools such as the Screener and Opioid Assessment for Patients With Pain; the Opioid Risk Tool; and the Diagnosis, Intractability, Risk, Efficacy instrument do have high validity and determine risk factors in clinical practice (Chou et al., 2009; Passik, Kirsh, & Casper, 2008).

e) Prior to the initiation of opioids, the clinician should evaluate the patient's propensity for addiction. A common and easy tool used routinely in clinical practice is the CAGE (Cutting down, Annoyance by criticism, Guilty feeling, and Eye-openers) questionnaire. A positive CAGE score (more than two positive answers) suggests an addictive risk factor.

f) Significant considerations when initiating opioids to manage chronic pain include the following:

        (1) History of alcohol, tobacco, or other substance (e.g., cannabis, benzodiazepines, anti-insomnia drugs, muscle relaxants) abuse

        (2) Presence of antisocial personality disorders, mood disorders, or psychotic disorders

g) If patients do not respond to nonpharmacologic and nonopioid analgesics and interventions, mild opioid analgesics (e.g., hydrocodone) can be considered. Prior to the initiation of opioid prescribing, there should be documentation of failure from all modalities.

h) Documentation should include a detailed assessment addressing substance abuse and psychiatric history. Using and documenting screening tools that assess for the presence of alcohol or drug abuse, depression, and the potential for opioid abuse is a valid and reliable method for ensuring best practice and implementation of the current guidelines.

i) The prescribing practitioner should request a baseline drug screen and, together with the patient, develop a specific care plan to direct optimal management of the patient's pain. The care plan should include a written patient–provider agreement regarding treatment goals and parameters, including having a single provider of opioids, using a single pharmacy, committing to follow-up visits, and agreeing to random urine drug screening (Jones, Mack, & Paulozzi, 2013).

j) Opioid prescribing should always be done with the focus of reducing opioid exposure for long-term use. Prolonged exposure to opioid intervention attenuates the risk for tolerance, addiction, and the untoward effects associated with withdrawal.

C. The WHO analgesic ladder is useful when considering the patient's pain intensity (numeric rating score) and type of medications.

D. The WHO analgesic ladder assists providers with the administration of multimodal analgesia by dividing analgesic prescribing into four groups: simple analgesics, weak opioids, strong opioids, and adjuvants.
   1. Each step of the WHO analgesic ladder consists of nonopioid analgesics as the basis for treatment; therefore, acetaminophen or an NSAID should be prescribed along with an opioid.
   2. A multimodal approach such as this serves to deliver more effective pain management that requires less amounts of opioids in addition to lessening the potential for side effects and adverse events related to prolonged opioid use (Pain Community Centre, n.d.).
E. In response to the opioid abuse epidemic, on September 10, 2013, FDA announced dramatic changes to the indications for the use of long-acting opioid analgesics.
   1. FDA revised its recommendations such that long-acting opioids are no longer indicated for chronic pain of moderate severity.
   2. Following FDA's revisions, the indication for long-acting opioids is for severe pain, as a second option, after other treatment modalities have failed to adequately relieve pain (U.S. FDA, 2013).
F. DHHS (2015) has addressed the issue of opioid abuse and opioid-related overdose and deaths as a high priority.
   1. DHHS has two broad goals pertaining to this priority: to decrease opioid-related overdoses along with decreasing overall mortality, and to decrease the prevalence of opioid use disorders.
   2. To reach these goals, the DHHS secretary is targeting three key areas to thwart abuse of opioids: use of appropriate opioid prescribing practices, expanded distribution and distribution of naloxone to treat opioid overdose, and expanded use of medication-assisted treatment to decrease opioid abuse disorders (U.S. DHHS, 2015).
G. Adjunct analgesics include a group of medications with a primary indication not related to analgesia but with physiologic properties that target the etiology of pain, particularly in neuropathic pain (e.g., duloxetine, gabapentin, pregabalin).
   1. These medications have analgesic properties used in the management of somatic and neuropathic pain.
   2. Examples of these medications include antidepressants, corticosteroids, neuroleptics, muscle relaxants, calcitonin, bisphosphonates, anticholinergics, biologics, chemotherapy, and radiopharmaceuticals (Carlson & Carlson, 2011).
   3. Use of a methylprednisolone dose pack can help to relieve extreme pain associated with neuropathic or somatic etiology.
   4. Patients should be cautioned to not use NSAIDs at the same time as the methylprednisolone dose pack and to resume the NSAID following completion of the corticosteroid.
   5. Caution should be used with patients with diabetes.
H. Nonpharmacologic interventions for chronic pain management should always be considered and combined with nonopioid, adjuvant, and, if needed, opioid analgesics.
   1. Because pain is a multidimensional symptom, all disciplines should collaborate on areas of consideration: physical, emotional, spiritual, pharmacologic, and nonpharmacologic.
   2. Disciplines and interventions include the following:
      a) Physical therapy or rehabilitation to promote physical functioning, mobility, and improved health through exercise, socialization, and strength training

    b) Occupational therapy for fine muscles in the hand and feet

    c) Chiropractor for facet relief in patients with spinal facet syndrome

    d) Massage to improve circulation and promote distraction from perception of pain

    e) Durable medical equipment, lumbar brace, wrist brace, sling

    f) Heat and cold modalities

    g) Topical lidocaine, capsaicin for neuropathic conditions

    h) Cognitive behavioral interventions

    i) Transcutaneous electrical nerve stimulation and ultrasound

    j) Trigger point injections with local anesthetic (e.g., 0.25% bupivacaine hydrochloride) injection (27-gauge needle) into the fascia of affected area (e.g., cervical scapular, lumbar, sacrum)

    k) Weight loss to achieve a body mass index of less than 29 kg/m^2

    l) Increased physical activity

 I. Interventional pain management should be considered in patients with an acute exacerbation of chronic pain or in those with chronic poorly managed pain primarily managed with opioid analgesics. These interventions should be considered to reduce opioid exposure and improve physical functioning.

   1. Spinal interventions for somatic and neuropathic conditions, such as intra-articular facet injections in patients with spinal facet effusion or hypertrophy of the facet ligaments

   2. Intralaminar or intrathecal epidural steroid injections targeting specific spinal dermatomes based on spinal pathophysiology and patient-specific symptoms

   3. Mesenchymal stem cells, which have been shown in animal models to attenuate chronic neuropathic pain

   4. Preliminary studies in the United States have shown positive outcomes for patients treated with stem cells for neuropathic pain (Vickers, Karsten, Flood, & Lilischkis, 2014).

Case Study

 M.K. is a 73-year-old African American woman who has a past medical history of osteoarthritis, diabetes mellitus with peripheral neuropathies, obesity, hypertension, and depression. She comes to the clinic after having a motor vehicle accident. She was rear-ended and her car was totaled. She was taken by ambulance to the local emergency department where she had a radiograph done of her lumbar spine and was given a prescription for hydrocodone 7.5 mg/acetaminophen 325 mg to take every six hours as needed for pain and cyclobenzaprine 5 mg every eight hours if needed for muscle spasm. Today she describes her pain as shooting, sharp, and intermittent to the point of taking her breath away. The pain is more prominent on her left leg, and she describes a radiculopathy that is posterior and lateral and radiates from her lower back into the anterior surface of her foot. She is having difficulty with ambulation and frequently awakens during sleep to reposition herself.

 Her last hemoglobin A1c was 7.5%. She was prescribed gabapentin 300 mg at bedtime in the past with good results for her peripheral neuropathies but has not been taking it because it makes her feel tired throughout the day. Because of her daily 81 mg dose of aspirin, she is not taking an NSAID. She is not taking anything for depression. Her hypertension is well managed.

 On physical examination of her lumbar spine, she has normal alignment and no atrophy or skin changes. She is unable to perform an active range of motion with hyperextension, flexion, and lateral bending. She has positive tenderness and swelling on her bilateral lumbar facets, positive posterior superior iliac spine tenderness bilaterally, and positive straight leg rise on the left and negative on the right. Patellar reflexes are non-brisk and symmetrical bilaterally. She has reduced proprioception on microfilament examination of her left plantar and medial side of her foot and normal findings on her right foot.

Based on these findings, the advanced practice registered nurse (APRN) promptly orders an MRI of her lumbar spine. The APRN also discusses the benefits of an antidepressant to aid in managing the neuropathic features of M.K.'s pain, support her depression, and help her to sleep. An initial dose of duloxetine 30 mg/day is prescribed. M.K. is discontinued from her daily aspirin and prescribed celecoxib 200 mg every morning. She is referred to physical therapy for strengthening and rehabilitation and to a registered dietitian for review her dietary choices and help in reducing her weight. Depending on the findings from her MRI, she may be a good candidate for a transforaminal epidural steroid injection to reduce her radiculopathy. She will return to the clinic following the results of her MRI.

Authors' note: Subsequent to the development of this chapter, the Centers for Disease Control and Prevention released new guidelines in the management of chronic nonmalignant pain. These guidelines and additional resources are available at www.cdc.gov/drugoverdose/prescribing/guideline.html.

References

American Chronic Pain Association. (2012). ACPA resource guide to chronic pain medication and treatment. Retrieved from https://www.theacpa.org/uploads/ACPA_Resource_Guide_2012_Update%20031912.pdf

Anxiety and Depression Association of America. (2015). Understand the facts: Chronic pain. Retrieved http://www.adaa.org/understanding-anxiety/related-illnesses/other-related-conditions/chronic-pain

Bruehl, S., Apkarian, A.V., Ballantyne, J.C., Berger, A., Borsook, D., Chen, W.G., … Lin, Y. (2013). Personalized medicine and opioid analgesic prescribing for chronic pain: Opportunities and challenges. *Journal of Pain, 14,* 103–113. doi:10.1016/j.jpain.2012.10.016

Canadian Institute for the Relief of Pain and Disability. (2016, January). What is chronic pain? Retrieved from http://www.cirpd.org/PainManagement/WhatIsChronicPain

Carlson, H., & Carlson, N. (2011). An overview of the management of persistent musculoskeletal pain. *Therapeutic Advances in Musculoskeletal Disease, 3,* 91–99. doi:10.1177/1759720X11398742

Chou, R., Fanciullo, G.J., Fine, P.G., Adler, J.A., Ballantyne, J.C., Davies, P., … Miaskowski, C. (2009). Clinical guidelines for the use of chronic opioid therapy in chronic noncancer pain. *Journal of Pain, 10,* 113–130.e22. doi:10.1016/j.jpain.2008.10.008

Cohen, S.P., & Mao, J. (2014). Neuropathic pain: Mechanisms and their clinical implications. *BMJ, 348,* S66–S73. doi:10.1136/bmj.f7656

Costigan, M., Scholz, J., & Woolf, C.J. (2009). Neuropathic pain: A maladaptive response of the nervous system to damage. *Annual Review of Neuroscience, 32,* 1–32. doi:10.1146/annurev.neuro.051508.135531

Dansie, E.J., & Turk, D.C. (2013). Assessment of patients with chronic pain. *British Journal of Anaesthesia, 111,* 19–25. doi:10.1093/bja/aet124

Dowell, D., Haegerich, T.M., & Chou, R. (2016). CDC guideline for prescribing opioids for chronic pain—United States, 2016. *MMWR Recommendations and Reports, 65,* 1–49. doi:10.15585/mmwr.rr6501e1

Harvard Men's Health Watch. (2015, July 1). Best bets for back pain. Retrieved from http://www.health.harvard.edu/pain/best-bets-for-back-pain?utm_source=mens&utm_medium=pressrelease&utm_campaign=Mens0715

Hooten, W.M., Timming, R., Belgrade, M., Gaul, J., Goertz, M., Haake, B., … Walker, N. (2013). *Institute for Clinical Systems Improvement health care guideline: Assessment and management of chronic pain.* Retrieved from https://www.icsi.org/_asset/bw798b/ChronicPain.pdf

Institute of Medicine. (2011). *Relieving pain in America: A blueprint for transforming prevention, care, education, and research.* Washington, DC: National Academies Press.

International Association for the Study of Pain. (2009). Task Force on Wait-Times: Summary and recommendations. Retrieved from http://www.iasp-pain.org/files/Content/NavigationMenu/EducationalResources/IASP_Wait_Times.pdf

Janssen, S.P., Truin, M., Van Kleef, M., & Joosten, E.A. (2011). Differential GABAergic disinhibition during the development of painful peripheral neuropathy. *Neuroscience, 184,* 183–194. doi:10.1016/j.neuroscience .2011.03.060

Jensen, T.S., & Finnerup, N.B. (2014). Allodynia and hyperalgesia in neuropathic pain: Clinical manifestations and mechanisms. *Lancet Neurology, 13,* 924–935. doi:10.1016/S1474-4422(14)70102-4

Jones, C.M., Mack, K.A., & Paulozzi, L.J. (2013). Pharmaceutical overdose deaths, United States, 2010. *JAMA, 309,* 657–659. doi:10.1001/jama.2013.272

Kroenke, K., Outcalt, S., Krebs, E., Bair, M.J., Wu, J., Chumbler, N., & Yu, Z. (2013). Association between anxiety, health-related quality of life and functional impairment in primary care patients with chronic pain. *General Hospital Psychiatry, 35,* 359–365. doi:10.1016/j.genhosppsych.2013.03.020

Lee, M., Silverman, S.M., Hansen, H., Patel, V.B., & Manchikanti, L. (2011). A comprehensive review of opioid-induced hyperalgesia. *Pain Physician, 14,* 145–161.

National Institute of Mental Health. (2015). Chronic illness and mental health. Retrieved from http://www .nimh.nih.gov/health/publications/chronic-illness-mental-health-2015/index.shtml

National Institute of Neurological Disorders and Stroke. (2015). Complex regional pain syndrome fact sheet. Retrieved from http://www.ninds.nih.gov/disorders/reflex_sympathetic_dystrophy/detail_reflex_sympathetic _dystrophy.htm

National Research Council Committee on Recognition and Alleviation of Pain in Laboratory Animals. (2009). *Recognition and alleviation of pain in laboratory animals.* Retrieved from http://www.ncbi.nlm.nih.gov/books/NBK32658

National Sleep Foundation. (2015). 2015 Sleep in America™ poll finds pain a significant challenge when it comes to Americans' sleep. Retrieved from https://sleepfoundation.org/media-center/press-release/2015 -sleep-america-poll

Pain Community Centre. (n.d.). WHO analgesic ladder. Retrieved from http://www.paincommunitycentre .org/article/who-analgesic-ladder

Passik, S.D., Kirsh, K.L., & Casper, D. (2008). Addiction-related assessment tools and pain management: Instruments for screening, treatment planning, and monitoring compliance. *Pain Medicine, 9*(Suppl. 2), S145–S166. doi:10.1111/j.1526-4637.2008.00486.x

Roddie, A. (2013). Sex and chronic pain. Retrieved from http://painconcern.org.uk/sex-and-chronic-pain

Rosenblum, A., Marsch, L.A., Joseph, H., & Portenoy, R.K. (2008). Opioids and the treatment of chronic pain: Controversies, current status, and future directions. *Experimental and Clinical Psychopharmacology, 16,* 405–416. doi:10.1037/a0013628

Smart, K.M., Blake, C., Staines, A., Thacker, M., & Doody, C. (2012a). Mechanisms-based classifications of musculoskeletal pain: Part 1 of 3: Symptoms and signs of central sensitisation in patients with low back (± leg) pain. *Manual Therapy, 17,* 336–344. doi:10.1016/j.math.2012.03.013

Smart, K.M., Blake, C., Staines, A., Thacker, M., & Doody, C. (2012b). Mechanisms-based classifications of musculoskeletal pain: Part 2 of 3: Symptoms and signs of peripheral neuropathic pain in patients with low back (± leg) pain. *Manual Therapy, 17,* 345–351. doi:10.1016/j.math.2012.03.003

Smart, K.M., Blake, C., Staines, A., Thacker, M., & Doody, C. (2012c). Mechanisms-based classifications of musculoskeletal pain: Part 3 of 3: Symptoms and signs of nociceptive pain in patients with low back (± leg) pain. *Manual Therapy, 17,* 352–357. doi:10.1016/j.math.2012.03.002

Theobald, M. (2013). Chronic pain curbing your sex drive? Retrieved from http://www.everydayhealth.com/ pain-management/1120/chronic-pain-curbing-your-sex-life.aspx

Throckmorton, D.C. (2014, October 6). Re-scheduling prescription hydrocodone combination drug products: An important step toward controlling misuse and abuse. *FDA Voice.* Retrieved from http://blogs.fda.gov/ fdavoice/index.php/2014/10/re-scheduling-prescription-hydrocodone-combination-drug-products-an -important-step-toward-controlling-misuse-and-abuse

Turk, D.C., & Robinson, J.P. (2011). Assessment of patients with chronic pain: A comprehensive approach. In D.C. Turk & R. Melzack (Eds.), *Handbook of pain assessment* (3rd ed., pp. 188–210). New York, NY: Guilford Press.

U.S. Department of Health and Human Services. (2015). Opioid abuse in the U.S. and HHS actions to address opioid-drug related overdoses and deaths. Retrieved from https://aspe.hhs.gov/basic-report/opioid-abuse -us-and-hhs-actions-address-opioid-drug-related-overdoses-and-deaths

U.S. Food and Drug Administration. (2013, September 10). FDA announces safety labeling changes and post-market study requirements for extended-release and long-acting opioid analgesics [News release]. Retrieved from http://www.fda.gov/NewsEvents/Newsroom/PressAnnouncements/ucm367726.htm

Vickers, E.R., Karsten, E., Flood, J., & Lilischkis, R. (2014). A preliminary report on stem cell therapy for neuropathic pain in humans. *Journal of Pain Research, 7,* 255–263. doi:10.2147/JPR.S63361

World Health Organization. (2008). Scoping document for WHO treatment guidelines on chronic non-malignant pain in adults. Retrieved from http://www.who.int/medicines/areas/quality_safety/Scoping _WHOGuide_non-malignant_pain_adults.pdf

CHAPTER 21

Constipation

Suzette Walker, DNP, FNP-BC, AOCNP®

I. Definition
   A. Constipation is defined as infrequent bowel movements, fewer than three a week, or as having a large amount of stool in the colon by clinical examination or abdominal x-ray.
   B. Patients often provide a broader definition including hard stools, the feeling of incomplete emptying, abdominal pain, straining to defecate, discomfort, and bloating. Patients experience a change in normal bowel function.
   C. Constipation leads to significant discomfort, anxiety, and often psychological preoccupation with bowel function (American Gastroenterological Association [AGA], 2013; Clark, Urban, & Currow, 2010).
II. Pathophysiology
   A. The colon absorbs water and electrolytes in the proximal half while the distal half stores and excretes waste. Stool transit time varies greatly in individuals and is affected by diet, fluid intake, exercise, time of day, and medications, as well as changes in lifestyle.
   B. Many endocrine or metabolic disorders can lead to constipation. Delayed gastric emptying or a decrease in colonic contractions of smooth muscles results in a slower transit time.
   C. Slow sluggish peristalsis leads to decreased fluid absorption within the bowel, resulting in bowel dysfunction. Constipation in palliative care is multifactorial, complex, and only partially understood (AGA, 2013; National Institute of Diabetes and Digestive and Kidney Diseases, 2015; Sykes, 2006).
   D. Functional constipation: Colonic inertia, delayed transit, pelvic floor dysfunction
      1. Diet: Dehydration, low fiber intake, anorexia
      2. Environmental: Assistance needed for care, lack of privacy, discomfort
      3. Older age, inactivity, confinement to bed, sedation, depression
   E. Organic factors
      1. Pharmacologic agents: Opioids, neuroleptics, chemotherapy, antiemetics, hypertensives, anticholinergics, antidiarrheals, iron, diuretics, antidepressants, antacids
      2. Metabolic disturbances: Dehydration, hypocalcemia, hypokalemia, hypothyroidism, diabetes
      3. Neurologic abnormalities: Spinal cord involvement, brain tumors, Parkinson disease, multiple sclerosis, gastroparesis, tumor involvement, bowel diseases
   F. Structural: Tumor compression, radiation fibrosis, anorectal conditions
III. Presenting symptoms

A. Constipation is underreported by patients and often overlooked by healthcare practitioners.
B. Vigilant assessment and implementation of preventive and treatment interventions are essential at every clinical evaluation.
C. Symptoms, precipitating factors, onset, location, and duration are all vital components for correct evaluation and appropriate diagnosis (McKay, Fravel, & Scanlon, 2009).
   1. Abdominal pain
   2. Increase or decrease in flatulence
   3. Bloating and abdominal distention
   4. Feeling of fullness or anorexia
   5. Increase in hardness of stool or difficulty in having bowel movement
   6. Decrease in frequency
   7. Malaise
   8. Anal pain
   9. Tenesmus
   10. Feeling of incomplete evacuation
   11. Nausea and vomiting
   12. Liquid stool, seen with impaction
IV. Physical examination
   A. Review of past medical history (Larkin et al., 2008; McHugh & Miller-Saultz, 2011)
      1. Bowel disease history
         a) Irritable bowel
         b) Ulcerative colitis
         c) Crohn disease
         d) Previous bowel surgery
      2. History of cancer or cancer treatment
         a) Bowel surgery
         b) Pelvic irradiation
         c) Chemotherapy
         d) Cancer in the pelvis or abdomen
      3. Current medical history: Many medical conditions and treatments can lead to bowel dysfunction.
      4. Current medications
         a) Prescription medications: Assess for medications that cause constipation.
         b) Over-the-counter medications (e.g., stool softeners, laxatives, antacids) and use of supplements such as iron or calcium
      5. Recent lifestyle changes or progressive worsening of chronic conditions
         a) Change in mobility
         b) Change in hydration or diet (Dahl & Stewart, 2015)
            (1) Decrease in fluid volume (need 30–35 ml/kg/day)
            (2) Decrease or change in fiber intake (need 20–35 g/day)
            (3) Change in foods that cause constipation, such as dairy products, bananas, and high-fat foods such as chips and red meat
         c) Fluid intake
         d) Fiber intake
         e) Amount of solid intake
         f) Evaluate the patient's diet and determine if it has an appropriate combination of protein, fat, and carbohydrates and types of foods consumed (e.g., fresh, processed).

      6. Usual pattern of elimination
         a) Frequency and amount; color, size, and consistency
         b) Recent changes in bowel function
         c) Incontinence
         d) Previous experience with constipation
         e) Specific interventions used in the past that were helpful
         f) Environmental changes
            (1) Privacy
            (2) Toileting patterns
            (3) Toilet accessibility
      7. Depression assessment
   B. Vital signs, weight, and body mass index
      1. Signs of infection
         a) Fever
         b) Chills or sweats
         c) Increase in pulse, decrease in blood pressure
      2. Signs of dehydration
         a) Poor skin turgor, skin tenting, dry skin, and dry, pale mucous membranes
         b) Increase in pulse or temperature, decrease in blood pressure, decrease in weight
         c) Concentrated urine with odor
   C. Cardiac and respiratory
      1. Dehydration; increase in pulse; thready, weak pulse; flat and thin vessels on top of hand; poor skin turgor
      2. Respiratory compromise, shallow breathing, acetone breath
   D. Abdominal
      1. Visual: Distention, bulging sides, visible peristalsis action
      2. Auscultation: Normal, hypoactive, hyperactive, or no bowel sounds
      3. Palpation: Mass, palpable stool, positive or negative Murphy sign—rebound tenderness, ascites
      4. Percussion: Air swallowing, increase in gas, ascites, wavelike motion in the presence of fluid
   E. Rectal (contraindicated if leukopenia or thrombocytopenia is present)
      1. Visual: Irritation, hemorrhoids, fissures, rash
      2. Rectal digital examination: Sphincter tone, internal hemorrhoids, mass, obstipation (severe constipation often due to obstruction), color and consistency of stool, test for occult blood using the recommended fecal immunochemical test (National Comprehensive Cancer Network®, 2015)
   F. Lower extremity: Evaluate for spinal cord dysfunction.
      1. Strength: Lower extremities, changes in gait, difficulty in changing positions from sitting to standing
      2. Sensation: May exhibit decrease in sensory evaluation (e.g., microfilament examination)
      3. Reflexes: Either flat or brisk, brachial, radial, patellar
V. Diagnostics
   A. An aggressive evaluation is determined by sudden onset or severe symptoms and overt presence of blood in stool (AGA, 2013; Clark & Currow, 2012).
   B. Laboratory analysis
      1. Complete blood count with differential

    2. Thyroid function test including thyroid-stimulating hormone (TSH), free T3, and free T4

    3. Comprehensive metabolic panel

    4. Stool sample for occult blood (e.g., fecal immunochemical test)

  C. Radiology: Evaluate for bowel obstruction with abdominal flat plate.

  D. Other

    1. Sigmoidoscopy, colonoscopy, or barium enema considered for bleeding or suspected obstruction

    2. Abdominal computed tomography scan if symptoms are sudden and patient reports significant pain

VI. Differential diagnosis

  A. Constipation, functional or drug induced

  B. Constipation, delayed transit

  C. Constipation, chronic or acute

  D. Constipation, outlet obstruction

  E. Bowel obstruction

  F. Colon impaction

  G. Gastroparesis

  H. Gastric outlet obstruction

  I. Irritable bowel syndrome, constipation type

VII. Interventions

  A. The goals of therapy are to improve colon function and to promote elimination comfort.

  B. Many patients are living with multiple chronic conditions and will require multiple interventions for optimal outcomes.

  C. Include prophylactic bowel management whenever patients are prescribed opioid analgesics.

    1. The combination of a stimulant laxative plus a stool softener is recommended with opioid prescribing.

    2. The doses used should be individually titrated for effectiveness according to bowel function, not opioid dose (National Comprehensive Cancer Network, 2015; Thorpe et al., 2015).

  D. The primary focus is on prevention: increasing fluids, dietary management, and physical activity.

  E. If appropriate, consider discontinuing supplements and specific medications that contribute to constipation, such as iron, calcium, anticholinergics, and other agents.

  F. Correct any metabolic etiology (e.g., hypocalcemia, hypothyroidism).

  G. Nonpharmacologic (Folden, 2002; Gallegos-Orozco, Foxx-Orenstein, Sterler, & Stoa, 2012; Hunt et al., 2014; McHugh & Miller-Saultz, 2011)

    1. Well-balanced diet

      a) Promote adequate fluid intake (30–35 ml/kg/day).

      b) Instruct patients to drink warm or hot fluids prior to their usual time for bowel movement to help stimulate peristalsis.

      c) Encourage regular timing of meals and snacks to increase episodes of peristalsis to promote gut motility.

      d) Advise patients to add soluble fiber such as oatmeal, applesauce, bananas, lentils, pears, and white rice.

      e) Advise patients to add insoluble fiber such as whole wheat and bran, nuts, seeds, fruits, and vegetables. Avoid these foods if symptoms of gas, nausea, or history of bowel obstructions or diverticulitis is noted.

       f) Instruct patients to eat 1–2 tablespoons of fruit paste (see University of Michigan Comprehensive Cancer Center, 2012, for recipes to help manage constipation) before bed followed by 8 oz of water.

  2. Physical activity

     a) Tailor activity recommendations to individuals' physical abilities and health condition.

     b) Recommend regular physical activity per patient tolerances. Patients should avoid more than two hours of sedentary activity. Encourage sitting up or additional movement every two hours if possible.

     c) Instruct patients to walk for 15–20 minutes once or twice a day.

  3. Toileting

     a) Ignoring or suppressing the urge to have a bowel movement contributes to constipation.

     b) Establishing a routine toileting regimen is helpful.

     c) Routine should include toileting 5–15 minutes after meals, especially after breakfast.

H. Pharmacologic therapy is indicated if symptoms of constipation do not resolve with lifestyle changes.

  1. Selection of agents should be based on patient characteristics, such as contraindications to a specific class, previous laxative use, and personal preference (AGA, 2013).

  2. Pharmacologic agents that require a large amount of fluid may not be best for many palliative care patients.

  3. In the instance of impending death, pharmacologic therapy often is not needed (Clark, Byfieldt, Dawe, & Currow, 2012).

  4. Include preventive measures with the implementation of opioids.

     a) The combination of a stimulant laxative plus a stool softener is better than either one alone.

     b) Doses should be individually titrated for effectiveness according to bowel function, not opioid dose (Camilleri et al., 2014).

       (1) Minimum fluid intake of 30–35 ml/kg/day

       (2) Docusate sodium 100–300 mg/day

       (3) Senna 2–6 tabs every 12 hours to begin and titrated as needed

I. Treatment of impactions

  1. Glycerin suppository

  2. Mineral oil retention enema

  3. Manual disimpaction if needed

J. Consider appetite stimulants if anorexia is a concurrent symptom (McHugh & Miller-Saultz, 2011).

  1. Megestrol acetate 400–800 mg/day

  2. Corticosteroids: Dexamethasone 4–100 mg/day

  3. Dronabinol 5–10 mg/day

  4. Metoclopramide 10–30 mg/day

K. The pharmacologic agents used for constipation can be classified into several categories. The goal of treatment is to have one bowel movement every 24–48 hours (AGA, 2013; Ford et al., 2014; McHugh & Miller-Saultz, 2011).

  1. Emollients: Docusate sodium 50–500 mg/day

  2. Lubricants: Mineral oil 10–30 ml/day

  3. Osmotic laxatives

        a) Polyethylene glycol 17 g in 8 oz of fluid/day
        b) Lactulose 15–30 ml 2–3 times a day and titrate
        c) Sorbitol 30–60 ml/day
   4. Stimulants
        a) Senna 1–6 tabs/day
        b) Bisacodyl 10–30 mg/day
   5. Chloride-channel stimulators: Lubiprostone 16–44 mcg/day
   6. Bulk-forming laxatives (must be taken with 8 oz of water): This class should not be used with patients at the end of life because of amount of fluid needed.
        a) Methylcellulose 2–6 g/day
        b) Polycarbophil 2–8 tabs/day
        c) Psyllium 3.4–10.2 g/day
   7. Metoclopramide 20 mg/day
   8. Methylnaltrexone 12 mg subcutaneously every other day in severe opioid-induced constipation
   9. Prokinetic agents: Tegaserod 2–6 mg PO BID
L. Non-oral pharmacologic interventions
   1. May be needed for patients who cannot swallow
   2. For those with concurrent nausea and vomiting
        a) Suppositories
           (1) Glycerin
           (2) Bisacodyl
        b) Enemas
           (1) Oil retention
           (2) Sodium phosphate
           (3) Bisacodyl
M. Evaluation and follow-up
   1. Assess patients within 24 hours to determine efficacy of pharmacologic and nonpharmacologic interventions.
   2. Modify the treatment plan if it is not working to promote bowel movement every 24–48 hours.
   3. Patients who are living with multiple chronic conditions need continued evaluation at every point of care.
   4. Consider diagnostic evaluation if interventions are ineffective.
N. Referrals
   1. Registered dietitian for diet and hydration recommendations for all palliative care patients
   2. Occupational and physical therapy for patients who require evaluation of their physical condition and support in gaining new skills to promote physical functioning

Case Study

W.A. is a 66-year-old Caucasian woman with chronic medical conditions including hypothyroidism, insulin-dependent type 2 diabetes, and hypertension. Sequelae of these multiple chronic conditions include gastroparesis, peripheral neuropathy, and renal dysfunction. She was diagnosed with non-small cell carcinoma of the lung just over a year ago. She was treated with chemotherapy and radiation. When metastatic disease was found, she received additional chemotherapy until disease progression and worsening symptom burden led her and her spouse to change the focus of care to palliative care. W.A. is an urgent add-on to the advanced practice registered nurse (APRN) clinic schedule with complaints of worsening severe back pain resulting in a pain crisis. Prior to W.A.'s arrival in the clinic, spine films were obtained. The radiologist has alerted the APRN that the films show new lytic lesions of T10 and T11 with a compression fracture.

On review of systems, the patient and her husband state that she has increased her pain medications without relief. Her pain had been well controlled with her current pain medications until 48 hours ago when she began to have severe back pain that came on suddenly when she was getting up from bed. She has been bedbound for two days because of pain. The husband reports that he thinks his wife is somewhat confused and wonders if it is the pain medications. He noted that the medication in her pill box did not look right to him. She is not eating or drinking well. She also reports decrease in appetite and constipation.

On physical examination, W.A. appears uncomfortable. Her pupils are equal and reactive to light, although sluggish to respond. Oral mucus is dry, and skin turgor is fair. Lungs are clear through all fields. Her heart rate is 112 beats per minute and regular. Her abdominal examination shows distention, diffuse tenderness, and quiet bowel sounds. She is point tender at T10. Neurologically, she is alert and oriented times three but slow to respond. She exhibits a decrease in sensory examination in both feet to her ankles. Examination found no edema and 2+ pulses.

W.A.'s current medications consist of metformin 1,000 mg BID; insulin glargine 24 units every night; amlodipine 10 mg daily; lisinopril 40 mg daily; levothyroxine 125 mcg daily; time-released morphine 60 mg every 8 hours, using up to 40 mg of morphine immediate-release within 24 hours; and calcium supplements of 1,200 mg BID.

Imaging results include spine films showing lytic lesions at T10 and T11 with new compression fracture; chest x-ray showing a 4 cm mass in the right lung with multiple smaller nodules; and abdominal films showing a large amount of stool in the lower colon with no sign of obstruction. Laboratory data include normal complete blood count, platelet count, and differential. TSH was 12.2 uIU/ml. Electrolyte abnormalities included calcium of 13.2 mg/dl, glucose of 158 mg/dl, sodium of 133 mmol/L, creatinine of 2.4 mg/dl, and blood urea nitrogen of 56 mg/dl. On assessment, the APRN notes dehydration, hypercalcemia, hypothyroidism, drug-induced constipation, renal dysfunction, pain crisis, bone metastasis (T10 and T11), diabetes, and lung cancer.

The treatment plan for W.A. includes sustained hydration with normal saline. Pain control is optimized using home medications of sustained-released morphine and morphine immediate-release for breakthrough pain. Sustained-released morphine during admission is increased to 100 mg every eight hours with morphine immediate-release as needed. A bowel program with stool softeners and laxatives is begun and titrated using docusate sodium 100 mg BID and senna 2 tabs BID. Two doses of polyethylene glycol are given over six hours with good success. Following institutional formulary, zoledronic acid 4 mg IV is given to correct calcium. Levothyroxine is increased to 137 mcg to correct TSH. W.A.'s diabetes is managed with home medications and the addition of a sliding scale with regular insulin. W.A.'s calcium supplement and amlodipine are discontinued. Dietary and physical therapy referrals are obtained. W.A. follows recommendations for an increase in oral fluids and fiber as well as for an exercise program initiated by physical therapy.

During admission, W.A.'s mental status improves with the normalization of the calcium. Pain crisis is resolved with the increase in the dose of time-released morphine, resulting in increasing mobility. Prior to discharge, the patient's pain is greatly improved, as is her function. She is having daily bowel movements with the prescribed bowel regimen. Electrolytes return to baseline with creatinine of 1.3 mg/dl, blood urea nitrogen of 24 mg/dl, and normalization of calcium and sodium. Blood pressure remains in good control. She no longer requires the addition of regular insulin. She is discharged home with a care plan and the addition of a palliative homecare service. She is given a return appointment to see the APRN in one week.

References

American Gastroenterological Association. (2013). American Gastroenterological Association medical position statement on constipation. *Gastroenterology, 144,* 211–217.

Camilleri, M., Drossman, D.A., Becker, G., Webster, L.R., Davies, A.N., & Mawe, G.M. (2014). Emerging treatments in neurogastroenterology: A multidisciplinary working group consensus statement on opioid-induced constipation. *Neurogastroenterology and Motility, 26,* 1386–1395. doi:10.1111/nmo.12417

Clark, K., Byfieldt, N., Dawe, M., & Currow, D.C. (2012). Treating constipation in palliative care: The impact of other factors aside from opioids. *American Journal of Hospice and Palliative Medicine, 29,* 122–125. doi:10.1177/1049909111409389

Clark, K., & Currow, D.C. (2012). Assessing constipation in palliative care within a gastroenterology framework. *Palliative Medicine, 26,* 834–841. doi:10.1177/0269216311414756

Clark, K., Urban, K., & Currow, D.C. (2010). Current approaches to diagnosing and managing constipation in advanced cancer and palliative care. *Journal of Palliative Medicine, 13,* 473–476. doi:10.1089/jpm.2009.0274

Dahl, W.J., & Stewart, M.L. (2015). Position of the Academy of Nutrition and Dietetics: Health implications of dietary fiber. *Journal of the Academy of Nutrition and Dietetics, 115,* 1861–1870. doi:10.1016/j.jand.2015.09.003

Folden, S.L. (2002). Practice guidelines for the management of constipation in adults. *Rehabilitation Nursing, 27,* 169–175. doi:10.1002/j.2048-7940.2002.tb02005.x

Ford, A.C., Moayyedi, P., Lacy, B.E., Lembo, A.J., Saito, Y.A., Schiller, L.R., … Quigley, E.M. (2014). American College of Gastroenterology monograph on the management of irritable bowel syndrome and chronic idiopathic constipation. *American Journal of Gastroenterology, 109*(Suppl. 1), S2–S26.

Gallegos-Orozco, J.F., Foxx-Orenstein, A.E., Sterler, S.M., & Stoa, J.M. (2012). Chronic constipation in the elderly. *American Journal of Gastroenterology, 107,* 18–25.

Hunt, R., Quigley, E., Abbas, Z., Eliakim, A., Emmanuel, A., Goh, K.-L., … LeMair, A. (2014). Coping with common gastrointestinal symptoms in the community: A global perspective on heartburn, constipation, bloating, and abdominal pain/discomfort May 2013. *Journal of Clinical Gastroenterology, 48,* 567–578. doi:10.1097/MCG.0000000000000141

Larkin, P.J., Sykes, N.P., Centeno, C., Ellershaw, J.E., Elsner, F., Eugene, B., … Zuurmond, W.W.A. (2008). The management of constipation in palliative care: Clinical practice recommendations. *Palliative Medicine, 22,* 796–807. doi:10.1177/0269216308096908

McHugh, M.E., & Miller-Saultz, D. (2011). Assessment and management of gastrointestinal symptoms in advanced illness. *Primary Care: Clinics in Office Practice, 38,* 225–246. doi:10.1016/j.pop.2011.03.005

McKay, S.L., Fravel, M., & Scanlon, C. (2009). Management of constipation. Iowa City, IA: University of Iowa Gerontological Nursing Interventions Research Center, Research Translation and Dissemination Core.

National Comprehensive Cancer Network. (2015). *NCCN Clinical Practice Guidelines in Oncology (NCCN Guidelines®): Palliative care* [v.1.2016]. Retrieved from http://www.nccn.org/professionals/physician_gls/pdf/palliative.pdf

National Institute of Diabetes and Digestive and Kidney Diseases. (2015). Constipation. Retrieved from http://www.niddk.nih.gov/health-information/health-topics/digestive-diseases/constipation/Pages/overview.aspx

Sykes, N.P. (2006). The pathogenesis of constipation. *Journal of Supportive Oncology, 4,* 213–218.

Thorpe, D.M., Byar, K.L., Conley, S., Davis, A.B., Drapek, L., Hays, A., … Kiker, E.S. (2015, July 29). Putting Evidence Into Practice: Constipation. Retrieved from https://www.ons.org/practice-resources/pep/constipation

University of Michigan Comprehensive Cancer Center. (2012, May). Nutritional management of constipation. Retrieved from http://www.cancer.med.umich.edu/files/nutritional-management-of-constipation.pdf

CHAPTER 22

Cough

Craig S. Conoscenti, MD, FCCP

I. Definition
   A. Cough is a common symptom that results in frequent healthcare provider visits in both the primary and secondary care settings.
   B. Cough can cause significant disruption to patients' daily lives.
   C. Acute cough, defined as one lasting less than three weeks (Morice, McGarvey, & Pavord, 2006), is generally something that is self-limiting and rarely requires the use of healthcare resources.
   D. Chronic cough can be an indicator of chronic respiratory disease or other nonrespiratory illnesses.
      1. Chronic cough is defined as one lasting more than eight weeks (Morice et al., 2006).
      2. The period between three and eight weeks is a gray zone that is marked by many patients with a postviral cough that can linger and still resolve spontaneously (Morice et al., 2006).
   E. In 2006, the British Thoracic Society released cough guidelines (Morice et al., 2006). These guidelines defined cough as a forced expulsive maneuver, usually against a closed glottis, that is associated with a characteristic sound.
II. Pathophysiology
   A. Early work in animal models of the cough reflex revealed that the basis for cough was a vagal reflex that resulted in the physical maneuver of cough (Morice, 2008).
   B. This early work also led to an understanding that two models of cough exist.
      1. The first model is a three-phase maneuver that is initiated with inspiration (inspiratory phase), followed by expiration against a closed glottis (compressive phase), followed by expiratory flow as the glottis opens (expiratory phase) (Morice, 2008).
      2. The second model of cough just involves an expiratory maneuver (Morice, 2008).
   C. The cough reflex is multifactorial.
      1. It is the result of modifications to normal breathing patterns as a reflex to certain stimuli (Widdicombe, 1998).
      2. Cough requires the accurately timed and sequential coordination of the activation of the diaphragm, chest wall, cervical spine, and abdominal and laryngeal muscles and input from the medullary and higher cortical regions within the brain (Morris et al., 2003; Poliacek et al., 2005).
         a) Sensory phase: Mechanosensory input

Any views expressed in this chapter represent the personal opinions of the author and not those of Boehringer Ingelheim Pharmaceuticals.

  (1) Mechanical stimulation, postnasal drip, and a water bolus placed into the pharynx will evoke coughing (Canning, 2007; Canning et al., 2004).

  (2) The mechanosensory cough is comprised of an inspiratory maneuver followed by an expiratory maneuver.

  (3) It can manifest as just a short expiratory maneuver, which is referred to as an *expiratory reflex* (Baekey et al., 2001; Polley et al., 2008; Tatar, Hanacek, & Widdicombe, 2008).

 b) Chemosensory input

  (1) The activation of C-fibers in the airways induces coughing, mucus production, and bronchoconstriction. C-fibers are found in the mucosa of airways, the lung parenchyma, and also in the spaces between epithelial cells.

  (2) They will respond to thermal stimuli, chemical stimuli (i.e., capsaicin), acid, cigarette smoke, and air pollutants (Rogerio, Andrade, & Calixto, 2011).

  (3) The sensation of an urge to cough is ostensibly associated with activation of bronchopulmonary C-fibers (Davenport, Vovk, Duke, Bolser, & Robertson, 2009; Mazzone, McLennan, McGovern, Egan, & Farrell, 2007).

 c) Motor phase (Brooks, 2011)

  (1) During the inspiratory phase of cough, the glottis is in abduction.

  (2) The laryngeal motor neurons that begin in the nucleus ambiguus follow vagal and superior laryngeal nerves to excite the motor neurons of the glottis, external intercostal muscles, diaphragm, and other major inspiratory and expiratory respiratory muscles.

  (3) The compressive phase of the cough reflex begins almost immediately after inspiration.

  (4) The laryngeal motor neurons are transiently hyperpolarized during the transition between the inspiratory and expiratory compressive phases of the cough, resulting in glottis closure.

  (5) Glottis closure is essential for the process of coughing because the maximal level of intrathoracic pressure is attained, and the efficiency of the expiratory cough depends in great part on the quality of glottic occlusion.

 d) Expiratory phase (Brooks, 2011)

  (1) The expiratory phase of the cough reflex begins as the laryngeal adductor muscles (thyroarytenoid and arytenoideus) contract.

  (2) A diaphragmatic force assists in producing the cough. Additionally, the laryngeal adductor motor neurons are inhibited, which is important in the generation of explosive expiratory airflow as the cough progresses.

  (3) The posterior cricoarytenoid muscles contract for a brief period, which enlarges the glottic opening to a lesser degree than during the inspiratory phase.

  (4) This leads to a strong positive swing of pleural pressure.

  (5) The cricothyroid muscle causes vocal fold elongation and increased size of the glottic opening.

  (6) A transiently relaxed glottis releases a burst of expired air, and the full expiratory cough phase ensues.

(7) Finally, the larynx constricts a bit, and the diaphragm relaxes after coughing stops.

D. Epidemiology

1. Cough is an important epidemiologic concern but has been neglected over the years in large controlled epidemiologic studies.

2. Studying cough from an epidemiologic perspective is important for several reasons.

   a) First, cough is a very common symptom that affects many people.

   b) Second, it is less complex to understand the symptom of cough than it is to explore the entire complex of respiratory diseases, such as asthma and chronic obstructive pulmonary disease (COPD), for which cough is one of many symptoms.

   c) Third, it is possible for cough to represent a specific disease entity, such as cough hypersensitivity syndrome, which would warrant further study (Kauffmann & Varraso, 2011).

   d) Addressing the heterogenic nature of cough allows for research in both disease-related cough, such as in asthma and COPD, as well as unexplained chronic cough, which affects many people and results in cough clinic visits (Chung & Pavord, 2008).

III. Presenting symptoms: Cough is a symptom, but patients will often present with the following additional symptoms (Morice & Kastelik, 2003; Morice et al., 2006):

A. Postnasal drip

B. Sinus congestion

C. Frequent clearing of throat

D. Sensation of secretions in posterior pharynx

E. Symptoms of gastroesophageal reflux disease (GERD)

F. Wheezing

G. Sputum production

H. Dyspnea

I. Malaise

J. Rhinorrhea

K. Fever

IV. Diagnostics

A. Standardized questionnaires are typically used to characterize cough in epidemiologic studies.

1. The first major questionnaire was developed for chronic bronchitis with an emphasis on cough and sputum production and derived from the British Medical Research Council questionnaire from the 1950s.

2. Those questions were then incorporated into the European Coal and Steel Community and the American Thoracic Society questionnaires, which were used into the 1970s.

3. As the prevalence of asthma increased, asthma-related questionnaires expanded the understanding of symptoms and led to two large international studies: the European Community Respiratory Health Survey for adults and the International Study on Asthma and Allergy in Children (Chung & Pavord, 2008).

4. More clinically oriented quality-of-life questionnaires have been designed and are now standardized and used in epidemiologic surveys.

   a) One example is the Asthma Quality of Life Questionnaire, which includes a specific question on cough.

    b) The problem with using data from a single item in a questionnaire is that the questionnaire is typically based on global scoring (Chung & Pavord, 2008; Juniper, Guyatt, Ferrie, & Griffith, 1993).

5. With the use of several different questionnaire surveys, the prevalence of cough in many cohorts in Europe and the United States is 9%–33%.

6. With cough being a predominant symptom in chronic smokers, its prevalence is three times higher in smokers than in nonsmokers or former smokers.

7. Exposure to particulate matter, especially particles 10 microns or smaller in diameter (referred to as PM10), often results in productive cough and nonproductive cough in adults and children (Chung & Pavord, 2008; Cook & Strachan, 1999; David, Koh, Lee, Yu, & London, 2005; Ho, Lam, Chung, & Lam, 2006; Ségala et al., 2004; Zemp et al., 1999).

B. Cough accounts for approximately 6% of all referrals to general practice clinics. Approximately 90% of these patients had either bronchial hyperresponsiveness or upper airway disease as the etiology of the cough (Morice & Kastelik, 2003).

1. In contrast to this, more than half of the patients referred to a general respiratory clinic had underlying lung disorders such as asthma, bronchiectasis, COPD, pulmonary fibrosis, or lung cancer.

2. Because of this referral pattern, many common causes of cough have been excluded by the time a patient is referred to a pulmonary clinic (Kardos & Gebhardt, 1996; McGarvey, Heaney, & MacMahon, 1998; Morice & Kastelik, 2003).

C. In a study by Palombini et al. (1999), patients with chronic cough underwent more than 12 diagnostic procedures during evaluation.

1. The patients were considered positive for a diagnosis if the result was abnormal.

2. This led to the finding that cough had multiple causes in more than 60% of the patients.

3. Even if the evaluation is tailored to just the presenting symptoms, multiple diagnoses still are made.

4. The three most common causes of chronic cough are asthma, esophageal disease, and rhinitis.

5. This so-called diagnostic triad accounts for the majority of patients who suffer from chronic cough (Palombini et al., 1999).

D. Defining asthma in epidemiologic studies has been quite problematic.

1. There is no single test that has sufficient sensitivity and specificity to allow for diagnosis of a disease with extensive symptoms and presentations.

2. This is particularly obvious when cough is the presenting symptom.

3. Asthma associated with cough has been termed *cough-variant asthma* or *variant asthma* and was originally described by Glauser (1972).

4. It was more clearly described by Corrao, Braman, and Irwin (1979) who reported on six patients with cough, bronchial hyperresponsiveness, and bronchodilator response but exhibited no wheezing or airflow obstruction.

5. Subsequently, Pratter, Bartter, Akers, and DuBois (1993) coined the term *cough-predominant asthma* to account for the fact that cough is part of the spectrum of asthma that includes wheezing, dyspnea, and airflow obstruction (Corrao et al., 1979; Glauser, 1972; Pratter et al., 1993; Siersted et al., 1996; Taylor, 1997).

6. The presence of eosinophilic inflammation in cough-predominant asthma and a variant, eosinophilic bronchitis, is characterized by airway eosinophilia but the absence of bronchial hyperresponsiveness.

E. Eosinophilic bronchitis can be identified in patients with a chronic cough when there is the availability of sputum induction and a reliable analytic process (Brightling, Ward, Goh, Wardlaw, & Pavord, 1999; Carney et al., 1997; Gibson, Denburg, Dolovich, Ramsdale, & Hargreave, 1989; Niimi et al., 1998). Eosinophilic bronchitis and cough-predominant asthma appear to be distinct entities, which are etiologies of chronic cough.

F. GERD can be found in up to 40% of patients with chronic cough (Morice & Kastelik, 2003).

   1. The exact mechanism of the relationship is not fully understood (Morice & Kastelik, 2003).

   2. Cough can result from the relationship between GERD, and cough may include microaspiration of esophageal contents into the perilaryngeal space or tracheobronchial tree.

   3. It also may be due to a localized inflammatory reaction of the cough receptors in the lower esophagus (Morice & Kastelik, 2003).

   4. Reports show that up to 75% of patients may have cough as their sole presenting symptom of GERD (Morice & Kastelik, 2003).

   5. Assuming the upright posture causes the lower esophageal sphincter to relax. This often precipitates a cough, which is a characteristic finding in GERD-associated cough. Although often a difficult symptom to elicit, it is an important finding (Dent et al., 1980).

   6. Even though a complete history and physical may show no indication of GERD, it may still be the etiology of the cough.

   7. In these circumstances, 24-hour ambulatory esophageal pH monitoring can be used.

      a) Not all patients who test positive on 24-hour monitoring will necessarily respond to antireflux therapy, and not all patients with a negative study fail to respond to antireflux treatment.

      b) Studies suggest that an empirical course of antireflux therapy should be used prior to testing because not all patients respond the same way to this type of therapy.

      c) Of note, it may take up to several months for a response and may require elevated doses of antireflux medications (Kiljander, Salomaa, Hietanen, & Terho, 2000; Ours, Kavuru, Schilz, & Richter, 1999; Vaezi & Richter, 1997; Waring, Lacayo, Hunter, Katz, & Suwak, 1995).

G. In opposition to the relatively direct way in which cough associated with asthma and GERD can be investigated, the relationship of cough with upper respiratory disease is much less objective and more difficult to prove.

H. Postnasal drip syndrome (PNDS) has been reported to be one of the most common causes of chronic cough (Morice & Kastelik, 2003).

   1. The main problem is that this "syndrome" has no objective identifying findings.

   2. The diagnosis relies on identifying one or more of the following: the sensation of something dripping in the throat, frequent throat clearing, nasal congestion, or nasal discharge.

   3. A major complication is that these symptoms are common in those without a cough (Irwin, Curley, & French, 1990; Palombini et al., 1999; Pratter et al., 1993; Smyrnios, Irwin, & Curley, 1995).

   4. The use of the term *PNDS* for cough is secondary to the fact that clinicians have observed clinical responses to the combination of antihistamines and decongestants.

     5. Pratter et al. (1993) used a stepwise therapy approach that started with the combination of a decongestant and antihistamine. This allowed for a diagnosis of PNDS in more than 80% of the patients. Some of these patients actually presented with only cough and were otherwise asymptomatic.

     6. For this group, it was proposed that the diagnosis be called *silent PNDS* (Morice & Kastelik, 2003; Pratter et al., 1993).

I. Other causes of chronic cough exist. Even though several distinct causes have been mentioned already, others cause diagnostic confusion when confronted.

J. Angiotensin-converting enzyme (ACE) inhibitors are frequently used as antihypertensive agents, and up to 15% of patients treated with ACE inhibitors have an associated cough response (Yeo, Chadwick, Kraskiewicz, Jackson, & Ramsay, 1995; Yeo, Foster, & Ramsay, 1991).

     1. This cough has a variable onset of action and also a variable occurrence of disappearing (Yeo et al., 1991, 1995).

     2. ACE inhibitors are known to alter the sensitivity of the cough reflex and can account for the cough (Morice, Brown, Lowry, & Higenbottam, 1987).

     3. In addition, those with subclinical cough due to GERD or PNDS may suddenly see the cough become apparent because of this alteration in the cough reflex (Morice et al., 2006).

     4. Although cessation of ACE inhibitors returns the cough reflex to normal, the variable of the reflex results in up to several months of continued coughing before it subsides (Ojoo, Kastelik, & Morice, 2001; Yeo et al., 1995).

K. A variety of agents have been shown to have a variable effect on the cough, such as sodium cromoglycate, nifedipine, and indomethacin (Fogari et al., 1992; Hargreaves & Benson, 1995).

L. Occupational diseases also can be an important cause of chronic cough.

     1. When cough occurs as an isolated finding, clinicians need to assess the potential for low-molecular-weight irritants as the etiology.

     2. An example is glass bottle workers exposed to hydrochloric acid and organic oils (Gordon, Curran, Fishwick, Morice, & Howard, 1998; Gordon et al., 1997).

M. For some patients, a minor respiratory tract infections results in a subsequent prolonged cough.

     1. Cough can remain for several weeks to months following an infection.

     2. It has been thought that viral infections are more likely to cause this response, yet cough also occurs in the presence of bacterial infection (Morice & Kastelik, 2003).

V. Interventions

A. In most instances, acute cough is of known etiology and requires symptomatic therapy.

     1. If the acute event is a viral infection, prescription therapy typically is not necessary.

     2. Patients have reported variable responses to over-the-counter preparations, although the specific pharmacologic effect remains unknown (Morice et al., 2006).

B. Opiate antitussives carry a significant adverse event profile and should be avoided (Morice et al., 2006).

C. Chronic cough poses a different circumstance.

     1. Care needs to be given to address not only the cough but the underlying etiology.

     2. If the underlying etiology is treated, the cough will equally be treated. Patients will vary in their time to resolution of cough.

D. All components of cough-variant asthma typically respond to inhaled corticosteroids.
   1. Although an early response to inhaled corticosteroids occurs in classical asthma, this response is often delayed in cough-variant asthma (Morice & Kastelik, 2003; Pratter et al., 1993).
   2. In cough associated with the variant of eosinophilic bronchitis, improvement in cough and sputum eosinophilia has been seen within four weeks of inhaled corticosteroid.
   3. Despite this finding, treatment may be required for several months to obtain maximum response (Brightling, Ward, Wardlaw, & Pavord, 2000; Morice & Kastelik, 2003).
   4. Some patients, despite moderate doses of inhaled corticosteroid, remain symptomatic with cough. No clear-cut evidence-based strategy is available to address this continued cough.
E. Leukotriene antagonists have not been shown to have an effect on cough as seen in classic asthma, but evidence supports their efficacy in cough-variant asthma (Dicpinigaitis & Dobkin, 1999; Dicpinigaitis, Dobkin, & Reichel, 2002).
F. Evidence suggests that lipoxygenase compounds, such as zileuton, may have a role in cough-variant asthma (Morice & Kastelik, 2003).
G. Fujimura and colleagues have shown a significant response to antihistamines in a syndrome they have called *eosinophilic tracheobronchitis* (Fujimura, Ogawa, Yasui, & Matsuda, 2000; Fujimura, Sakamoto, & Matsuda 1992; Fujimura, Songür, Kamio, & Matsuda, 1997).
H. In the treatment of chronic cough associated with GERD, conservative measures are often helpful.
   1. Some measures that have been identified include weight reduction; high-protein, low-fat diets; elevation of the head of the bed; and avoidance of smoking, caffeine, and chocolate.
   2. There is no basis for this positive response despite frequent use of treatment rendered (Morice & Kastelik, 2003).
I. GERD-associated chronic cough frequently responds to antireflux therapy.
   1. H_2 antagonists, proton pump inhibitors (PPIs), and prokinetic medications have been used (Irwin, Corrao, & Pratter, 1981; Irwin et al., 1990; Irwin, Zawacki, Curley, French, & Hoffman, 1989; McGarvey, Heaney, Lawson, et al., 1998; O'Connell, Thomas, Pride, & Fuller, 1994; Smyrnios et al., 1995; Waring et al., 1995). PPIs, particularly at high doses, seem superior in treating cough (Pratter et al., 1993; Vaezi & Richter, 1997).
   2. PPIs also appear to be effective in patients with abnormal esophageal manometry but normal 24-hour pH monitoring (Kastelik et al., 2003).
J. Cough associated with PNDS has responded to the combination of antihistamines and decongestants. Pratter et al. (1993) used a stepwise therapy approach that started with the combination of a decongestant and antihistamine and resulted in a significant treatment response.
K. Typical over-the-counter treatments such as nasal saline sprays have been shown to be very helpful but with very short response time and frequent use.
L. Although cessation of ACE inhibitors helps to resolve cough associated with these agents, it can take up to several months of continued coughing before it subsides (Ojoo et al., 2001; Yeo et al., 1995).
M. A variety of agents such as sodium cromoglycate, nifedipine, and indomethacin have been shown to have variable effects on the cough (Fogari et al., 1992; Hargreaves

& Benson, 1995). Alternative agents that provide similar beneficial antihypertensive actions should be considered as substitutes for ACE inhibitors.

N. Follow-up

1. The heterogeneity of cough, especially chronic cough, remains partially understood.

2. More research needs to be done regarding the findings of cough in large populations.

3. In addition, better characterization of environmental aspects of chronic cough needs to be established.

    a) When patients present with chronic cough, they have evidence of the significant morbidity associated with the cough.

    b) Although lengthy, the investigation of the chronic cough is often successful in determining the underlying etiology.

    c) A standard approach should be used including a full history and physical, simple diagnostic investigations, and therapeutic trials aimed at the underlying cause.

    d) Failure of therapy should lead to further investigation for an alternate etiology.

Case Study

A.K. is a 34-year-old Caucasian man who works as a heating and refrigeration technician. For the past several days, he has experienced progressive discomfort associated with near-continuous postnasal dripping and frequent awakening at night from a dry nonproductive cough. He is feeling fatigued and frustrated by his inability to get a full night's sleep and experiences a nagging sore throat with occasional cough during the day.

A.K. reports to the clinic, stating, "I have been having a runny nose, sniffling, and sore throat." History of present illness reveals intermittent symptoms for about one month but more frequent in the past 7–10 days. The drainage is clear, and his sore throat is worse upon awakening. A.K. has disturbed sleep and frequent awakening. He has not experienced febrile episodes but occasionally experiences dysphagia. He has been using an over-the-counter sinus product with acetaminophen and phenylephrine at bedtime. The patient is not using prescribed medication because of the cost.

A.K.'s current medications consist of the acetaminophen-phenylephrine 2 tabs every evening, albuterol HFA 2 puffs every three to four hours PRN, and fluticasone propionate-salmeterol 250 mcg/50 mcg dry powder inhaler BID. He reports allergies to pollen, ragweed, mites, and dust but no medication or food allergies. His past medical history includes seasonal allergies, exercise-induced asthma diagnosed when he was a child, and asthma exacerbation about twice a year, usually in the spring and fall. Past surgical history is unremarkable. The family history reveals that his mother has asthma, hypertension, and hyperlipidemia; his father died of motor vehicle accident; and all four grandparents died of myocardial infarction. A.K.'s social history reveals he is a 5-pack-year smoker and drinks a 12-pack of light beer per week. He lives with his girlfriend and has a dog.

The advanced practice registered nurse (APRN) performs a review of systems, finding that A.K. is not in acute distress. Head, eyes, ears, nose, and throat (HEENT) examination finds no purulent mucus, ophthalmic drainage, itchy eyes, or loss of hearing. Pulmonary examination finds no wheezing, dyspnea, purulent mucus on cough, or exercise intolerance.

Physical examination findings include blood pressure of 146/88 mm Hg, pulse rate of 86 beats per minute, respiratory rate of 22 breaths per minute, temperature of 99°F (37.2°C), and body mass index of 32 kg/m². His general appearance is older than stated age, and he appears sleepy with apathy and occasional sniffling.

HEENT examination finds pupils equal and reactive to light and accommodation, bilateral conjunctivae innervated and pale, tympanic membranes intact and nonbulging bilaterally, nasal turbinates intact and erythematous, and no polyps. Oropharynx appears erythematous, and uvula uncrowded. Right posterior auricular lymphadenopathy is noted. Chest examination finds heart rate and rhythm with S_1 and S_2, no S_3 or S_4. Lungs have bilateral wheezing in the lower lobes with deep inspiration that clears with cough. No hyperresonance or dullness to percussion is noted. Abdominal examination was deferred, as the patient is morbidly obese. Peripheral vascular examination finds no edema or claudication and strong pedal pulses. The APRN's assessment findings include cough secondary to postnasal drip syndrome, allergic rhinitis, asthma, conjunctivitis, sleep apnea, obesity, and GERD.

The APRN draws a complete blood count with differential and comprehensive metabolic panel (the patient's last laboratory tests were two years ago), as well as lipids and spirometry (forced expiratory volume in one second, or FEV_1, baseline) postbronchodilator. The nurse educates A.K. on bronchodilator use and increased prevalence of an asthmatic exacerbation. A.K. receives education on smoking cessation, weight loss, and increased physical activity. He is prescribed mometasone furoate nasal spray 50 mcg/spray 2 sprays each nostril every day and instructed to initiate albuterol inhalation 2 puffs four times a day, especially prior to physical activity. Follow-up will take place depending on laboratory results or if symptoms worsen. A prophylactic macrolide antibiotic is prescribed as needed for exacerbation (azithromycin 500 mg day 1, then 250 mg PO every 24 hours for four days), as well as prednisone taper 40 mg for two days, 20 mg for two days, and 10 mg for two days, and discontinue. A.K. is instructed to call the APRN prior to filling the prescription. The APRN may need to evaluate for GERD if symptoms persist.

References

Baekey, D.M., Morris, K.F., Gestreau, C., Li, Z., Lindsey, B.G., & Shannon, R. (2001). Medullary respiratory neurones and control of laryngeal motoneurones during fictive eupnoea and cough in the cat. *Journal of Physiology, 534*, 565–581. doi:10.1111/j.1469-7793.2001.t01-1-00565.x

Brightling, C.E., Ward, R., Goh, K.L., Wardlaw, A.J., & Pavord, I.D. (1999). Eosinophilic bronchitis is an important cause of chronic cough. *American Journal of Respiratory and Critical Care Medicine, 160*, 406–410. doi:10.1164/ajrccm.160.2.9810100

Brightling, C.E., Ward, R., Wardlaw, A.J., & Pavord, I.D. (2000). Airway inflammation, airway responsiveness and cough before and after inhaled budesonide in patients with eosinophilic bronchitis. *European Respiratory Journal, 15*, 682–686. doi:10.1034/j.1399-3003.2000.15d10.x

Brooks, S.M. (2011). Perspective on the human cough reflex. *Cough, 7*, 10. doi:10.1186/1745-9974-7-10

Canning, B.J. (2007). Encoding of the cough reflex. *Pulmonary Pharmacology and Therapeutics, 20*, 396–401. doi:10.1016/j.pupt.2006.12.003

Canning, B.J., Mazzone, S.B., Meeker, S.N., Mori, N., Reynolds, S.M., & Undem, B.J. (2004). Identification of tracheal and laryngeal afferent neurones mediating cough in anaesthetized guinea-pigs. *Journal of Physiology, 557*, 543–558. doi:10.1113/jphysiol.2003.057885

Carney, I.K., Gibson, P.G., Murree-Allen, K., Saltos, N., Olson, L.G., & Hensley, M.J. (1997). A systematic evaluation of mechanisms in chronic cough. *American Journal of Respiratory and Critical Care Medicine, 156*, 211–216. doi:10.1164/ajrccm.156.1.9605044

Chung, K.F., & Pavord, I.D. (2008). Prevalence, pathogenesis, and causes of chronic cough. *Lancet, 371*, 1364–1374. doi:10.1016/S0140-6736(08)60595-4

Cook, D.G., & Strachan, D.P. (1999). Summary of effects of parental smoking on the respiratory health of children and implications for research. *Thorax, 54*, 357–366. doi:10.1136/thx.54.4.357

Corrao, W.M., Braman, S.S., & Irwin, R.S. (1979). Chronic cough as the sole presenting manifestation of bronchial asthma. *New England Journal of Medicine, 300,* 633–637. doi:10.1056/NEJM197903223001201

Davenport, P.W., Vovk, A., Duke, R.K., Bolser, D.C., & Robertson, E. (2009). The urge-to-cough and cough motor response modulation by the central effects of nicotine. *Pulmonary Pharmacology and Therapeutics, 22,* 82–89. doi:10.1016/j.pupt.2008.11.013

David, G.L., Koh, W.-P., Lee, H.-P., Yu, M.C., & London, S.J. (2005). Childhood exposure to environmental tobacco smoke and chronic respiratory symptoms in non-smoking adults: The Singapore Chinese Health Study. *Thorax, 60,* 1052–1058. doi:10.1136/thx.2005.042960

Dent, J., Dodds, W.J., Friedman, R.H., Sekiguchi, T., Hogan, W.J., Arndorfer, R.C., & Petrie, D.J. (1980). Mechanism of gastroesophageal reflux in recumbent asymptomatic human subjects. *Journal of Clinical Investigation, 65,* 256–267. doi:10.1172/JCI109667

Dicpinigaitis, P.V., & Dobkin, J.B. (1999). Effect of zafirlukast on cough reflex sensitivity in asthmatics. *Journal of Asthma, 36,* 265–270. doi:10.3109/02770909909075410

Dicpinigaitis, P.V., Dobkin, J.B., & Reichel, J. (2002). Antitussive effect of the leukotriene receptor antagonist zafirlukast in subjects with cough-variant asthma. *Journal of Asthma, 39,* 291–297. doi:10.1081/JAS-120002285

Fogari, R., Zoppi, A., Tettamanti, F., Malamani, G.D., Tinelli, C., & Salvetti, A. (1992). Effects of nifedipine and indomethacin on cough induced by angiotensin-converting enzyme inhibitors: A double-blind, randomized, cross-over study. *Journal of Cardiovascular Pharmacology, 19,* 670–673.

Fujimura, M., Ogawa, H., Yasui, M., & Matsuda, T. (2000). Eosinophilic tracheobronchitis and airway cough hypersensitivity in chronic non-productive cough. *Clinical and Experimental Allergy, 30,* 41–47. doi:10.1046/j.1365-2222.2000.00698.x

Fujimura, M., Sakamoto, S., & Matsuda, T. (1992). Bronchodilator-resistive cough in atopic patients: Bronchial reversibility and hyperresponsiveness. *Internal Medicine, 31,* 447–452. doi:10.2169/internalmedicine.31.447

Fujimura, M., Songür, N., Kamio, Y., & Matsuda, T. (1997). Detection of eosinophils in hypertonic saline-induced sputum in patients with chronic nonproductive cough. *Journal of Asthma, 34,* 119–126. doi:10.3109/02770909709075656

Gibson, P.G., Denburg, J., Dolovich, J., Ramsdale, E.H., & Hargreave, F.E. (1989). Chronic cough: Eosinophilic bronchitis without asthma. *Lancet, 333,* 1346–1348. doi:10.1016/S0140-6736(89)92801-8

Glauser, F.L. (1972). Variant asthma. *Annals of Allergy, 30,* 457–459.

Gordon, S.B., Curran, A.D., Fishwick, D., Morice, A.H., & Howard, P. (1998). Respiratory symptoms among glass bottle workers—Cough and airways irritancy syndrome? *Occupational Medicine, 48,* 455–459. doi:10.1093/occmed/48.7.455

Gordon, S.B., Curran, A.D., Turley, A., Wong, C.-H., Rahman, S.N., Wiley, K., & Morice, A.H. (1997). Glass bottle workers exposed to low-dose irritant fumes cough but do not wheeze. *American Journal of Respiratory and Critical Care Medicine, 156,* 206–210. doi:10.1164/ajrccm.156.1.9610042

Hargreaves, M.R., & Benson, M.K. (1995). Inhaled sodium cromoglycate in angiotensin-converting enzyme inhibitor cough. *Lancet, 345,* 13–16. doi:10.1016/S0140-6736(95)91151-0

Ho, S.Y., Lam, T.H., Chung, S.F., & Lam, T.P. (2006). Cross-sectional and prospective associations between passive smoking and respiratory symptoms at the workplace. *Annals of Epidemiology, 17,* 126–131. doi:10.1016/j.annepidem.2006.06.010

Irwin, R.S., Corrao, W.M., & Pratter, M.R. (1981). Chronic persistent cough in the adult: The spectrum and frequency of causes and successful outcome of specific therapy. *American Review of Respiratory Disease, 123,* 413–417.

Irwin, R.S., Curley, F.J., & French, C.L. (1990). Chronic cough: The spectrum and frequency of causes, key components of the diagnostic evaluation, and outcome of specific therapy. *American Review of Respiratory Disease, 141,* 640–647. doi:10.1164/ajrccm/141.3.640

Irwin, R.S., Zawacki, J.K., Curley, F.J., French, C.L., & Hoffman, P.J. (1989). Chronic cough as the sole presenting manifestation of gastroesophageal reflux. *American Review of Respiratory Disease, 140,* 1294–1300. doi:10.1164/ajrccm/140.5.1294

Juniper, E.F., Guyatt, G.H., Ferrie, P.J., & Griffith, L.E. (1993). Measuring quality of life in asthma. *American Review of Respiratory Disease, 147,* 832–838. doi:10.1164/ajrccm/147.4.832

Kardos, P., & Gebhardt, T. (1996). [Chronic persistent cough in general practice: Diagnosis and therapy in 329 patients over the course of 2 years]. *Pneumologie, 50,* 437–441.

Kastelik, J.A., Redington, A.E., Aziz, I., Buckton, G.K., Smith, C.M., Dakkak, M., & Morice, A.H. (2003). Abnormal esophageal motility in patients with chronic cough. *Thorax, 58,* 699–702. doi:10.1136/thorax.58.8.699

Kauffmann, F., & Varraso, R. (2011). The epidemiology of cough. *Pulmonary Pharmacology and Therapeutics, 24,* 289–294. doi:10.1016/j.pupt.2010.10.012

Kiljander, T.O., Salomaa, E.R., Hietanen, E.K., & Terho, E.O. (2000). Chronic cough and gastro-oesophageal reflux: A double-blind placebo-controlled study with omeprazole. *European Respiratory Journal, 16,* 633–638. doi:10.1034/j.1399-3003.2000.16d11.x

Mazzone, S.B., McLennan, L., McGovern, A.E., Egan, G.F., & Farrell, M.J. (2007). Representation of capsaicin-evoked urge-to-cough in the human brain using functional magnetic resonance imaging. *American Journal of Respiratory and Critical Care Medicine, 176,* 327–332. doi:10.1164/rccm.200612-1856OC

McGarvey, L.P.A., Heaney, L.G., Lawson, J.T., Johnston, B.T., Scally, C.M., Ennis, M., ... MacMahon, J. (1998). Evaluation and outcome of patients with chronic non-productive cough using a comprehensive diagnostic protocol. *Thorax, 53,* 738–743. doi:10.1136/thx.53.9.738

McGarvey, L.P.A., Heaney, L.G., & MacMahon, J. (1998). A retrospective survey of diagnosis and management of patients presenting with chronic cough to a general chest clinic. *International Journal of Clinical Practice, 52,* 158–161.

Morice, A.H. (2008). Rebuttal: Cough is an expiratory sound. *Lung, 186*(Suppl. 1), 7–9. doi:10.1007/s00408-007-9039-5

Morice, A.H., Brown, M.J., Lowry, R., & Higenbottam, T. (1987). Angiotensin-converting enzyme and the cough reflex. *Lancet, 330,* 1116–1118. doi:10.1016/S0140-6736(87)91547-9

Morice, A.H., & Kastelik, J.A. (2003). Chronic cough in adults. *Thorax, 58,* 901–907. doi:10.1136/thorax.58.10.901

Morice, A.H., McGarvey, L., & Pavord, I. (2006). Recommendations for the management of cough in adults. *Thorax, 61*(Suppl. 1), i1–i24. doi:10.1136/thx.2006.065144

Morris, K.F., Baekey, D.M., Nuding, S.C., Dick, T.E., Shannon, R., & Lindsey, B.G. (2003). Invited review: Neural network plasticity in respiratory control. *Journal of Applied Physiology, 94,* 1242–1252. doi:10.1152/japplphysiol.00715.2002

Niimi, A., Amitani, R., Suzuki, K., Tanaka, E., Murayama, T., & Kuze, F. (1998). Eosinophilic inflammation in cough variant asthma. *European Respiratory Journal, 11,* 1064–1069. doi:10.1183/09031936.98.11051064

O'Connell, F., Thomas, V.E., Pride, N.B., & Fuller, R.W. (1994). Capsaicin cough sensitivity decreases with successful treatment of chronic cough. *American Journal of Respiratory and Critical Care Medicine, 150,* 374–380. doi:10.1164/ajrccm.150.2.8049818

Ojoo, J.C., Kastelik, J.A., & Morice, A.H. (2001). Duration of angiotensin converting enzyme inhibitor induced cough. *Thorax, 56*(Suppl. III), iii72.

Ours, T.M., Kavuru, M.S., Schilz, R.J., & Richter, J.E. (1999). A prospective evaluation of esophageal testing and a double-blind, randomized study of omeprazole in a diagnostic and therapeutic algorithm for chronic cough. *American Journal of Gastroenterology, 94,* 3131–3138.

Palombini, B.C., Villanova, C.A.C., Araújo, E., Gastal, O.L., Alt, D.C., Stolz, D.P., & Palombini, C.O. (1999). A pathogenic triad in chronic cough: Asthma, postnasal drip syndrome, and gastroesophageal reflux disease. *Chest, 116,* 279–284. doi:10.1378/chest.116.2.279

Poliacek, I., Stránsky, A., Szereda-Przestaszewska, M., Jakus, J., Baráni, H., Tomori, Z., & Halasová, E. (2005). Cough and laryngeal muscle discharges in brainstem lesioned anaesthetized cats. *Physiological Research, 54,* 645–654.

Polley, L., Yaman, N., Heaney, L., Cardwell, C., Murtagh, E., Ramsey, J., ... McGarvey, L. (2008). Impact of cough across different chronic respiratory diseases: Comparison of two cough-specific health-related quality of life questionnaires. *Chest, 134,* 295–302. doi:10.1378/chest.07-0141

Pratter, M.R., Bartter, T., Akers, S., & DuBois, J. (1993). An algorithmic approach to chronic cough. *Annals of Internal Medicine, 119,* 977–983. doi:10.7326/0003-4819-119-10-199311150-00003

Rogerio, A.P., Andrade, E.L., & Calixto, J.B. (2011). C-fibers, but not the transient potential receptor vanilloid 1 (TRPV1), play a role in experimental allergic airway inflammation. *European Journal of Pharmacology, 662,* 55–62. doi:10.1016/j.ejphar.2011.04.027

Ségala, C., Poizeau, D., Neukirch, F., Aubier, M., Samson, J., & Gehanno, P. (2004). Air pollution, passive smoking, and respiratory symptoms in adults. *Archives of Environmental Health, 59,* 669–676. doi:10.1080/00039890409602952

Siersted, H.C., Mostgaard, G., Hyldebrandt, N., Hansen, H.S., Boldsen, J., & Oxhøj, H. (1996). Interrelationships between diagnosed asthma, asthma-like symptoms, and abnormal airway behaviour in adolescence: The Odense Schoolchild Study. *Thorax, 51,* 503–509. doi:10.1136/thx.51.5.503

Smyrnios, N.A., Irwin, R.S., & Curley, F.J. (1995). Chronic cough with a history of excessive sputum production: The spectrum and frequency of causes, key components of the diagnostic evaluation, and outcome of specific therapy. *Chest, 108,* 991–997. doi:10.1378/chest.108.4.991

Tatar, M., Hanacek, J., & Widdicombe, J.G. (2008). The expiration reflex from the trachea and bronchi. *European Respiratory Journal, 31,* 385–390. doi:10.1183/09031936.00063507

Taylor, D.R. (1997). Making the diagnosis of asthma. *BMJ, 315,* 4–5. doi:10.1136/bmj.315.7099.4

Vaezi, M.F., & Richter, J.E. (1997). Twenty-four-hour ambulatory esophageal pH monitoring in the diagnosis of acid reflux-related chronic cough. *Southern Medical Journal, 90,* 305–311.

Waring, J.P., Lacayo, L., Hunter, J., Katz, E., & Suwak, B. (1995). Chronic cough and hoarseness in patients with severe gastroesophageal reflux disease: Diagnosis and response to therapy. *Digestive Disease and Sciences, 40,* 1093–1097. doi:10.1007/BF02064205

Widdicombe, J.G. (1998). Afferent receptors in the airways and cough. *Respiratory Physiology, 114,* 5–15. doi:10.1016/S0034-5687(98)00076-0

Yeo, W.W., Chadwick, I.G., Kraskiewicz, M., Jackson, P.R., & Ramsay, L.E. (1995). Resolution of ACE inhibitor cough: Changes in subjective cough and responses to inhaled capsaicin, intradermal bradykinin and substance-P. *British Journal of Clinical Pharmacology, 40,* 423–429.

Yeo, W.W., Foster, G., & Ramsay, L.E. (1991). Prevalence of persistent cough during long-term enalapril treatment: Controlled study versus nifedipine. *Quarterly Journal of Medicine, 80,* 763–770.

Zemp, E., Elsasser, S., Schindler, C., Künzli, N., Perruchoud, A.P., Domenighetti, G., ... Zellweger, J.P. (1999). Long-term ambient air pollution and respiratory symptoms in adults (SAPALDIA study). *American Journal of Respiratory and Critical Care Medicine, 159,* 1257–1266. doi:10.1164/ajrccm.159.4.9807052

CHAPTER 23

Dehydration

Kelly Browning, MSN, RN, FNP

I. Definition
   A. Dehydration is a condition that occurs when the body lacks the adequate amount of water or fluids to function properly. This imbalance is due to inadequate fluid intake or loss of fluid from activities such as perfuse sweating, vomiting, fever, or diarrhea (U.S. National Library of Medicine, 2015).
   B. Patients living with multiple chronic conditions, young children, and older adults are most susceptible to developing severe complications such as dehydration (Centers for Disease Control and Prevention [CDC], 2012).
   C. Contributing factors include decreased fat storage or the body's inability to store water or fluid in fat cells (due to age), inadequate thermoregulation, and even medications (CDC, 1996).
      1. In these patients, the condition can become severe, leading to a life-threatening situation (U.S. National Library of Medicine, 2015).
      2. An example of a patient with increased risk for dehydration is a patient with uncontrolled type 2 diabetes mellitus. This patient is prone to fluid loss due to excessive urination.
      3. Other concomitant conditions that often accompany diabetes, such as hypertension, may further compound the fluid loss if the patient is taking diuretic medications (U.S. National Library of Medicine, 2015).
      4. These patients face increased risk for morbidity and mortality, experience decreased quality of life, incur increased health costs, and require frequent hospitalizations (Institute of Medicine [IOM], 2012).
      5. Therefore, it is important to recognize patients who are at risk.
II. Key aspects
   A. Various federal services acknowledge dehydration and its potential disease complications as a public health concern. The information includes current data such as healthcare expenditures related to complications of dehydration and statistics pertaining to those at risk for increased morbidity and mortality due to dehydration and disease complication.
   B. One in four adults have two or more chronic diseases such as diabetes, which can lead to dehydration and kidney failure (CDC, 2016).
   C. Dehydration is directly related to a majority of conditions, such as the following listed by CDC as the leading causes of death (Heron, 2016):
      1. Heart disease
      2. Cancer
      3. Chronic lower respiratory diseases

    4. Accidents (unintentional injuries)
    5. Stroke (cerebrovascular diseases)
    6. Alzheimer disease
    7. Diabetes
    8. Influenza and pneumonia
    9. Nephritis, nephrotic syndrome, and nephrosis
    10. Intentional self-harm (suicide)

  D. Poor nutrition is among the four health risk behaviors known to cause illness, suffering, and early death related to chronic disease and conditions (CDC, 2013).

III. Current findings

  A. The nutrition objective for Healthy People 2020 emphasizes the health benefits of behaviors aimed at maintaining a healthy diet.

    1. Limitation of sodium intake is a recommended goal for helping to reduce the risks for fluid imbalance–related health conditions such as hypertension, malnutrition, oral disease, constipation, diabetes, and some cancers (U.S. Department of Health and Human Services Office of Disease Prevention and Health Promotion, n.d.).

    2. Social and physical determinants are factors that influence healthful diets.

    3. For example, immobility due to age-related arthritic disease may limit access to water and food.

    4. In addition, diets can be influenced by demographic and economic factors (U.S. Department of Health and Human Services Office of Disease Prevention and Health Promotion, n.d.).

  B. Hospitalization for acute illnesses such as dehydration and readmissions for worsening chronic conditions such as congestive heart failure may be preventable if managed correctly (Moy, Chang, & Barrett, 2013).

    1. Conditions leading to potentially preventable hospitalizations in 2009 (Moy et al., 2013)

      a) Diabetes
      b) Congestive heart failure
      c) Angina
      d) Hypertension
      e) Asthma
      f) Dehydration
      g) Pneumonia
      h) Urinary tract infections

    2. Hospitalizations for these conditions are costly (Moy et al., 2013). It is important to manage symptoms of these fluid-imbalance conditions that contribute to readmission rates (see Figure 23-1).

IV. Relevance to practice

  A. It is predicted that people aged 65 years and older will make up the largest portion of the American population (IOM, 2012; Kuebler, 2015).

  B. Self-management is directly linked to successful outcomes regarding health promotion and prevention of chronic disease exacerbation (Kuebler, 2015; Ryan, 2009).

  C. It is important to stay current with resources available to support this initiative.

    1. Additional resources and information are illustrated in Chapter 1.

    2. The programs are each funded by the Patient Protection and Affordable Care Act of 2010.

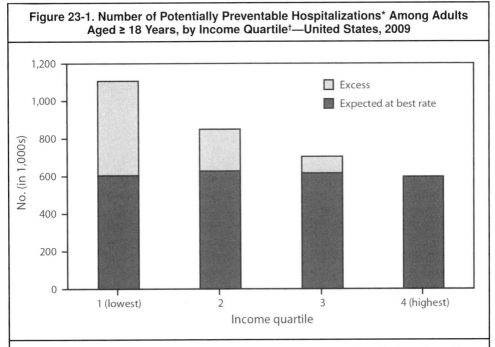

Figure 23-1. Number of Potentially Preventable Hospitalizations* Among Adults Aged ≥ 18 Years, by Income Quartile†—United States, 2009

* For diabetes, hypertension, congestive heart failure, angina without procedure, asthma, dehydration, bacterial pneumonia, and urinary infections

† Area income was divided into quartiles based on the mean household income by the patient's zip code. Quartile 1 refers to the lowest income communities, and quartile 4 refers to the wealthiest communities.

Data source: Agency for Healthcare Research and Quality, Healthcare Cost and Utilization Project, Nationwide Inpatient Sample, 2009.

Note. From "Potentially Preventable Hospitalizations—United States, 2001–2009," by E. Moy, E. Chang, and M. Barrett, 2013, *Morbidity and Mortality Weekly Report, 62,* p. 141. Retrieved from http://www.cdc.gov/mmwr/preview/mmwrhtml/su6203a23.htm.

    3. Federal programs such as the National Institute of Nursing Research, Agency for Health and Research Quality, the IOM, Centers for Medicare and Medicaid Services, and National Council on Aging have created programs to meet the U.S. Department of Health and Human Services' goals to improve self-management of an aging population with multiple chronic conditions (Kuebler, 2015).

    4. The goals serve as a guideline for healthcare providers in caring for these patients and include the following (Kuebler, 2015):

        a) Implement changes in healthcare systems to improve the health of patients living with multiple chronic diseases.

        b) Utilize self-management services to their maximal potential.

        c) Increase public awareness by providing better tools and information regarding self-management.

        d) Facilitate further research.

V. Role of the advanced practice registered nurse (APRN)

    A. APRNs play a key role in influencing self-management techniques that help prevent disease complications such as dehydration. To do so, they must first understand the basic pathophysiologic processes involved with fluid imbalance and the symptoms that often accompany the condition.

B. Pathophysiology
   1. Fluid imbalance disrupts homeostasis (Bardgett et al., 2014).
      a) If imbalance is severe, the sympathetic nervous system becomes hyperactive, resembling the autonomic responses that occur in hypertension and congestive heart failure (Bardgett et al., 2014).
      b) In addition, this activity may produce neurologic effects such as confusion, neurosensory disturbance, or seizures (Bardgett et al., 2014).
      c) For the body to make urine, water and blood must be present in the kidneys. Disruption of this process causes acute renal failure (Cunha, 2014).
      d) Dehydration is the number-one cause of this type of renal failure and is due to nausea, vomiting, diuretic medications, and blood loss (Cunha, 2014).
   2. Symptoms that present with dehydration (CDC, 2014)
      a) Moderate dehydration
         (1) Restlessness and irritability
         (2) Sunken eyes
         (3) Dry mouth and tongue
         (4) Increased thirst
         (5) Poor skin turgor
         (6) Decreased urine
      b) Severe dehydration
         (1) Lethargy
         (2) Unconsciousness
         (3) Extreme dry mouth and tongue
         (4) Skin turgor demonstrates little or no elasticity
         (5) Weak or absent pulse
         (6) Hypotension
         (7) Minimal or no urine output
VI. Integration of palliative care
   A. According to the World Health Organization (WHO, 2004), palliative care includes symptom management during both acute and chronic illness and care at the end of life.
      1. The integration of palliative care into symptom management for dehydration is important for preventing disease and helping patients maximize health and function (Mentes, 2012).
      2. Homecare interventions help relieve patients' symptoms and prevent further complications (WHO, 2004).
   B. WHO (2004) guidelines for good palliative care according to symptoms that may lead to dehydration
      1. Fever: Consider the cause, treat with antibiotic if applicable, and prevent dehydration by increasing fluid intake.
      2. Diarrhea: Increase fluid intake to make up for fluid loss, and check for blood in stool.
      3. Mouth ulcers: Treat thrush or other cause, implement a softened diet to help patients tolerate swallowing and reduce discomfort, and use topical anesthetics for pain.
      4. Nausea and vomiting: Manage with antiemetics; instruct patients to eat small, frequent meals and drink slowly; and avoid cooking smells next to sick person.
      5. Constipation: Encourage high-fiber foods, fruits, and vegetables, increase fluid intake, and treat with laxative medications.

6. Constipating medications and medications that cause dry mouth: Instruct patients to take frequent sips of fluids and moisten mouth regularly.

C. Nonpharmacologic treatments for symptoms that accompany dehydration and multiple chronic conditions include psychological, emotional, and support counseling; anxiety relief measures such as deep breathing; and relaxation techniques for reducing stress such as distraction, imaging, and calm music (WHO, 2004).

D. Self-management support is effective in meeting the needs of patients, families, and communities living with multiple chronic conditions (Agency for Health Care Research and Quality, 2015).

E. The quality of life of patients and their families who suffer with chronic illness can be improved by palliative care interventions that focus on management of common symptoms associated with dehydration (WHO, 2015).

F. Early palliative care reduces unnecessary hospital admissions and the use of health services (WHO, 2015).

G. Training and awareness of palliative care among healthcare professionals help to meet the growing need for access to palliative care associated with the aging population (WHO, 2015).

H. Symptom management is achieved by early identification and correct assessment of symptoms associated with chronic conditions (WHO, 2015).

I. Healthcare professionals help overcome significant barriers to symptom management and relieve suffering of patients and families with symptomatic chronic conditions (WHO, 2015).

J. Optimal symptom management and quality of life is achieved by a team approach that uses palliative care for addressing the physical, psychological, and spiritual needs of patients with chronic conditions.

Case Study

L.S. is an 82-year-old Caucasian woman with a past medical history of ulcerative colitis, cardiovascular disease, and hypertension. She was brought to the clinic today by her daughter, who describes that L.S. became confused two days ago after suffering abdominal pain and several bouts of diarrhea. The confusion has worsened over the past 24 hours. Symptoms are described as intermittent periods of restlessness, rambling, and wandering. Additionally, she is experiencing disorientation to time and familiar people.

The APRN performs an assessment, noting a presentation that includes lethargic appearance, inattentiveness, disorientation to time and place, and dry skin and mucous membranes. Vital signs revealed tachypnea and tachycardia. The patient's body mass index is below normal at 17.5 kg/m². Laboratory values showed increased blood urea nitrogen, creatinine, and hematocrit and low sodium (132 mEq/L). The assessment findings and symptoms are suggestive of delirium and dehydration secondary to exacerbation of ulcerative colitis.

Management for this patient should be aimed at restoring fluid loss from diarrhea and educating the patient and family about complications associated with ulcerative colitis. Current guidelines direct the APRN's approach to managing this patient. The National Institute for Health and Care Excellence (2010) provides guidelines for treating delirium. The recommendations include treating the underlying cause, providing frequent reorientation and reassurance to patients and their families, ensuring adequate hydration, preventing constipation, and considering short-term antipsychotic use for patients at risk to themselves or others (National Institute for Health and Care Excellence, 2010).

Primary prevention and management for ulcerative colitis includes probiotic use with antibiotics to decrease the incidence of antibiotic-associated diarrhea (Surawicz et al., 2013). Management of dehydration requires identification of risk factors for acute situations such as diarrhea, vomiting, and fever. Additionally, input and output should be monitored, and education should be given to patients and their families regarding ongoing fluid hydration. Follow-up monitoring of the condition is important and can be accomplished by a 24-hour intake recording or urine-specific gravity checks (Mentes, 2012).

References

Agency for Health Care Research and Quality. (2015). Prevention and chronic care. Retrieved from http://www.ahrq.gov/professionals/prevention-chronic-care

Bardgett, M.E., Chen, Q.-H., Guo, Q., Calderon, A.S., Andrade, M., & Toney, G.M. (2014). Coping with dehydration: Sympathetic activation and regulation of glutamatergic transmission in the hypothalamic PVN. *American Journal of Physiology—Regulatory, Integrative and Comparative Physiology, 306,* 804–813. doi:10.1152/ajpregu.00074.2014

Centers for Disease Control and Prevention. (1996). *Physical activity and health: A report of the Surgeon General.* Retrieved from http://www.cdc.gov/nccdphp/sgr/pdf/sgrfull.pdf

Centers for Disease Control and Prevention. (2012). Influenza (flu): Information for specific groups. Retrieved from http://www.cdc.gov/flu/groups.htm

Centers for Disease Control and Prevention. (2013). Preventing chronic diseases and reducing health risk factors. Retrieved from http://www.cdc.gov/nccdphp/dch/programs/healthycommunitiesprogram/overview/diseasesandrisks.htm

Centers for Disease Control and Prevention. (2014). Rehydration therapy. Retrieved from http://www.cdc.gov/cholera/treatment/rehydration-therapy.html

Centers for Disease Control and Prevention. (2016). Chronic disease overview. Retrieved from http://www.cdc.gov/chronicdisease/overview/index.htm

Cunha, J.P. (2014). Acute kidney failure facts. Retrieved from http://www.emedicinehealth.com/acute_kidney_failure/article_em.htm#acute_kidney_failure_facts

Heron, M. (2016). Deaths: Leading causes for 2013. *National Vital Statistics Reports, 65*(2). Retrieved from http://www.cdc.gov/nchs/data/nvsr/nvsr65/nvsr65_02.pdf

Institute of Medicine. (2012). *Living well with chronic illness: A call for public health action.* Retrieved from http://www.iom.edu/Reports/2012/Living-Well-with-Chronic-Illness.aspx

Kuebler, K. (2015). Federal initiatives in self-management for patients with multiple chronic conditions: Implications for the doctor of nursing practice. *Clinical Scholars Review, 8,* 139–144.

Mentes, J.C. (2012). Managing oral hydration. In M. Boltz, E. Capezuti, T. Fulmer, & D. Zwicker (Eds.), *Evidence-based geriatric nursing protocols for best practice* (4th ed., pp. 419–438). New York, NY: Springer.

Moy, E., Chang, E., & Barrett, M. (2013). Potentially preventable hospitalizations—United States, 2001–2009. *Morbidity and Mortality Weekly Report, 62,* 139–143. Retrieved from http://www.cdc.gov/mmwr/preview/mmwrhtml/su6203a23.htm

National Institute for Health and Care Excellence. (2010, July). *Delirium: Prevention, diagnosis and management* (Clinical guideline). Retrieved from http://www.nice.org.uk/guidance/cg103/chapter/1-recommendations

Ryan, P. (2009). Integrated theory of health behavior change: Background and intervention development. *Clinical Nurse Specialist, 23,* 161–170. doi:10.1097/NUR.0b013e3181a42373

Surawicz, C.M., Brandt, L.J., Binion, D.G., Ananthakrishnan, A.N., Curry, S.R., Gilligan, P.H., … Zuckerbraun, B.S. (2013). Guidelines for diagnosis, treatment, and prevention of *Clostridium difficile* infections. *American Journal of Gastroenterology, 108,* 478–498. Retrieved from http://gi.org/guideline/diagnosis-and-management-of-c-difficile-associated-diarrhea-and-colitis

U.S. Department of Health and Human Services Office of Disease Prevention and Health Promotion. (n.d.). 2020 topics and objectives: Nutrition and weight status. Retrieved from http://healthypeople.gov/2020/topics-objectives/topic/nutrition-and-weight-status

U.S. National Library of Medicine. (2015, August). Dehydration. Retrieved from http://www.nlm.nih.gov/medlineplus/ency/article/000982.htm

World Health Organization. (2004). *Palliative care: Symptom management and end-of-life care* (Interim guidelines for first-level facility health workers). Retrieved from http://www.who.int/hiv/pub/imai/primary_palliative/en

World Health Organization. (2015, July). Palliative care (Fact sheet No. 402). Retrieved from http://www.who.int/mediacentre/factsheets/fs402/en

CHAPTER 24

Dementia

Helene M. Holbrook, DNP, FNP-C

I. Definition
  A. Dementia is defined by the Alzheimer's Association (2015) as a disease that affects 5%–10% of the population older than 65 years of age and 45%–50% of the population older than 85 years of age and is associated with serious forms of cognitive impairment.
    1. The Alzheimer's Association (2015) estimates that nearly 16 million Americans will have dementia of the Alzheimer type by 2050.
    2. Percent of nursing home residents with Alzheimer diagnosis: 50.4% (Harris-Kojetin et al., 2016)
  B. The fifth edition of the *Diagnostic and Statistical Manual of Mental Disorders* (American Psychiatric Association, 2013) defines dementia as the development of multiple cognitive deficits as a result of the direct physiologic effects of general medical condition, the persisting effects of a substance, or multiple etiologies, for example, cerebrovascular accident or cardio-cerebral vascular disease, and Alzheimer disease (American Psychiatric Association, 2013).
  C. The trajectory and transition states of normal aging to mild cognitive impairment are expected, but the progression to dementia is demonstrated in this group with a risk of progression at a rate of 10%–15% a year (Albert et al., 2011).
  D. The most common forms of dementia are Alzheimer disease and vascular dementia, affecting 80%–90% of all dementias in older adults (Alzheimer's Association, 2015).
II. Presenting symptoms
  A. In patients with dementia, the early symptoms of progressive memory loss develop and affect speech, which becomes halting as the patient seeks to remember a word and eventually loses comprehension of the spoken word.
    1. Patients lose literacy skills, including reading and writing ability, and have difficulty in reckoning change and dealing with financial affairs (Shaik & Varma, 2012).
    2. Visual impairment affects ability to write, button clothes, negotiate stairs, and eventually recognize faces (Bauer & Moquist, 2009).
  B. Key characteristics
    1. Disturbance in attention (reduced ability to direct, sustain, and shift focus and attention) and awareness
    2. The disturbance develops over a short period of time (usually hours to days), represents a change from baseline, and tends to fluctuate during the course of the day.

   3. The disturbances are not better explained by another preexisting, evolving, or established neurocognitive disorder and do not occur in the context of a severely reduced level of arousal, such as coma.
   4. Evidence from the history, physical examination, or laboratory findings supports that the disturbance is caused by a medical condition, substance intoxication or withdrawal, or medication side effect (American Psychiatric Association, 2013).
C. Alzheimer disease predominantly affects the medial temporal and temporal parietal cortex (Weintraub, Wicklund, & Salmon, 2012).
   1. The symptoms of Alzheimer disease worsen over time, although the rate at which the disease progresses varies.
   2. On average, a person with Alzheimer disease lives four to eight years after diagnosis.
D. In patients with a diagnosis of advanced dementia, research supports palliative care as a means to offer a better quality of life than continued aggressive or burdensome medical interventions (Mitchell et al., 2009).
   1. Changes in the brain related to Alzheimer disease begin years before any signs of the disease.
   2. This time period, which can last for years, is referred to as *preclinical Alzheimer disease.*
E. According to the Alzheimer's Association (n.d.), Alzheimer disease typically has a slow progression through three general stages of mild (early stage), moderate (middle stage), and severe (late stage). Because Alzheimer disease affects people differently, each person will experience symptoms and progress through the stages (Alzheimer's Association, n.d.).
   1. The Functional Assessment Staging (FAST) criteria were developed as a tool for assessment and consist of the following seven stages (Reisberg, 1988):
      a) Normal adult
      b) Normal older adult
      c) Early dementia
      d) Mild dementia
      e) Moderate dementia
      f) Moderately severe dementia
      g) Severe dementia
   2. On physical examination, patients with Alzheimer-type dementia are differentiated into the following stages (Reisberg, 1988):
      a) Mild (early stage)
         (1) Patients have some degree of independent function.
         (2) Patients are able to drive, work, and attend social functions but will be affected by memory lapses associated with loss of familiar words, names, and location of familiar objects, such as keys or glasses.
         (3) Impairment occurs in planning and accomplishing tasks. The defects are apparent to those in contact with patients.
      b) Moderate (middle stage)
         (1) Typically the longest stage and can last for many years
         (2) As the disease progresses, patients will require a greater level of care.
         (3) Patients may confuse words, get frustrated or angry, or act in unexpected ways, such as refusing to bathe.

    (4) Safety is an issue, as patients are at risk for failing to dress appropriately for the weather, failing to remember a street address or phone number, or wandering away and becoming lost.

   c) Severe (late stage)

    (1) Patients are unable to respond to their environment.

    (2) Patients may use neologisms in conversations.

    (3) On assessment, patients would be functioning at an Adapted FAST stage 6 (moderately severe dementia), reflecting the need for full-time (24/7) assistance with personal care and observation for infections, as they are vulnerable, especially for pneumonia, as their ability to swallow may be compromised.

  3. Advancing age represents an independent risk factor for dysphagia, as even with healthy aging there is a physical toll on head and neck anatomy and changes to the physiologic and neural mechanisms that support swallowing (Ney, Weiss, Kind, & Robbins, 2009).

 F. Risk factors: Worldwide, Alzheimer dementia cases were attributable to seven potentially modifiable risk factors: low education (21%), smoking (14%), physical inactivity (13%), depression (11%), mid-life hypertension (6%), obesity (6%), and diabetes (2%) (Barnes & Yaffe, 2011).

III. Diagnostics

 A. Diagnosing a patient with dementia involves examining prognostic factors.

  1. FAST system or the Mortality Risk Index, a score based on 12 risk factor criteria using the Minimum Data Set. An assessment can arrive at a six-month prognosis (Levy et al., 2015).

  2. Use of such tools creates a point system for determining the advanced chronic condition. In dementia, that includes categories such as mild, moderate, severe (see Figures 24-1, 24-2, and 24-3), and terminal.

  3. *Terminal dementia* is defined as a loss of communication, ambulation, swallowing, and continence (Mitchell et al., 2009).

  4. Use of biomarkers and diagnostic imaging

 B. Such staging assists a palliative care team in the evaluation of interventions offered and appropriate referral to hospice teams (Schonwetter et al., 2003).

  1. These evaluations inform patients of how their condition affects their body.

  2. This awareness removes the component of fear, and patients and families can incorporate this knowledge into the plan associated with disease progression when physical episodes occur or symptoms worsen.

  3. Prearranged contact for the patient and the caretaker exists and has been encouraged to initiate the appropriate next step.

 C. A coordinated, patient-centered care plan prevents exacerbation of the dementia to reduce the need for hospitalization or the risk of readmission if hospitalization is deemed necessary.

 D. Stewart et al. (2012) demonstrated in patients with congestive heart failure that home-based interventions were associated with significantly lower healthcare costs, attributable to fewer days of hospitalization, and were perceived as patient centered and consumer friendly.

 E. The approach to dementia as a chronic disease and one across the older adult life span must differentiate the reversible forms of memory impairment and help patients and their families understand what type and stage of dementia is affecting the patient (Levy et al., 2015).

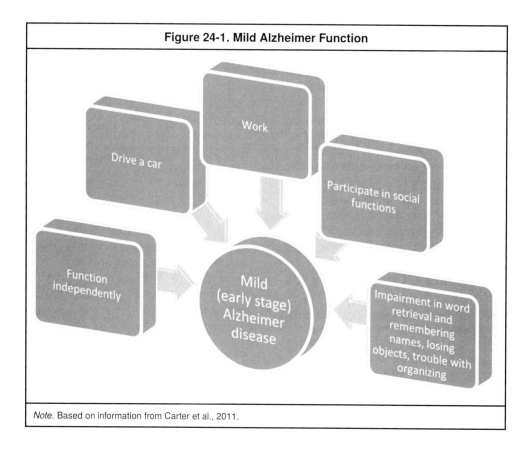

Figure 24-1. Mild Alzheimer Function

Note. Based on information from Carter et al., 2011.

1. The differentiation helps providers, patients, and families understand the progression of dementia and the appropriate best practice, support, and treatment (Petersen et al., 2014).
2. Truth telling with the dementia diagnosis and providing a realistic view of the anticipated disease trajectory help inform patients, families, and caretakers of realistic and truthful expectations of the stages of dementia (Levy et al., 2015).

IV. Interventions
  A. Palliative care begins with the diagnosis of dementia.
  B. All management efforts should be directed toward improving comfort and quality of life for patients with dementia.
    1. The management of dementia depends on the stage of the disease.
    2. The integrated team identifies the treatment goals of the correctable factors that might be interfering with the accomplishment of activities of daily living (Harris-Kojetin et al., 2016).
    3. The integration of palliative care early in the diagnosis stage informs patients of what to expect and allows them to input personal wishes.
    4. Building on a model for staged disease management, patients and their caregivers have a clear understanding of the diagnosis and the stages the disease can progress through (Minkman, Vermeulen, Ahaus, & Huijsman, 2011).
  C. As the disease transitions, early anticipatory guidance is integrated into the patient's care plan with the primary provider, specialist, and palliative care health services

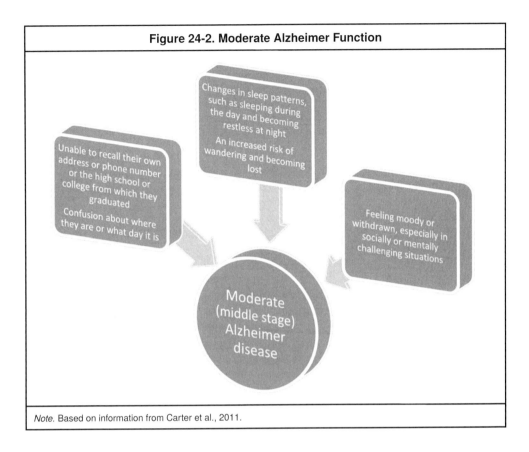

Figure 24-2. Moderate Alzheimer Function

Changes in sleep patterns, such as sleeping during the day and becoming restless at night

An increased risk of wandering and becoming lost

Unable to recall their own address or phone number or the high school or college from which they graduated

Confusion about where they are or what day it is

Feeling moody or withdrawn, especially in socially or mentally challenging situations

Moderate (middle stage) Alzheimer disease

Note. Based on information from Carter et al., 2011.

able to come into play, thus fostering patient-centered outcomes of comfort, reduction of hospitalizations and emergency department visits, and patient and family and caretaker satisfaction (Meier, 2011; Stewart et al., 2012).

D. Timely referrals for palliative care early in the dementia diagnosis bridge the stages of disease. Studies show that patients with chronic conditions such as chronic cardiopulmonary disease follow a less predictable course than patients with an incurable cancer (Hoefer, Johnson, & Bender, 2013; Murray, Kendall, Boyd, & Sheikh, 2005; Sachs, Shega, & Cox-Hayley, 2004; Shaik & Varma, 2012).

E. The natural progression of dementia contributes to a need for institutionalization for some and home management for others.

V. Integration of palliative care

A. Palliative care is well suited to meet the needs of patients with dementia.

B. Because dementia is progressive and irreversible, palliative care will support family members and assist patients in attaining quality of life and maintaining comfort at home or in a supportive environment (Mehta, Giorgini, Ellison, & Roth, 2012).

Case Study

In a small rural community, C.M. lives at home with her husband. She has a diagnosis of Alzheimer dementia and is in good health except for poor memory and wandering. She is able

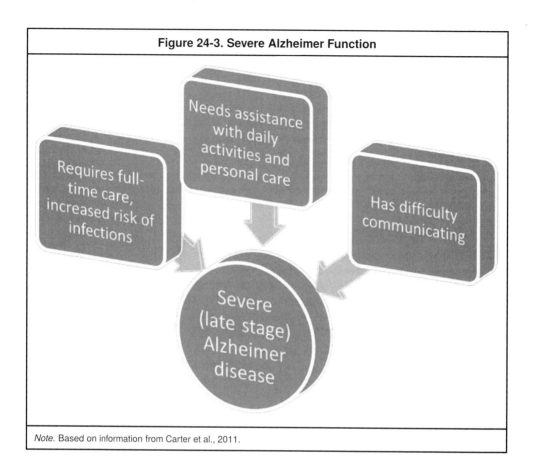

Figure 24-3. Severe Alzheimer Function

Note. Based on information from Carter et al., 2011.

to dress and feed herself and has success with familiar tasks, such as folding clothes and weeding, with minimal supervision or reminders. The family wanted C.M. to spend more time outside.

Taking information from the Alzheimer's Society (n.d.), the family developed a dementia-friendly garden design to make a suitable, safe area for C.M. They used wide paths with raised beds to minimize the risk of falls and improve visibility for caretakers from the house. The garden was enclosed with sturdy, mesh wire fencing and a gate with an alarm that sounded when opened and closed. Approaches to the garden on a path from the house had signs of vegetables and fruits along the way with arrows pointing to the garden entrance. Inside the enclosure, the family had installed a few benches, baskets for trash, and a garden hose with a pressure-activated nozzle to minimize the risk of water being left on. They left lightweight, handheld garden tools on a small table near the entrance gate. C.M. reported many hours of enjoyment and satisfaction spent in the garden. The caretaker and extended family expressed satisfaction in C.M.'s improved outlook and better attention span.

The physical environment influences outcomes among patients, their family, and caregivers in three main areas: (a) quality of life, (b) safety, and (c) caretaker stress. The physical environment has been shown to affect both patients' and caretakers' outcomes in long-term care settings and contributes to a better quality of life (Desai, Kim, Fall, & Wang, 2007; Joseph, Zimring, Harris-Kojetin, & Kiefer, 2006).

References

Albert, M.S., DeKosky, S.T., Dickson, D., Dubois, B., Feldman, H.H., Fox, N.C., … Phelps, C.H. (2011). The diagnosis of mild cognitive impairment due to Alzheimer's disease: Recommendations from the National Institute on Aging-Alzheimer's Association workgroups on diagnostic guidelines for Alzheimer's disease. *Alzheimer's and Dementia, 7,* 270–279. doi:10.1016/j.jalz.2011.03.008

Alzheimer's Association. (n.d.). Stages of Alzheimer's. Retrieved from http://www.alz.org/alzheimers_disease _stages_of_alzheimers.asp

Alzheimer's Association. (2015). *2015 Alzheimer's disease facts and figures.* Retrieved from https://www.alz.org/facts/downloads/facts_figures_2015.pdf

Alzheimer's Society. (n.d.). Sample sections from *Taking Part: Activities for People With Dementia.* Retrieved from https://www.alzheimers.org.uk/site/scripts/documents_info.php?documentID=2592&pageNumber=2

American Psychiatric Association. (2013). *Diagnostic and statistical manual of mental disorders* (5th ed.). Washington, DC: American Psychiatric Publishing.

Barnes, D., & Yaffe, K. (2011). The projected impact of risk factor reduction on Alzheimer's disease prevalence [Abstract]. *Alzheimer's and Dementia, 7*(Suppl. 4), S511. doi:10.1016/j.jalz.2011.05.1429

Bauer, D., & Moquist, D.C. (Eds.). (2009). *Family practice curriculum in neurology* (2nd ed.). Minneapolis, MN: American Academy of Neurology.

Carter, S.F., Caine, D., Burns, D., Herholz, K., & Ralph, M.A.L. (2011). Staging of the cognitive decline in Alzheimer's disease: Insights from a detailed neuropsychological investigation of mild cognitive impairment and mild Alzheimer's disease. *International Journal of Geriatric Psychiatry, 27,* 423–432. doi:10.1002/gps.2738

Desai, M.J., Kim, A., Fall, P.C., & Wang, D. (2007). Optimizing quality of life through palliative care. *Journal of the American Osteopathic Association, 107*(Suppl. 7), ES9–ES14.

Harris-Kojetin, L., Sengupta, M., Park-Lee, E., Valverde, R., Caffrey, C., Rome, V., & Lendon, J. (2016). Long-term care providers and services users in the United States: Data from the National Study of Long-Term Care Providers, 2013–2014. National Center for Health Statistics. *Vital and Health Statistics, 3*(38). Retrieved from http://www.cdc.gov/nchs/data/series/sr_03/sr03_038.pdf

Hoefer, D.R., Johnson, S.K., & Bender, M. (2013). Development and preliminary evaluation of an innovative advanced chronic disease care model. *Journal of Clinical Outcomes Management, 20,* 408–418. Retrieved from http://www.turner-white.com/pdf/jcom_sep13_chronic.pdf

Joseph, A., Zimring, C., Harris-Kojetin, L., & Kiefer, K. (2006). Presence and visibility of outdoor and indoor physical activity features and participation in physical activity among older adults in retirement communities. *Journal of Housing for the Elderly, 19,* 141–165. doi:10.1300/J081v19n03_08

Levy, C., Kheirbek, K., Alemi, F., Wojtusiak, J., Sutton, B., Williams, A.R., & Williams, A. (2015). Predictors of six-month mortality among nursing home residents: Diagnoses may be more predictive than functional disability. *Journal of Palliative Medicine, 18,* 100–106. doi:10.1089/jpm.2014.0130

Mehta, Z., Giorgini, K., Ellison, N., & Roth, M.E. (2012). Integrating palliative medicine with dementia care. *Aging Well, 5*(2), 18. Retrieved from http://www.todaysgeriatricmedicine.com/archive/031912p18.shtml

Meier, D.E. (2011). Increased access to palliative care and hospice services: Opportunities to improve value in health care. *Milbank Quarterly, 89,* 343–380. doi:10.1111/j.1468-0009.2011.00632.x

Minkman, M.M.N., Vermeulen, R.P., Ahaus, K.T.B., & Huijsman, R. (2011). The implementation of integrated care: The empirical validation of the Development Model for Integrated Care. *BMC Health Services Research, 11,* 177. doi:10.1186/1472-6963-11-177

Mitchell, S.L., Teno, J.M., Kiely, D.K., Shaffer, M.L., Jones, R.N., Prigerson, H.G., … Hamel, M.B. (2009). The clinical course of advanced dementia. *New England Journal of Medicine, 361,* 1529–1538. doi:10.1056/NEJMoa0902234

Murray, S.A., Kendall, M., Boyd, K., & Sheikh, A. (2005). Illness trajectories and palliative care. *BMJ, 330,* 1007–1011. doi:10.1136/bmj.330.7498.1007

Ney, D.M., Weiss, J.M., Kind, A.J.H., & Robbins, J. (2009). Senescent swallowing: Impact, strategies, and interventions. *Nutrition in Clinical Practice, 24,* 395–413. doi:10.1177/0884533609332005

Petersen, R.C., Caracciolo, B., Brayne, C., Gauthier, S., Jelic, V., & Fratiglioni, L. (2014). Mild cognitive impairment: A concept in evolution (Key Symposium). *Journal of Internal Medicine, 275,* 214–228. doi:10.1111/joim.12190

Reisberg, B. (1988). Functional assessment staging (FAST). *Psychopharmacology Bulletin, 24,* 653–659.

Sachs, G.A., Shega, J.W., & Cox-Hayley, D. (2004). Barriers to excellent end-of-life care for patients with dementia. *Journal of General Internal Medicine, 19,* 1057–1063. doi:10.1111/j.1525-1497.2004.30329.x

Schonwetter, R.S., Han, B., Small, B.J., Martin, B., Tope, K., & Haley, W.E. (2003). Predictors of six-month survival among patients with dementia: An evaluation of hospice Medicare guidelines. *American Journal of Hospice and Palliative Care, 20,* 105–113.

Shaik, S.S., & Varma, A.R. (2012). Differentiating the dementias: A neurological approach. *Progress in Neurology and Psychiatry, 16,* 11–18. doi:10.1002/pnp.224

Stewart, S., Carrington, M.J., Marwick, T.H., Davidson, P.M., Macdonald, P., Horowitz, J.D., … Scuffham, P.A. (2012). Impact of home versus clinic-based management of chronic heart failure: The WHICH? (Which Heart Failure Intervention Is Most Cost-Effective and Consumer Friendly in Reducing Hospital Care) multicenter, randomized trial. *Journal of the American College of Cardiology, 60,* 1239–1248. doi:10.1016/j.jacc.2012.06.025

Weintraub, S., Wicklund, A.H., & Salmon, D.P. (2012). The neuropsychological profile of Alzheimer disease. *Cold Spring Harbor Perspectives in Medicine, 2*(4), a006171. doi:10.1101/cshperspect.a006171

CHAPTER 25

Depression

Terry A. Badger, PhD, PMHCNS-BC, FAAN, FAPOS, Laura McRee, DNP, ACNP-BC,
and Mark Lazenby, PhD, APRN, AOCNP®, FAPOS

I. Definition
   A. Depression is difficult to define because it ranges on a continuum from feelings of sadness and unhappiness about a particular event to a clinical diagnosis.
   B. The criteria for clinical diagnosis are as follows: Depression can be categorized as major depressive disorder or persistent depressive disorder (formerly called dysthymia) (American Psychiatric Association [APA], 2013).
      1. Major depressive disorder is described as having five or more of the criterion symptoms (see Figure 25-1) (APA, 2013).
         a) These symptoms must be present nearly every day and for almost all day, for at least two weeks, and must represent a change from previous functioning.
         b) At least one of the criterion symptoms must be either depressed mood or loss of interest or pleasure in usual activities.
      2. Persistent depressive disorder can be diagnosed when an individual has depressed mood for most of the day and for more days than not, for at least two years in adults and one year in children, plus two of the criterion symptoms when depressed (APA, 2013).
   C. In both major depressive disorder and persistent depressive disorder, the symptoms cause clinically significant distress and impairment in social, occupational, or other important areas of functioning.
   D. The prevalence of depression in palliative care patients is 1%–69%, depending on the study reviewed (Mitchell et al., 2011).

Figure 25-1. Criterion Symptoms for Diagnosing Major Depressive Disorder

- Depressed mood (irritable mood in children and adolescents)
- Marked diminished interest or pleasure in usual activities
- Weight loss or gain without dieting, or decrease or increase in appetite
- Insomnia or hypersomnia
- Psychomotor agitation or retardation
- Fatigue or loss of energy
- Feelings of worthlessness or excessive or inappropriate guilt
- Difficulty thinking, concentrating, and making decisions
- Recurrent thoughts of death or suicidal ideation

Note. Based on information from American Psychiatric Association, 2013.

    E. Both nurses (McCabe, Mellor, Davison, Hallford, & Goldhammer, 2012) and palliative care patients (Baile, Palmer, Bruera, & Parker, 2011) report that psychological distress is highly prevalent, yet undetected and untreated.

    F. Strong evidence exists that depression causes serious suffering and distress, reduces quality of life and survival, reduces participation and adherence with medical care, prolongs the duration of the hospital stay, and is a predictor of desire for death in terminally ill patients (Badger & Lazenby, 2015; Mitchell et al., 2011; Rayner, Lee, et al., 2011).

    G. Less than half of those with depression in palliative care ever receive treatment (Goodwin et al., 2012; Mellor, McCabe, Davison, Goldhammer, & Hallford, 2012).

II. Pathophysiology

    A. Depression is currently recognized as having a neuroanatomic, neuroendocrinologic, or neurophysiologic basis, although more research is needed before a biologic diagnostic test is developed for this disorder.

    B. Strong evidence suggests that factors such as temperament (negative affectivity), adverse childhood experiences, stressful life events, genetic predisposition, or having a chronic or disabling medical condition can all place a person at risk for depression (APA, 2013).

    C. Evidence is increasing from genetic studies on the genetic inheritance of depression. Burkhouse, Gibb, Coles, Knopik, and McGeary (2011) found that, under the same environmental influences, children carrying two copies of certain alleles involved in the genes that help control serotonin transport were more likely to exhibit signs of depression than children who did not.

    D. Biologic marker studies have focused on growth hormone, serotonergic and other neurotransmitter receptors, sleep, and hypothalamic-pituitary-adrenal (HPA) function (Giese-Davies, Sephton, Abercrombie, Durán, & Spiegel, 2004; Giese-Davies et al., 2006; Spiegel, 2012; Spiegel, Giese-Davis, Taylor, & Kraemer, 2006). Chronic stress can cause changes in HPA axis function that contribute to depression (Booij, Bouma, de Jonge, Ormel, & Oldehinkel, 2013).

    E. Raison and Miller (2011) have proposed that inflammatory processes may play a role in causing depression. Inflammation as a cause of depression is receiving more attention in recent years.

    F. An individual with first-degree relatives with major depression has a two- to four-fold higher risk than that of the general population. The risk of depression during illness is higher in individuals who had a more severe episode of depression when younger or who have had recurrent episodes (APA, 2013).

    G. Evidence suggests that abnormalities in biologic markers persist throughout the life span and that these depression-causing abnormalities may worsen when individuals are facing life-threatening illnesses such as cancer (Reyes-Gibby et al., 2013).

    H. Medications used for treating life-threatening illness (e.g., cancer) have been implicated as the cause of depression symptoms. Medications include chemotherapy agents (especially vinca alkaloids), immunomodulatory agents (thalidomide), biologics (interferon), and corticosteroids. Indeed, many antidepressant medications may interact with antineoplastic drugs (Miguel & Albuquerque, 2011). When cancer medications are added to medications prescribed for another illness and these medications have been implicated in causing depressive symptoms, patients require additional evaluation for depression to determine the additive effect of multiple medications.

III. Presenting symptoms

    A. Symptoms (APA, 2013)

1. Depressed mood (irritable mood in children and adolescents)
2. Marked diminished interest or pleasure in usual activities
3. Weight loss or gain without dieting, or decrease or increase in appetite
4. Insomnia or hypersomnia
5. Psychomotor agitation or retardation
6. Fatigue or loss of energy
7. Feelings of worthlessness or excessive or inappropriate guilt
8. Difficulty thinking, concentrating, and making decisions
9. Recurrent thoughts of death or suicidal ideation

B. However, these presenting symptoms of depression also could be attributable to decreased functional status or symptoms related to the primary illness. Thus, diagnosing depression can be complex.

IV. Physical examination

A. A physical examination provides information about other illnesses or medications that may be causing or exacerbating depressive symptoms. Depending on the diagnostic picture, providers may be able to adjust or change the treatment regimen to alleviate symptoms of depression.

B. To date, no physical examination or routine diagnostic tests exist to diagnose depression.

V. Diagnostics

A. Diagnosing depression in patients can be complex, and using the diagnostic criteria can create false positives (i.e., diagnosing depression when it is, in fact, not present). When assessing patients for depression, nurses must evaluate physical symptoms, as well as emotional, psychological, and behavioral clues. Physical symptoms in patients with life-threatening illnesses may include fatigue, lack of energy, inability to concentrate, insomnia or drowsiness, subjectively described restlessness, or appetite changes (either loss of appetite or carbohydrate craving). It is important to differentiate which symptoms are from the life-threatening illness rather than from depression.

B. The following alternative approaches to assessing depression in patients with advanced disease are commonly used: inclusive, etiologic, substitutive, exclusive, and increased thresholds (Badger, 2005; Marks & Heinrich, 2013; Passik & Lowery, 2011).

1. The inclusive approach uses all the symptoms of depression, regardless of whether they are secondary to medical illness. Most depression screening tools use the inclusive approach.

2. The etiologic approach counts only symptoms that are not the result of physical illness. The advantage of the etiologic approach is fewer false positives, but a major disadvantage is that many depressed patients may be missed. Furthermore, this approach does not take into account that some groups (e.g., older adults and culturally and racially diverse groups) use somatic symptoms to describe depression.

3. The substitutive approach replaces symptoms that may be related to illness (e.g., fatigue) and includes additional psychological symptoms (e.g., social withdrawal) (Asghar-Ali, Wagle, & Braun, 2013). This approach requires use of assessment tools that are not readily available in the literature. Endicott (1984) suggested substituting somatic symptoms when assessing for depression in those with terminal illness. His approach uses a clinical interview rather than questionnaire approach to assessment. Previous research showed that "fearfulness and brooding" were suggestive of mild depression, "social withdrawal" with

moderate-severity major depression, and "cannot be cheered up" with severe major depression (Akechi et al., 2009).

4. The exclusive approach eliminates two common symptoms of depression (fatigue and weight or appetite changes). This approach increases the chances that clinicians will identify potentially depressed patients but also increases the chance that clinicians will screen patients who are not depressed.

5. The final approach is to increase the threshold score (e.g., set a higher score than is typically used to indicate significant depressive symptoms). The issue with this approach is that there have been insufficient studies to determine what the new threshold score should be.

C. Of these approaches, we recommend the inclusive method, as it allows for maximum sensitivity in assessing depression in patients with life-threatening illness.

1. Two barriers to the use of screening tools for nurses and other healthcare professionals are lack of training and lack of confidence in use of self-report tools (McCabe et al., 2012).

2. The use of self-report measures for screening has several advantages, such as ease of administration, scoring of the measure by individuals who have not had extensive training, and the speed in which the tools can be completed by patients (Badger, 2005; Jacobsen & Donovan, 2015). Furthermore, self-report screening measures can provide a relatively quick assessment of depression before a clinical interview is conducted, quantifying the severity of the depression and identifying changes over time (Passik & Lowery, 2011). A lengthier evaluation should be scheduled for those who score above the established cutoff scores on depression screening tools.

3. Standardized easy-to-use tools with established cutoff scores to indicate depression or significant depressive symptoms include the following:

   a) Beck Depression Inventory (BDI) and Beck Depression Inventory–Short Form (BDI-SF): Available online for purchase only; see www.pearson clinical.com/psychology.html

   b) Center for Epidemiologic Studies Depression Scale and Center for Epidemiologic Studies Depression Scale Revised (CES-D and CESD-R): http://cesd-r.com

   c) Hamilton Rating Scale for Depression: http://healthnet.umassmed.edu/mhealth/HAMD.pdf

   d) Patient Health Questionnaire (PHQ)-2: www.commonwealthfund.org/usr_doc/phq2.pdf; PHQ-9: www.phqscreeners.com

   e) Zung Self-Rating Depression Scale (ZSDS): http://healthnet.umassmed.edu/mhealth/ZungSelfRatedDepressionScale.pdf

   f) The National Comprehensive Cancer Network® (NCCN®) Distress Thermometer with emotional problem list: www.nccn.org/professionals/physician_gls/PDF/distress.pdf (accessible after registration on the site)

4. These tools have evidence of reliability, validity, sensitivity, and specificity in patients with cancer or other terminal illnesses. *Reliability* refers to the consistency of the responses, and *validity* refers to its correlation with an accepted gold standard (e.g., clinical interview). *Sensitivity* is the ability to correctly identify those who are depressed, and *specificity* is the ability to correctly identify those who are not depressed.

5. Although the PHQ-9 (Kroenke, Spitzer, & Williams, 2001, 2003) and the Distress Thermometer (NCCN, 2015) have been used more frequently in

the past few years to screen for depression and distress in patients with life-threatening illnesses, there have been too few studies validating the PHQ-9 in palliative care (e.g., Chilcot et al., 2013).

6. The nurse may find that using the short forms of various instruments or the Distress Thermometer is an efficient way to screen for depression within a busy practice (Lazenby, Dixon, Bai, & McCorkle, 2014). Another important new tool comes from the Patient-Reported Outcomes Measurement Information System initiative of the National Institutes of Health. This initiative allows for screening using computer-adaptive testing, which reduces the number of items needed in order to determine depression and reduces measurement error to increase confidence in the findings (Badger, Heitkemper, Lee, & Bruner, 2014).

7. In the course of caring for patients, nurses develop relationships with their patients and engage in talking with them during care episodes. Thus, it would be normal for nurses to ask screening questions as part of a larger conversation.
    a) Using the Kroenke et al. (2003) PHQ-2 scale as a foundation, the nurse could ask two simple questions: "Over the past few weeks, have you been feeling sad, down, depressed, or hopeless?" and "Over the past few weeks, have you had little interest or pleasure in doing your usual activities?"
    b) If the patient answers yes to one or both of the questions, the nurse can follow with another simple question about frequency: "How many days of this past week have you felt this way?" If the patient tells the nurse this feeling was present several days of the past week, there is a 37% chance that the patient suffers from a depressive disorder (Kroenke et al., 2003).
    c) Although this two-question screening was designed for the general population and is not specific to cancer, it can easily be included in conversations with patients (Lazenby et al., 2014) and may serve to cultivate a more in-depth evaluation from other members of the healthcare team.

8. Chochinov, Wilson, Enns, and Lander (1997) found that a single screening question—"Have you felt depressed most of the day, nearly every day, for two or more weeks?"—correctly identified the diagnosis of major depression with high specificity and sensitivity in 197 terminally ill patients. Taylor, Lovell, Ward, Wood, and Hosker (2013) used a similar question with similarly high sensitivity (0.8) and specificity (0.85) in palliative care patients. The positive predictive value was 0.57 and the negative predictive value was 0.94. In both studies, the screening question correctly identified those who needed further evaluation.

9. Specifically, nurses can use simple screening tools to identify potentially depressed patients; refer to the advanced practice registered nurse (APRN), physician assistant, or physician for further comprehensive assessment; and work with the healthcare team to establish routine screening procedures within their practices (Lazenby et al., 2014).

10. APRNs have an important role in diagnosing and treating depression in palliative care patients, which will influence patient outcomes such as patient satisfaction, healthcare costs, and system improvements (Brooten, Youngblut, Deosires, Singhala, & Guido-Sanz, 2012). APRNs who are qualified to treat patients with depression include clinical nurse specialists and nurse practitioners based on the Consensus Model for APRN Regulation (APRN Consensus Work Group & National Council of State Boards of Nursing APRN Advisory Committee, 2008).

VI. Differential diagnosis
   A. Central nervous system disorders
      1. Parkinson disease
      2. Dementia
      3. Multiple sclerosis
   B. Neoplastic lesions
   C. Endocrine
      1. Hyperthyroidism
      2. Hypothyroidism
   D. Sleep disorders
VII. Interventions
   A. Pharmacologic interventions are recommended for patients with depression in palliative care (Rayner, Price, et al., 2011). Antidepressants have been found to be effective in reducing depressive symptoms in patients with milder mood disorders as well as major depressive disorder.
      1. The first antidepressants, which have been available for more than 50 years, were the tricyclics, such as amitriptyline and imipramine, and the monoamine oxidase inhibitors, such as phenelzine. The newer antidepressants (e.g., selective serotonin reuptake inhibitors [SSRIs], such as escitalopram and citalopram; serotonin–norepinephrine reuptake inhibitors, such as milnacipran; atypical antidepressants, such as mirtazapine) are preferable over older antidepressants because of their safety profile among patients receiving chemotherapy (Kelly et al., 2010) or with life-threatening illnesses (Rayner, Price, et al., 2011).
      2. The medications used in palliative care patients with depression should be selected and dosed based on a number of factors, including comorbid conditions, current treatments and medications, side effect profile, potential toxicities, hepatic and renal function, and published indications (Badger & Lazenby, 2015). For example (Rodin et al., 2007):
         a) Patients with neuropathic pain may benefit from tricyclic antidepressants (Grassi, Nanni, Uchitomi, & Riba, 2011).
         b) Patients with comorbid cardiovascular disease may benefit from medications that cause the least orthostatic hypotension (such as fluoxetine and sertraline).
         c) Patients with slow intestinal motility may benefit from antidepressants that have the least anticholinergic effects (such as the SSRIs). Patients who cannot swallow pills may use liquid formulations (available for some SSRIs and tricyclic antidepressants).
         d) Patients with impaired hepatic or renal function may benefit from antidepressants with short half-lives (such as sertraline and paroxetine).
      3. Methylphenidate, a central nervous system stimulant, has been used most often for its mood-elevating properties, to negate the effect of opioid-induced somnolence, and to improve cognitive functioning (Prommer, 2012). In a review of psychostimulants in the treatment of depression, Sinita and Coghill (2014) reported that, among older adult patients, when added to escitalopram, methylphenidate was found to be useful in treating depression, with 80% of the patients having a favorable response.
      4. Kerr et al. (2012) found that methylphenidate reduced symptoms of fatigue and depression when compared to placebo. Patients who presented with clinically significant depression at baseline showed a significant reduction in

depressed mood following a trial with methylphenidate. Berger, Yennu, and Million (2013) found similar results when using methylphenidate in patients with advanced cancer.

5. Major depression is a well-known side effect of interferon-alpha, which is used to treat malignant melanoma. The lack of randomized controlled trials among patients with cancer on interferon-alpha treatment notwithstanding, a meta-analysis of seven clinical trials of patients with hepatitis C receiving interferon-alpha showed that prophylactic treatment with an SSRI lowered the incidence of interferon-alpha–induced depression (Jiang et al., 2014).

6. Nonpharmacologic treatment of depression at the end of life should be selected based on the stage of disease of the individual (Stagg & Lazenby, 2012). For individuals with more than six months to live, psychotherapeutic interventions remain first-line treatment. For individuals with less than six months to live, semipsychotherapeutic techniques (e.g., life review therapies) are the most promising.

a) Psychotherapy interventions with the strongest evidence include cognitive therapy or cognitive behavioral therapy (CBT) (Andersen, Dorfman, & Godiwala, 2015; Stagg & Lazenby, 2012). Over the past several decades, cognitive therapy or CBT and its derivatives (e.g., problem-solving therapy, acceptance and commitment therapy) have been among the most widely used types of counseling with physically ill patients with depressive symptoms (Hart et al., 2012; Kissane, Levin, Hales, Lo, & Rodin, 2011; Mohr et al., 2012). This type of therapy is based on the premise that it is not a specific situation that causes the emotional disturbance but rather how the person perceives the situation (Beck, 2011). CBT is used to help patients recognize and change cognitive distortions (for example, how screening is viewed) that cause or exacerbate psychological distress (depression). CBT is guided by a therapist who works collaboratively with patients to uncover how cognitions (thoughts), emotions, and behavior interrelate and how experiences or other external stimuli influence perceptions (Beck, 2011). The therapist assists patients in evaluating their cognitive distortions and reformulating or changing their thoughts and perceptions to reduce negative outcomes (e.g., depression, stress). CBT is goal oriented and based on the principles of behavior change (Beck, 2011). Several studies of short-term CBT delivered by nurses have found that CBT was effective for reducing depressive symptoms and general stress and distress. Pitceathly et al. (2009) found that a short CBT intervention delivered by nurses trained in CBT significantly reduced depressive symptoms in patients who were at high risk for depression but were not depressed at baseline. Moorey et al. (2009) taught homecare nurses to use CBT techniques in their practice with patients in palliative care and found that the use of CBT was effective in reducing anxiety.

b) Supportive-expressive group therapy is the second most commonly used with those with terminal illnesses (Kissane & Ngan, 2015; Stagg & Lazenby, 2012). Most studies have been done with women with breast cancer, which limits generalizability.

(1) Meaning-centered group psychotherapy (MCGP) (Breitbart et al., 2010; Lichtenthal, Applebaum, & Breitbart, 2015) was established to help patients with advanced cancer to sustain or enhance

      a sense of meaning, peace, and purpose in their lives, even as they approached the end of life.

    (2) In a 2010 randomized clinical trial, Breitbart et al. (2010) compared MCGP to supportive group psychotherapy. MCGP resulted in significantly greater improvements in spiritual well-being, sense of meaning, anxiety, and desire for death (p < 0.05). No such improvements were seen in the supportive group.

    (3) In a 2015 randomized clinical trial comparing MCGP to supportive group psychotherapy, Breitbart et al. (2015) replicated the 2010 findings: MCGP improved spiritual well-being and quality of life and reduced depression, hopelessness, desire for hastened death, and physical symptom distress (p < 0.05) compared with those receiving supportive group psychotherapy.

c) Psychotherapeutic interventions range in the number of sessions, length of treatment (average of 8–12 weeks), method of delivery (face to face, web based, telephone), and target of intervention (individual versus group, dyad, couple, or family). Yet, despite the variability in type and format, psychosocial interventions have resulted in symptom improvements. Psychoeducational and psychosocial interventions generally require advanced education and training and usually are performed by professionals other than nurses. These professionals may not always be readily available without referral. In palliative care, these types of interventions generally are 8–12 weeks long, and many palliative care patients at the end of life are not able to complete the treatment. Furthermore, these treatments have not been shown to be effective in those with limited life expectancy (Kissane et al., 2011).

d) Psychoeducational interventions have been shown to reduce depressive symptoms. The focus of these interventions is education, such as teaching the patient about advanced cancer, distress, or specific symptom management strategies. Unlike counseling and psychotherapeutic interventions, psychoeducational interventions generally do not require specialized training. In a nurse-led, palliative care–focused intervention (Project ENABLE [Educate, Nurture, Advise, Before Life Ends]) with 322 patients with advanced cancer compared to the usual care group, those receiving the ENABLE intervention had improved quality of life (p = 0.02) and mood (p = 0.02) (Bakitas et al., 2009).

e) Psychoeducation often is part of a larger intervention package.

    (1) For example, in the Improving Mood-Promoting Access to Collaborative Treatment (IMPACT) program, education, support of a depression care manager, and a brief, structured problem-solving psychosocial intervention were combined to treat older patients with cancer, including advanced cancer (N = 215) (Fann, Fan, & Unützer, 2009). At 6 and 12 months, 55% and 39% of intervention patients had at least 50% reduction in depressive symptoms from baseline, versus 34% and 20% of usual care patients (p = 0.003 and p = 0.029).

    (2) The benefits of education are clear, and nurses routinely teach patients as an integral part of patient care. Nurses can decrease depressive symptoms and distress by talking with patients and families about psychological and physical symptoms, and strategies to deal with

the symptoms, along with other topics relevant to palliative and end-of-life care.

    (3) During this teaching, nurses can assess for depression and refer for additional assessment as needed.

f) Couples therapy models have also been explored at end of life, but the efficacy of such models has yet to be determined.

    (1) The inclusion of family members in palliative care interventions yields positive effects on caregiving burden, depression, and anxiety (Northouse, Katapodi, Song, Zhang, & Mood, 2010); the strongest effects are evident when the intervention targets social support and relationship issues.

    (2) In a study of focused grief therapy among families before and after a family member has died from cancer, Zaider and Kissane (2015) found that more effective communication, enhanced cohesion, and adaptive resolution of conflict reduced depression and encouraged mourning.

    (3) Relationship-focused interventions such as interpersonal psychotherapy, interpersonal counseling, and couples or family therapy can effectively strengthen family functioning amid illness-related changes, reduce the risk for psychiatric morbidity, and enhance the quality of life of patients and their families.

g) Semipsychotherapeutic techniques that have been studied in end-of-life populations include dignity therapy, short-term life review, life completion discussions, and meaning-making discussions (Stagg & Lazenby, 2012).

    (1) Most techniques have not had sufficient study to highly recommend them for practice; however, it is likely that these techniques would benefit palliative care patients at the end of life.

    (2) Dignity therapy, pioneered by Chochinov and colleagues, is a week-long therapy of three or four sessions that results in a document that records the person's life accomplishments and includes a ceremony to pass this document on to family members (Chochinov & Kredentser, 2015). Results of early clinical trials of this type of therapy are promising, but effectiveness has not been definitively established.

    (3) Short-Term Life Review was developed by Ando, Morita, Akechi, and Takashi (2012) to be a time-effective treatment of depression, as it has only two sessions; however, it has not been tested with Western populations and thus requires further research before it can be recommended for practice.

    (4) Steinhauser, Alexander, Byock, George, and Tulsky in 2009 tested a version of life review in which participants discussed getting their affairs in order and completing unfinished business. Life completion discussions may well assist terminally ill patients in decreasing their symptoms of depression in the final months of life (Stagg & Lazenby, 2012).

h) Complementary and alternative therapies include massage therapy (Falkensteiner, Mantovan, Müller, & Them, 2011), hypnotherapy (Lew, Kravits, Garberoglio, & Williams, 2011), and guided imagery or relaxation (Chaoul et al., 2015; Rajasekaran, Edmonds, & Higginson, 2005; Stagg & Lazenby, 2012).

    (1) These interventions may be useful, but insufficient randomized controlled trials have been conducted to support the level of effectiveness.

    (2) However, anecdotally, patients at the end of life have reported benefit from these alternative techniques.

i) Exercise is documented to be beneficial in improving mood, coping, and energy and decreasing depressive symptoms (Carek, Laibstain, & Carek, 2011).

    (1) Increased interest but little evidence exists in using exercise as an adjuvant intervention with established methods of treatment for depression such as pharmaceuticals in palliative care.

    (2) A review of 37 trials provided evidence to support that those who exercised demonstrated a greater reduction in depression symptoms compared to those who received no treatment, a placebo, or active control interventions, including relaxation or meditation (Cooney, Dwan, & Mead, 2014).

    (3) A critical feature in managing depression is to guide patients to accept their condition and focus on functioning and quality of life (Keitner & Mansfield, 2012).

    (4) Exercise provides distraction for patients not to dwell on the symptoms of depression and requires focus, which contributes to their active participation in improving their quality of life.

    (5) The biophysical mechanisms associated with exercise, such as the increase in beta-endorphins and a decrease in depression, are documented but not conclusive (Dinas, Koutedakis, & Flouris, 2011).

    (6) The challenge of using exercise as part the treatment plan for palliative care patients with depression is that the evidence of the type, frequency, and duration is not established (Vina, Sanchis-Gomar, Martinez-Bello, & Gomez-Cabrera, 2012).

j) Spiritual support at the end of life is important to address for patients who may find it helpful.

    (1) APRNs should include assessing spiritual and religious needs as part of the patients' treatment plan (Miller et al., 2012).

    (2) Religion, spirituality, and belief in God have been identified in the literature as providing well-being and positive treatment outcomes (Corn, Chochinov, & Vachon, 2012; Rosmarin et al., 2013; Vallurupalli et al., 2012; Vieten et al., 2013).

    (3) The National Consensus Project for Quality Palliative Care (2013), a consortium of U.S. palliative care organizations that sets palliative care quality standards, includes spiritual and religious aspects of care as one of the eight domains of quality palliative care provision.

B. Evaluation

  1. Patients' response to treatment is an essential part of the evaluation, although it typically takes four to six weeks for most patients to report response to antidepressants.

  2. Often, patients report improvements in initial bothersome symptoms (such as sleep and pain) prior to alleviation of mood.

3. Rayner, Price, et al. (2011) suggested that the length of time for antidepressants to alleviate symptoms is why assessment and early diagnosis are so critical in palliative care patients. If depression is diagnosed early in treatment, clinicians are able to intervene earlier to improve life quality at the end of life.

C. Current guidelines (e.g., NCCN, 2015) suggest that patients should be routinely screened upon admission and monthly thereafter or when a significant change in health is present.

D. Referrals
   1. After initial screening: APRN, physician assistant, or physician for further comprehensive assessment
   2. Consultation from the supportive care services if available

Case Study

A.T. is a 47-year-old mother of three children, aged 16, 18, and 23, and has been married 25 years to her high school sweetheart. Her recent mammogram revealed a 3 cm spiculated mass in her right breast. A biopsy and positron-emission tomography–computed tomography scan revealed a stage 4 ductal infiltrating carcinoma, with metastases to her ribs and spine. She will receive chemotherapy first, followed by a bilateral mastectomy and radiation. She sits in the infusion center receiving the third dose of every-two-week dose-dense ACT (doxorubicin, cyclophosphamide, and paclitaxel). Each session, the nurse has observed that A.T. is more disheveled, her posture is slumped, and she is withdrawn. During the infusion, the nurse asks A.T. how she has been feeling over the two weeks since her last treatment. A.T. replies, "I am very tired. I feel as if it takes everything out of me just to get out of bed. When will I get my energy back?" The nurse probes a bit more, and A.T. reveals that she is having trouble thinking and gets upset at every little thing. She begins to cry. "How will my family cope? I am just a burden now. And what will they do when I am no longer here?"

This patient would be best managed with an interdisciplinary plan of treatment. The RN is the first on the healthcare team to identify the problem. The RN needs to acknowledge the patient because what the patient is communicating is critical in timing for treatment. The RN could use active listening and reflective language to clarify what A.T. has just shared, including her fatigue, inability to think, feelings of irritability and anger, and concerns and fears about the future. The RN can suggest to the patient that she might be experiencing depression, which is common among patients who are in treatment for cancer, and give the patient a referral to the APRN who can address the patient's emotional distress. The clinical team (in this case, the RN who did the initial screening and the APRN who received the referral) should collaboratively develop the plan of care with other members of the healthcare team to include behavioral health and medicine.

References

Akechi, T., Ietsugu, T., Sukigara, M., Okamura, H., Tomohito, N., Akizuki, N., … Uchitomi, Y. (2009). Symptom indicator of severity of depression in cancer patients: A comparison of *DSM-IV* criteria with alternative diagnostic criteria. *General Hospital Psychiatry, 31,* 225–232. doi:10.1016/j.genhosppsych.2008.12.004

American Psychiatric Association. (2013). *Diagnostic and statistical manual of mental disorders* (5th ed.). Washington, DC: Author.

Andersen, B.L., Dorfman, C.S., & Godiwala, N. (2015). Cognitive and behavioral interventions. In J.C. Holland, W.S. Breitbart, P.N. Butow, P.B. Jacobsen, M.J. Loscalzo, & R. McCorkle (Eds.), *Psycho-oncology* (3rd ed., pp. 449–457). New York, NY: Oxford University Press.

Ando, M., Morita, T., Akechi, T., & Takashi, K. (2012). Factors in narratives to question in the Short-Term Life Review interviews of terminally ill cancer patients and utility of the questions. *Palliative and Supportive Care, 10,* 83–90. doi:10.1017/S1478951511000708

APRN Consensus Work Group & National Council of State Boards of Nursing APRN Advisory Committee. (2008). Consensus Model for APRN Regulation: Licensure, Accreditation, Certification & Education. Retrieved from https://www.ncsbn.org/Consensus_Model_for_APRN_Regulation_July_2008.pdf

Asghar-Ali, A., Wagle, K.C., & Braun, U.K. (2013). Depression in terminally ill patients: Dilemmas in diagnosis and treatment. *Journal of Pain and Symptom Management, 45,* 926–933. doi:10.1016/j.jpainsymman.2012.12.011

Badger, T.A. (2005). *Measuring nursing-sensitive patient outcomes: Evidenced-based summary for depression.* Pittsburgh, PA: Oncology Nursing Society.

Badger, T.A., Heitkemper, M., Lee, K.A., & Bruner, D.W. (2014). An experience with the Patient-Reported Outcomes Measurement Information System: Pros and cons and unanswered questions. *Nursing Outlook, 62,* 332–338. doi:10.1016/j.outlook.2014.06.009

Badger, T.A., & Lazenby, M. (2015). Depression. In C.G. Brown (Ed.), *A guide to oncology symptom management* (2nd ed., pp. 239–264). Pittsburgh, PA: Oncology Nursing Society.

Baile, W.F., Palmer, J.L., Bruera, E., & Parker, P.A. (2011). Assessment of palliative care cancer patients' most important concerns. *Supportive Care in Cancer, 19,* 475–481. doi:10.1007/s00520-010-0839-4

Bakitas, M., Lyons, K.D., Hegel, M.T., Balan, S., Brokaw, F.C., Seville, J., … Ahles, T.A. (2009). Effects of a palliative care intervention on clinical outcomes in patients with advanced cancer: The Project ENABLE II randomized controlled trial. *JAMA, 302,* 741–749. doi:10.1001/jama.2009.1198

Beck, J.S. (2011). *Cognitive behavior therapy: Basics and beyond* (2nd ed.). New York, NY: Guildford Press.

Berger, A.M., Yennu, S., & Million, R. (2013). Update on interventions focused on symptom clusters: What has been tried and what have we learned? *Current Opinion in Supportive and Palliative Care, 7,* 60–66. doi:10.1097/SPC.0b013e32835c7d88

Booij, S.H., Bouma, E.M.C., de Jonge, P., Ormel, J., & Oldehinkel, A.J. (2013). Chronicity of depressive problems and the cortisol response to psychosocial stress in adolescents: The TRAILS study. *Psychoneuroendocrinology, 38,* 659–666. doi:10.1016/j.psyneuen.2012.08.004

Breitbart, W., Rosenfeld, B., Gibson, C., Pessin, H., Poppito, S., Nelson, C., … Olden, M. (2010). Meaning-centered group psychotherapy for patients with advanced cancer: A pilot randomized controlled trial. *Psycho-Oncology, 19,* 21–28. doi:10.1002/pon.1556

Breitbart, W., Rosenfeld, B., Pessin, H., Applebaum, A., Kulikowski, J., & Lichtenthal, W.G. (2015). Meaning-centered group psychotherapy: An effective intervention for improving psychological well-being in patients with advanced cancer. *Journal of Clinical Oncology, 33,* 749–754. doi:10.1200/jco.2014.57.2198

Brooten, D., Youngblut, J.A., Deosires, W., Singhala, K., & Guido-Sanz, F. (2012). Global considerations in measuring effectiveness of advanced practice nurses. *International Journal of Nursing Studies, 49,* 906–912 doi:10.1016/j.ijnurstu.2011.10.022

Burkhouse, K.L., Gibb, B.E., Coles, M.E., Knopik, V.S., & McGeary, J.E. (2011). Serotonin transporter genotype moderates the link between children's reports of overprotective parenting and their behavioral inhibition. *Journal of Abnormal Child Psychology, 39,* 783–790. doi:10.1007/s10802-011-9526-2

Carek, P.J., Laibstain, S.E., & Carek, S.M. (2011). Exercise for the treatment of depression and anxiety. *International Journal of Psychiatry in Medicine, 41,* 15–28. doi:10.2190/PM.41.1.c

Chaoul, A., Lopez, G., Lee, R.T., Garcia, M.K., Frenkel, M., & Cohen, L. (2015). Integrative oncology. In J.C. Holland, W.S. Breitbart, P.N. Butow, P.B. Jacobesen, M.J. Loscalzo, & R. McCorkle (Eds.), *Psycho-oncology* (3rd ed., pp. 509–514). New York, NY: Oxford University Press.

Chilcot, J., Rayner, L., Lee, W., Price, A., Goodwin, L., Monroe, B., … Hotopf, M. (2013). The factor structure of the PHQ-9 in palliative care. *Journal of Psychosomatic Research, 75,* 60–64. doi:10.1016/j.jpsychores.2012.12.012

Chochinov, H.M., & Kredentser, M.S. (2015). Dignity in the terminally ill: Empirical findings and clinical applications. In J.C. Holland, W.S. Breitbart, P.N. Butow, P.B. Jacobsen, M.J. Loscalzo, & R. McCorkle (Eds.), *Psycho-oncology* (3rd ed., pp. 480–486). New York, NY: Oxford University Press.

Chochinov, H.M., Wilson, K.G., Enns, M., & Lander, S. (1997). "Are you depressed?" Screening for depression in the terminally ill. *American Journal of Psychiatry, 154,* 674–676. doi.org/10.1176/ajp.154.5.674

Cooney, G., Dwan, K., & Mead, G. (2014). Exercise for depression. *JAMA, 311,* 2432–2433. doi:10.1001/jama.2014.4930

Corn, B.W., Chochinov, H.M., & Vachon, M. (2012). Integrating spiritual care into the practice of oncology. *Current Opinion in Supportive and Palliative Care, 6,* 226–227. doi:10.1097/SPC.0b013e328353b8e6

Dinas, P.C., Koutedakis, Y., & Flouris, A.D. (2011). Effects of exercise and physical activity on depression. *Irish Journal of Medical Science, 180,* 319–325. doi:10.1007/s11845-010-0633-9

Endicott, J. (1984). Measurement of depression in patients with cancer. *Cancer, 53,* 2243–2249.

Falkensteiner, M., Mantovan, F., Müller, I., & Them, C. (2011). The use of massage therapy for reducing pain, anxiety, and depression in oncological palliative care patients: A narrative review of the literature. *ISRN Nursing, 2011,* Article ID 929868. doi:10.5402/2011/929868

Fann, J.R., Fan, M.-Y., & Unützer, J. (2009). Improving primary care for older adults with cancer and depression. *Journal of General Internal Medicine, 24,* 417–424. doi:10.1007/s11606-009-0999-4

Giese-Davis, J., Sephton, S.E., Abercrombie, H.C., Durán, R.E.F., & Spiegel, D. (2004). Repression and high anxiety are associated with aberrant diurnal cortisol rhythms in women with metastatic breast cancer. *Health Psychology, 23,* 645–650. doi:10.1037/0278-6133.23.6.645

Giese-Davis, J., Wilhelm, F.H., Conrad, A., Abercrombie, H.C., Sephton, S., Yutsis, M., … Spiegel, D. (2006). Depression and stress reactivity in metastatic breast cancer. *Psychosomatic Medicine, 68,* 675–683. doi:10.1097/01.psy.0000238216.88515.e5

Goodwin, L., Lee, W., Price, A., Rayner, L., Monroe, B., Sykes, N., Hansford, P., … Hotopf, M. (2012). Predictors of non-remission of depression in a palliative care population. *Palliative Medicine, 26,* 683–695. doi:10.1177/0269216311412230

Grassi, L., Nanni, M.G., Uchitomi, Y., & Riba, M. (2011). Pharmacotherapy of depression in people with cancer. In D.W. Kissane, M. Maj, & N. Sartorius (Eds.), *Depression and cancer* (pp. 151–176). Oxford, United Kingdom: Wiley-Blackwell.

Hart, S.L., Hoyt, M.A., Diefenbach, M., Anderson, D.R., Kilbourn, K.M., Craft, L.L., … Stanton, A.L. (2012). Meta-analysis of efficacy of interventions for elevated depressive symptoms in adults diagnosed with cancer. *Journal of the National Cancer Institute, 104,* 990–1004. doi:10.1093/jnci/djs256

Jacobsen, P.B., & Donovan, K.A. (2015). Assessment and screening for anxiety and depression. In J.C. Holland, W.S. Breitbart, P.N. Butow, P.B. Jacobsen, M.J. Loscalzo, & R. McCorkle (Eds.), *Psycho-oncology* (3rd ed., pp. 378–383). New York, NY: Oxford University Press.

Jiang, H.-Y., Deng, M., Zhang, Y.-H., Chen, H.-Z., Chen, Q., & Ruan, B. (2014). Specific serotonin reuptake inhibitors prevent interferon-α–induced depression in patients with hepatitis C: A meta-analysis. *Clinical Gastroenterology and Hepatology, 12,* 1452–1460.e3. doi:10.1016/j.cgh.2013.04.035

Keitner, G.I., & Mansfield, A.K. (2012). Management of treatment-resistant depression. *Psychiatric Clinics of North America, 35,* 249–265. doi:10.1016/j.psc.2011.11.004

Kelly, C.M., Juurlink, D.N., Gomes, T., Duong-Hua, M., Pritchard, K.I., Austin, P.C., & Paszat, L.F. (2010). Selective serotonin reuptake inhibitors and breast cancer mortality in women receiving tamoxifen: A population based cohort study. *BMJ, 340,* c693. doi:10.1136/bmj.c693

Kerr, C.W., Drake, J., Milch, R.A., Brazeau, D.A., Skretny, M.A., Brazeau, G.A., & Donnelly, J.P. (2012). Effects of methylphenidate on fatigue and depression: A randomized, double-blind, placebo-controlled trial. *Journal of Pain and Symptom Management, 43,* 68–77. doi:10.1016/j.jpainsymman.2011.03.026

Kissane, D.W., Levin, T., Hales, S., Lo, C., & Rodin, G. (2011). Psychotherapy for depression in cancer and palliative care. In D.W. Kissane, M. Maj, & N. Sartorius (Eds.), *Depression and cancer* (pp. 177–206). Oxford, United Kingdom: Wiley-Blackwell.

Kissane, D.W., & Ngan, C. (2015). Supportive-expressive and other forms of group psychotherapy in cancer care. In J.C. Holland, W.S. Breitbart, P.N. Butow, P.B. Jacobsen, M.J. Loscalzo, & R. McCorkle (Eds.), *Psycho-oncology* (3rd ed., pp. 532–540). New York, NY: Oxford University Press.

Kroenke, K., Spitzer, R.L., & Williams, J.B.W. (2001). The PHQ-9. *Journal of General Internal Medicine, 16,* 606–613. doi:10.1046/j.1525-1497.2001.016009606.x

Kroenke, K., Spitzer, R.L., & Williams, J.B.W. (2003). The Patient Health Questionnaire-2: Validity of a two-item depression screener. *Medical Care, 41,* 1284–1292. Retrieved from http://journals.lww.com/lww-medicalcare/Abstract/2003/11000/The_Patient_Health_Questionnaire_2__Validity_of_a.8.aspx

Lazenby, M., Dixon, J., Bai, M., & McCorkle, R. (2014). Comparing the Distress Thermometer (DT) with the Patient Health Questionnaire (PHQ)-2 for screening for possible cases of depression among patients newly diagnosed with advanced cancer. *Palliative and Supportive Care, 12,* 63–68. doi:10.1017/S1478951513000394

Lew, M.W., Kravits, K., Garberoglio, C., & Williams, A.C. (2011). Use of preoperative hypnosis to reduce postoperative pain and anesthesia-related side effects. *International Journal of Clinical and Experimental Hypnosis, 59,* 406–423. doi:10.1080/00207144.2011.594737

Lichtenthal, W.G., Applebaum, A.J., & Brietbart, W.S. (2015). Meaning-centered psychotherapy. In J.C. Holland, W.S. Breitbart, P.N. Butow, P.B. Jacobsen, M.J. Loscalzo, & R. McCorkle (Eds.), *Psycho-oncology* (3rd ed., pp. 475–479). New York, NY: Oxford University Press.

Marks, S., & Heinrich, T. (2013). Assessing and treating depression in palliative care patients. *Current Psychiatry, 12*(8), 35–40.

McCabe, M.P., Mellor, D., Davison, T.E., Hallford, D.J., & Goldhammer, D.L. (2012). Detecting and managing depressed patients: Palliative care nurses' self-efficacy and perceived barriers to care. *Journal of Palliative Medicine, 15,* 463–467. doi:10.1089/jpm.2011.0388

Mellor, D., McCabe, M.P., Davison, T.E., Goldhammer, D.L., & Hallford, D.J. (2012). Barriers to the detection and management of depression by palliative care professional carers among their patients: Perspectives from professional carers and patients' family members. *American Journal of Hospice and Palliative Medicine, 30,* 12–20. doi:10.1177/1049909112438705

Miguel, C., & Albuquerque, E. (2011). Drug interaction in psycho-oncology: Antidepressants and antineoplastics. *Pharmacology, 88,* 333–339. doi:10.1159/000334738

Miller, L., Wickramaratne, P., Gameroff, M.J., Sage, M., Tenke, C.E., & Weissman, M.M. (2012). Religiosity and major depression in adults at high risk: A ten-year prospective study. *American Journal of Psychiatry, 169,* 89–94. doi:10.1176/appi.ajp.2011.10121823

Mitchell, A.J., Chan, M., Bhatti, H., Halton, M., Grassi, L., Johansen, C., & Meader, N. (2011). Prevalence of depression, anxiety, and adjustment disorder in oncological, haematological, and palliative-care settings: A meta-analysis of 94 interview-based studies. *Lancet Oncology, 12,* 160–174. doi:10.1016/S1470-2045(11)70002-X

Mohr, D.C., Ho, J., Duffecy, J., Reifler, D., Sokol, L., Burns, M.N., … Siddique, J. (2012). Effect of telephone-administered vs face-to-face cognitive behavioral therapy on adherence to therapy and depression outcomes among primary care patients: A randomized trial. *JAMA, 307,* 2278–2285. doi:10.1001/jama.2012.5588

Moorey, S., Cort, E., Kapari, M., Monroe, B., Hansford, P., Mannix, K., … Hotopf, M. (2009). A cluster randomized controlled trial of cognitive behaviour therapy for common mental disorders in patients with advanced cancer. *Psychological Medicine, 39,* 713–723. doi:10.1017/S0033291708004169

National Comprehensive Cancer Network. (2015). *NCCN Clinical Practice Guidelines in Oncology (NCCN Guidelines®): Distress management* [v.3.2015]. Retrieved from http://www.nccn.org/professionals/physician_gls/PDF/distress.pdf

National Consensus Project for Quality Palliative Care. (2013). *Clinical practice guidelines for quality palliative care* (3rd ed.). Retrieved from https://www.hpna.org/multimedia/NCP_Clinical_Practice_Guidelines_3rd_Edition.pdf

Northouse, L.L., Katapodi, M.C., Song, L., Zhang, L., & Mood, D.W. (2010). Interventions with family caregivers of cancer patients: Meta-analysis of randomized trials. *CA: A Cancer Journal for Clinicians, 60,* 317–339. doi:10.3322/caac.20081

Passik, S.D., & Lowery, A.E. (2011). Recognition of depression and methods of depression screening in people with cancer. In D.W. Kissane, M. Maj, & N. Sartorius (Eds.), *Depression and cancer* (pp. 81–100). Oxford, United Kingdom: Wiley-Blackwell.

Pitceathly, C., Maguire, P., Fletcher, I., Parle, M., Tomenson, B., & Creed, F. (2009). Can a brief psychological intervention prevent anxiety or depressive disorders in cancer patients? A randomised controlled trial. *Annals of Oncology, 20,* 928–934. doi:10.1093/annonc/mdn708

Prommer, E. (2012). Methylphenidate: Established and expanding roles in symptom management. *American Journal of Hospice and Palliative Medicine, 29,* 483–490. doi:10.1177/1049909111427029

Raison, C.L., & Miller, A.H. (2011). Is depression an inflammatory disorder? *Current Psychiatry Reports, 13,* 467–475. doi:10.1007/s11920-011-0232-0

Rajasekaran, M., Edmonds, P.M., & Higginson, I.L. (2005). Systematic review of hypnotherapy for treating symptoms in terminally ill adult cancer patients. *Palliative Medicine, 19,* 418–426. 10.1191/0269216305pm1030oa

Rayner, L., Lee, W., Price, A., Monroe, B., Sykes, N., Hansford, P., … Hotopf, M. (2011). The clinical epidemiology of depression in palliative care and the predictive value of somatic symptoms: Cross-sectional survey with four-week follow-up. *Palliative Medicine, 25,* 229–241. doi:10.1177/0269216310387458

Rayner, L., Price, A., Evans, A., Valsraj, K., Hotopf, M., & Higginson, I.J. (2011). Antidepressants for the treatment of depression in palliative care: Systematic review and meta-analysis. *Palliative Medicine, 25,* 36–51. doi:10.1177/0269216310380764

Reyes-Gibby, C.C., Wang, J., Spitz, M., Wu, X., Yennurajalingam, S., & Shete, S. (2013). Genetic variations in interleukin-8 and interleukin-10 are associated with pain, depressed mood, and fatigue in lung cancer patients. *Journal of Pain and Symptom Management, 46,* 161–172. doi:10.1016/j.jpainsymman.2012.07.019

Rodin, G., Lloyd, N., Katz, M., Green, E., Mackay, J.A., & Wong, R.K.S. (2007). The treatment of depression in cancer patients: A systematic review. *Supportive Care in Cancer, 15,* 123–136. doi:10.1007/s00520-006-0145-3

Rosmarin, D.H., Bigda-Peyton, J.S., Kertz, S.J., Smith, N., Rauch, S.L., & Björgvinsson, T. (2013). A test of faith in God and treatment: The relationship of belief in God to psychiatric treatment outcomes. *Journal of Affective Disorders, 146,* 441–446. doi:10.1016/j.jad.2012.08.030

Sinita, E., & Coghill, D. (2014). The use of stimulant medications for non-core aspects of ADHD and in other disorders. *Neuropharmacology, 87,* 161–172. doi:10.1016/j.neuropharm.2014.06.014

Spiegel, D. (2012). Mind matters in cancer survival. *Psycho-Oncology, 21,* 588–593. doi:10.1002/pon.3067

Spiegel, D., Giese-Davis, J., Taylor, C.B., & Kraemer, H. (2006). Stress sensitivity in metastatic breast cancer: Analysis of hypothalamic-pituitary-adrenal axis function. *Psychoneuroendocrinology, 31,* 1231–1244. doi:10.1016/j.psyneuen.2006.09.004

Stagg, E.K., & Lazenby, M. (2012). Best practices for the nonpharmacological treatment of depression at the end of life. *American Journal of Hospice and Palliative Medicine, 29,* 183–194. doi:10.1177/1049909111413889

Steinhauser, K.E., Alexander, S.C., Byock, I.R., George, L.K., & Tulsky, J.A. (2009). Seriously ill patients' discussions of preparation and life completion: An intervention to assist with transition at the end of life. *Palliative and Supportive Care, 7,* 393–404. doi:10.1017/S147895150999040X

Taylor, L., Lovell, N., Ward, J., Wood, F., & Hosker, C. (2013). Diagnosis of depression in patients receiving specialist community palliative care: Does using a single screening question identify depression otherwise diagnosed by clinical interview? *Journal of Palliative Medicine, 16,* 1140–1142. doi:10.1089/jpm.2012.0569

Vallurupalli, M., Lauderdale, K., Balboni, M.J., Phelps, A.C., Block, S.D., Ng, A., ... Balboni, T.A. (2012). The role of spirituality and religious coping in the quality of life of patients with advanced cancer receiving palliative radiation therapy. *Journal of Supportive Oncology, 10,* 81–87. Retrieved from http://www.ncbi.nlm.nih.gov/pmc/articles/PMC3391969

Vieten, C., Scammell, S., Pilato, R., Ammondson, I., Pargament, K.I., & Lukoff, D. (2013). Spiritual and religious competencies for psychologists. *Psychology of Religion and Spirituality, 5,* 129–144. doi:10.1037/a0032699

Vina, J., Sanchis-Gomar, F., Martinez-Bello, V., & Gomez-Cabrera, M.C. (2012). Exercise acts as a drug; the pharmacological benefits of exercise. *British Journal of Pharmacology, 167,* 1–12. doi:10.1111/j.1476-5381.2012.01970.x

Zaider, T.I., & Kissane, D.W. (2015). Psychosocial interventions for couples and families coping with cancer. In J.C. Holland, W.S. Breitbart, P.N. Butow, P.B. Jacobsen, M.J. Loscalzo, & R. McCorkle (Eds.), *Psycho-oncology* (3rd ed., pp. 526–531). New York, NY: Oxford University Press.

CHAPTER 26

Dyspnea

Craig S. Conoscenti, MD, FCCP

I. Definition
   A. Dyspnea is "a subjective experience of breathing discomfort that consists of qualitatively distinct sensations that vary in intensity" (American Thoracic Society, 1999).
      1. Distinct mechanisms and afferent pathways are reliably associated with different sensory qualities (notably work and effort, tightness, and air hunger and unsatisfied inspiration).
      2. Distinct sensations most often do not occur in isolation.
      3. Dyspnea sensations also vary in their unpleasantness and their emotional and behavioral significance (Parshall et al., 2012).
   B. When someone experiences dyspnea, the condition "derives from interactions among multiple physiological, psychological, social, and environmental factors, and may induce secondary physiological and behavioral responses" (American Thoracic Society, 1999, p. 322).
   C. The perception of dyspnea requires conscious awareness and interpretation of numerous sensory stimuli; therefore, dyspnea requires self-reporting on the part of the patient.
   D. Dyspnea is a symptom, and this needs to be clearly distinguished from the signs that a healthcare practitioner will identify.
   E. Dyspnea is not only a symptom with great complexity, but it also is often a sign of a threat to the stability of a person's underlying health. This condition often leads to the person seeking medical help, which often leads to specific activities taking place to better characterize the dyspnea and its cause. Dyspnea causes not only distress to the patient, but also impaired quality of life.
   F. Dyspnea most often begins with physiologic impairment. This subsequently leads to stimulation of both pulmonary and extrapulmonary afferent receptors, transmission of information to the cerebral cortex, and perception of the sensation as uncomfortable (Lee, 2009; Undem & Nassenstein, 2009; Widdicombe, 2009).
   G. Because numerous afferent pathways are involved, it is unlikely that any laboratory stimulus used to study dyspnea will reproduce exactly what the patient perceives (Simon et al., 1990; Williams, Garrard, Cafarella, Petkov, & Frith, 2009).
   H. Each person perceives dyspnea differently. This can vary from day to day or even hour to hour.

Any views expressed in this chapter represent the personal opinions of the author and not those of Boehringer Ingelheim Pharmaceuticals.

1. Dyspnea often is associated with anxiety, depression, and fear and is viewed as a threat to the person's well-being. This often results in anxiety, fear, and depression, leading to thoughts of serious illness.
2. Because of this, the person often identifies particular activities that initiate the dyspnea and avoids these activities, resulting in muscle wasting and an overall state of decreased fitness, contributing to the overall disability that is often seen with dyspnea (Kunik et al., 2005; Sassi-Dambron, Eakin, Ries, & Kaplan, 1995; Williams, Cafarella, Olds, Petkov, & Frith, 2010).

II. Pathophysiology
   A. Dyspnea produces several different sensations dependent on patient interpretation. They are very different when the patient is asked to describe them. This suggests that the sensations arise from several different sensory mechanisms (Elliott et al., 1991; Harver, Mahler, Schwartzstein, & Baird, 2000; Mahler et al., 1996; Simon et al., 1989, 1990).
   B. Several sensory afferent sources can potentially play a role in dyspnea. In addition to traditionally defined sensory pathways, sensory information also is available from respiratory motor areas in the brain.
   C. In a multidirectional pathway, these areas can send copies of the motor activity that they transmit to perceptual areas of the brain.
   D. This is termed *corollary discharge*. Because of the unusual nature of the respiratory system having both automatic sources of motor command from the brain stem and voluntary sources from the cortex, corollary discharge from each of these leads to a hypothesis as to why different sensations are associated with dyspnea (Lee, 2009; Parshall et al., 2012; Undem & Nassenstein, 2009; Widdicombe, 2009).
   E. For several decades, it was thought that the sensations of effort and work were responsible for the feeling of dyspnea. Under periods of excess demand, the effort needed to maximize the muscle output to breathe at a ventilatory rate commensurate with need might in fact cause muscle fatigue, and this increased effort and work leading to fatigue would also lead to dyspnea (Altose, Cherniack, & Fishman, 1985).
   F. However, several groups have disproved this theory. Banzett et al. (1990) have shown that after alteration and raising of partial pressure of carbon dioxide (PCO_2) followed by muscle paralysis, study participants described typical air hunger or shortness of breath.
   G. Despite this, patients with diseases such as chronic obstructive pulmonary disease (COPD), asthma, and respiratory muscle dysfunction all do report dyspnea (O'Donnell, Bertley, Chau, & Webb, 1997; Simon et al., 1990).

III. Presenting symptoms
   A. *Chest tightness* is a common term asked of the person experiencing dyspnea and often is used by patients to describe what they are experiencing. This is a common component of bronchoconstriction, such as that seen in asthma. This results in not only chest tightness but also increased work of breathing and increased effort (Lougheed, Fisher, & O'Donnell, 2006; Lougheed, Lam, Forkert, Webb, & O'Donnell, 1993; Moy, Lantin, Harver, & Schwartzstein, 1998).
   B. Evidence has shown that patients with asthma who have the sensation of increased work and effort do not have as rapid a response to nebulized beta-agonists as those who report tightness. This points to the increased work effort being related to increased motor input to overcome bronchoconstriction, and the sensation of chest tightness being related to the stimulation of airway receptors. This all points to the

likelihood that tightness arises from pulmonary afferents and not a work-related sensation (Parshall et al., 2012).

C. *Air hunger* is another common term associated with dyspnea. As demand exceeds capacity, an imbalance develops between the motor-induced drive to breathe (corollary discharge) and afferent receptor feedback. This leads to the unpleasant feeling of air hunger (Parshall et al., 2012).

D. Wright and Branscomb (1955) proposed the term *air hunger* to describe severe respiratory discomfort evoked by strapping the chest and abdomen with broad adhesive tape during exercise and subsequently by using a device that limited tidal volume and respiratory rate during hypoxia.

E. Air hunger can be intensified by applying stimuli that inherently increase spontaneous ventilator drive. This can be attained through stimuli such as hypoxia, hypercapnia, and acidosis (Lane & Adams, 1993; Lane, Adams, & Guz, 1990; Moosavi et al., 2003).

F. Although all of these sensations can occur separately, they usually occur in multiple combinations that all result in an uncomfortable feeling for patients. This constellation of sensations is what is referred to most often as dyspnea. Very specific stimuli generated in the laboratory seem to stimulate more than one pathway. General reports of dyspnea are not as consistent as other sensations (Parshall et al., 2012).

IV. Physical examination

A. Patients typically fit into two categories with respect to dyspnea. The first is those who have new onset of dyspnea and no known etiology at the time of evaluation, and the second is those patients who have known respiratory, cardiovascular, or neuromuscular disease who have progressive dyspnea.

1. When evaluating the first group, clinicians will begin an investigation into finding the etiology of the dyspnea (Parshall et al., 2012; Schwartzstein & Adams, 2010).

2. When evaluating the second group, clinicians evaluate the underlying disorder to understand its progression.

B. When evaluating a patient with new-onset dyspnea, it is best to follow a standard procedure to evaluate the symptom thoroughly, as the mechanisms and the clinical conditions associated with dyspnea are extensive (Parshall et al., 2012; Schwartzstein & Adams, 2010).

C. This should start with an inclusive history and include all subjective components of the dyspnea. The evaluation also should include an extensive past medical history and a history of potential occupational and social exposures.

D. Although the combination of examination, laboratory, radiographic, and clinical studies elucidate much about dyspnea, the patient's own words often are able to provide significant information about the underlying cause of the dyspnea (Elliott et al., 1991; Killian, Watson, Otis, St. Amand, & O'Byrne, 2000; Mahler et al., 1996; Simon et al., 1990).

E. When a patient uses the term *chest tightness*, this most often refers to dyspnea due to bronchoconstriction, such as might be seen in asthma (Killian et al., 2000).

F. The sensations of air hunger or inability to take a deep breath often refer to the feeling of increased respiratory drive and a limited tidal volume and inspiratory capacity as seen in dynamic hyperinflation with COPD and restrictive lung disease (pulmonary fibrosis) (O'Donnell et al., 1997).

G. Occasionally the initial evaluation is unrevealing as to the etiology of the dyspnea or the patient may have multiple conditions compounding the evaluation. In these circumstances, cardiopulmonary exercise testing can be very helpful. Identifying nonrespiratory causes of exercise limitation (e.g., leg discomfort, fatigue, weakness) is important because they often coexist with breathing discomfort (Martinez et al., 1994).

H. A small number of blood tests are useful in the evaluation of dyspnea. Anemia should be ruled out by obtaining a hemoglobin and hematocrit because these may identify reduced oxygen-carrying capacity. Arterial blood gas measurements often are helpful for patients presenting with dyspnea associated with severe cardiopulmonary disease (e.g., acute respiratory distress syndrome, acute respiratory failure) but are not as helpful for stable patients with dyspnea (Parshall et al., 2012).

I. Measurement of dyspnea
1. To adequately assess dyspnea and its impact, it should be measured. The American Thoracic Society (1999) addressed several validated measures but gave no direct guidance on which tools should be used in different circumstances.
2. Each instrument measures a different domain or aspect of dyspnea. It may address what breathing feels like or whether it affects quality of life or performance of activities of daily living (Parshall et al., 2012).
3. Several systematic reviews have looked at dyspnea measures. Dorman, Byrne, and Edwards (2007) identified and then appraised 29 breathlessness scales used in palliative care: 6 measured breathlessness, 4 assessed breathlessness descriptions, and 19 measured impact.
4. The numeric rating scale, modified Borg, Chronic Respiratory Questionnaire dyspnea subscale, and the Japanese Cancer Dyspnea Scale appear most suitable for use in palliative care, but further evaluation is required before adopting any scale as standard either in palliative care or any other specialty (Dorman et al., 2007).
5. Bausewein, Farquhar, Booth, Gysels, and Higginson (2007) performed a systematic review with the aim of identifying all measures available and evaluating their usefulness in patients with advanced disease. They identified 33 tools: 29 were multidimensional in nature, with 11 being breathlessness specific and 18 disease specific; and 4 tools were one dimensional and measured severity. The majority of the tools were validated for COPD. Their conclusion was that no one scale was adequate and that the combination of a one-dimensional scale such a visual analog scale with a disease-specific scale (if available) or a multidimensional scale with an additional qualitative scale was the best approach (Bausewein et al., 2007).
6. Johnson and colleagues completed a systematic review attempting to establish which tools have been used in research looking at the severity of dyspnea in patients with congestive heart failure (CHF). They found 19 studies that used a one-dimensional tool, which included the Borg or Likert scales and a visual analog scale, alone or with a quality-of-life scale. Five used the CHF questionnaire and two used the Baseline Dyspnea Index and Transitional Dyspnea Index. Unfortunately, the review resulted in no consensus on a consistent tool that should be used in CHF (Johnson, Oxberry, Cleland, & Clark, 2010).
7. It has been suggested that dyspnea measurements should be looked at as either sensory–perceptual experience, affective distress, or symptom impact or burden (Parshall et al., 2012).
   a) Sensory–perceptual would relate to what breathing feels like to the patient. This measure would concentrate on intensity and quality of the sensation.

These measures would include separate single-item scales, such as the Borg scale or a visual analog scale.

b) Affective distress is based in perception. This may be either the perception of immediate unpleasantness or to the response around possible consequences of the perceived dyspnea. These measures may use single-item ratings of severity of distress or unpleasantness; multiple-item ratings of emotional responses such as anxiety; or unidimensional ratings of disability or activity limitation, for example, the Medical Research Council scale.

c) Measures of symptom impact or burden refer to how dyspnea may affect behavior or beliefs of what may occur with a behavior, functional ability, employment, quality of life, or health status. They may use unidimensional or multidimensional ratings of functional ability or multidimensional ratings of quality of life and health status.

d) Usually these measures involve multiple-item scales. These scales usually cross several areas of patient assessment. These may include functional performance and disability, quality of life, and psychosocial behavior.

e) It is important to note that these measures do not assess the sensation of dyspnea but rather its impact on the patient's life. To understand the changes in dyspnea in these measures, nurses need to assess the changes in impact or burden and make an assumption from that. The one concern is that changes in other concomitant parameters (e.g., depression, pain) may not make this assumption valid (Craig, 2003; Parshall et al., 2012; Price, 2000).

V. Interventions

A. The initial approach to the treatment of patients with dyspnea should be to optimize the treatment of the underlying condition. This may include the use of inhaled bronchodilators or inhaled corticosteroids in patients with COPD and asthma, or diuretics and afterload reduction for people with CHF. Although several U.S. Food and Drug Administration–approved treatments are available for diseases where dyspnea is a prominent component, no approved treatments for dyspnea currently exist (Parshall et al., 2012).

B. Supplemental oxygen has been shown to reduce mortality in patients with chronic hypoxemia secondary to COPD. This response has not been consistently shown when evaluated for the relief of breathlessness (Cranston, Crockett, & Currow, 2008).

C. In some instances, helium-containing gas mixtures may help to reduce the resistance to airflow and work of breathing. This may lead to improved hyperinflation and improved dyspnea. This is sometimes a very useful approach in obstructive lung disease (Eves, Petersen, Haykowsky, Wong, & Jones, 2006).

D. Opioids have been widely studied in the management of dyspnea. Some studies have shown that short-term administration has reduced dyspnea in several underlying conditions, such as COPD, interstitial lung disease, cancer, and chronic CHF. No evidence exists of long-term efficacy, so its usefulness is limited (Abernethy et al., 2003; Johnson, McDonagh, Harkness, McKay, & Dargie, 2002; Mahler et al., 2010; Poole, Veale, & Black, 1998; Qaseem et al., 2008).

1. Side effects are a concern and some occur frequently (e.g., constipation).

2. Although it is always a concern, there have been no reports of clinically significant respiratory depression.

3. Evidence-based guidelines have recommended to consider opioids on an individual basis for the relief of dyspnea when the underlying illness has been treated adequately (Marciniuk et al., 2011; Qaseem et al., 2008).

E. Although the mechanism has not been fully proved, inhaled furosemide has been shown to reduce breathlessness that is induced in normal volunteers, possibly related to vagal afferent nerves (Moosavi et al., 2007; Nishino, Ide, Sudo, & Sato, 2000). Although it should continue to be studied, no indication exists for its use at the present time (Parshall et al., 2012).

F. Pulmonary rehabilitation has been shown to be beneficial in patients with chronic lung disease by reducing exertional dyspnea during daily activity and with exercise, improving exercise tolerance, and resulting in less self-reported dyspnea during activity (Nici et al., 2006; Ries et al., 2007; Troosters, Casaburi, Gosselink, & Decramer, 2005).

G. Although the main approach used in pulmonary rehabilitation is exercise, the exact mechanism that leads to this improvement is not clear. It is unclear whether it is due to reduced oxygen requirements resulting from improved conditioning of the muscles used in the exercise; the pacing of activities guided by symptoms; or desensitization to the sensations of dyspnea. In fact, it may be a combination of these effects (Nici et al., 2006; Ries et al., 2007).

H. Patients with chronic respiratory disease often have a high ventilatory demand with a limited capacity of the respiratory muscles. This often leads to dyspnea caused by the increased respiratory muscle effort and oxygen requirements under this stress. If the demand of the respiratory muscles is decreased, this may lead to decreased dyspnea. Noninvasive ventilation can help reduce the demand in many patients with chronic respiratory disease. Unfortunately, very little information exists for dyspnea as an endpoint in studies. Several studies have shown that long-term and short-term use of nocturnal noninvasive ventilation has led to a reduction in dyspnea in patients with COPD (Casanova et al., 2000; Clini et al., 2002; Meduri, Conoscenti, Menashe, & Nair, 1989).

I. Follow-up
   1. Although the goal of medical research is often to find the cure for diseases, it cannot be forgotten that symptom control and palliative care often are as important as treating the underlying disease.
   2. With regard to dyspnea, much is known about the mechanism of dyspnea and how to evaluate it, but there has not been equal success in defining therapy.
   3. Future research needs to continue to study possible treatments for dyspnea. At this stage, where little directed therapy exists, the primary goal initially must be to stabilize any underlying diseases to begin to address the foundation of dyspnea for many patients.

Case Study

T.C. is a 61-year-old woman who presents with a complaint of increasing dyspnea with exertion that is limiting her ability to carry out some of her activities of daily living. She has developed a bilateral peripheral neuropathy secondary to long-standing type 2 diabetes mellitus, which has led to difficulty in her ambulation. She has bilateral osteoarthritis of both knees that has decreased her physical activity and daily exercise. She denies any chest pain, palpitations, wheezing, cough, or sputum production.

Her past medical history is positive for type 2 diabetes mellitus, osteoarthritis, hypertension, obesity, and seasonal allergies. She denies any history of cardiac disease, respiratory disease, or vascular disease. Her medications include metformin 500 mg BID, hydrochlorothiazide 25 mg daily, and lisinopril 20 mg daily. Ibuprofen 800 mg every eight hours is used PRN for arthritis pain.

On physical examination, T.C. has clear lungs through all fields with no wheezing, rales, or rhonchi. Cardiac auscultation reveals normal heart sounds with no murmur or gallop. Rhythm was regular. She has no peripheral edema but does have decreased quadriceps and hamstring strength with arthritic deformity of her knees. She has decreased popliteal and pedal pulses bilaterally with decreased sensation bilaterally.

Diagnostic testing shows normal complete blood count, chemistry, and urinalysis. Her chest x-ray is normal except minimal cardiomegaly. Electrocardiogram is normal. She had an echocardiogram that is normal except for mild left ventricular enlargement. Ambulatory oxygen saturation testing is completed. The patient has to stop her ambulation because of dyspnea and lower-extremity weakness. Her oxygen saturation was 96% on room air at rest and fell to 93% at the time she needed to stop ambulating.

It is decided, given T.C.'s normal cardiac function, lack of findings suggestive of pulmonary disease, and muscle weakness and concurrent need to stop ambulating, that she has muscle deconditioning secondary to increasing sedentary lifestyle due to a combination of peripheral neuropathy associated with debilitating arthritis. The therapeutic plan includes treatment of her neuropathy with continued control of her diabetes. Referral to physical therapy concentrating on lower-extremity strengthening and conditioning will allow for greater activity and less oxygen requirement to the debilitated muscle.

References

Abernethy, A.P., Currow, D.C., Frith, P., Fazekas, B.S., McHugh, A., & Bui, C. (2003). Randomised, double blind, placebo controlled crossover trial of sustained release morphine for the management of refractory dyspnoea. *BMJ, 327,* 523–528. doi:10.1136/bmj.327.7414.523

Altose, M., Cherniack, N., & Fishman, A.P. (1985). Respiratory sensations and dyspnea. *Journal of Applied Physiology, 58,* 1051–1054. Retrieved from http://jap.physiology.org/content/58/4/1051.long

American Thoracic Society. (1999). Dyspnea: Mechanisms, assessment, and management: A consensus statement. *American Journal of Respiratory and Critical Care Medicine, 159,* 321–340. doi:10.1164/ajrccm.159.1.ats898

Banzett, R.B., Lansing, R.W., Brown, R., Topulos, G.P., Yager, D., Steele, S.M., … Adams, L. (1990). 'Air hunger' from increased PCO_2 persists after complete neuromuscular block in humans. *Respiration Physiology, 81,* 1–17. doi:10.1016/0034-5687(90)90065-7

Bausewein, C., Farquhar, M., Booth, S., Gysels, M., & Higginson, I.J. (2007). Measurement of breathlessness in advanced disease: A systematic review. *Respiratory Medicine, 101,* 399–410. doi:10.1016/j.rmed.2006.07.003

Casanova, C., Celli, B.R., Tost, L., Soriano, E., Abreu, J., Velasco, V., & Santolaria, F. (2000). Long-term controlled trial of nocturnal nasal positive pressure ventilation in patients with severe COPD. *Chest, 118,* 1582–1590. doi:10.1378/chest.118.6.1582

Clini, E., Sturani, C., Rossi, A., Viaggi, S., Corrado, A., Donner, C.F., & Ambrosino, N. (2002). The Italian multicentre study on noninvasive ventilation in chronic obstructive pulmonary disease patients. *European Respiratory Journal, 20,* 529–538. doi:10.1183/09031936.02.02162001

Craig, A.D. (2003). Interoception: The sense of the physiological condition of the body. *Current Opinion in Neurobiology, 13,* 500–505. doi:10.1016/S0959-4388(03)00090-4

Cranston, J.M., Crockett, A., & Currow, D. (2008). Oxygen therapy for dyspnoea in adults. *Cochrane Database of Systematic Reviews, 2008*(3). doi:10.1002/14651858.CD004769.pub2

Dorman, S., Byrne, A., & Edwards, A. (2007). Which measurement scales should we use to measure breathlessness in palliative care? A systematic review. *Palliative Medicine, 21,* 177–191. doi:10.1177/0269216307076398

Elliott, M.W., Adams, L., Cockcroft, A., MacRae, K.D., Murphy, K., & Guz, A. (1991). The language of breathlessness: Use of verbal descriptors by patients with cardiopulmonary disease. *American Review of Respiratory Disease, 144,* 826–832. doi:10.1164/ajrccm/144.4.826

Eves, N.D., Petersen, S.R., Haykowsky, M.J., Wong, E.Y., & Jones, R.L. (2006). Helium-hyperoxia, exercise, and respiratory mechanics in chronic obstructive pulmonary disease. *American Journal of Respiratory and Critical Care Medicine, 174,* 763–771. doi:10.1164/rccm.200509-1533OC

Harver, A., Mahler, D.A., Schwartzstein, R.M., & Baird, J.C. (2000). Descriptors of breathlessness in healthy individuals: Distinct and separable constructs. *Chest, 118,* 679–690. doi:10.1378/chest.118.3.679

Johnson, M.J., McDonagh, T.A., Harkness, A., McKay, S.E., & Dargie, H.J. (2002). Morphine for the relief of breathlessness in patients with chronic heart failure—A pilot study. *European Journal of Heart Failure, 4,* 753–756. doi:10.1016/S1388-9842(02)00158-7

Johnson, M.J., Oxberry, S.G., Cleland, J.G.F., & Clark, A.L. (2010). Measurement of breathlessness in clinical trials in patients with chronic heart failure: The need for a standardized approach. A systematic review. *European Journal of Heart Failure, 12,* 137–147. doi:10.1093/eurjhf/hfp194

Killian, K.J., Watson, R., Otis, J., St. Amand, T.A., & O'Byrne, P.M. (2000). Symptom perception during acute bronchoconstriction. *American Journal of Respiratory and Critical Care Medicine, 162,* 490–496. doi:10.1164/ajrccm.162.2.9905079

Kunik, M.E., Roundy, K., Veazey, C., Souchek, J., Richardson, P., Wray, N.P., & Stanley, M.A. (2005). Surprisingly high prevalence of anxiety and depression in chronic breathing disorders. *Chest, 127,* 1205–1211. doi:10.1378/chest.127.4.1205

Lane, R., & Adams, L. (1993). Metabolic acidosis and breathlessness during exercise and hypercapnia in man. *Journal of Physiology, 461,* 47–61. doi:10.1113/jphysiol.1993.sp019500

Lane, R., Adams, L., & Guz, A. (1990). The effects of hypoxia and hypercapnia on perceived breathlessness during exercise in humans. *Journal of Physiology, 428,* 579–593. doi:10.1113/jphysiol.1990.sp018229

Lee, L.-Y. (2009). Respiratory sensations evoked by activation of bronchopulmonary C-fibers. *Respiratory Physiology and Neurobiology, 167,* 26–35. doi:10.1016/j.resp.2008.05.006

Lougheed, M.D., Fisher, T., & O'Donnell, D.E. (2006). Dynamic hyperinflation during bronchoconstriction in asthma: Implications for symptom perception. *Chest, 130,* 1072–1081. doi:10.1378/chest.130.4.1072

Lougheed, M.D., Lam, M., Forkert, L., Webb, K.A., & O'Donnell, D.E. (1993). Breathlessness during acute bronchoconstriction in asthma: Pathophysiologic mechanisms. *American Review of Respiratory Disease, 148,* 1452–1459. doi:10.1164/ajrccm.148.6_Pt_1.1452

Mahler, D.A., Harver, A., Lentine, T., Scott, J.A., Beck, K., & Schwartzstein, R.M. (1996). Descriptors of breathlessness in cardiorespiratory diseases. *American Journal of Respiratory and Critical Care Medicine, 154,* 1357–1363. doi:10.1164/ajrccm.154.5.8912748

Mahler, D.A., Selecky, P.A., Harrod, C.G., Benditt, J.O., Carrieri-Kohlman, V., Curtis, J.R., ... Waller, A. (2010). American College of Chest Physicians consensus statement on the management of dyspnea in patients with advanced lung or heart disease. *Chest, 137,* 674–691. doi:10.1378/chest.09-1543

Marciniuk, D., Goodridge, D., Hernandez, P., Rocker, G., Balter, M., Bailey, P., ... Brown, C. (2011). Managing dyspnea in patients with advanced chronic obstructive pulmonary disease: A Canadian Thoracic Society clinical practice guideline. *Canadian Respiratory Journal, 18,* 69–78. doi:10.1155/2011/745047

Martinez, F.J., Stanopoulos, I., Acero, R., Becker, F.S., Pickering, R., & Beamis, J.F. (1994). Graded comprehensive cardiopulmonary exercise testing in the evaluation of dyspnea unexplained by routine evaluation. *Chest, 105,* 168–174. doi:10.1378/chest.105.1.168

Meduri, G.U., Conoscenti, C.C., Menashe, P., & Nair, S. (1989). Noninvasive face mask ventilation in patients with acute respiratory failure. *Chest, 95,* 865–870. doi:10.1378/chest.95.4.865

Moosavi, S.H., Binks, A.P., Lansing, R.W., Topulos, G.P., Banzett, R.B., & Schwartzstein, R.M. (2007). Effect of inhaled furosemide on air hunger induced in healthy humans. *Respiratory Physiology and Neurobiology, 156,* 1–8. doi:10.1016/j.resp.2006.07.004

Moosavi, S.H., Golestanian, E., Binks, A.P., Lansing, R.W., Brown, R., & Banzett, R.B. (2003). Hypoxic and hypercapnic drives to breathe generate equivalent levels of air hunger in humans. *Journal of Applied Physiology, 94,* 141–154. doi:10.1152/japplphysiol.00594.2002

Moy, M.L., Lantin, M.L., Harver, A., & Schwartzstein, R.M. (1998). Language of dyspnea in assessment of patients with acute asthma treated with nebulized albuterol. *American Journal of Respiratory and Critical Care Medicine, 158,* 749–753. doi:10.1164/ajrccm.158.3.9707088

Nici, L., Donner, C., Wouters, E., Zuwallack, R., Ambrosino, N., Bourbeau, J., ... Troosters, T. (2006). American Thoracic Society/European Respiratory Society statement on pulmonary rehabilitation. *American Journal of Respiratory and Critical Care Medicine, 173,* 1390–1413. doi:10.1164/rccm.200508-1211ST

Nishino, T., Ide, T., Sudo, T., & Sato, J. (2000). Inhaled furosemide greatly alleviates the sensation of experimentally induced dyspnea. *American Journal of Respiratory and Critical Care Medicine, 161,* 1963–1967. doi:10.1164/ajrccm.161.6.9910009

O'Donnell, D.E., Bertley, J.C., Chau, L.K., & Webb, K.A. (1997). Qualitative aspects of exertional breathlessness in chronic airflow limitation: Pathophysiologic mechanisms. *American Journal of Respiratory and Critical Care Medicine, 155,* 109–115. doi:10.1164/ajrccm.155.1.9001298

Parshall, M.B., Schwartzstein, R.M., Adams, L., Banzett, R.B., Manning, H.L., Bourbeau, J., … O'Donnell, D.E. (2012). An official American Thoracic Society statement: Update on the mechanisms, assessment, and management of dyspnea. *American Journal of Respiratory and Critical Care Medicine, 185*, 435–452. doi:10.1164/rccm.201111-2042ST

Poole, P.J., Veale, A.G., & Black, P.N. (1998). The effect of sustained-release morphine on breathlessness and quality of life in severe chronic obstructive pulmonary disease. *American Journal of Respiratory and Critical Care Medicine, 157*, 1877–1880. doi:10.1164/ajrccm.157.6.9711061

Price, D.D. (2000). Psychological and neural mechanisms of the affective dimension of pain. *Science, 288*, 1769–1772. doi:10.1126/science.288.5472.1769

Qaseem, A., Snow, V., Shekelle, P., Casey, D.E., Jr., Cross, J.T., Jr., & Owens, D.K. (2008). Evidence-based interventions to improve the palliative care of pain, dyspnea, and depression at the end of life: A clinical practice guideline from the American College of Physicians. *Annals of Internal Medicine, 148*, 141–146. doi:10.7326/0003-4819-148-2-200801150-00009

Ries, A.L., Bauldoff, G.S., Carlin, B.W., Casaburi, R., Emery, C.F., Mahler, D.A., … Herrerias, C. (2007). Pulmonary rehabilitation: Joint ACCP/AACVPR evidence-based clinical practice guidelines. *Chest, 131*(Suppl. 5), 4S–42S. doi:10.1378/chest.06-2418

Sassi-Dambron, D.E., Eakin, E.G., Ries, A.L., & Kaplan, R.M. (1995). Treatment of dyspnea in COPD: A controlled clinical trial of dyspnea management strategies. *Chest, 107*, 724–729. doi:10.1378/chest.107.3.724

Schwartzstein, R.M., & Adams, L. (2010). Dyspnea. In R.J. Mason, V.C. Broaddus, T.R. Martin, T.E. King Jr., D.E. Schraufnagel, J.F. Murray, & J.A. Nadel (Eds.), *Murray and Nadel's textbook of respiratory medicine* (5th ed.) [Electronic edition]. Philadelphia, PA: Elsevier Saunders.

Simon, P.M., Schwartzstein, R.M., Weiss, J.W., Fencl, V., Teghtsoonian, M., & Weinberger, S.E. (1990). Distinguishable types of dyspnea in patients with shortness of breath. *American Review of Respiratory Disease, 142*, 1009–1014. doi:10.1164/ajrccm/142.5.1009

Simon, P.M., Schwartzstein, R.M., Weiss, J.W., Lahive, K., Fencl, V., Teghtsoonian, M., & Weinberger, S.E. (1989). Distinguishable sensations of breathlessness induced in normal volunteers. *American Review of Respiratory Disease, 140*, 1021–1027. doi:10.1164/ajrccm/140.4.1021

Troosters, T., Casaburi, R., Gosselink, R., & Decramer, M. (2005). Pulmonary rehabilitation in chronic obstructive pulmonary disease. *American Review of Respiratory Disease, 172*, 19–38. doi:10.1164/rccm.200408-1109SO

Undem, B.J., & Nassenstein, C. (2009). Airway nerves and dyspnea associated with inflammatory airway disease. *Respiratory Physiology and Neurobiology, 167*, 36–44. doi:10.1016/j.resp.2008.11.012

Widdicombe, J. (2009). Lung afferent activity: Implications for respiratory sensation. *Respiratory Physiology and Neurobiology, 167*, 2–8. doi:10.1016/j.resp.2008.09.012

Williams, M., Cafarella, P., Olds, T., Petkov, J., & Frith, P. (2010). Affective descriptors of the sensation of breathlessness are more highly associated with severity of impairment than physical descriptors in people with COPD. *Chest, 138*, 315–322. doi:10.1378/chest.09-2498

Williams, M., Garrard, A., Cafarella, P., Petkov, J., & Frith, P. (2009). Quality of recalled dyspnoea is different from exercise-induced dyspnoea: An experimental study. *Australian Journal of Physiotherapy, 55*, 177–183. doi:10.1016/S0004-9514(09)70078-9

Wright, G.W., & Branscomb, B.V. (1955). The origin of the sensations of dyspnea? *Transactions of the American Clinical and Climatological Association, 66*, 116–125. Retrieved from http://www.ncbi.nlm.nih.gov/pmc/articles/PMC2248903

CHAPTER 27

Insomnia

Suzette Walker, DNP, FNP-BC, AOCNP®

I. Definition
   A. Insomnia is defined as difficulty in initiating and maintaining sleep, as well as suffering from nonrestorative sleep.
   B. Sleep disturbance and associated daytime fatigue result in significant distress and impairment in social, occupational, or other important areas of functioning.
   C. Criteria to meet the definition of insomnia from the *International Statistical Classification of Diseases and Related Health Problems, 10th Revision* (World Health Organization, 2016) and the *Diagnostic and Statistical Manual of Mental Disorders* (American Psychiatric Association, 2013)
      1. Difficulty initiating sleep at least three times a week
      2. Difficulty maintaining sleep
         a) Waking three or more times a night
         b) Problems staying asleep at least three times a week
         c) Taking at least 30 minutes to get back to sleep
         d) Waking too early in the morning at least three times a week
      3. Complaining of nonrestorative sleep
         a) Feeling unrefreshed in the morning at least three times a week
         b) Interference with daytime activities
II. Pathophysiology
   A. Restorative sleep is one of the essential needs of all humans. Sleep is critical for optimal mental and physical health for all patients.
   B. There is a growing body of knowledge regarding the pathophysiology of insomnia in the general public.
   C. The pathophysiology of sleep disorders in chronic illness and palliative care is not fully understood.
   D. Sleep disorders often are part of a symptom cluster that affects patients in the palliative care setting. Insomnia often goes hand in hand with depression, anxiety, fatigue, decreased sense of well-being, and pain. In many cases, it is impossible to know which symptom came first (Delgado-Guay, Yennurajalingam, Parsons, Palmer, & Bruera, 2011).
   E. Despite great advances in symptom management overall, sleep disturbances often go unrecognized by providers and underreported by patients.
   F. The pathophysiology of insomnia centers on hyperarousal during sleep.
      1. The production of cortisol and adrenocorticotropic hormone can cause disruptions in rapid eye movement sleep (REMS) and non-rapid eye movement sleep (NREMS).

2. Sleep typically occurs in 90-minute cycles of NREMS/REMS. Disruption in this cycle can have negative effects on health.

G. Patients with sleep disorders are more likely to develop hypertension, obesity, metabolic syndrome, depression, cardiovascular disease, and cerebrovascular disease (Bloom et al., 2009).

III. Presenting symptoms
  A. Daytime fatigue
    1. Inability to perform normal tasks
    2. Great effort required for routine endeavors
    3. Need for naps during the day
    4. Poor performance at work or school
  B. Sleep disturbances
    1. Lie awake for a long time prior to falling asleep
    2. Sleep for short periods of time
    3. Awaken early in the morning
    4. Wake several times in the night
  C. Trouble focusing
    1. Inability to complete tasks
    2. Cognitive impairment
  D. Depression
  E. Anxiety
  F. Irritability
  G. Headaches

IV. Physical examination
  A. Screening should occur at every point of care (Davis, Khoshknabi, Walsh, Lagman, & Platt, 2014; Schutte-Rodin, Broch, Buysse, Dorsey, & Sateia, 2008).
    1. Guidelines from the National Institutes of Health published within the Pan-Canadian practice guideline recommend the following two questions for screening (Howell et al., 2013):
      a) Do you have problems with your sleep or sleep disturbances three or more times a week?
      b) Does the problem with your sleep negatively affect your daytime function?
    2. If the patient answers the two questions positively, the clinician should initiate further screening.
  B. Screening tools are recommended if initial screening is positive (Davis et al., 2014; Schutte-Rodin et al., 2008).
    1. The Edmonton Symptom Assessment System (ESAS) is a validated tool that consists of visual analog scales for the assessment of nine symptoms.
    2. The Insomnia Severity Index is a validated tool with five questions regarding sleep and a visual analog scale.
    3. The "BEARS" tool covers five domains of sleep: Bedtime problems, Excessive sleepiness, Awakenings, Regularity of sleep, and Sleep-disorder breathing.
    4. Two-week sleep diary: This record should include sleep quality, daytime impairment, medications, caffeine, and alcohol consumption for each 24-hour period.
    5. Screening for depression and psychiatric illness should be performed.
  C. Health, substance, and psychiatric history (Schutte-Rodin et al., 2008)
    1. Insomnia is primarily diagnosed by clinical evaluation through a thorough sleep history and detailed medical, substance, and psychiatric history.

2. A wide range of medical and psychiatric illnesses can be comorbid with insomnia (Schutte-Rodin et al., 2008). A survey among older adults found that those with more than two chronic conditions were more likely to complain of difficulty sleeping.
3. Sleep history (Schutte-Rodin et al., 2008)
    a) Primary insomnia complaint: Characterization of complaint, onset, duration, frequency, severity, course, perpetuation factors, treatments tried and responses
    b) Pre-sleep conditions: Activities before bedtime, environment, physical and mental status
    c) Sleep–wake schedule: Bedtime, time to fall asleep, awakenings, wake time versus time out of bed, amount of sleep
    d) Nocturnal symptoms: Respiratory, motor, medical, behavioral and psychological
    e) Daytime activities and function: Sleepiness versus fatigue, napping, employment, lifestyle, travel, daytime consequences (e.g., quality of life, mood, cognitive function, effect on comorbidities)
4. Medications and substances: Many can contribute to sleep disorders. Consider stopping or changing medications if possible.
    a) Antidepressants
        (1) Selective serotonin reuptake inhibitors
        (2) Monoamine oxidase inhibitors
    b) Stimulants
        (1) Caffeine
        (2) Methylphenidate
        (3) Amphetamine derivatives
        (4) Cocaine
        (5) Ephedrine and derivatives
    c) Decongestants
        (1) Pseudoephedrine
        (2) Phenylephrine
        (3) Phenylpropanolamine
    d) Analgesics
        (1) Oxycodone
        (2) Codeine
        (3) Propoxyphene
    e) Cardiovascular
        (1) Beta-blockers
        (2) Alfa-receptor agonists and antagonists
        (3) Diuretics
        (4) Lipid-lowering agents
    f) Pulmonary
        (1) Beta-2 agonist
        (2) Anticholinergics
        (3) Steroids
    g) Antiemetic
        (1) Prochlorperazine
        (2) Metoclopramide
        (3) Granisetron
    h) Corticosteroids

    i) Alcohol

  5. Physical and mental status examination (Bloom et al., 2009; Schutte-Rodin et al., 2008)

    a) Insomnia is not associated with any specific physical or mental status findings.

    b) The examination may provide essential information regarding comorbid conditions and differential diagnosis.

    c) The physical must evaluate for risk of sleep apnea, including neck size and obesity. The examination should include the evaluation for comorbid conditions such as cardiac, pulmonary, endocrine, gastrointestinal, rheumatologic, and neurologic disorders.

    d) The mental examination focuses on mood, anxiety, memory, concentration, and alertness.

 V. Diagnostics (Schutte-Rodin et al., 2008)

  A. Polysomnography is indicated when reasonable clinical evidence exists of breathing or movement disorders.

  B. Laboratory testing is not indicated for the routine evaluation of insomnia unless suspicion for comorbid disorders exists.

  C. Sleep scale data

  D. Sleep diary data

 VI. Differential diagnosis

  A. Insomnia associated with sleep disorders

   1. Central sleep apnea

   2. Movement disorders

   3. Circadian rhythm sleep disorder

  B. Insomnia due to medical condition

  C. Insomnia due to psychiatric disorders

  D. Insomnia due to substance abuse

  E. Insomnia due to medication

  F. Primary insomnia

   1. Psychophysiologic

   2. Idiopathic

   3. Paradoxical

 VII. Interventions

  A. A goal of treatment is to improve quality of life by improving sleep quality and quantity, as well as daytime function.

  B. Stop or change any medications that may be causing sleep issues.

  C. Recognize and treat any comorbid condition that may be contributing to sleep issues. Depression, fatigue, and pain are common.

  D. Identify and modify behaviors that inhibit sleep.

  E. Nonpharmacologic interventions

   1. Behavioral and psychological interventions should be employed prior to adding pharmacologic therapies.

   2. It often is necessary to use more than one cognitive behavioral therapy intervention (CBTI).

   3. The most common components of CBTI are sleep restriction, sleep hygiene, stimulus control, and cognitive therapy.

   4. Sleep hygiene: Although sleep hygiene itself is generally inadequate for the treatment of chronic insomnia, this education should be provided for all patients. Combining sleep hygiene and other nonpharmacologic interventions has been

found to be helpful (Induru & Walsh, 2014). Behaviors and habits that can improve sleep include the following:

    a) Avoid daytime napping.

    b) Do not spending too much time in bed. Use the bed only for sleeping.

    c) Have a fixed bedtime and wake time.

    d) Limit caffeine, alcohol, and heavy evening meals.

    e) Do not exercise late in the day.

    f) Avoid clock watching.

    g) Perform simple relaxation techniques such as deep breathing or positive thinking.

    h) Take a warm bath prior to bedtime.

    i) Maintain a comfortable sleep environment. Minimize noise, ensure a comfortable temperature, and minimize the brightness of the room.

F. Sleep restriction
   1. This component of CBTI limits the amount of time spent in bed to consolidate actual sleeping time.
   2. If the patient reports spending 10 hours in bed but only sleeps 6 hours, the patient would be counseled to only spend 6 hours in bed.
   3. This reduction increases the homeostatic sleep drive through mild sleep deprivation, which will result in improved sleep quality and decrease the time it takes to fall asleep.

G. Stimulus control: Many patients who suffer from chronic insomnia have adopted poor coping strategies that have exacerbated the problem. The bedroom should be used only for sleep and sexual activities. Sleep hygiene and stimulus control go hand in hand. Helpful practices for stimulus control include the following:
   1. Develop a sleep ritual. Have a 30-minute relaxation time or take a hot bath prior to bedtime.
   2. Ensure that the bedroom is comfortable.
   3. Go to bed only when feeling sleepy.
   4. Do not watch TV or use computers or other electronics in bed.
   5. If unable to fall asleep in 30 minutes, get up.
   6. Maintain the same sleep and wake schedule.

H. Relaxation therapy
   1. The goal of relaxation therapy is to have the patient reach a relaxed state.
   2. Some patients find guided imagery, progressive muscle relaxation, deep breathing, and meditation helpful.

I. Exercise therapy
   1. Several studies have shown that walking, yoga, and tai chi will improve sleep for some individuals; however, of the studies that showed improvement, not all of the improvements showed a statistical difference (Howell et al., 2013).
   2. Nevertheless, many good reasons support suggesting this to patients to help with relaxation and sleep.

J. Pharmacologic interventions
   1. Pharmacologic therapy should always be used in combination with nonpharmacologic modalities.
   2. The choice of treatment should be driven by symptom pattern, treatment goals, past treatment, patient preference, cost, other concurrent medications, and medical conditions.

3. All patients should be educated on the prescribed medication, including goals, side effects, and safety concerns.

   a) Benzodiazepines: Use with caution in older adults because of side effect profile.

      (1) Alprazolam 0.25–2 mg at bedtime

      (2) Lorazepam 0.5–2 mg at bedtime

      (3) Clonazepam 0.5–4 mg at bedtime

      (4) Temazepam 15–30 mg at bedtime

   b) Nonbenzodiazepines

      (1) Zolpidem 5–10 mg at bedtime

      (2) Zolpidem extended release 6.25–12.5 mg at bedtime

      (3) Eszopiclone 1–2 mg at bedtime

   c) Antihistamines

      (1) Diphenhydramine 25–100 mg at bedtime

      (2) Hydroxyzine 10–100 mg at bedtime

   d) Antidepressants

      (1) Amitriptyline 10–15 mg at bedtime

      (2) Nortriptyline 10–50 mg at bedtime

      (3) Trazodone 25–200 mg at bedtime; shown to be useful for patients suffering from nightmares or terrors (Tanimukai et al., 2013)

      (4) Mirtazapine 7.5–45 mg at bedtime

   e) Antipsychotics

      (1) Quetiapine 25–100 mg at bedtime

      (2) Chlorpromazine 10–50 mg at bedtime

      (3) Olanzapine 5–20 mg at bedtime

   f) Melatonin receptor agonist: Ramelteon 8 mg at bedtime

K. Evaluation and follow-up

   1. Follow-up is recommended to occur at frequent intervals. Initially, weekly follow-up may be needed, moving to monthly until stable. Once stable, the patient should be assessed at least every six months. Patients can be encouraged to continue keeping a sleep diary and bringing it to follow-up appointments.

   2. Repeat assessment surveys may be helpful in assessing treatment and guiding further treatment as needed.

   3. If treatment is ineffective, add other nonpharmacologic options prior to trying other medications. Reassess for other comorbid causes as needed.

L. Referrals

   1. Sleep medicine: If the patient does not respond to medical management, consider referral to rule out sleep apnea or movement disorder.

   2. Dietitian: Consider referral for all patients. Caffeine and other products that can affect sleep often are hidden in foods and drinks. Dietitians also can offer other dietetic options for relaxation.

   3. Mental health: Many sleeping disorders are rooted in psychological issues such as depression, stress, and grief. Social work is a valuable resource as well as a gateway if other psychological interventions are needed. Mental health professionals can provide guidance and education for behavioral and relaxation techniques.

   4. Physical therapy: Exercise can be helpful for some patients. Teaching patients gentle stretching, yoga, and other forms of exercise can assist in providing stress reduction and improving sleep.

Case Study

S.L. is a 62-year-old Caucasian woman with multiple chronic medical conditions including moderate-stage chronic obstructive pulmonary disease (COPD), hypertension, and hypothyroidism. Recently she began using oxygen 2 L continuous to maintain partial pressure of oxygen (PO_2) above 94%. She recently was discharged from the hospital for an exacerbation of COPD and has had a total of eight hospital admissions this year because of dyspnea and exercise intolerance.

The advanced practice registered nurse (APRN) makes a home visit to evaluate S.L. following hospital discharge. During the clinical encounter, S.L. complains of fatigue. She is spending 20 hours a day in bed or her recliner. She complains of not being able to sleep; she has a difficult time falling asleep and awakens frequently. She is anxious about her breathing and unable to lie flat. She is having trouble focusing and informs the APRN that she is unable to do the dishes because she is too tired. She has dyspnea on exertion but not at rest. She admits that she has refused pulmonary rehabilitation many times, as she does not see the point. She denies pain. She has decreased appetite, no nausea, no constipation or diarrhea, and no abdominal pain. She has been drinking 10–12 cups of coffee a day in an attempt to not feel so tired. She admits to feeling sad and depressed because of her failing health. She worries about her husband and the burden she is placing on him for her care. She states that she lies awake worrying about him. She continues to smoke one pack of cigarettes a day and is an 84-pack-year smoker.

On physical examination, the APRN notes S.L. is thin and cachectic, is well hydrated and alert, and appears fatigued. She has O_2 at 2 L per nasal cannula. On oximetry, S.L.'s oxygen saturation is 96% resting and 86% after two-minute walk test. Her heart rate is 80 beats per minute and regular at rest, and 150 beats per minute while walking. Oral mucosa is moist. Nares are dry with dried blood. Lung sounds are coarse with scattered wheezing throughout all lobes. Abdomen is soft and nontender, with normal bowel sounds in all four quadrants. Digital clubbing is noted bilaterally in the hands and feet, and no pedal edema is present. Neurologically, she is alert and oriented. Current medications consist of levothyroxine 75 mcg PO daily, lisinopril 20 mg PO daily, tiotropium dry powder inhalation daily, albuterol inhaler 4 puffs four times a day rescue inhaler, and prednisone 10 mg every morning for four days.

The APRN's assessment findings for S.L. are depression, insomnia, hypothyroidism, hypertension, COPD, oxygen dependence, smoking addiction, and environmental allergies.

The APRN determines the plan for S.L.'s care as the following:

- Hypertension and hypothyroidism: Continue current medications.
- COPD
  - Add inhaled corticosteroids.
  - Encourage pulmonary rehabilitation.
  - Continue other COPD medications.
  - Add moisturizer to oxygen therapy.
- Smoking addiction
  - Strongly encourage patient to stop smoking.
  - Provide educational material.
  - Offer support in the form of both medication and counseling.
- Environmental allergies
  - Change medication to fexofenadine with the pseudoephedrine.
  - Add nasal steroid spray.
- Insomnia

– Ask the patient to complete a sleep diary in the next two weeks.
– Discuss sleep hygiene and stimulus control with the patient and provide educational material.
– Instruct the patient to limit caffeine intake.
• Depression
– Refer the patient to behavioral health.
– Discuss antidepressant therapy. (Patient declined at this time.)

On two-week follow-up, S.L. says the education on sleep hygiene and stimulus control was helpful, but she is still struggling to sleep and is feeling depressed. The social worker has instructed her on relaxation techniques, including pursed-lip breathing and progressive muscle relaxation. The patient's sleep diary is consistent with insomnia. She agrees to try an antidepressant. The APRN confirms the diagnosis of depression and that S.L. would benefit from medication. The APRN selects bupropion sustained release 150 mg PO daily for the indications of depression and smoking cessation.

Another follow-up in two weeks finds improvement in both sleep and depression. S.L. states she is now sleeping seven hours a night without waking frequently. She is able to do more during the day, such as cooking meals and washing the dishes. She can leave her home without worrying about not having enough oxygen. Her dyspnea has improved. At the end of the clinical encounter, she announces that she has not smoked for 10 days. She is motivated to attend eight weeks of pulmonary rehabilitation.

References

American Psychiatric Association. (2013). *Diagnostic and statistical manual of mental disorders* (5th ed.). Washington, DC: Author.

Bloom, H.G., Ahmed, I., Alessi, C.A., Ancoli-Israel, S., Buysse, D.J., Kryger, M.H., … Zee, P.C. (2009). Evidence-based recommendations for the assessment and management of sleep disorders in older persons. *Journal of the American Geriatrics Society, 57,* 761–789. doi:10.1111/j.1532-5415.2009.02220.x

Davis, M.P., Khoshknabi, D., Walsh, D., Lagman, R., & Platt, A. (2014). Insomnia in patients with advanced cancer. *American Journal of Hospice and Palliative Care, 31,* 365–373. doi:10.1177/1049909113485804

Delgado-Guay, M., Yennurajalingam, S., Parsons, H., Palmer, J.L., & Bruera, E. (2011). Association between self-reported sleep disturbance and other symptoms in patients with advanced cancer. *Journal of Pain and Symptom Management, 41,* 819–827. doi:10.1016/j.jpainsymman.2010.07.015

Howell, D., Oliver, T.K., Keller-Olaman, S., Davidson, J., Garland, S., Samuels, C., … Taylor, C. (2013). A Pan-Canadian practice guideline: Prevention, screening, assessment, and treatment of sleep disturbances in adults with cancer. *Supportive Care in Cancer, 21,* 2695–2706. doi:10.1007/s00520-013-1823-6

Induru, R.R., & Walsh, D. (2014). Cancer-related insomnia. *American Journal of Hospice and Palliative Medicine, 31,* 777–785. doi:10.1177/1049909113508302

Schutte-Rodin, S., Broch, L., Buysse, D., Dorsey, C., & Sateia, M. (2008). Clinical guideline for the evaluation and management of chronic insomnia in adults. *Journal of Clinical Sleep Medicine, 4,* 487–504. Retrieved from http://www.ncbi.nlm.nih.gov/pmc/articles/PMC2576317/pdf/jcsm.4.5.487.pdf

Tanimukai, H., Murai, T., Okazaki, N., Matsuda, Y., Okamoto, Y., Kabeshita, Y., … Tsuneto, S. (2013). An observational study of insomnia and nightmare treated with trazodone in patients with advanced cancer. *American Journal of Hospice and Palliative Medicine, 30,* 359–362. doi:10.1177/1049909112452334

World Health Organization. (2016). *International statistical classification of diseases and related health problems, 10th revision* (ICD-10). Geneva, Switzerland: Author.

CHAPTER 28

Pruritus

Mary E. Murphy, MS, AOCN®, ACHPN, CNS,
and Jackie Matthews, RN, MS, AOCN®, ACHPN, CNS

I. Definition
   A. A cutaneous sensation or itch that provokes scratching, itching, or rubbing of an affected part or complete systemic area caused by a variety of metabolic, pathologic, or psychiatric disorders
   B. The most common symptom in dermatology
   C. Symptoms may be both acute and chronic (defined as lasting over six weeks in duration) (Grundmann & Ständer, 2011).
II. Pathophysiology
   A. Transmission of signals along unelated, histamine-sensitive C-fibers that is produced by a variety of neural mediators of the epidermis
   B. Pathophysiology: Dermal–epidermal junction
      1. Mediators and major contributors include histamine, cathepsins, gastrin-releasing peptides, opioids, substance P nerve growth factor, interleukins, and prostaglandins.
      2. Itch results from transmission of affecting C neurons that cross the contralateral spinothalamic tract, ascending to the thalamus. Sensation is from the cerebral cortex and activation of multiple sites including sensory function, motor function, and emotion.
      3. No single area is primarily responsible for the itch stimulus, which contributes to the multifaceted aspects of the symptom (Grundmann & Ständer, 2011; McNeil & Dong, 2012; Reamy, Bunt, & Fletcher, 2011).
III. Presenting symptoms (Grundmann & Ständer, 2011; McNeil & Dong, 2012; Reamy et al., 2011)
   A. Localized
      1. Scaling, cracking, red patches on skin
      2. Rash—location, features, and findings
      3. Pustules with or without exudate
      4. Macules
      5. Hives, welts
      6. Dryness
      7. Itching (local)
      8. Excoriation
      9. Scratch marks
      10. Pain (local)
   B. Systemic

       1. Erythema
       2. Pain (systemic)
       3. Itching (systemic)
       4. Jaundice
       5. Anxiety

IV. Physical examination
  A. Physical—complete skin inspection including skin folds
       1. Distribution (local or generalized)
       2. Type of skin concern
       3. Onset
       4. Longevity
       5. Precipitating factors
       6. Relieving factors
       7. Effect on sleep patterns and activities of daily living
       8. Grading
  B. Systemic—medical history specific for pruritus
       1. Hepatomegaly
       2. Splenomegaly
       3. Scleral icterus
       4. Lymphadenopathy
       5. Infections (recent)
       6. Hypothyroidism and hyperthyroidism
       7. Shingles
       8. Exposure to infestation and travel history (lice, scabies, bed bugs, rodents)
       9. Weight loss (constitutional symptoms: fever, weight loss, night sweats)
      10. Psychiatric history
      11. Medication history (prescribed and over the counter)
      12. Exposure history (chemicals, animals, plants)
      13. Contact with people with fever or rash
  C. Assessment: Currently, no reliable tool exists to assess pruritus.
       1. Determination of the location, character, and timing of symptoms assists with the diagnosis and management.
       2. The pruritus grading system (PGS) can be used to determine pruritus grade based on distribution, frequency, and severity of itching and sleep-cycle disturbance (Al-Qarqaz, Al Aboosi, Al-Shiyab, & Bataineh, 2012).
         a) Mild grade: Total score of 0–5
         b) Moderate grade: Total score of 6–11
         c) Severe grade: Total score of 12–19
       3. Despite a lack of a designated gold standard, the PGS offers an opportunity to assist with evaluation of symptoms and its severity (Al-Qarqaz et al., 2012).

V. Diagnostics
  A. Laboratory testing is based on history, intensity of symptoms, and suspected pathophysiology.
       1. Complete blood count and differential (for malignancies, myeloproliferative disease, anemia, polycythemia vera)
       2. Serum bilirubin, transaminases, and alkaline phosphatase (liver disease)
       3. Thyroid-stimulating hormone (thyroid disorders)
       4. Blood urea nitrogen (BUN) and creatinine (renal disease)

      5. Serum protein electrophoresis (gammopathies or malignancies)
      6. Erythrocyte sedimentation rate (inflammation and infection)
      7. Chemical profile (renal, hepatic, or pancreatic disorders, cholestasis, dietary deficiencies)
      8. Fasting blood sugar (hypoglycemia and hyperglycemia)
      9. HIV antibody test (HIV infection)
     10. Antinuclear antibody (rheumatoid arthritis factors)
  B. Radiology: Chest x-ray (adenopathy, malignancies, infection, inflammation)
  C. Other
      1. Skin biopsy
      2. Skin scrapings (malignancies or scabies)
      3. Cultures (bacterial, viral, or fungal)
  D. Consider psychogenic evaluation if all tests are negative and symptoms and patient history indicate a concern (Fazio & Yosipovitch, 2015).

VI. Differential diagnosis
  A. Gathering a detailed medical history and performing a physical examination will assist clinicians with identification of the underlying cause and determination of a focused treatment plan (Patel & Yosipovitch, 2010).
  B. Evaluation should determine the presence or absence of a primary skin lesion, the presence of which suggests a dermatologic condition.
  C. Pruritus can be attributed to a primary dermatologic condition or to any number of underlying disease processes, with or without a primary skin eruption into these major categories (Fazio & Yosipovitch, 2015):
      1. Dermatologic: Xerostomia, atopic dermatitis (eczema), contact dermatitis, urticaria, psoriasis, infestation (lice, scabies), lichen simplex chronicus
      2. Systemic: Infection, renal, cholestatic, hematologic, endocrine (thyroid), malignancy, paraneoplastic syndromes, autoimmune, HIV
      3. Neurologic: Postherpetic neuralgia, multiple sclerosis, neuropathy and nerve compression
      4. Psychogenic: Stress induced, delusional parasitosis, mood or anxiety disorders
      5. Mixed: One or more of these conditions
      6. Other: Medication induced, such as opioids; keloids; burns; advanced age; idiopathic

VII. Interventions
  A. Treatment is dependent on the differential and treatment of the underlying cause, as well as symptomatic relief.
  B. Despite the various available therapeutic options, evidence is limited as to the efficacy of many interventions.
  C. A combination approach using pharmacologic and nonpharmacologic therapy should be considered.
      1. Nonpharmacologic interventions for generalized care
         a) Prevent dry skin. Moisturize daily and after bathing; use gentle cleansers with soaps and moisturizers with a mild or low pH.
         b) Apply cool, moist compresses.
         c) Wear loose, cotton clothing; avoid wool.
         d) Trim fingernails.
         e) Wear gloves or mitts.
         f) Avoid perfumes, lotions, and alcohol-based products.
         g) An air-conditioned environment may reduce the sensation of itching.

　　　h) Bathe or shower in cool or tepid water; avoid using hot water.
　　　i) Reduce stress.
　2. Pharmacologic interventions
　　　a) Local therapy: Topical agents are the mainstay of therapy for mild or localized itch, whereas systemic therapy should be considered for severe or generalized itch (Patel & Yosipovitch, 2010).
　　　　(1) Recommendations for the use of topical corticosteroids are for use with an inflammatory skin component and are not indicated without skin inflammation, for generalized chronic itch, or for a prolonged period because of side effects (Patel & Yosipovitch, 2010).
　　　　(2) Topical moisturizers and emollients: Sarna®, Aveeno®, Bag Balm®, Eucerin®, Cetaphil®
　　　　(3) Topical anesthetics: Pramoxine 1% cream, lidocaine 2.5%, prilocaine 2.5%, menthol 1%–3%
　　　　(4) Topical antihistamines: Doxepin, diphenhydramine
　　　　(5) Topical corticosteroids: Hydrocortisone 2.5%, dexamethasone, prednisone
　　　　(6) Topical calcineurin inhibitors: Pimecrolimus 1% cream, tacrolimus 0.03%/0.1% ointment
　　　　(7) Topical capsaicin: 0.025%–0.1% Cream may be useful in pruritus with neuropathic component
　　　b) Systemic therapy: Although commonly used as first-line systemic therapy for pruritus, systemic antihistamines have limited data supporting their use (Fazio & Yosipovitch, 2016).
　　　　(1) The exception is with use in urticaria or other disorders in which histamine is known to play an important role (Fazio & Yosipovitch, 2016).
　　　　(2) Consider sedating antihistamines for use at night; use cautiously during hours of activity and with older patients (Fazio & Yosipovitch, 2016).
　　　　(3) Generalized
　　　　　(a) Antihistamines
　　　　　　i. H_1: Diphenhydramine, hydroxyzine, loratadine, cetirizine
　　　　　　ii. H_2: Cimetidine
　　　　　(b) Corticosteroids: Dexamethasone, prednisone
　　　　　(c) Opioid receptor antagonists: Naltrexone, naloxone
　　　　　(d) Opioid receptor agonists: Butorphanol
　　　　　(e) Antidepressants: Sertraline (selective serotonin reuptake inhibitor), mirtazapine (serotonin–norepinephrine reuptake inhibitor), doxepin (tricyclic with antihistamine properties)
　　　　　(f) Anticonvulsants: Gabapentin, pregabalin
　　　　(4) Opioid induced
　　　　　(a) Diphenhydramine and hydroxyzine (rotate opioid, yet may decrease in few days because of tolerance)
　　　　　(b) Cholestatic: Cholestyramine, ursodiol acid
　　　　(5) Uremic
　　　　　(a) Dialysis modification and optimization
　　　　　(b) Oral antihistamine

         (c) Topical emollients

         (d) Topical anesthetics

         (e) Gabapentin in refractory pruritus after each dialysis session

      (6) Tumor-related: corticosteroids, treatment directed to underlying pathology

  3. Other

    a) If symptom is thought to be medication induced, stop the medication.

    b) Paroxetine, ondansetron, or naloxone also may be effective in select patients (von Gunten & Ferris, 2015).

    c) Phototherapy may be considered in patients with psoriasis, eczema, vitiligo, and diffuse T-cell cutaneous lymphoma.

D. Referrals

  1. Dermatology consult for chronic, progressive symptoms or primary lesion

  2. Specialty referral for patients with primary dermatologic condition, systemic etiology, or psychogenic causes that require evaluation and treatment

  3. Enterostomal therapy

Case Study

J.T. is a 65-year-old Caucasian man with a past history of hypertension. He presents to his primary care provider with insomnia, early fatigue, and generalized pruritus ongoing for three months. He did not report any fever, night sweats, or weight loss.

Physical examination demonstrates no primary cutaneous lesions, yet the patient does have secondary skin excoriation and inflammation on his bilateral lower extremities from scratching. The itch–scratch pattern is frequent and occurs at night. Based on generalized distribution pattern of itch (score 3), frequency (score 3), severity (score 1 and 3), and sleep disturbance (score 4), symptom grading was severe with a score of 14.

No presence of rash, lymphadenopathy, or hepatosplenomegaly is found on examination. Complete blood count with differential shows mild anemia, and a comprehensive metabolic panel shows some elevation of BUN and creatinine consistent with dehydration. A combination trial of topical steroids and oral antihistamines scheduled at bedtime with every-six-hours PRN daily dosing provided initial relief for approximately 10–14 days. However, one month from his initial office contact, J.T.'s clinical condition worsens. The patient returns to the office presenting with significant low back pain; bilateral, radiating hip pain of 8/10; progressive early fatigue; generalized weakness; fever; and continued generalized pruritus. Laboratory evaluation reveals hypercalcemia with an elevated calcium of 13 mg/dl, as well as renal failure with a BUN of 100 mg/dl and creatinine of 4 mg/dl. He is admitted with referral to oncology for a more extensive evaluation to look for systemic illness, including underlying malignancies. The results are consistent with a diagnosis of multiple myeloma.

With rehydration and initiation of cancer treatments, the patient's laboratory values normalize and he improves clinically. Symptom-directed therapies for pruritus and pain optimize the plan of care. Although opioid antagonists have been found to be effective in pruritus, management of intractable pain for this patient is a priority; therefore, other agents are considered. Gabapentin is used as an adjuvant to opioid therapy and for the management of pruritus. Antihistamines continue to provide some nocturnal relief. After two months of combined cancer- and symptom-directed therapies, the patient continues to respond and is doing well.

References

Al-Qarqaz, F., Al Aboosi, M., Al-Shiyab, D., & Bataineh, A. (2012). Using pruritus grading system for measurement of pruritus in patients with diseases associated with itch. *Jordan Medical Journal, 46,* 39–44. Retrieved from http://journals.ju.edu.jo/JMJ/article/view/3023/2655

Fazio, S.B., & Yosipovitch, G. (2015, January 21). Pruritus: Etiology and patient evaluation [Literature review current through April 2016]. Retrieved from http://www.uptodate.com/contents/pruritus-etiology-and-patient-evaluation

Fazio, S.B., & Yosipovitch, G. (2016, January 13). Pruritus: Overview of management [Literature review current through April 2016]. Retrieved from http://www.uptodate.com/contents/pruritus-overview-of-management

Grundmann, S., & Ständer, S. (2011). Chronic pruritus: Clinics and treatment. *Annals of Dermatology, 23,* 1–11. doi: 10.5021/ad.2011.23.1.1

McNeil, B., & Dong, X. (2012). Peripheral mechanisms of itch. *Neuroscience Bulletin, 28,* 100–110. doi:10.1007/s12264-012-1202-1

Patel, T., & Yosipovitch, G. (2010). Therapy of pruritus. *Expert Opinion on Pharmacotherapy, 11,* 1673–1682. doi:10.1517/14656566.2010.484420

Reamy, B.V., Bunt, C.W., & Fletcher, S. (2011). A diagnostic approach to pruritus. *American Family Physician, 84,* 195–202. Retrieved from http://www.aafp.org/afp/2011/0715/p195.html

von Gunten, C., & Ferris, F. (2015). Fast Facts and Concepts #37: Pruritus. Retrieved from http://www.mypcnow.org/#!blank/sk9ni

Section V.

Oncologic Emergencies

CHAPTER 29

Hypercalcemia of Malignancy

Marcelle Kaplan, MS, RN, CBCN®, CNS

I. Definition
   A. Hypercalcemia of malignancy (HCM) is a metabolic complication that occurs in up to 30% of patients with cancer (Fallah-Rad & Morton, 2013).
   B. Patients at highest risk for HCM are those with squamous cell lung cancer, breast cancer with bone metastases, or multiple myeloma (Fallah-Rad & Morton, 2013; Morton & Lipton, 2014). Figure 29-1 lists malignancies associated with increased risk of HCM.
   C. Hypercalcemia is considered to exist when serum calcium levels become elevated above the upper laboratory reference range of normal (generally 10.5 mg/dl) (Agraharkar, Dellinger, & Gangakhedkar, 2015).
   D. The appearance of HCM typically indicates cancer recurrence or disease progression and portends a poor prognosis for survival, often measured in weeks (Siddiqui & Weissman, 2010).
   E. HCM may go unrecognized because the symptoms are nonspecific and may be attributed to effects of disease or treatment (Fallah-Rad & Morton, 2013; Morton & Lipton, 2014).
   F. Nurses caring for patients with cancer should have an understanding of which patients are at risk for HCM and be alert to the early manifestations.
   G. Prompt recognition and treatment initiation can help prevent HCM from becoming a life-threatening emergency and improve the patient's quality of life and length of survival.

Figure 29-1. Malignancies Associated With Increased Risk of Hypercalcemia

- Breast cancer with bone metastases
- Lung cancer, especially squamous cell type
- Multiple myeloma
- Renal cell cancer
- Squamous cell cancers of the head and neck, esophagus, cervix
- Cancers of the ovary, vulva, endometrium, liver, pancreas
- Lymphomas: non-Hodgkin, Hodgkin, adult T-cell

Note. Based on information from Fallah-Rad & Morton, 2013; Kaplan, 2013; Santarpia et al., 2010.

II. Pathophysiology
   A. HCM most frequently results from cancer-induced disruption of the normal balance between bone breakdown (resorption) and bone formation in concert with impaired renal excretion of calcium (Coleman & Holen, 2014; Kaplan, 2013).
      1. Pathologic destruction of bone (Fojo, 2015; Reagan, Pani, & Rosner, 2014; Wright & Guise, 2014)
         a) Tumor cells from certain cancers are able to secrete a humoral substance that inappropriately acts on tissue receptors for parathyroid hormone and thus is called parathyroid hormone–related protein (PTHrP).
         b) The abnormal systemic and local actions of PTHrP on the bone microenvironment disrupt normal bone metabolism and cause destruction of bone.
         c) Increased bone destruction coupled with decreased bone formation leads to increased serum calcium.
      2. Renal contributions to the development of hypercalcemia
         a) The kidneys can excrete excess calcium until compensatory mechanisms become overwhelmed and renal failure develops (Morton & Lipton, 2014; Rosner & Dalkin, 2012).
         b) Renal failure potentiates or exacerbates hypercalcemia in a vicious circle.
            (1) Fluid volume depletion and dehydration develop because of a combination of factors: the adverse effects of disease, treatment, or existing hypercalcemia (e.g., anorexia, vomiting, dysphagia, mucositis, fever, confusion) (Kaplan, 2013).
            (2) Acute renal failure occurs as renal perfusion decreases; renal calcium excretion decreases and calcium reabsorption increases.
            (3) The kidneys also become resistant to the action of antidiuretic hormone and lose the ability to concentrate urine. Excretion of large volumes of dilute urine occurs and is a hallmark sign of HCM (Fojo, 2015).
   B. Vitamin D activation
      1. A less common initiator of HCM that develops in the absence of bone destruction
      2. Tumor cells of certain lymphomas, notably lymphoma disease and non-Hodgkin lymphoma, can inappropriately stimulate the metabolism of vitamin D to its active form (1,25-dihydroxyvitamin D_3, called calcitriol) (Reagan et al., 2014).
      3. Increased calcitriol stimulates increased calcium absorption from the gut, resulting in HCM (Hariri, Mount, & Rastegar, 2013).
III. Presenting symptoms
   A. Presenting symptoms of HCM often are vague and nonspecific (e.g., nausea, anorexia, fatigue, lethargy) and are frequently unrecognized (Agraharkar et al., 2015; Kaplan, 2013)
   B. Signs and symptoms of HCM reflect the depressant effects of elevated calcium levels on nerve conduction and contractility of all types of muscles (Kaplan, 2013).
   C. Clinical manifestations vary among patients regardless of measured serum calcium levels (Kaplan, 2013; Santarpia, Koch, & Sarlis, 2010).
   D. Multiple organ systems are affected (Agraharkar et al., 2015; Fojo, 2015; Khosla, 2015; LeGrand, 2011; Maier & Levine, 2015; Morton & Lipton, 2014; Reagan et al., 2014).

1. Renal: Hallmark signs of HCM—polyuria (large volumes of dilute urine), polydipsia (thirst), and nocturia
2. Central nervous system: Altered mental status—lethargy, depression, cognitive changes, confusion; hyporeflexia
3. Gastrointestinal: Anorexia, nausea, vomiting, constipation
4. Cardiac: Bradycardia, hypertension
5. Musculoskeletal: Muscle weakness, fatigue, hypotonia

E. Rapidly increasing serum calcium levels produce more severe symptoms than measured calcium concentrations may indicate (Agraharkar et al., 2015; Rosner & Dalkin, 2012). Table 29-1 presents grade classifications for hypercalcemia often used in the clinical setting and based on serum calcium levels.

F. Patients who display symptoms are considered to have severe hypercalcemia regardless of measured serum calcium and need emergency treatment (Morton & Lipton, 2014; Santarpia et al., 2010).

IV. Physical examination
   A. Patient history (Agraharkar et al., 2015; Kaplan, 2013; Morton & Lipton, 2014; Rosner & Dalkin, 2012)
      1. Known history of cancer, tumor type (see Figure 29-1), treatments
      2. Medications: Prescribed and over the counter
      3. Presenting symptoms: Rapidity of onset, duration, severity
      4. Changes in activities of daily living, mental status, renal function
      5. Preexisting conditions: Granulomatous conditions (e.g., sarcoidosis), endocrine disorders (e.g., hyperthyroidism), renal failure
      6. Concurrent conditions: Anorexia, vomiting, diarrhea, fever, confusion that can lead to dehydration, prolonged immobility
      7. Dietary review: Deficient intake of phosphorus-containing foods that can lead to increased serum calcium
      8. Risk factors for undiagnosed cancer: Family history (e.g., premenopausal breast cancer), lifestyle behaviors (e.g., smoking, excessive alcohol consumption), environmental exposure (e.g., radon gas), occupational exposure (e.g., asbestos, benzene products)
      9. Cancer screening tests: Dates and results
   B. Physical assessment
      1. Renal findings: Signs of dehydration (e.g., orthostatic hypotension, poor skin turgor), renal insufficiency or failure (Fojo, 2015; Rosner & Dalkin, 2012)

Table 29-1. Grade Classifications for Hypercalcemia		
Grade	**Corrected Calcium Level (mg/dl)**	**Comments**
Mild	10.5–11.9	Patient is generally asymptomatic. Routine laboratory testing may reveal mild calcium elevation.
Moderate	12–14	Patient may be asymptomatic. Calcium can increase rapidly and symptoms appear.
Severe	> 14	This is an oncologic emergency. Patient is invariably symptomatic. Immediate intervention is required.

Note. Based on information from Agraharkar et al., 2015; Maier & Levine, 2015; Morton & Lipton, 2014.

2. Neurologic findings: Changes in mental status (e.g., lethargy, confusion, coma), diminished deep tendon reflexes, and decreased muscle strength and tone (Agraharkar et al., 2015; Fallah-Rad & Morton, 2013; LeGrand, 2011; Maier & Levine, 2015)

3. Gastrointestinal findings: Constipation and signs of malignancy (e.g., enlarged liver or abdominal masses) (Agraharkar et al., 2015; Morton & Lipton, 2014)

4. Cardiac findings: Hypertension, bradycardia, or arrhythmias causing feelings of light-headedness or fainting (Agraharkar et al., 2015; Fallah-Rad & Morton, 2013; Green, 2014)

V. Diagnostics
   A. Laboratory tests
      1. Serum calcium is the most important test (Agraharkar et al., 2015; Hariri et al., 2013; Khosla, 2015).
      2. Serum albumin should be measured concurrently with calcium (Kaplan, 2013; Khosla, 2015; Santarpia et al., 2010). Figure 29-2 presents an algorithm used when serum albumin is low to estimate corrected serum calcium concentration.
      3. Serum electrolytes: Phosphorus, potassium, magnesium, chloride (Green, 2014; Khosla, 2015; Morton & Lipton, 2014)
      4. Blood urea nitrogen and creatinine (Khosla, 2015; Morton & Lipton, 2014)
      5. Intact parathyroid hormone and PTHrP levels (Maier & Levine, 2015; Rosner & Dalkin, 2012)
      6. Thyroid-stimulating hormone (Green, 2014; Soyfoo, Brenner, Paesmans, & Body, 2013)
      7. Serum and urine protein electrophoresis and serum free light chains to assess for multiple myeloma (Maier & Levine, 2015; Rosner & Dalkin, 2012)
      8. Vitamin D (calcitriol) (Maier & Levine, 2015; Santarpia et al., 2010)

Figure 29-2. Formula for Estimating Corrected Ionized Serum Calcium Adjusted for Decreases in Serum Albumin

Patients with cancer often have low serum albumin levels. Calcium ions circulate in the serum in two forms: bound to albumin (biologically inactive) or unbound and free (biologically active). When serum albumin is below normal, more free calcium circulates. When hypoalbuminemia is present, laboratory reports generally underreport serum calcium by 0.8 mg/dl for every 1 g/dl decrease in normal serum albumin. A calcium correction formula is used to arrive at an estimation of the actual serum calcium concentration.

Calcium correction formula: Corrected serum calcium (mg/dl) = measured serum calcium (mg/dl) + [(normal albumin (4.0 g/dl) – patient's measured albumin in g/dl)] × 0.8

Example
Laboratory results: Calcium = 10.0 mg/dl; albumin = 1.8 g/dl
Step 1: Determine decrease in albumin from normal: 4.0 g/dl – 1.8 g/dl = 2.2 g/dl.
Step 2: Estimate underreported serum calcium: 2.2 g/dl × 0.8 mg/dl = 1.76 mg/dl.
Step 3: Correct measured serum calcium: 10.0 mg/dl + 1.76 mg/dl = 11.76 mg/dl.
Step 4: Corrected serum calcium = 11.76 mg/dl (ULN = 10.5 mg/dl)
Conclusion: Hypercalcemia is present.

ULN—upper level of normal

Note. Based on information from Agraharkar et al., 2015; Kaplan, 2013.

    B. An electrocardiogram to assess for slowed conduction through the heart, bradycardia, and arrhythmias (Green, 2014; Khosla, 2015; Morton & Lipton, 2014)

    C. Imaging studies such as x-ray, computed tomography, magnetic resonance imaging, ultrasound; mammography; and skeletal survey to assess for presence of undiagnosed or recurrent malignancy (e.g., cancers of lung, breast, or kidney; bone metastases; multiple myeloma) (Agraharkar et al., 2015; Santarpia et al., 2010)

VI. Differential diagnosis

    A. It is important to differentiate between benign and tumor-induced etiologies for HCM in a patient with cancer.

    B. Nonmalignant causes that can coexist with malignancy

        1. Primary hyperparathyroidism: Most common cause of hypercalcemia in the general population; usually found incidentally (Agraharkar et al., 2015; Pallan, Rahman, & Khan, 2012; Soyfoo et al., 2013)

        2. Granulomatous conditions: Sarcoidosis, tuberculosis, histoplasmosis, coccidiomycosis (Green, 2014; Soyfoo et al., 2013)

        3. Endocrine disorders: Hyperthyroidism, adrenal insufficiency, pheochromocytoma, acromegaly (Soyfoo et al., 2013)

        4. Drug-induced etiologies: Excessive ingestion of vitamin D or vitamin A supplements or antacids containing calcium, use of thiazide diuretics, lithium, thyroid hormone replacement (Agraharkar et al., 2015; Green, 2014; Soyfoo et al., 2013)

        5. Tamoxifen therapy (Green, 2014; Kaplan, 2013)

        6. Renal disease (Kaplan, 2013)

        7. Genetic disorders: Multiple endocrine neoplasia type 1 or type 2 (Agraharkar et al., 2015; Green, 2014)

        8. Prolonged immobilization and lack of weight-bearing activity (Green, 2014; Kaplan, 2013)

        9. Dietary phosphate deficiency (Kaplan, 2013; Morton & Lipton, 2014)

VII. Interventions

    A. Initial considerations

        1. Treatment depends on the severity of symptoms and the patient's survival prognosis and quality of life.

        2. When HCM presents in patients with recurrent or advanced cancer, difficult decisions may need to be made about whether to initiate aggressive antihypercalcemic therapies or instead provide palliative measures (Fallah-Rad & Morton, 2013).

           a) End-of-life discussions with the patient and caregivers regarding the risks and benefits of treatment and prognosis for survival may help them arrive at care goals appropriate to the patient's stage of disease.

           b) The decision to institute palliative care aimed at relieving the distressing symptoms of severe hypercalcemia and to allow the patient to succumb without discomfort to the central nervous system effects of HCM (i.e., central nervous system depression or coma) may be deemed most appropriate.

        3. Patients for whom HCM is the first sign of malignancy and those with a history of a cancer that is likely to respond to antineoplastic treatments should receive immediate antihypercalcemic therapy (LeGrand, 2011; Potts & Jüppner, 2015).

           a) Patients with mild hypercalcemia often can be treated at home.

    b) Patients with moderate and severe hypercalcemia are hospitalized to receive aggressive treatment.

B. Interventions

  1. Preventive measures for patients with malignancies associated with increased risk for HCM include the following (see Figure 29-1) (Fallah-Rad & Morton, 2013; Kaplan, 2013; Maier & Levine, 2015; Santarpia et al., 2010):

    a) Maintain oral fluid intake at 3 L/day.

    b) Avoid drugs and supplements that increase serum calcium levels.

    c) Identify and report conditions that can contribute to dehydration.

    d) Minimize sedating medications.

    e) Maintain weight-bearing activities.

    f) Calcium-containing foods are not restricted unless HCM is caused by cancers associated with increased synthesis of vitamin D.

    g) Encourage adequate salt intake to help expand fluid volume.

    h) Monitor for appearance of signs or symptoms that indicate increasing calcium levels.

  2. Initial therapies

    a) Vigorous rehydration to rapidly expand depleted fluid volume and increase renal excretion of calcium

      (1) IV normal saline

        (a) Initial doses of 200–500 ml/hr depending on cardiovascular and renal status and individual patient factors until patient is rehydrated (Fojo, 2015; LeGrand, 2011; Morton & Lipton, 2014; Potts & Jüppner, 2015; Rosner & Dalkin, 2012; Santarpia et al., 2010)

        (b) Daily maintenance infusion of 3 L of normal saline following restoration of normal fluid volume (Morton & Lipton, 2014)

        (c) Close monitoring of fluid and electrolyte status throughout treatment (LeGrand, 2011; Maier & Levine, 2015; Morton & Lipton, 2014)

      (2) Forced diuresis with a loop diuretic (e.g., furosemide) following rehydration

        (a) Only used after the patient has been adequately rehydrated to promote further renal excretion of calcium (Fojo, 2015; Khosla, 2015; Santarpia et al., 2010)

        (b) Current recommendations are to reserve use of loop diuretics for patients who develop fluid overload due to aggressive rehydration (LeGrand, 2011; Morton & Lipton, 2014; Potts & Jüppner, 2015).

        (c) Furosemide dose is 20–40 mg IV every 12 hours (Fojo, 2015).

        (d) Electrolytes are monitored and replaced as needed, especially potassium, phosphorus, and magnesium, which are excreted along with calcium; their losses can be life threatening (Maier & Levine, 2015; Potts & Jüppner, 2015).

        (e) Thiazide diuretics are avoided because they promote calcium absorption (Green, 2014).

    b) Calcitonin, a hormone produced by cells in the thyroid gland that inhibits renal reabsorption of calcium

(1) May be used in combination with hydration in patients with severe symptoms as a rapid-acting temporary therapy (LeGrand, 2011)

(2) Dose is 4–8 IU/kg body weight administered every 12 hours either subcutaneously or intramuscularly (LeGrand, 2011; Rosner & Dalkin, 2012; Santarpia et al., 2010).

(3) Side effects include facial flushing, nausea, and vomiting (Potts & Jüppner, 2015; Rosner & Dalkin, 2012).

(4) Resistance to calcitonin (tachyphylaxis) develops within 48 hours (Potts & Jüppner, 2015; Rosner & Dalkin, 2012).

c) Drugs inhibiting bone resorption

(1) IV bisphosphonates (Novartis Pharmaceuticals Corp., 2016a, 2016b)

(a) Used after initial hydration. Action is delayed but the drugs produce long-lasting effects.

(b) All drugs in this class have potential for renal toxicity; thus, measurement of creatinine levels is mandatory before treatment initiation and each dose.

(c) Hydration is maintained at 2 L/day throughout bisphosphonate therapy.

(d) Adverse side effects typically are transient and may include flu-like syndrome (i.e., aches, chills, fever), bone pain, and infusion-site reaction.

(e) Uncommon but severe side effects that may occur with prolonged bisphosphonate use

　i. Osteonecrosis of the jaw (ONJ), which is persistent non-healing exposed necrotic bone in the jaw

　ii. Atypical fracture of the femur (AF), occurring with little or no trauma

(2) IV bisphosphonates approved in the United States to treat HCM

(a) Zoledronic acid: Single IV dose of 4 mg infused over no less than 15 minutes (Novartis Pharmaceuticals Corp., 2016b)

(b) Pamidronate: Single IV dose of 60–90 mg infused over 2–24 hours (Novartis Pharmaceuticals Corp., 2016a)

(3) IV bisphosphonates licensed outside the United States to treat HCM

(a) Ibandronate (Genentech, Inc., 2015; von Moos et al., 2008)

　i. 6 mg infusion over one to two hours every three to four weeks

　ii. Drug does not affect renal function; therefore, mandatory creatinine monitoring prior to each infusion is not required.

　iii. Side effects seen with use for osteoporosis include hypocalcemia; anaphylaxis; severe bone, joint, or muscle pain; ONJ; and AF.

(b) Clodronate (Cancer Care Ontario, 2013)

　i. Initially: IV infusion of 300 mg over at least two to six hours, repeated on days 2–5 if necessary

　ii. Maintenance: Oral doses of 1,600–2,400 mg taken on an empty stomach daily, not to exceed 3,200 mg/day

　iii. Side effects include mild local reaction with the IV route. ONJ and AF are rare.

    (4) Denosumab (Amgen Inc., 2016)

        (a) Monoclonal antibody approved in the United States for treatment of HCM refractory to bisphosphonate therapy

        (b) Administered as a subcutaneous injection of 120 mg every four weeks; additional doses of 120 mg on days 8 and 15 of the first month of therapy

        (c) Adverse side effects are similar to the bisphosphonates; risk for severe symptomatic hypocalcemia, hypersensitivity, ONF, and AF.

C. Antineoplastic treatments (Kaplan, 2013; Morton & Lipton, 2014)

  1. Most effective therapy for providing long-term suppression of HCM

  2. Initiated in appropriate patients to control the underlying malignancy precipitating HCM

  3. Therapy is selected based on individual patient factors and may include chemotherapy, targeted biologic agents, radiation therapy, or surgery.

D. Other interventions

  1. Corticosteroids (Agraharkar et al., 2015; Morton & Lipton, 2014; Rosner & Dalkin, 2012)

    a) Therapy of choice for HCM caused by cancers that activate vitamin D (lymphomas) and for treating multiple myeloma. Not used for HCM caused by solid tumors.

    b) Dosage: IV hydrocortisone 200–300 mg/day for three to five days. Maintenance therapy: Oral prednisone 10–30 mg/day if needed.

    c) Adverse effects seen with prolonged steroid use include hyperglycemia, immunosuppression, cushingoid symptoms, gastritis, osteoporosis, and muscle wasting.

  2. Dialysis (Fallah-Rad & Morton, 2013; Potts & Jüppner, 2015)

    a) Especially safe for patients with renal failure or congestive heart failure who cannot tolerate saline rehydration with large volumes of fluid

    b) Occasionally used emergently in patients with severe symptomatic hypercalcemia to rapidly reduce serum calcium

    c) Phosphate levels are measured along with calcium after each dialysis session because large quantities of phosphate are lost during treatment and require replacement.

  3. Phosphate replacement (Kaplan, 2013; Potts & Jüppner, 2015; Santarpia et al., 2010)

    a) Phosphate loss is common in patients with HCM. Calcium and phosphorus are regulated in inverse proportion to one another; increases in calcium concentration lead to decreases in phosphorus.

    b) Thus, hypophosphatemia needs to be corrected so that it does not contribute to increased calcium levels.

        (1) Patients with adequate renal function are given phosphate orally or through a nasogastric tube as neutral phosphate until serum phosphorus reaches low normal range (2.5–3 mg/dl).

        (2) Most common adverse effect is diarrhea.

        (3) IV administration of phosphate is considered only for patients with severe, life-threatening HCM. It is very dangerous and can lead to sudden death.

4. Dietary calcium restriction (Kaplan, 2013): Only necessary for patients with HCM due to increased intestinal absorption of calcium associated with malignancies that stimulate increased synthesis of vitamin D

5. Patient mobilization (Kaplan, 2013)
   a) Weight-bearing activities are encouraged as tolerated to help reduce bone breakdown that releases calcium into circulation.
   b) Patients who are bedbound can receive active resistive exercises in conjunction with pain management to help limit calcium loss from bone.

E. Evaluation and follow-up
   1. Assess for increasing symptom severity.
   2. Assess for treatment efficacy and side effects.
   3. Monitor laboratory values.
   4. Monitor fluid balance.
   5. Monitor renal and cardiac function.
   6. Provide pain relief and comfort measures and assess efficacy.
   7. Provide teaching and instruction to patients and caregivers so that they understand the need to:
      a) Maintain oral fluid intake of 3 L/day and adequate salt intake.
      b) Recognize and report clinical manifestations of increasing serum calcium.
      c) Recognize and report conditions that lead to fluid loss.
      d) Understand the medical regimen, drug side effects, and laboratory follow-up schedule.
      e) Avoid use of drugs and supplements that potentiate HCM.
      f) Avoid use of sedating drugs.
      g) Manage pain and confusion.
      h) Perform weight-bearing activities, as appropriate.
      i) Follow safety precautions and use of assistive devices.
   8. Provide emotional support to patient and caregivers.
   9. Assess coping mechanisms.
   10. Support the decision to initiate palliative or hospice care as end of life nears.

F. Referrals
   1. Professional psychological counseling, as indicated
   2. Home hospice palliative care nursing services

Case Study

P.D. is a 78-year-old widower who lives with his daughter and was diagnosed with advanced renal cell carcinoma in the left kidney after undergoing a workup for hematuria and severe pain in the left flank. He underwent a palliative left radical nephrectomy. One month later, he began a course of systemic therapy with sunitinib, a tyrosine-kinase inhibitor targeted against angiogenesis.

P.D. has been taking sunitinib by mouth for about three months when his daughter notices that he is getting up several times during the night to urinate, his appetite is poor, and he is becoming increasingly lethargic and confused and appeared short of breath. At his office visit later in the week, P.D.'s daughter describes his symptoms to his oncologist and the oncology advanced practice registered nurse (APRN).

Imaging tests and blood work are ordered emergently. Computed tomography scans of the chest and abdomen reveal a new tumor mass in the left lung, most likely representing renal cancer metastatic to the lung. Blood test results reveal a mildly elevated serum calcium level of 11.5 mg/dl and below-normal levels of phosphorus (1.8 mg/dl) and albumin (3 g/dl). Based on the finding of low albumin, the serum protein that binds with calcium, the oncology APRN performs a correction calculation and finds that the estimated level of serum calcium is actually 12.5 mg/dl, indicating that P.D. has moderate hypercalcemia. The patient also reports that he urinates frequently and always feels thirsty.

P.D. is admitted to the hospital to receive aggressive antihypercalcemic treatment. IV normal saline is administered at a rate of 300 ml/hr to expand his intravascular fluid volume and increase renal calcium excretion. He subsequently develops fluid overload and is administered IV furosemide 20 mg along with calcitonin 4 IU/kg every 12 hours for two days. His electrolytes are carefully monitored during this period to detect losses and he receives oral phosphate replacement.

P.D.'s laboratory results normalize in three days, after which his oral fluid intake is maintained at 2 L/day and he is started on bisphosphonate therapy with a dose of IV zoledronic acid. A biopsy done via thoracotomy reveals that the lung mass is metastatic renal cell carcinoma, and P.D. is started on antineoplastic therapy with sorafenib, another oral targeted agent.

He is sent home to his daughter's care after five days in the hospital. The APRN provides verbal and written instructions to P.D. and his daughter regarding the importance of maintaining adequate fluid and salt intake, performing weight-bearing activity as feasible, avoiding the use of sedating drugs and supplements that contain calcium, and recognizing and reporting conditions that lead to fluid loss, such as vomiting and diarrhea, which could be related to sorafenib therapy.

Three weeks later, P.D.'s daughter finds him comatose in bed and he is readmitted to the hospital. His corrected calcium level is calculated to be 13.9 mg/dl. The palliative care team visits his daughter in P.D.'s room and discusses possible options on how to proceed. The decision is made to stop aggressive antihypercalcemic and antineoplastic therapies and send P.D. home to receive end-of-life care from the hospice team designed to provide comfort and ameliorate the symptoms associated with severe hypercalcemia. Team members provide P.D.'s daughter with emotional support and support her anticipatory grieving. Three days later, still comatose, P.D. passes away peacefully at home from the effects of hypercalcemia-induced central nervous system depression with his hospice nurse and daughter by his bedside.

References

Agraharkar, M., Dellinger, D., III, & Gangakhedkar, A.K. (2015, June 23). Hypercalcemia. Retrieved from http://emedicine.medscape.com/article/240681-overview

Amgen Inc. (2016, March). *Xgeva® (denosumab)* [Package insert]. Thousand Oaks, CA: Author.

Cancer Care Ontario. (2013, May). Drug formulary: Clodronate (Bonefos®). Retrieved from https://www.cancercare.on.ca/cms/one.aspx?portalId=1377&pageId=10760

Coleman, R.E., & Holen, I. (2014). Bone metastases. In J.E. Niederhuber, J.O. Armitage, J.H. Doroshow, M.B. Kastan, & J.E. Tepper (Eds.), *Abeloff's clinical oncology* (5th ed., pp. 739–763). Philadelphia, PA: Elsevier Saunders.

Fallah-Rad, N., & Morton, A.R. (2013). Managing hypercalcaemia and hypocalcaemia in cancer patients. *Current Opinion in Supportive and Palliative Care, 7,* 265–271. doi:10.1097/SPC.0b013e3283640f5f

Fojo, A.T. (2015). Metabolic emergencies. In V.T. DeVita Jr., T.S. Lawrence, & S.A. Rosenberg (Eds.), *Cancer: Principles and practice of oncology* (10th ed., pp. 1822–1831). Philadelphia, PA: Wolters Kluwer Health/ Lippincott Williams & Wilkins.

Genentech, Inc. (2015, October). *Boniva® (ibandronate)* [Package insert]. South San Francisco, CA: Author.

Green, T.E. (2014, July 8). Hypercalcemia in emergency medicine. Retrieved from http://emedicine.medscape.com/article/766373-overview

Hariri, A., Mount, D.B., & Rastegar, A. (2013). Disorders of calcium, phosphate, and magnesium metabolism. In D.B. Mount, M.H. Sayegh, & A.K. Singh (Eds.), *Core concepts in the disorders of fluid, electrolytes and acid-base balance* (pp. 103–146). New York, NY: Springer Science and Business Media.

Kaplan, M. (2013). Hypercalcemia of malignancy. In M. Kaplan (Ed.), *Understanding and managing oncologic emergencies: A resource for nurses* (2nd ed., pp. 103–155). Pittsburgh, PA: Oncology Nursing Society.

Khosla, S. (2015). Hypercalcemia and hypocalcemia. In D.L. Longo, A.S. Fauci, D.L. Kasper, S.L. Hauser, J.L. Jameson, & J. Loscalzo (Eds.), *Harrison's principles of internal medicine* (19th ed.). New York, NY: McGraw-Hill. Retrieved from http://accessmedicine.mhmedical.com/Content.aspx?bookid=1130&Sectionid=79726855

LeGrand, S.B. (2011). Modern management of malignant hypercalcemia. *American Journal of Hospice and Palliative Medicine, 28,* 515–517. doi:10.1177/1049909111141164

Maier, J.D., & Levine, S.N. (2015). Hypercalcemia in the intensive care unit: A review of pathophysiology, diagnosis, and modern therapy. *Journal of Intensive Care Medicine, 30,* 235–252. doi:10.1177/0885066613507530

Morton, A.R., & Lipton, A. (2014). Hypercalcemia. In J.E. Niederhuber, J.O. Armitage, J.H. Doroshow, M.B. Kastan, & J.E. Tepper (Eds.), *Abeloff's clinical oncology* (5th ed., pp. 581–590). Philadelphia, PA: Elsevier Saunders.

Novartis Pharmaceuticals Corp. (2016a, March). *Aredia® (pamidronate)* [Package insert]. East Hanover, NJ: Author.

Novartis Pharmaceuticals Corp. (2016b, March). *Zometa® (zoledronic acid)* [Package insert]. East Hanover, NJ: Author.

Pallan, S., Rahman, M.O., & Khan, A.A. (2012). Diagnosis and management of primary hyperparathyroidism. *BMJ, 344,* e1013. doi:10.1136/bmj.e1013

Potts, J.T., Jr., & Jüppner, H. (2015). Disorders of the parathyroid gland and calcium homeostasis. In D.L. Longo, A.S. Fauci, D.L. Kasper, S.L. Hauser, J.L. Jameson, & J. Loscalzo (Eds.), *Harrison's principles of internal medicine* (19th ed.). New York, NY: McGraw-Hill. Retrieved from http://accessmedicine.mhmedical.com/content.aspx?bookid=1130&Sectionid=79753597

Reagan, P., Pani, A., & Rosner, M.H. (2014). Approach to diagnosis and treatment of hypercalcemia in a patient with malignancy. *American Journal of Kidney Diseases, 63,* 141–147. doi:10.1053/j.ajkd.2013.06.025

Rosner, M.H., & Dalkin, A.C. (2012). Onco-nephrology: The pathophysiology and treatment of malignancy-associated hypercalcemia. *Clinical Journal of the American Society of Nephrology, 7,* 1722–1729. doi:10.2215/CJN.02470312

Santarpia, L., Koch, C.A., & Sarlis, N.J. (2010). Hypercalcemia in cancer patients: Pathobiology and management. *Hormone and Metabolic Research, 42,* 153–164. doi:10.1055/s-0029-1241821

Siddiqui, F., & Weissman, D.E. (2010). Hypercalcemia of malignancy. *Journal of Palliative Medicine, 13,* 77–78. doi:10.1089/jpm.2010.9894

Soyfoo, M.S., Brenner, K., Paesmans, M., & Body, J.J. (2013). Non-malignant causes of hypercalcemia in cancer patients: A frequent and neglected occurrence. *Supportive Care in Cancer, 21,* 1415–1419. doi:10.1007/s00520-012-1683-5

von Moos, R., Caspar, C.B., Thürlimann, B., Angst, R., Inauen, R., Greil, R., … Pecherstorfer, M. (2008). Renal safety profiles of ibandronate 6 mg infused over 15 and 60 min: A randomized, open-label study. *Annals of Oncology, 19,* 1266–1270. doi:10.1093/annonc/mdn038

Wright, L.E., & Guise, T.A. (2014). The role of PTHrP in skeletal metastases and hypercalcemia of malignancy. *Clinical Reviews in Bone and Mineral Metabolism, 12,* 119–129. doi:10.1007/s12018-014-9160-y

CHAPTER 30

Malignant Pleural Effusion

Marcelle Kaplan, MS, RN, CBCN®, CNS

I. Definition
   A. Malignant pleural effusion (MPE) is the abnormal collection of fluid in the pleural space and is a common complication of the malignant process (Yu, 2011; Zarogoulidis et al., 2013).
   B. Approximately 1.5 million pleural effusions are diagnosed in the United States each year (Rubins, 2014), of which about 150,000 cases are due to MPE (Nguyen & Manning, 2015).
   C. MPE occurs most often in patients with cancers of the lung (40%) and breast (25%) that metastasize to the pleura and in patients with lymphoma (10%) (Nguyen & Manning, 2015; Zarogoulidis et al., 2013).
   D. Other cancers that contribute to the incidence of MPE include mesothelioma, a primary cancer of the pleura (about 10%); ovarian and gastric cancer (5% each); and cancers of unknown origin (less than 10%) (Nguyen & Manning, 2015; Zarogoulidis et al., 2013).
   E. Patients with cancer can concomitantly develop pleural effusions not related to the disease process. Common nonmalignant causes of pleural effusion include congestive heart failure, pneumonia, pulmonary embolism, liver cirrhosis, and malnutrition with low serum albumin (National Cancer Institute [NCI], 2015; Rubins, 2014; Yu, 2011).
   F. MPE typically heralds advanced incurable disease (Davies & Lee, 2013) but also may be the first sign of cancer (NCI, 2015; Nguyen & Manning, 2015).
   G. MPE can result from the disease process or be caused by cancer treatments, such as systemic chemotherapy and radiation therapy to the chest and mediastinum (NCI, 2015; Story, 2013).
   H. MPE is a life-threatening complication because it can lead to respiratory and cardiac arrest (Story, 2013).
   I. Prognosis for survival following the occurrence of MPE is poor and generally is limited to a few months depending on the type and extent of the underlying malignancy (Heffner, 2016; Nguyen & Manning, 2015).
   J. Therapy focuses on the patient's needs at the end of life: providing palliation of symptoms (dyspnea predominantly) and comfort measures, avoiding invasive procedures, and improving quality of life while allowing the patient to avoid hospitalization and remain at home (Davies & Lee, 2013; Heffner, 2016; Muduly, Deo, Subi, Kallianpur, & Shukla, 2011).
II. Pathophysiology
   A. The lungs and their pleural sacs are located in the thorax. Two layers of pleura form the pleural sac: one adheres to the lungs (the visceral pleura), and the other covers

the inner surface of the thoracic cavity (the parietal pleura), including the mediastinum, diaphragm, and chest wall (Cope, 2011; Rubins, 2014) (see Figure 30-1).

B. The space between the two layers of pleura is the pleural space. It normally contains a small amount of fluid (about 5–15 ml) that serves to reduce friction during
inspiration and expiration (Rubins, 2014; Story, 2013; Zarogoulidis et al., 2013).

C. Normal pleural fluid contains about 2 g/dl of protein (NCI, 2015; Rubins, 2014).

D. The volume of fluid in the pleural space is maintained through a balance between
fluid secretion and reabsorption through lymphatic channels (Cope, 2011). Pleural effusions result when this balance is disrupted.

E. Certain cancers can metastasize to the pleura via lymphatic channels or the blood-
stream or can directly invade the pleura and lead to development of MPE (Davies
& Lee, 2013).

F. Two mechanisms commonly contribute to the formation of MPE.

Figure 30-1. Malignant Pleural Effusion

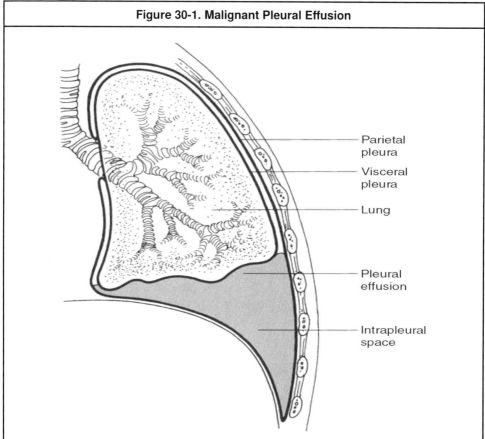

In the lung, fluid is constantly being filtered across the intrapleural space from the parietal pleural surface and reabsorbed through the visceral pleura. When obstruction by malignant processes prevents
reabsorption, fluid accumulates in the intrapleural space and a pleural effusion results.

Note. From "Malignant Effusions" (p. 864), by D.G. Cope in C.H. Yarbro, D. Wujcik, and B.H. Gobel (Eds.), *Cancer
Nursing: Principles and Practice* (7th ed.), 2011, Burlington, MA: Jones & Bartlett Learning, www.jbpub.com. Copyright 2011 by Jones & Bartlett Learning. Reprinted with permission.

   1. Increased production and accumulation of fluid occurs within the pleural space because of the presence of tumor cells that inflame or irritate pleural membranes and cause increased membrane and vascular permeability (Davies & Lee, 2013; Rubins, 2014). This mechanism is seen most often in patients with lung cancer (Cope, 2011).
   2. Impaired lymphatic drainage occurs because of obstruction of lymphatic channels draining the pleura or the lungs by the tumor, resulting in accumulation of fluid within the pleural space (Davies & Lee, 2013; Rubins, 2014). This mechanism occurs most often with metastases from lung and breast cancer and lymphoma (Story, 2013).
   G. Pleural effusions are classified into two types based on the mechanism of fluid formation and the composition of pleural fluid (Rubins, 2014; Wilcox et al., 2014; Yu, 2011).
   1. Transudative effusion: Clear fluid; usually not due to malignancy; associated with congestive heart failure and liver cirrhosis
   2. Exudative effusion: Cloudy fluid with a high cell count and protein content; associated with malignancy and a variety of nonmalignant infectious or inflammatory conditions
   H. MPEs are typically exudates rather than transudates (NCI, 2015; Zarogoulidis et al., 2013).
III. Presenting symptoms
   A. Symptom severity is related to the volume and speed of fluid accumulation in the pleural space (Story, 2013).
   B. Patients with small MPEs may be asymptomatic and the effusions found incidentally (Heffner, 2016).
   C. Dyspnea, occurring with exertion or at rest, is the most predominant symptom in patients with MPE (Davies & Lee, 2013; Heffner, 2016).
   D. Pleuritic chest pain is common and may range from a dull ache to a sharp or stabbing pain that increases with deep inspiration or coughing (Muduly et al., 2011; Nguyen & Manning, 2015; Rubins, 2014).
   E. Dry, nonproductive cough is common (Muduly et al., 2011).
   F. Weight loss, chills, and malaise may be reported (NCI, 2015; Yu, 2011).
   G. Sensation of heaviness or pressure in the chest (Nguyen & Manning, 2015) that is relieved by splinting the affected area and sleeping on the affected side may be reported (Story, 2013).
   H. Feelings of suffocation and anxiety may be reported (Story, 2013).
IV. Physical examination
   A. History
   1. History of cancer, including tumor type, stage, and treatments, is elicited. MPE can develop many years after initial diagnosis (Rubins, 2014).
   2. Cancer risk factors and screening test dates and results, including history of smoking and mammogram results, are evaluated. MPE may be the first indication of cancer (NCI, 2015).
   3. Occupational and environmental history is explored. Exposure to asbestos can lead to mesothelioma, a primary cancer of the pleura (Rubins, 2014; Zarogoulidis et al., 2013).
   4. Preexisting respiratory conditions, such as chronic obstructive pulmonary disease, pulmonary embolus, tuberculosis, or interstitial lung disease, are noted as potential causes of dyspnea (Davies & Lee, 2013; Glennon, 2015).

5. Cardiac conditions related to cancer therapies, such as chemotherapy-induced cardiomyopathy or radiation-induced pericardial disease, as well as congestive heart failure, are noted as potential causes of dyspnea (Glennon, 2015).

6. Severity of dyspnea and chest pain and their characteristics are elicited (Held-Warmkessel & Schiech, 2008).

B. Physical assessment

1. Physical examination of the lungs includes visual inspection of the chest during inspiration and expiration, auscultation to assess the pattern and volume of airflow, and palpation and percussion to detect differences in sound transmission from the lungs through the chest wall (Hildreth, Lynm, & Glass, 2009) (see Figure 30-2).

2. Physical assessment findings with MPE depend on the effusion volume.

   a) Effusions smaller than 300 ml generally produce subtle or normal findings (Rubins, 2014; Yu, 2011).

   b) Effusions larger than 300 ml may produce the following physical assessment findings:

Figure 30-2. Clinical Features of Malignant Pleural Effusion Symptoms

Symptoms
- May be asymptomatic
- Dyspnea on exertion or at rest
- Shortness of breath
- Dry, nonproductive cough
- Chest pain—may be achy and heavy or pleuritic
- Malaise
- Weight loss
- Anxiety, fear of suffocation
- Desire to lie on affected side

Signs
- Tachypnea
- Labored breathing
- Decreased or absent breath sounds
- Bronchial breath sounds
- Pleuritic rub over affected area
- Restricted chest wall expansion
- Decreased tactile fremitus
- Dullness to percussion
- Egophony
- Larger effusions also may exhibit:
  - Splinting of chest
  - Cyanosis
  - Chest tenderness
  - Tracheal deviation to the unaffected side
  - Bulging of intercostal spaces
  - Lymphadenopathy
  - Shift in point of maximal impulse
  - Use of accessory muscles of breathing

Note. Based on information from Camp-Sorrell, 2006; Cope, 2011; Heffner, 2011a; Porcel & Light, 2006.

From "Malignant Pleural Effusion" (p. 265), by K.T. Story in M. Kaplan (Ed.), *Understanding and Managing Oncologic Emergencies: A Resource for Nurses* (2nd ed.), 2013, Pittsburgh, PA: Oncology Nursing Society. Copyright 2013 by Oncology Nursing Society. Reprinted with permission.

        (1) Diminished or absent breath sounds, dullness to percussion, and decreased tactile fremitus (Nguyen & Manning, 2015; Rubins, 2014)

        (2) Asymmetrical chest expansion during breathing, with restricted chest expansion observed on the side of the effusion (Rubins, 2014)

    c) Massive pleural effusions (greater than 1,000 ml) may cause the mediastinum to shift away from the effusion and lead to tracheal deviation from the midline and low cardiac output (Nguyen & Manning, 2015; Story, 2013).

3. Pleural friction rub and alterations in breath and heart sounds may be present on auscultation over the effusion (Story, 2013) (see Figure 30-2).

    a) Pleuritic chest pain may be localized to the chest wall or referred to the shoulder on the side of the MPE (Rubins, 2014).

    b) Vital signs may reveal elevated temperature and blood pressure, tachypnea, and tachycardia (Stark, 2014; Story, 2013).

    c) Certain physical findings may suggest causes other than malignancy for a pleural effusion.

        (1) Peripheral edema, distended neck veins, and S_3 gallop heart sound may reflect congestive heart failure (Rubins, 2014; Story, 2013).

        (2) Ascites suggests liver disease, whereas hepatosplenomegaly suggests malignancy (Rubins, 2014; Story, 2013).

V. Diagnostics

  A. Imaging studies

    1. Chest x-ray is the primary diagnostic test used to image a pleural effusion (Yu, 2011). Upright and lateral decubitus (side-lying) views can confirm an effusion and provide an estimate of the amount of pleural fluid (Muduly et al., 2011; Stark, 2014).

    2. Chest computed tomography (CT) scans with IV contrast can detect pleural effusions that are quite small (less than 10 ml) or loculated (encapsulated). Chest CT scans are the preferred study to reveal pathology within the thorax, including the presence of mesothelioma, involvement of mediastinal or hilar lymph nodes, pleural masses, and underlying lung disease (Nguyen & Manning, 2015; Stark, 2014; Yu, 2011).

    3. Other imaging tests used in select cases include the following:

      a) Ultrasonography, which can detect small pleural effusions (less than 5 ml), identify the presence of loculations, and provide guidance for thoracentesis for small effusions or for placement of drainage catheters (Stark, 2014; Yu, 2011)

      b) Magnetic resonance imaging, which can provide details about pleural effusions and the extent of invasion of pleural tumors (Stark, 2014)

  B. Invasive diagnostic procedures

    1. Thoracentesis involves placing a catheter into the pleural space to obtain fluid for laboratory analysis and diagnosis. It also provides symptom relief by removing excess fluid (Muduly et al., 2011). Thoracentesis can be performed at the bedside with use of local anesthesia and ultrasound guidance (Heffner, 2016; Yu, 2011).

    2. Thoracoscopy involves placing a fiber-optic scope (pleuroscope) into the pleural space with the patient under local anesthesia to evaluate exudative effu-

sions of unknown cause through direct viewing and pleural biopsy (Rubins, 2014; Story, 2013).

C. Evaluation of pleural fluid
  1. Pleural fluid is collected via thoracentesis and examined for color (e.g., straw, bloody, milky, black, green), character (e.g., viscous, contains pus or debris), and odor (e.g., putrid, ammonia) (Heffner, 2016).
  2. Results of laboratory tests are used to distinguish between pleural effusions that are transudates, which are not typically associated with malignancy, and exudates, which are most typical of malignancy (Heffner, 2016; Rubins, 2014; Wilcox et al., 2014).
  3. Tests commonly performed on pleural fluid include cell count, pH, protein concentration, lactate dehydrogenase (LDH), cholesterol, triglycerides, albumin, and glucose (Heffner, 2016; Rubins, 2014; Wilcox et al., 2014).
  4. The Light Criteria Rule is the traditional method for distinguishing between transudative and exudative effusions. Pleural fluid is classified as an exudate if at least one of the following three criteria is met. If none of the criteria are met, the fluid is considered a transudate (Light, Macgregor, Luchsinger, & Ball, 1972; Wilcox et al., 2014; Zarogoulidis et al., 2013).
    a) Pleural fluid protein/serum protein ratio greater than 0.5
    b) Pleural fluid LDH level higher than two-thirds of the upper limit of normal for serum LDH
    c) Pleural fluid LDH/serum LDH ratio greater than 0.6
  5. Pleural fluid from an MPE frequently contains blood, white blood cells (mostly lymphocytes and monocytes), reactive mesothelial cells, and cancer cells shed from the tumor (Nguyen & Manning, 2015).
  6. Pleural fluid cytology is a simple and effective method for diagnosing mesothelioma, which arises in the pleura (Rubins, 2014).

VI. Differential diagnosis
  A. Exudative effusions are typical of malignancy (more than 90% of MPEs are exudates) (Zarogoulidis et al., 2013).
  B. However, exudative effusions also are associated with many nonmalignant etiologies, especially heart and lung disorders, and a wide variety of other pathologic conditions (see Figure 30-3).

Figure 30-3. Differential Diagnosis of Exudative Pleural Effusion

- Malignancy: metastatic and primary (mesothelioma), chylothorax (obstruction of thoracic duct by tumor causes chyle to leak into pleural space)
- Infections: pneumonias (bacterial, viral, mycoplasma), tuberculosis, pulmonary fungal disease, abdominal abscesses (liver, spleen), hepatitis
- Inflammatory disorders: pulmonary embolism; pancreatitis; chest irradiation; pleuritis associated with rheumatoid arthritis, lupus erythematosus, or uremia; sarcoidosis; postcardiac injury syndrome; acute respiratory distress syndrome; hemothorax; asbestos exposure
- Iatrogenic: drug-induced pleural disease; central venous catheter displacement; esophageal perforation; feeding tube in pleural space; ovarian hyperstimulation syndrome
- Other: trapped lung (lung unable to expand due to restricting "peel"); yellow nail syndrome (presence of yellow nails, peripheral edema, and pleural effusions); Meigs syndrome (presence of pleural effusion and ascites associated with benign ovarian tumor)

Note. Based on information from Rubins, 2014; Stark, 2014; Story, 2013.

VII. Interventions
  A. Treatment considerations are based on patients' disease and performance status, symptom severity, expected length of survival, and goals of care (NCI, 2015; Story, 2013).
  B. Improving quality of life by palliating symptoms (especially dyspnea) through interventions to drain fluid from the pleural space and prevent reaccumulation is the primary treatment goal for most patients (Muduly et al., 2011; Yu, 2011; Zarogoulidis et al., 2013).
  C. Factors considered in the choice of methods to drain an MPE include rapid and effective symptom relief with minimum invasiveness, discomfort, morbidity, cost, and time spent in the hospital (Davies & Lee, 2013; Heffner, 2016; Muduly et al., 2011) (see Table 30-1).
  D. Therapeutic thoracentesis may be the initial and simplest intervention used to drain the MPE and palliate dyspnea.
    1. However, it provides short-term relief, as rapid fluid reaccumulation is common with MPE and requires repeated procedures.
    2. Thus, thoracentesis may be an appropriate treatment for patients expected to have a brief survival or to respond to systemic therapy (Muduly et al., 2011; Yu, 2011; Zarogoulidis et al., 2013).
    3. It can be performed at the bedside with local anesthesia and ultrasound guidance (Held-Warmkessel & Schiech, 2008).
  E. Tube thoracostomy involves the insertion of a chest tube to drain recurrent or massive pleural effusions (Muduly et al., 2011; Story, 2013).
    1. The procedure is performed with general anesthesia and video guidance (Cope, 2011; Nguyen & Manning, 2015).
    2. It may be used for patients with expected survival of three months or less (Muduly et al., 2011).
  F. Chemical pleurodesis is a more permanent method to manage MPE in patients with good performance status and life expectancy of more than three months.
    1. After complete drainage of the MPE through the chest tube, a sclerosing agent (frequently talc) is introduced into the pleural space via the chest tube as talc slurry or through a thoracoscope in aerosol form (insufflation) as talc poudrage (Heffner, 2016; Nguyen & Manning, 2015; Zarogoulidis et al., 2013).
    2. The procedure prevents reaccumulation of fluid by damaging and inflaming the pleura, thereby resulting in fibrosis and obliteration of the pleural space (Rubins, 2014).
  G. An indwelling pleural catheter (also known as a tunneled pleural catheter) permits long-term management of MPE in the home.
    1. The PleurX® catheter is the preferred catheter for this purpose in the United States (Story, 2013; Yu, 2011).
    2. It can be inserted in a minimally invasive outpatient procedure with local anesthesia and imaging guidance (Story, 2013).
    3. Use of the tunneled pleural catheter may be the most appropriate method to treat MPEs in patients with brief life expectancy or when chemical pleurodesis is contradicted or has failed (Davies & Lee, 2013; Heffner, 2016; Nguyen & Manning, 2015).
  H. Pleuroperitoneal shunting is a rarely used surgical option to treat patients with MPE that has not been controlled with other methods or those who cannot perform inter-

mittent drainage via an indwelling pleural catheter (Davies & Lee, 2013; Heffner, 2016; Nguyen & Manning, 2015). Shunt placement allows fluid to be drained from the pleural space into the peritoneal cavity, where it is absorbed (Held-Warmkessel & Schiech, 2008).

Table 30-1. Treatment Interventions for Malignant Pleural Effusion		
Treatment	**Indications**	**Methodology**
Observation	Asymptomatic effusions; most will progress and require therapy.	Frequent reassessments with serial chest x-ray
Therapeutic thoracentesis	First line of treatment; rapid relief of dyspnea; obtain pleural fluid for analysis.	Catheter is inserted into pleural space, and fluid is withdrawn and sent to laboratory for analysis.
Chest tube drainage only	Loculated effusions, massive effusions, poor performance status, treatment failures	Large-bore chest tube or indwelling catheter is placed into the pleural space for long-term drainage.
Pleurodesis	Control of effusion; demonstrated benefit from therapeutic thoracentesis	Large-bore or small-bore chest tube is placed, fluid is drained, and sclerosant is administered into the tube. The tube is left in place until drainage volume is less than 100 ml/day.
Thoracoscopy with talc poudrage	Control of effusion; demonstrated benefit from therapeutic thoracentesis	Thoracoscope is inserted into pleural space, fluid is drained, and talc is administered as a spray using an atomizer.
Pleuroperitoneal shunt	When other options have failed or are not indicated; may be useful with chylothorax	Denver® shunt is implanted into the abdomen with drainage catheters in the pleural and peritoneal space and drains fluid into the abdomen.
Indwelling pleural catheter	Control of effusion for outpatient management	PleurX® or Tenckhoff® catheter is inserted into the pleural space and sutured in place; patient or caregiver can drain with special equipment. Implanted catheter may be intermittently accessed similar to other implanted ports.
Pleurectomy and pleural abrasion	Good performance status; used only if other measures have failed and good life expectancy	Requires thoracoscopy or thoracotomy; pleural membrane is resected and abraded; prevents reaccumulation of pleural fluid.

Note. Based on information from Heffner, 2011b; Lombardi et al., 2010; Musani, 2009; Uzbeck et al., 2010.

From "Malignant Pleural Effusion" (p. 271), by K.T. Story in M. Kaplan (Ed.), *Understanding and Managing Oncologic Emergencies: A Resource for Nurses* (2nd ed.), 2013, Pittsburgh, PA: Oncology Nursing Society. Copyright 2013 by Oncology Nursing Society. Reprinted with permission.

I. Pleurectomy is a lengthy surgical procedure involving removal of the parietal pleura to prevent recurrent effusions.
   1. It is reserved for patients who have not benefited from other less invasive interventions and have a longer life expectancy.
   2. It is associated with acute and chronic pain and other morbidity (23%) and a mortality risk of 5%–10% at one month (NCI, 2015; Nguyen & Manning, 2015).
J. Antineoplastic treatment with chemotherapy or radiation therapy may be used to treat the underlying cancer, although these therapies are unlikely to control symptomatic MPE (Heffner, 2016).
   1. However, systemic chemotherapy is likely to provide a good response in patients with newly diagnosed small cell lung cancer or lymphoma (NCI, 2015; Zarogoulidis et al., 2013).
   2. MPEs related to lymphomas involving mediastinal lymph nodes may respond to chest radiation therapy (Heffner, 2016).
K. Evaluation and follow-up
   1. Nurses have a crucial role in the care of patients with MPE that includes providing symptom management, emotional support, and education; evaluating response to treatments; and managing side effects.
   2. Key nursing interventions (Cope, 2011; Held-Warmkessel & Schiech, 2008; Hildreth et al., 2009; Story, 2013; Walker & Bryden, 2010)
      a) Assess respiratory, cardiac, and neurologic status.
      b) Institute measures to promote oxygenation and palliate dyspnea.
      c) Manage pain and promote comfort.
      d) Teach breathing techniques and positioning to help relieve breathlessness.
      e) Provide information and instructions about diagnostic measures and invasive procedures.
      f) Care for drainage tubes and surgical sites.
      g) Record the amount and quality of drainage fluid and monitor for catheter air leaks.
      h) Monitor treatment efficacy, and assess and manage side effects.
      i) Provide instructions to patients and caregivers about managing drainage systems at home and recording drainage amounts.
      j) Teach patients and caregivers to recognize and report signs and symptoms of fluid reaccumulation.
      k) Provide emotional support to patients and caregivers to decrease anxiety about the symptoms and significance of MPE, and assess coping methods.
      l) Support the decision to decline aggressive cancer therapies and prepare to address end-of-life issues, as appropriate.
      m) Provide referrals to palliative care, home care, hospice, and pain management specialists, social workers, psychologists, clergy, and others, as appropriate.
L. Referrals and consultations
   1. Pulmonologist
   2. Interventional radiologist
   3. Thoracic surgeon
   4. Palliative care team
   5. Home care or hospice services
   6. Pain management team
   7. Social worker

Case Study

A.J. is a 69-year-old married woman who was diagnosed with estrogen receptor– and progesterone receptor–positive stage IIB (T2 N1 M0) cancer of the left breast seven years ago. Her surgical treatment included a lumpectomy and axillary lymph node biopsy (after a sentinel node biopsy tested positive). Pathology results reported a 3.5 cm breast mass and four positive lymph nodes. She received adjuvant combination chemotherapy followed by whole breast irradiation. A.J. was also started on antiestrogen hormone therapy with an aromatase inhibitor. However, she stopped taking the drug after five months because of what she felt were intolerable side effects, including bone and joint pain, hot flashes, and nausea. No signs of breast cancer recurrence have occurred since she completed the initial treatments.

A.J. is now being seen at the medical oncologist's office for her annual visit and reports increasing shortness of breath with activity and even at rest, feelings of breathlessness relieved by sleeping elevated on two pillows, a dry nonproductive cough, and a dull ache on the left side of her chest. The oncology advanced practice registered nurse (APRN) orders an immediate chest x-ray including upright and lateral decubitus views to help distinguish between radiation-related lung fibrosis and pleural effusion. Chest x-ray results report the presence of a large pleural effusion on the left estimated to be about 500 ml in volume. A follow-up chest CT scan with IV contrast reveals lesions in both lungs and enlarged mediastinal lymph nodes on the left, most likely due to metastases from A.J.'s breast cancer.

In performing a physical examination of A.J.'s lungs, the oncology APRN notes absent breath sounds, dullness to percussion, and decreased tactile fremitus in the lower left lung. No peripheral edema, neck vein distension, or abnormal heart sounds are noted. A thoracentesis of the left lung with ultrasound guidance is scheduled to remove pleural fluid to send for laboratory analysis and to help relieve A.J.'s dyspnea.

Laboratory test results on the pleural fluid show that the levels of protein and LDH are elevated beyond the extent needed to meet the Light criteria for an exudate: (a) pleural fluid protein/serum protein ratio greater than 0.5; (b) pleural fluid LDH level is greater than two-thirds of the upper limit of normal for serum LDH; and (c) pleural fluid LDH/serum LDH ratio is greater than 0.6. Cell cytology demonstrates the presence of breast cancer cells with pathologic features consistent with that of the original breast tumor. The diagnosis is MPE due to metastatic breast cancer.

The oncology APRN is aware that an MPE generally signals an advanced stage of cancer and a life expectancy measured in months. The nurse schedules an office visit with A.J. and her husband to discuss test results, treatment options, symptom palliation measures, and goals of care. A.J. tells the nurse that she and her husband are greatly saddened that the breast cancer returned and have arrived at the decision to spare her the side effects and discomfort of aggressive antitumor therapy. Maintaining A.J.'s comfort is their primary treatment goal. They desire that A.J.'s quality of life be kept as good as possible with relief of dyspnea and chest pain.

After the oncology nurse explains the various options for draining the MPE, they decide that the most appropriate intervention for A.J. is placement of an indwelling pleural catheter because it can be inserted in an outpatient procedure so that she does not have to spend time in the hospital. It will be emptied at home every few days as needed based on her symptoms.

After the indwelling catheter has been placed, the homecare nurse visits A.J. and her husband and teaches them catheter care and how to empty the drainage and record the amounts and provides written instructions. They also are taught to recognize and report signs and symptoms of fluid reaccumulation. Supplemental oxygen is provided in the home, and analgesia is prescribed at the levels appropriate to meet A.J.'s increasing needs for pain relief. The homecare nurse provides strategies to help relieve A.J.'s shortness of breath, including using pursed-lip breathing, sleeping with the head of the bed elevated, and pacing her activities to reduce energy expenditure. The nurse visits A.J. daily at home to assess her vital signs and respiratory, cardiac, and neurologic status and monitor drain care and the amount of drainage and pain relief.

With the pleural fluid being drained intermittently by her husband through the indwelling catheter, A.J. becomes more comfortable. Her dyspnea, cough, and chest pain diminish for the first few weeks. However, after eight weeks, as the amount of MPE increases and A.J. becomes more breathless and weaker and requires more frequent pain palliation, the hospice team is called in to evaluate her care and comfort needs at the end of life. She is seen daily in her home by a member of the hospice team and dies peacefully 10 days later.

References

Camp-Sorrell, D. (2006). Pleural effusion. In D. Camp-Sorrell & R.A. Hawkins (Eds.), *Clinical manual for the oncology advanced practice nurse* (2nd ed., pp. 189–194). Pittsburgh, PA: Oncology Nursing Society.

Cope, D.G. (2011). Malignant effusions. In C.H. Yarbro, D. Wujcik, & B.H. Gobel (Eds.), *Cancer nursing: Principles and practice* (7th ed., pp. 863–878). Burlington, MA: Jones & Bartlett Learning.

Davies, H.E., & Lee, Y.C.G. (2013). Management of malignant pleural effusions: Questions that need answers. *Current Opinion in Pulmonary Medicine, 19,* 374–379. doi:10.1097/MCP.0b013e3283615b67

Glennon, C. (2015). Dyspnea. In C.G. Brown (Ed.), *A guide to oncology symptom management* (2nd ed., pp. 283–317). Pittsburgh, PA: Oncology Nursing Society.

Heffner, J.E. (2011a, December 21). Diagnostic evaluation of a pleural effusion in adults [Literature review current through May 2012]. Retrieved from http://www.uptodate.com/contents/diagnostic-evaluation-of-a-pleural-effusion-in-adults-initial-testing

Heffner, J.E. (2011b). Management of malignant pleural effusions [Literature review current through May 2012]. Retrieved from http://www.uptodate.com/contents/management-of-malignant-pleural-effusions

Heffner, J.E. (2016, February 24). Management of malignant pleural effusions [Literature review current through April 2016]. Retrieved from http://www.uptodate.com/contents/management-of-malignant-pleural-effusions

Held-Warmkessel, J., & Schiech, L. (2008). Caring for a patient with malignant pleural effusion. *Nursing, 38*(11), 43–47. doi:10.1097/01.NURSE.0000341079.53082.b1

Hildreth, C.J., Lynm, C., & Glass, R.M. (2009). JAMA patient page: Pleural effusion. *JAMA, 301,* 344. doi:10.1001/jama.301.3.344

Light, R.W., Macgregor, M.I., Luchsinger, P.C., & Ball, W.C. (1972). Pleural effusions: The diagnostic separation of transudates and exudates. *Annals of Internal Medicine, 77,* 507–513. doi:10.7326/0003-4819-77-4-507

Lombardi, G., Zustovich, F., Nicoletto, M.O., Donach, M., Artioli, G., & Pastorelli, D. (2010). Diagnosis and treatment of malignant pleural effusion: A systematic literature review and new approaches. *American Journal of Clinical Oncology, 33,* 420–423. doi:10.1097/COC.0b013e3181aacbbf

Muduly, D.K., Deo, S.V.S., Subi, T.S., Kallianpur, A.A., & Shukla, N.K. (2011). An update in the management of malignant pleural effusion. *Indian Journal of Palliative Care, 17,* 98–103. doi:10.4103/0973-1075.84529

Musani, A.I. (2009). Treatment options for malignant pleural effusion. *Current Opinion in Pulmonary Medicine, 15,* 380–387. doi:10.1097/MCP.0b013e32832c6a8a

National Cancer Institute. (2015, August 31). Cardiopulmonary syndromes (PDQ®) [Health professional version]. Retrieved from http://www.cancer.gov/cancertopics/pdq/supportivecare/cardiopulmonary/HealthProfessional/page4

Nguyen, D.M., & Manning, E.W. (2015). Malignant pleural and pericardial effusions. In V.T. DeVita Jr., T.S. Lawrence, & S.A. Rosenberg (Eds.), *Cancer: Principles and practice of oncology* (10th ed., pp. 1880–1886). Philadelphia, PA: Lippincott Williams & Wilkins.

Porcel, J.M., & Light, R.W. (2006). Diagnostic approach to pleural effusion in adults. *American Family Physician, 73,* 1211–1220.

Rubins, J. (2014, September 4). Pleural effusion. Retrieved from http://emedicine.medscape.com/article/299959-overview

Stark, P. (2014, January 7). Imaging of pleural effusions in adults [Literature review current through April 2016]. Retrieved from http://www.uptodate.com/contents/imaging-of-pleural-effusions-in-adults

Story, K.T. (2013). Malignant pleural effusion. In M. Kaplan (Ed.), *Understanding and managing oncologic emergencies: A resource for nurses* (2nd ed., pp. 257–286). Pittsburgh, PA: Oncology Nursing Society.

Uzbeck, M.H., Almeida, F.A., Sarkiss, M.G., Morice, R.C., Jimenez, C.A., Eapen, G.A., & Kennedy, M.P. (2010). Management of malignant pleural effusions. *Advances in Therapy, 27,* 334–347. doi:10.1007/S12325 -010-0031-8

Walker, S.J., & Bryden, G. (2010). Managing pleural effusions: Nursing care of patients with a Tenckhoff catheter. *Clinical Journal of Oncology Nursing, 14,* 59–64. doi:10.1188/10.CJON.59-64

Wilcox, M.E., Chong, C.A., Stanbrook, M.B., Tricco, A.C., Wong, C., & Straus, S.E. (2014). Does this patient have an exudative pleural effusion? The Rational Clinical Examination systematic review. *JAMA, 311,* 2422–2431. doi:10.1001/jama.2014.5552

Yu, H. (2011). Management of pleural effusion, empyema, and lung abscess. *Seminars in Interventional Radiology, 28,* 75–86. doi:10.1055/s-0031-1273942

Zarogoulidis, K., Zarogoulidis, P., Darwiche, K., Tsakiridis, K., Machairiotis, N., Kougioumtzi, I., … Spyratos, D. (2013). Malignant pleural effusion and algorithm management. *Journal of Thoracic Disease, 5,* S413–S419. doi:10.3978/j.issn.2072-1439.2013.09.04

CHAPTER 31

Spinal Cord Compression

Marcelle Kaplan, MS, RN, CBCN®, CNS

I. Definition
  A. Spinal cord compression (SCC) is a true oncologic emergency.
    1. SCC occurs in patients with cancer when a tumor mass or fragments from a pathologically collapsed vertebra impinge on and compress the spinal cord.
    2. SCC annually affects about 20,000 patients with cancer (Becker & Baehring, 2015; Weinstein, 2013) and is the second most common neurologic complication of cancer, after brain metastasis (Hammack, 2012; McCurdy & Shanholtz, 2012).
    3. SCC most often occurs in patients who have a prior history of cancer but also may be the first indication of malignancy (Lewis, Hendrickson, & Moynihan, 2011; Schiff, 2015).
  B. Life expectancy following SCC typically is a few months (Becker & Baehring, 2015; Hammack, 2012; Weinstein, 2013).
  C. Cancers commonly associated with increased incidence of SCC are solid tumors that have a propensity to metastasize to vertebral bone, including cancers of the lung (especially), breast, and prostate (see Figure 31-1).
  D. Renal carcinoma, multiple myeloma, non-Hodgkin lymphoma, Hodgkin lymphoma, and cancers of unknown origin also contribute to SCC incidence (Huff, 2015; Kaplan, 2013; Weinstein, 2013).
  E. Rarely, primary tumors may arise within the spinal cord and cause SCC (Weinstein, 2013).
  F. Early recognition and intervention are critical to preserving patients' quality of life and functional independence.
  G. If unrelieved, SCC results in neurologic impairment that typically follows a sequence beginning with back pain and progressing to motor weakness, sensory loss, sphincter dysfunction (bladder and colon), and ultimately, irreversible paralysis (Becker & Baehring, 2015; Kaplan, 2013).

Figure 31-1. Cancers Most Often Associated With Increased Risk for Spinal Cord Compression

• Lung cancer	• Non-Hodgkin lymphoma
• Breast cancer	• Hodgkin lymphoma
• Prostate cancer	• Renal carcinoma
• Multiple myeloma	• Unknown primary

Note. Based on information from Kaplan, 2013.

II. Pathophysiology

A. The spinal column consists of 33 vertebrae divided into 5 segments, each with a varying number of vertebrae. In descending order, the segments are the following (Sugerman, 2013):

1. Cervical—7 vertebrae
2. Thoracic—12 vertebrae
3. Lumbar—5 vertebrae
4. Sacral—5 fused vertebrae (the sacrum)
5. Coccyx—4 fused vertebrae (the coccyx)

B. The vertebrae form the vertebral canal that encloses and protects the spinal cord.

1. The spinal cord is a long column of nervous tissue that extends from the brain stem to the level of the first or second lumbar vertebra.
2. The lumbar and sacral spinal nerve roots extend below the level of the cord and are called the cauda equina because they resemble a horse's tail (Sugerman, 2013).

    a) The spinal cord is covered and protected by three membranes (meninges).

    (1) The inner membrane that adheres to the spinal cord is the pia mater.
    (2) The middle membrane is the arachnoid membrane; the subarachnoid space exists between these two membranes and contains the cerebrospinal fluid.
    (3) The outermost membrane, to which the spinal nerves are attached, is the dura mater.

    b) The space between the dura mater and the vertebral column is the epidural space. The size of the epidural space varies among the different spinal segments (Sugerman, 2013).

C. SCC most often is caused by tumor metastasis to vertebral bone; the enlarging tumor mass invades the epidural space and compresses the spinal cord (Weinstein, 2013).

D. Less frequently, local tumor (e.g., lung cancer) or enlarged lymph nodes associated with lymphoma may extend through openings between vertebrae into the epidural space and cause SCC (Hammack, 2012).

E. Fragments from pathologically collapsed vertebrae also can compress the spinal cord (Kaplan, 2013).

F. The location of cord compression generally correlates with the volume of vertebral bone in the spinal region (Hammack, 2012; Kaplan, 2013).

1. Thus, the thoracic spine is the most frequent site for SCC (60%) because it is composed of 12 vertebrae and has the largest volume of bone.
2. Next in frequency is the lumbosacral spine (25%) followed by the cervical spine (10%–15%).

G. Interruption of blood flow secondary to cord compression leads to cord edema and the release of neurotoxins, causing neurologic injury (Huff, 2015; Kaplan, 2013).

H. More than one area of the spinal cord may be compressed at diagnosis (Hammack, 2012; Huff, 2015; Weinstein, 2013).

III. Presenting symptoms

A. Vary with the location and severity of the compression

B. Generally follow a similar sequence in all patients (see Figure 31-2)

1. Back pain is the initial presenting symptom in 90% of patients and may precede other symptoms by several months (Hammack, 2012; Huff, 2015; Kaplan, 2013; Weinstein, 2013).

Figure 31-2. Signs and Symptoms of Spinal Cord Compression

Cervical Spine
- Breathing difficulties
- Loss of sensation in arms
- Headache, neck, shoulder, or arm pain
- Muscle weakness in neck, trunk, arms, and hands
- Paralysis involving neck, trunk, arms, and hands

Thoracic Spine
- Paralysis
- Muscle weakness
- Chest or back pain
- Positive Babinski reflex
- Bladder, bowel, and sexual dysfunction
- Loss of sensation below the tumor level
- Increased sensation above the tumor level

Lumbar-Sacral Spine
- Paralysis
- Foot drop
- Weakness in the legs and feet
- Loss of sensation in the legs and feet
- Decreased or absent reflexes in the legs
- Bladder, bowel, and sexual dysfunction
- Lower back pain that may radiate down the legs or into the perineal area

Note. Based on information from Becker & Baehring, 2011; Flaherty, 2011; Kaplan, 2013.

From "Structural Oncologic Emergencies" (p. 713), by M. Kaplan in B.H. Gobel, S. Triest-Robertson, and W. Vogel (Eds.), *Advanced Oncology Nursing Certification Review and Resource Manual* (2nd ed.), 2016, Pittsburgh, PA: Oncology Nursing Society. Copyright 2016 by Oncology Nursing Society. Reprinted with permission.

---

    a) Pain localized over the area of the cord compression is the most common initial symptom. It is described as dull, aching, and constant and increases greatly in the supine position.

    b) Radicular pain that radiates into the extremities or across the chest or abdomen is less common. It may be described as a dull ache or a burning, shooting pain or as a tight band across the chest or abdomen.

    c) Both local and radicular pain are exacerbated by coughing, sneezing, movement, and straining at stool.

    d) Pain also may be referred to an area distant from the site of cord compression and thus is difficult to localize (see Figure 31-3).

2. Motor weakness is the second most common symptom at presentation and follows pain by weeks to months (Becker & Baehring, 2015; Hammack, 2012; Kaplan, 2013).

    a) Weakness generally begins in the legs. It may be described as leg stiffness or heaviness and reflects muscle spasticity (Becker & Baehring, 2015; Kaplan, 2013).

    b) The association with SCC may be missed because weakness is a common symptom in patients with advanced cancer (Kaplan, 2013).

3. Sensory deficits may be present and generally relate to the level of cord compression.

Figure 31-3. Types of Pain Associated With Spinal Cord Compression

Local Pain
- Definition: pain perceived within 1–2 spinal segments of the cord compression
- Location: back pain is localized near the midline near the site of the cord compression
- Quality: constant dull ache; may be worse in the morning; increases in intensity over time
- Exacerbating factors: reclining position; actions that increase intra-abdominal and intrathoracic pressures (e.g., coughing, sneezing, straining at stool, Valsalva maneuver)
- Relieving factors: sitting or standing positions; sleeping upright

Radicular Pain
- Definition: radiating pain triggered by compression of spinal nerve roots or the cauda equina
- Location: pain radiates in a band like pattern from back to front across the chest or abdomen, or down an extremity along dermatomes supplied by the affected nerve roots
- Quality: varies; may be constant dull ache that is difficult to localize or an easy-to-localize sharp shooting pain provoked by movement of the spine
- Exacerbating factors: movement, coughing, sneezing, Valsalva maneuver, reclining position
- Relieving factors: sitting or standing positions

Referred Pain
- Definition: pain that is perceived in an area distant from the site of spinal cord compression
- Location: pain is poorly localized due to involvement of multiple dermatomes
- Examples: Compression at first lumbar vertebra: pain may be experienced in the iliac crests, hips, or sacroiliac region. Compression at seventh cervical vertebra: pain may be referred to the area between the scapulae.

Note. Based on information from Kaplan, 2006.

From "Back Pain: Is It Spinal Cord Compression?" by M. Kaplan, 2009, *Clinical Journal of Oncology Nursing, 13,* p. 594. Copyright 2009 by the Oncology Nursing Society. Reprinted with permission.

---

    a) Loss of sensation to touch, pinprick, temperature, and of vibration and position sense may occur early (Huff, 2015).

    b) Numbness and paresthesias may be present in the toes and ascend upward over time (Weinstein, 2013).

    c) Loss of sensation in the "saddle" area (buttocks and perineal region) reflects compression of the cauda equina and is called *saddle anesthesia* (Dawodu et al., 2016; Lewis et al., 2011).

4. Reflexes may be hyperactive or hypoactive depending on the level of cord compression (Kaplan, 2013; Sun & Nemecek, 2009).

5. Autonomic dysfunction involving the bowel and bladder usually is a late finding but often is present at diagnosis. Dysfunction is due to loss of sphincter and reflex control (Hammack, 2012; Huff, 2015; Kaplan, 2013).

    a) Urinary retention and incontinence may be present. The patient may be unaware of urinary retention because of reduced bladder sensation (Sun & Nemecek, 2009).

    b) Difficulty expelling stool may progress to constipation and fecal incontinence (Flaherty, 2011).

    c) Sexual dysfunction, loss of sweating below the lesion, and orthostatic hypotension may be present (Hammack, 2012).

6. The ability to walk at presentation is an important indicator of the patient's neurologic status and the most important predictor of functional outcome (Hammack, 2012; Huff, 2015; Weinstein, 2013).

7. Difficulty walking may rapidly progress to irreversible paralysis. The longer SCC goes untreated, the lower the chances for neurologic recovery (Becker & Baehring, 2015; Weinstein, 2013).

IV. Physical examination
  A. Patient history
     1. Known history of cancer, tumor type (see Figure 31-1), date and stage at diagnosis, treatments received and outcome, history of metastatic disease
     2. Assessment of cancer risk factors in patients without a cancer history (i.e., family history, lifestyle behaviors, environmental exposures, history of cancer screening tests with dates and results)
     3. Assessment of back pain: Onset and duration, location and distribution, quality and intensity, and aggravating and alleviating factors. Level of suspicion for SCC increases if patient reports the following (Becker & Baehring, 2015; Flaherty, 2011; Huff, 2015):
        a) Lying supine during the night exacerbates back pain, and sitting or standing relieves it.
        b) Pain increases with coughing, sneezing, or straining at stool.
     4. Preexisting pain conditions: Prior history of acute neck or back pain related to benign degenerative conditions or muscle spasm (Kaplan, 2013)
     5. Motor history: Reports of leg weakness or heaviness, clumsiness, difficulty rising from seated position or climbing stairs, episodes of falling (Becker & Baehring, 2015; Weinstein, 2013)
     6. Bowel changes: Reports of difficulty passing stool or constipation (Flaherty, 2011)
     7. Urination history
        a) Reports of frequent, small voids of urine, stress incontinence, and new-onset nocturia may represent urinary retention (Flaherty, 2011; Weinstein, 2013).
        b) Urinary retention is a more reliable indicator of sphincter dysfunction than urinary incontinence, which often occurs with age (Sun & Nemecek, 2009).
     8. Sexual function: Reports of new-onset impotence in men (Kaplan, 2013)
     9. Changes in activities of daily living
     10. Preexisting health conditions
     11. Current medications and supplements: Prescription and over the counter
  B. Physical assessment (Becker & Baehring, 2015; Flaherty, 2011; Huff, 2015; Kaplan, 2013; Weinstein, 2013)
     1. Pain assessment
        a) Patient can point to site of pain and rank pain intensity via a visual analog scale.
        b) Gentle percussion and palpation of the vertebral column may elicit tenderness over the involved area.
        c) Neck flexion is done with great care to avoid exacerbating injury and may elicit sudden, electric shock–like pain termed the *Lhermitte sign*.
        d) Straight leg raises may cause pain that radiates from the back down the leg and increases on foot dorsiflexion.
     2. Motor function
        a) Evaluate posture, gait, and coordination. Ask the patient to walk and turn around, and observe for smoothness of gait and coordinated arm swinging.
        b) Observe for balance during heel-to-toe walking in a straight line to evaluate for presence of ataxia. Ask the patient to stand on one leg at a time.

  c) Assess coordination by asking the patient to touch the thumb of each hand with each finger in that hand in rapid sequence and to touch his or her nose with the index finger of each hand.

  d) Assess leg strength by observing the patient's ability to rise from a seated position and perform deep knee bends. Ask the patient to resist plantar flexion of each foot.

 3. Sensory perception

  a) Evaluate the patient's ability to sense pain, light touch, temperature, vibration, and proprioception.

  b) Ask the patient to keep eyes closed, and touch the patient's skin on the extremities and trunk with a sharp and then a dull object to localize pain. Light touch is evaluated in this manner using a wisp of cotton or cotton-tipped applicator.

  c) Test temperature sensitivity touching the patient's skin with a metal tuning fork that has been chilled and heated.

  d) Test vibration sensation by holding a tuning fork against the patient's bony prominences.

 4. Proprioception

  a) Ask the patient to stand with feet together and eyes closed. Observe how well this posture is maintained or if swaying or falling occurs.

  b) Move the patient's fingers or toes up or down and ascertain responses about direction of the movements.

 5. Bladder and bowel function

  a) Palpate the patient's abdomen to assess for bladder or bowel distension.

  b) Measure residual urine volume to determine the presence of urinary retention. Ask the patient to void completely, then catheterize the bladder. A residual urine volume greater than 200 ml suggests a neurogenic bladder (Huff, 2015).

 6. Reflex evaluation

  a) Assess tendon reflexes in elbows, knees, and ankles, and test abdominal reflexes and plantar reflexes (known as the *Babinski sign*).

  b) Perform digital rectal examination to assess anal sphincter reflex.

V. Diagnostics

 A. Magnetic resonance imaging (MRI) is currently the gold standard to evaluate SCC and is performed urgently. The entire spine is imaged to assess whether multiple areas are compressed (Becker & Baehring, 2015; Hammack, 2012; McCurdy & Shanholtz, 2012).

 B. Myelography, in conjunction with computed tomography (CT) scanning, is an acceptable alternative for patients in whom MRI is contraindicated (Hammack, 2012; McCurdy & Shanholtz, 2012; Weinstein, 2013).

 C. Plain x-ray, bone scan, CT of the spine, and positron-emission tomography–CT are not effective as the sole imaging modalities for diagnosing early SCC because they cannot adequately visualize the tumor, spinal cord, and paraspinal region (Hammack, 2012; Weinstein, 2013).

VI. Differential diagnosis

 A. Differentiate mechanical back pain related to trauma, arthritis, muscle strain, old vertebral injury, or degenerative disc disorders from SCC-related pain (Kaplan, 2013).

 B. Rule out conditions that can mimic SCC, including spinal inflammation, infection, and benign tumors (e.g., meningiomas) of the cord (Huff, 2015; Schiff, 2015).

    C. Patients with cancer also can experience back pain from vertebral osteoporosis resulting from spinal radiation therapy or corticosteroid use (Weinstein, 2013).

    D. Pain that worsens when the patient lies in the supine position should be considered malignant until proved otherwise (Schiff, 2015).

VII. Interventions

    A. Supportive care

        1. Corticosteroids (Loblaw, Mitera, Ford, & Laperriere, 2012)

           a) Initial supportive therapy administered immediately to patients with SCC who are symptomatic

           b) Dexamethasone is the most widely used corticosteroid for this indication. No standardized dose regimen exists, but two have been recommended depending on the severity of the patient's neurologic symptoms.

               (1) Minimal symptoms: Low-dose regimen is an IV bolus of 10 mg followed by 16 mg daily in divided doses. Dose is gradually tapered over weeks once definitive treatment is underway.

               (2) Severe symptoms: High-dose regimen starts with an IV bolus of 100 mg followed by maintenance doses of up to 96 mg/day with taper over weeks.

           c) Proton pump inhibitor drugs are used prophylactically while the patient is receiving corticosteroids because of increased risk for gastrointestinal ulceration and bleeding (Hammack, 2012).

           d) Patients diagnosed with SCC without neurologic deficits do not require steroids (Loblaw et al., 2012).

        2. Pain management: Administer opioid analgesics on a routine basis and on demand for breakthrough and incident pain. Anticonvulsants, antidepressants, and corticosteroids are adjuvant analgesics that may be effective for neuropathic pain (Flaherty, 2011; Hammack, 2012; Kaplan, 2013).

        3. Anticoagulation to prevent deep vein thrombosis and pulmonary embolism in immobilized patients

           a) Low-molecular-weight heparin is administered daily to immobilized patients with no contraindications (Hammack, 2012; Schiff, Brown, & Shaffrey, 2016).

           b) Immobilized patients should always wear compression stockings (Hammack, 2012).

        4. Bladder function (Flaherty, 2011; Kaplan, 2013)

           a) Monitor fluid intake and output. Increase daily fluid intake to 2 L to prevent urinary tract infection (UTI).

           b) Assess for bladder distension and presence of UTI secondary to urinary retention.

           c) Institute intermittent bladder catheterization if required to help fully empty the bladder.

           d) Perform daily catheter care and perineal hygiene for patients with an indwelling urinary catheter.

        5. Bowel regimen: Opiate analgesics and immobility can exacerbate the constipation that results from autonomic dysfunction (Hammack, 2012).

           a) Treat constipation effectively because straining at stool increases the pain of SCC (Becker & Baehring, 2015).

           b) Establish a daily elimination regimen using stool softeners and bulking agents, intestinal lubricants, and osmotic laxatives as necessary (Kaplan, 2013).

c) Incorporate high-fiber foods into diet, including fresh fruits and vegetables, legumes, and grains.

d) Maintain fluid intake greater than 2 quarts/day and include hot drinks.

6. Skin care: Immobility can lead to skin breakdown over pressure points.

a) Implement a safe, regular turning schedule.

b) Inspect the patient's skin daily.

c) Provide good perineal hygiene.

7. Safety and mobility

a) Place patients with spinal instability on total bedrest and position and move them with great care (Weinstein, 2013).

b) Orthotics, such as a cervical collar or a body brace, can be used to provide nonsurgical stabilization of the bony spine and reduce the pain of movement (Weinstein, 2013).

c) Evidence-based practice guidelines are lacking regarding the role of spinal bracing and proper positioning and transfers for patients with spinal instability due to SCC (Kilbride, Cox, Kennedy, Lee, & Grant, 2010).

d) Mobilize patients following surgery as soon as their condition safely allows.

8. Emotional support and counseling should begin at diagnosis with patients and caregivers. Topics discussed include the risks and benefits of each type of definitive therapy, the patient's prognosis for preserving or restoring functional abilities and for life expectancy following SCC, and referrals to specialists, as appropriate.

B. Definitive therapies: Radiation therapy or surgery (Hammack, 2012)

1. The optimal sequence of first-line therapy has not been established. Individual patient factors influence whether radiation or surgery will be the initial treatment (see Figure 31-4).

2. Indications for radiation as the initial therapy include the presence of radiosensitive tumors (i.e., lymphoma, multiple myeloma, seminoma, small cell lung cancer, prostate, breast), a brief life expectancy, loss of ambulation for more than 48 hours, multiple areas of cord compression, and surgery contraindications (McCurdy & Shanholtz, 2012; Prewett & Venkitaraman, 2010; Schiff et al., 2016)

Figure 31-4. Indications for Surgery or Radiation as First-Line Therapy for Spinal Cord Compression

Indications for Surgery	Indications for Radiation Therapy
• Spinal instability requiring correction	• Unable to tolerate surgery
• Life expectancy greater than 3–4 months	• Life expectancy less than 3 months
• Radioresistant tumor	• Radiosensitive tumor
• Single area of cord compression	• Multiple areas of cord compression
• Prior radiation to area	• Spine is stable
• Loss of ambulation less than 48 hours	• Loss of ambulation more than 48 hours
• Biopsy to determine pathology of unknown tumor	
• Good performance status	

Note. Based on information from Hammack, 2012; Kaplan, 2013; McCurdy & Shanholtz, 2012; Prewett & Venkitaraman, 2010; Schiff et al., 2016.

        a) External beam radiation therapy is used most frequently in a schedule of 30 Gy delivered in 10 fractions. Treatment may be accelerated for patients in severe pain; a single 8 Gy fraction is used (Hammack, 2012; Loblaw et al., 2012; Schiff et al., 2016).

        b) Radiation therapy provides pain relief and inhibits tumor growth (Kaplan, 2013; Weinstein, 2013).

        c) Patients who are ambulatory when radiation begins will most likely remain ambulatory. Of patients who are paraplegic at the start of radiation therapy, only about 5% regain ambulation (Hammack, 2012).

   3. Surgery typically is reserved for patients with a good prognosis or who have spinal instability that needs correction or with radioresistant tumors, such as sarcoma, renal cell, and melanoma (Hammack, 2012; McCurdy & Shanholtz, 2012; Prewett & Venkitaraman, 2010; Schiff et al., 2016) (see Figure 31-4).

   4. Surgical approaches (Becker & Baehring, 2015; McCurdy & Shanholtz, 2012; Schiff et al., 2016; Weinstein, 2013)

        a) Anterior approach with mechanical stabilization is the most common surgical technique.

           (1) Removal of the tumor mass relieves cord compression, and installation of materials and devices reconstructs and stabilizes the spine.

           (2) Bone filler cement (polymethyl methacrylate [PMMA]) is used to fill the surgical bone defect, and a variety of metallic internal fixation devices (e.g., pins, rods, plates) are applied.

           (3) Radiation therapy may be delivered postoperatively to provide better control of local disease (Weinstein, 2013).

        b) Laminectomy was used in the past but currently is indicated only for certain situations because it does not remove the entire tumor mass and increases spinal instability (Hammack, 2012; Schiff et al., 2016).

   5. Vertebroplasty and kyphoplasty (Hammack, 2012; Kaplan, 2013; Schiff et al., 2016)

        a) Both procedures are minimally invasive percutaneous techniques.

        b) They are used for patients who have pain without neurologic manifestations and who cannot tolerate more radical surgery.

        c) PMMA is injected into collapsed vertebrae to provide stability.

        d) Procedures are very effective for reducing pain and can be done on an outpatient basis.

        e) Radiation therapy to the affected area can begin one week after use of PMMA.

   6. Chemotherapy (Hammack, 2012; Kaplan, 2013)

        a) May be used as an adjunct to radiation therapy in treating SCC caused by chemosensitive tumors (i.e., breast, non-Hodgkin lymphoma, myeloma, small cell carcinoma, or germ cell tumors)

        b) May be used to treat recurrent tumors at a site of previous radiation in patients who cannot tolerate surgery

C. Evaluation and follow-up: Nursing care and evaluation are individualized to each patient depending on their neurologic status and spinal stability (see Figure 31-5).

   1. Pain control: Assess pain on a regular basis, provide pain relief and comfort measures, and assess efficacy.

   2. Safety and mobility

Figure 31-5. Nursing Interventions in the Care of Patients With Cancer and Spinal Cord Compression

- Institute pain relief measures, and evaluate effectiveness.
- Conduct ongoing assessment of sensory and motor functions.
- Measure vital signs, with attention to respiration, and fluid intake and output.
- Provide education and reassurance related to treatment modalities.
- Evaluate objective and subjective responses to therapy.
- Institute safety measures to prevent injury and further neurologic damage.
- Mobilize patients, and assist them with weight-bearing activities and proper body mechanics as appropriate.
- Manage preventive skincare regimen.
- Monitor nutrition and fluid status.
- Assess for bladder distension and need for urinary catheter.
- Assess bowel function, and establish an elimination program.
- Coordinate activity regimen and rehabilitation program.
- Assess coping mechanisms related to cancer diagnosis, altered body image, and changes in sexual function.
- Facilitate adaptation to neurologic deficits and advancing disease.
- Support patients and caregivers in accepting functional limitations and addressing end-of-life issues.

Note. Based on information from Brumbaugh, 2009; Flaherty, 2011; Miaskowski, 2009; Myers, 2007; Osowski, 2002.

From "Spinal Cord Compression" (p. 371), by M. Kaplan in M. Kaplan (Ed.), *Understanding and Managing Oncologic Emergencies: A Resource for Nurses* (2nd ed.), 2013, Pittsburgh, PA: Oncology Nursing Society. Copyright 2013 by Oncology Nursing Society. Reprinted with permission.

---

    a) Assess motor and sensory function routinely to detect changes from baseline. Mobilize patients according to findings of stable or unstable spine.

    b) Assess immobilized patients routinely for the presence of pressure ulcers, deep vein thromboses, respiratory infections, and joint contractures.

    c) Postoperatively, provide nursing care that includes serial neurologic assessments, pain assessment and management, wound care, body alignment, and maintenance of spinal stability.

    d) Mobilize patients following surgery as soon as their condition safely allows.

3. Skin care (Dawodu et al., 2016; Stubblefield, 2015)

    a) Meticulous skin assessment and skin care begin on admission and are ongoing.

    b) Place immobilized patients on high-airflow mattress; apply heel protectors.

    c) Implement safe position changes for immobilized patients every two hours as feasible.

    d) Monitor patients receiving radiation therapy for skin changes in the treated area and instructions regarding skin care provided per institution protocols.

4. Bladder dysfunction

    a) Monitor intake and output. Encourage daily fluid intake greater than 2 L.

    b) Assess for bladder distension and UTI.

5. Bowel regimen

    a) Institute a bowel regimen to achieve daily stool output.

    b) Assess abdomen for signs of distension and presence of bowel sounds.

    c) Check daily for presence of stool impaction.

6. Functional status

a) Monitor functional status on a regular basis to identify changes that may indicate progressive disease or recurrent SCC.

b) Monitor for signs of autonomic dysreflexia that can be triggered by a distended bladder or bowel in patients with cord compression at T6 or higher.

c) Classic signs of autonomic dysreflexia include elevated blood pressure, pounding headache, bradycardia, flushing, and profuse sweating above the level of the spinal block (Yadav, Shin, Guo, & Konzen, 2009).

7. Rehabilitation
   a) Goals
      (1) Maximize and restore function where feasible.
      (2) Protect patients from injury and further neurologic damage.
      (3) Promote safety and comfort.
   b) A multidisciplinary team approach is used. Team members may include physical and occupational therapists, social workers, homecare and palliative care nurses, and the patients and caregivers.
   c) Evaluate patients' needs for assistive devices, such as specialized hospital bed, wheelchair, or ramps in the home.
   d) Coordinate an activity regimen and rehabilitation program.
   e) Provide strength training or passive range-of-motion exercises.

8. Patient and caregiver education: Patients are prepared for discharge to home or hospice by receiving written and verbal instructions regarding the following:
   a) Proper positioning, safe transfer methods, falls prevention, use of assistive devices
   b) Daily strength training or passive range-of-motion exercises
   c) Adherence to medication schedules
   d) Treatment modalities and recognition and reporting of side effects
   e) Self-catheterization at home, if indicated, and recognition and reporting of signs of UTI
   f) Pain management techniques
   g) Regular skin assessment and use of products to protect the skin and bony prominences
   h) Regular bowel regimen

9. Emotional support
   a) Assess patient and caregiver coping mechanisms regarding dealing with patients' limitations in function, changes in life roles (at work and in the family and community), changes in sexuality and self-image, increased dependence, altered living arrangements, and impending mortality.
   b) Encourage expression of feelings, fears, and concerns.
   c) Provide support for decision making regarding end-of-life issues and anticipatory grieving.
   d) Provide referrals to specialists as appropriate.

D. Referrals
   1. Pain specialists are consulted early.
   2. Physiatrist to prescribe a rehabilitation program of physical or occupational therapy
   3. Social worker to plan for the patients' discharge home or to hospice care
   4. Palliative care team consult

Case Study

M.J. is a 67-year-old man who completed treatment for stage IIB non-small cell lung cancer nine months ago. He calls his oncologist's office to report pain in his mid-back of about three weeks' duration. He has recently noticed tingling in his toes. The oncology advanced practice registered nurse (APRN) sets up an appointment for M.J. to be seen in the office the following day. At the office, M.J. reports that the back pain feels like a dull ache that increases when he lies down and is worst on awakening in the morning. He rates the pain as a 7 on a visual analog scale of 0–10. He feels better sitting upright. He reports that his legs feel heavy and that it takes a lot of effort to climb the stairs to his bedroom. He also reports that he has to get up several times during the night to void small amounts of urine and has had trouble expelling stool.

The APRN performs a neurologic examination and notes that M.J. has weakness in both legs with hyperactive reflexes. A positive Babinski sign is present bilaterally. Vibration and joint position sense are reduced in his legs. Pinprick testing reveals a sensory level to T8. On palpation, M.J.'s bladder appears distended, which indicates retained urine.

An MRI of M.J.'s entire spine is ordered emergently. He is given 100 mg of dexamethasone IV as a loading dose. MRI results confirm the presence of direct extension of the lung tumor into the epidural space causing cord compression at the level of T9. M.J. is referred for consults with neurosurgery and radiation oncology.

After discussions with the specialists and M.J. and his wife, surgical intervention is selected as the initial treatment to relieve the cord compression with radiation therapy to follow. M.J. undergoes a surgical decompression through an anterior approach with vertebral fusion to stabilize the spine. Pathologic evaluation of the excised tumor reveals the same pathology as the original non-small cell lung tumor. Three weeks following surgery, M.J. begins a 10-day course of external beam radiation therapy to a total dose of 30 Gy. Throughout the definitive treatments, M.J. receives dexamethasone in tapered doses along with omeprazole, a proton pump inhibitor drug, to protect against gastrointestinal adverse events.

During this period, the APRN meets with M.J. and his wife to provide written and verbal instructions about performing wound and skin care, managing bladder dysfunction and avoiding UTIs, promoting bowel evacuation, managing medication administration and side effects, and pain control strategies. A physical therapist visits M.J. and his wife at home regularly to do strength training exercises and recommended falls safety precautions for the home environment.

M.J. recovers well from his treatments and regains his leg strength and sensation within four weeks of treatment completion. Fortunately, the SCC was recognized and treated before he lost the ability to walk. He also begins systemic therapy for his advanced lung cancer using erlotinib, a biologic agent targeted against the epidermal growth factor receptor. M.J.'s prognosis for survival related to lung cancer is limited, but his current quality of life and functional independence have been restored with the successful management of his SCC.

References

Becker, K.P., & Baehring, J.M. (2011). Oncologic emergencies: Spinal cord compression. In V.T. DeVita Jr., S. Hellman, & S.A. Rosenberg (Eds.), *Cancer: Principles and practice of oncology* (9th ed., pp. 2136–2141). Philadelphia, PA: Wolters Kluwer Health/Lippincott Williams & Wilkins.

Becker, K.P., & Baehring, J.M. (2015). Oncologic emergencies: Spinal cord compression. In V.T. DeVita Jr., S. Hellman, & S.A. Rosenberg (Eds.), *Cancer: Principles and practice of oncology* (10th ed., pp. 1816–1821). Philadelphia, PA: Wolters Kluwer Health/Lippincott Williams & Wilkins.

Brumbaugh, H.L. (2009). Structural oncologic emergencies. In B.H. Gobel, S. Triest-Robertson, & W.H. Vogel (Eds.), *Advanced oncology nursing certification review and resource manual* (pp. 599–636). Pittsburgh, PA: Oncology Nursing Society.

Dawodu, S.T., Beeson, M.S., Bechtel, K.A., Kellam, J.F., Hodges, S.D., & Humphreys, S.C. (2016, May 6). Cauda equina and conus medullaris syndromes. Retrieved from http://emedicine.medscape.com/article/1148690-overview

Flaherty, A.M. (2011). Spinal cord compression. In C.H. Yarbro, D. Wujcik, & B.H. Gobel (Eds.), *Cancer nursing: Principles and practice* (7th ed., pp. 979–994). Burlington, MA: Jones & Bartlett Learning.

Hammack, J.E. (2012). Spinal cord disease in patients with cancer. *Continuum, 18,* 312–327. doi:10.1212/01.CON.0000413660.58045.ae

Huff, J.S. (2015, February 9). Spinal cord neoplasms. Retrieved from http://emedicine.medscape.com/article/779872-overview

Kaplan, M. (2006). Spinal cord compression. In M. Kaplan (Ed.), *Understanding and managing oncologic emergencies: A resource for nurses* (pp. 219–259). Pittsburgh, PA: Oncology Nursing Society.

Kaplan, M. (2013). Spinal cord compression. In M. Kaplan (Ed.), *Understanding and managing oncologic emergencies: A resource for nurses* (2nd ed., pp. 337–383). Pittsburgh, PA: Oncology Nursing Society.

Kilbride, L., Cox, M., Kennedy, C.M., Lee, S.H., & Grant, R. (2010). Metastatic spinal cord compression: A review of practice and care. *Journal of Clinical Nursing, 19,* 1767–1783. doi:10.1111/j.1365-2702.2010.03236.x

Lewis, M.A., Hendrickson, A.W., & Moynihan, T.J. (2011). Oncologic emergencies: Pathophysiology, presentation, diagnosis, and treatment. *CA: A Cancer Journal for Clinicians, 61,* 287–314. doi:10.3322/caac.20124

Loblaw, D.A., Mitera, G., Ford, M., & Laperriere, N.J. (2012). A 2011 updated systematic review and clinical practice guideline for the management of malignant extradural spinal cord compression. *International Journal of Radiation Oncology, Biology, Physics, 84,* 312–317. doi:10.1016/j.ijrobp.2012.01.014

McCurdy, M.T., & Shanholtz, C.B. (2012). Oncologic emergencies. *Critical Care Medicine, 40,* 2212–2222. doi:10.1097/CCM.0b013e31824e1865

Miaskowski, C. (2009). Spinal cord compression. In C.C. Chernecky & K. Murphy-Ende (Eds.), *Acute care oncology nursing* (2nd ed., pp. 492–498). St. Louis, MO: Elsevier Saunders.

Myers, J.S. (2007). Structural oncologic complications. In M.E. Langhorne, J.S. Fulton, & S.E. Otto (Eds.), *Oncology nursing* (5th ed., pp. 412–417). St. Louis, MO: Mosby.

Osowski, M. (2002, October 14). Spinal cord compression: An obstructive oncologic emergency. *Topics in Advanced Practice Nursing eJournal, 2*(4). Retrieved from http://www.medscape.com/viewarticle/442735

Prewett, S., & Venkitaraman, R. (2010). Metastatic spinal cord compression: Review of the evidence for a radiotherapy dose fractionation schedule. *Clinical Oncology, 22,* 222–230. doi:10.1016/j.clon.2010.01.006

Schiff, D. (2015, November 9). Clinical features and diagnosis of neoplastic epidural spinal cord compression, including cauda equina syndrome [Literature review current through May 2016]. Retrieved from http://www.uptodate.com/contents/clinical-features-and-diagnosis-of-neoplastic-epidural-spinal-cord-compression-including-cauda-equina-syndrome

Schiff, D., Brown, P., & Shaffrey, M.E. (2016, February 22). Treatment and prognosis of neoplastic epidural spinal cord compression, including cauda equina syndrome [Literature review current through April 2016]. Retrieved from http://www.uptodate.com/contents/treatment-and-prognosis-of-neoplastic-epidural-spinal-cord-compression-including-cauda-equina-syndrome

Stubblefield, M.D. (2015). Rehabilitation of the cancer patient. In V.T. DeVita Jr., T.S. Lawrence, & S.A. Rosenberg (Eds.), *Cancer: Principles and practice of oncology* (10th ed., pp. 2141–2162). Philadelphia, PA: Wolters Kluwer Health/Lippincott Williams & Wilkins.

Sugerman, R.A. (2013). Structure and function of the neurologic system. In K.L. McCance & S.E. Huether (Eds.), *Pathophysiology: The biologic basis for disease in adults and children* (7th ed., pp. 447–483). St. Louis, MO: Elsevier Mosby.

Sun, H., & Nemecek, A.N. (2009). Optimal management of malignant epidural spinal cord compression. *Emergency Medicine Clinics of North America, 27,* 195–208. doi:10.1016/j.emc.2009.02.001

Weinstein, S.M. (2013). Management of spinal cord and cauda equina compression. In A.M. Berger, J.L. Shuster Jr., & J.H. Von Roenn (Eds.), *Principles and practice of palliative care and supportive oncology* (4th ed., pp. 514–528). Philadelphia, PA: Wolters Kluwer Health/Lippincott Williams & Wilkins.

Yadav, R., Shin, K.Y., Guo, Y., & Konzen, B. (2009). Cancer rehabilitation. In S.-C.J. Yeung, C.P. Escalante, & R.F. Gagel (Eds.), *Medical care of cancer patients* (pp. 563–570). Shelton, CT: BC Decker.

CHAPTER 32

Superior Vena Cava Syndrome

Marcelle Kaplan, MS, RN, CBCN®, CNS

I. Definition
   A. Superior vena cava syndrome (SVCS) is a spectrum of signs and symptoms that occur when obstruction of the superior vena cava (SVC) reduces venous blood return from the upper body to the right side of the heart (National Cancer Institute [NCI], 2015).
   B. SVC obstruction can be caused by extrinsic malignant masses or intrinsic thrombus or tumor (Kaplan, 2016; Shelton, 2013).
   C. SVCS affects about 15,000 people per year in the United States (Feng & Pennell, 2012). Most cases are due to malignancy, but nonmalignant conditions, especially thrombus formation related to the presence of intravascular devices, are increasingly associated with SVCS incidence (Beeson, 2014; Drews & Rabkin, 2016; Feng & Pennell, 2012).
   D. The appearance of SVCS may be the first indication of an unsuspected lung cancer (Feng & Pennell, 2012).
      1. Patients with right-sided lung cancers, especially men, have the highest risk for SVCS.
      2. However, the risk is low, affecting less than 10% of patients with lung cancer (Escalante, Manzullo, & Weiss, 2015; Nickloes et al., 2015; Theodore & Jablons, 2010).
   E. Enlarged mediastinal lymph nodes from non-Hodgkin lymphoma (NHL) and, less commonly, tumors (thymoma or germ cell tumor) or metastatic disease in the mediastinum (from breast, thyroid, and melanoma) also contribute to the incidence of SVCS (Drews & Rabkin, 2016; Feng & Pennell, 2012; Nickloes et al., 2015).
   F. SVCS does not often lead directly to death. Rather, survival depends on the status of the patient's underlying malignancy and response to antineoplastic therapies (NCI, 2015).
   G. SVCS becomes an emergency when venous blood return to the heart is compromised to the extent that cardiac output becomes inadequate to meet the needs of the body or complete obstruction of the SVC leads to cerebral edema and increased intracranial pressure (Shelton, 2013; Theodore & Jablons, 2010).
II. Pathophysiology
   A. The SVC is the major vessel that returns venous blood from the upper body (head, neck, arms, upper thorax) to the right atrium of the heart.

B. It is a thin-walled vein with low-pressure blood flow that is surrounded tightly by several structures in the mediastinum, including the sternum, trachea, right bronchus, aorta, pulmonary artery, vertebrae, and lymph node chains (Kaplan, 2016).

C. Because of its location and characteristics, the SVC is vulnerable to compression by space-occupying masses in the middle mediastinum, such as tumor masses or enlarged lymph nodes (Kaplan, 2016).

D. SVC obstruction that is partial and develops gradually (usually due to enlarging external tumor mass) allows time for collateral circulation to develop through the azygous venous system and is less severe (Shelton, 2013; Theodore & Jablons, 2010) (see Figure 32-1).

E. Intravascular thrombus formation plus external compression by tumor are factors most often responsible for sudden complete SVC obstruction; collateral venous circulation has not had time to develop (Ahmann, 1984).

F. Severe obstruction of the SVC leads to elevated venous pressure in the upper body and decreased cardiac filling and cardiac output due to reduced blood return to the heart can ultimately progress to respiratory distress and cerebral edema (Drews & Rabkin, 2016; Shelton, 2013).

III. Presenting symptoms

A. The clinical manifestations of SVCS depend on how rapidly and completely the SVC becomes obstructed and whether collateral blood vessels have had time to develop (Drews & Rabkin, 2016; Feng & Pennell, 2012; NCI, 2015).

B. Partial SVC obstruction may be asymptomatic or produce subtle signs and symptoms that reflect venous engorgement and edema, such as nasal congestion (Kaplan, 2016; Nickloes et al., 2014). See Figure 32-2 for early manifestations of SVCS.

C. Symptoms often progress gradually over a period of weeks and subside as collateral circulation develops (Drews & Rabkin, 2016; Shelton, 2013).

D. Presenting symptoms that patients may report
   1. Dyspnea, most commonly (Beeson, 2014; Nickloes et al., 2015)
   2. Nasal stuffiness (Beeson, 2014; Nickloes et al., 2015)
   3. Rings and shirt collars feel tight due to swelling of the face, neck, and arms (Stoke sign) (Shelton, 2013).
   4. Sense of "fullness" in the head, which may increase on bending to tie shoelaces, stooping, coughing, or lying down (Escalante et al., 2015; Nickloes et al., 2015; Shelton, 2013)
   5. Symptoms increase when lying down; sleeping in an upright position increases comfort (Escalante et al., 2015; Shelton, 2013).
   6. Nonproductive cough, hoarseness and dysphagia, visual changes, chest pain (Drews & Rabkin, 2016; Feng & Pennell, 2012)
   7. Mental status changes, including irritability, headaches, lethargy, and confusion (Drews & Rabkin, 2016; Feng & Pennell, 2012)

E. SVCS that develops rapidly can produce severe effects on the respiratory, cardiac, and central nervous systems (Kaplan, 2016). See Figure 32-3 for late manifestations of SVCS.

F. Yu, Wilson, and Detterbeck (2008) have proposed a system to classify the severity of SVCS based on symptom presentation to help differentiate patients who require urgent intervention from those who can begin treatment first for the precipitating malignancy. In this system, symptom grading progresses from asymptomatic to mild

---

Figure 32-1. Superior Vena Cava Obstruction With Azygos Venous System

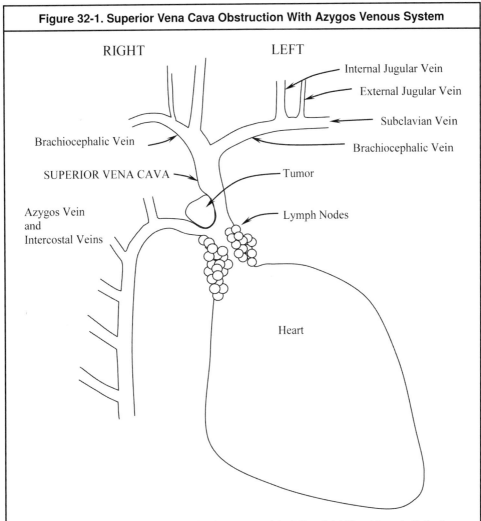

The superior vena cava (SVC) is formed by the merger of the left and right brachiocephalic (or innominate) veins in the upper mediastinum. They are the major veins returning blood to the SVC and are formed by the convergence of the corresponding internal jugular and subclavian veins.

Note. From "Superior Vena Cava Syndrome" (p. 389), by B.K. Shelton in M. Kaplan (Ed.), *Understanding and Managing Oncologic Emergencies: A Resource for Nurses* (2nd ed.), 2013, Pittsburgh, PA: Oncology Nursing Society. Copyright 2013 by Oncology Nursing Society. Reprinted with permission.

(head and neck edema, cyanosis, and ruddy face), moderate (cough, mild dysphagia, and ocular edema), severe (cerebral edema with headache and dizziness), and finally, fatal (Yu et al., 2008).

IV. Physical examination

    A. A careful history is important to identify the underlying etiology of SVCS, including risk factors for cancer (either as initial presentation or recurrence): history of prior cancer, smoking, and environmental and occupational risk factors; the presence of central venous catheters or pacemakers; and history of thoracic radiation and infections.

Figure 32-2. Early Manifestations of Superior Vena Cava Syndrome

- Dyspnea
- Feeling of fullness in head or neck
- Nasal congestion
- Face and neck edema
- Shirt collar becomes tight
- Upper extremity edema
- Thoracic and breast edema (in women)

- Cyanosis of face and arms
- Nonproductive cough
- Periorbital and conjunctival edema
- Plethora (ruddy facial complexion)
- Dilated veins in neck and upper chest
- Chest pain

Note. Based on information from Escalante et al., 2015; Feng & Pennell, 2012; Kaplan, 2016; Shelton, 2013; Yu et al., 2008.

Figure 32-3. Late Manifestations of Superior Vena Cava Syndrome

Respiratory System	**Cardiac System**	**Central Nervous System (related to cerebral edema)**
• Respiratory distress (dyspnea, orthopnea) • Tachypnea • Laryngeal or glossal edema causing hoarseness, stridor, dysphagia • Aspiration due to paralysis of the true vocal cord secondary to pressure on cranial nerve X (recurrent laryngeal nerve) • Pleural effusion (mainly right-sided)	• Tachycardia • Hypotension, syncope • Congestive heart failure • Hypoxia • Hemodynamic compromise causing dizziness, renal insufficiency	• Severe headache • Irritability • Visual disturbances • Mental status changes reflecting increased intracranial pressure: lethargy, confusion, obtundation, seizures, coma, death • Horner syndrome due to pressure on cervical sympathetic nerves

Note. Based on information from Drews & Rabkin, 2016; Escalante et al., 2015; Feng & Pennell, 2012; Kaplan, 2016; Shelton, 2013; Yahalom, 2011; Yu et al., 2008.

B. The physical examination alone is often sufficient to make the diagnosis of SVCS (Drews & Rabkin, 2016; Nickloes et al., 2015; Theodore & Jablons, 2010).

C. The patient may have the classic SVCS appearance resulting from edema involving the face and periorbital area and the upper thorax and upper extremities, facial plethora and cyanotic skin discoloration due to venous engorgement, and distended veins in the neck and upper extremities (Drews & Rabkin, 2016; Escalante et al., 2015; Feng & Pennell, 2012; Nickloes et al., 2015; Theodore & Jablons, 2010).

  1. Prominent veins on the chest wall and abdomen represent collateral circulation (Feng & Pennell, 2012; Theodore & Jablons, 2010).

  2. Breast swelling in women may be apparent (Kaplan, 2016)

  3. Papilledema may be noted (Nickloes et al., 2015).

  4. Cardiac symptoms may include tachycardia, hypotension, and congestive heart failure. Blood pressure may be high in the right arm and low in the legs (Shelton, 2013).

  5. Manifestations of respiratory distress, including stridor, tachypnea, and even pleural effusion, may be present (Theodore & Jablons, 2010; Yahalom, 2011).

D. Horner syndrome (ptosis and constricted pupil in one eye with loss of sweating on the same side of the face), a marker of lung cancer, may rarely be present (Beeson, 2014; Shelton, 2013).

V. Diagnostics
  A. SVCS diagnosis usually is made on the basis of the presenting symptoms and physical examination (Drews & Rabkin, 2016; Nickloes et al., 2015; Theodore & Jablons, 2010).
  B. Imaging tests and tissue diagnosis confirm the diagnosis and determine the etiology (Drews & Rabkin, 2016; Feng & Pennell, 2012; Nickloes et al., 2015).
  C. Imaging tests
    1. Chest x-ray: Often the initial imaging method
      a) Most commonly reveals a tumor mass, widened mediastinum, and pleural effusion (Yahalom, 2011)
      b) Thrombus formation within the SVC cannot be imaged by chest x-ray (Nickloes et al., 2015).
    2. Chest computed tomography (CT) scan with contrast: Provides details about the SVC obstruction and collateral venous circulation and guides biopsy procedures to attain tissue samples (Nickloes et al., 2015)
    3. MRI: May be used for patients who are allergic to contrast agents or have renal failure, or who will undergo SVC stenting (Nickloes et al., 2015)
    4. Contrast venography: Useful when thrombus formation is the cause of SVC obstruction (Drews & Rabkin, 2016) and when surgical interventions such as SVC stenting or bypass are planned (Nickloes et al., 2015)
  D. Tissue diagnosis is needed before initiation of SVCS treatment unless symptom severity prompts emergency intervention (Drews & Rabkin, 2016; Nickloes et al., 2015).
  E. Tissue diagnosis is made using the least invasive techniques (Drews & Rabkin, 2016; Feng & Pennell, 2012; Yahalom, 2011).
    1. Cytology examination of sputum or pleural fluid to diagnose lung cancer
    2. Biopsy of superficial masses or palpable lymph nodes in the cervical or supraclavicular areas
    3. Bone marrow biopsy to diagnose lymphoma or small cell lung cancer
    4. Percutaneous CT-guided fine needle biopsy of lung lesions
    5. If other methods are not successful, more invasive procedures to acquire tissue for a definitive diagnosis include mediastinoscopy, bronchoscopy, and video-assisted thoracoscopy or conventional thoracotomy.
VI. Differential diagnosis
  A. Apart from cancer, several nonmalignant conditions can cause SVCS (see Figure 32-4).
  B. Other conditions that can cause changes in the mediastinum and lead to symptoms similar to SVCS are listed in Figure 32-5.

Figure 32-4. Nonmalignant Causes of Superior Vena Cava Syndrome

- Thrombosis related to the presence of central venous catheter (most common cause in patients with cancer)
- Fibrosis in the mediastinum secondary to radiation therapy or tuberculosis
- Substernal thyroid goiter
- Vascular conditions: aortic aneurysm, arteriovenous fistulas, vasculitis
- Infections: actinomycosis, aspergillosis, histoplasmosis, syphilis
- Benign mediastinal tumors: teratoma, thymoma, dermoid cyst
- Granulomatous conditions, such as sarcoidosis or silicosis

Note. Based on information from Beeson, 2014; Drews & Rabkin, 2016; Escalante et al., 2015; Nickloes et al., 2015; Theodore & Jablons, 2010.

Figure 32-5. Differential Diagnoses for Superior Vena Cava Syndrome

- Acute respiratory distress syndrome
- Aortic dissection
- Cardiac tamponade
- Chronic obstructive pulmonary disease
- Congestive heart failure
- Constrictive pericarditis
- Pneumonia
- Postradiation mediastinal fibrosis
- Syphilis
- Tuberculosis

Note. Based on information from Beeson, 2014; Drews & Rabkin, 2016; Feng & Pennell, 2012; Nickloes et al., 2015; Theodore & Jablons, 2010.

VII. Interventions
    A. In general, SVCS does not require immediate emergency treatment unless severe or life-threatening symptoms are present because of upper airway obstruction or cerebral edema (Drews & Rabkin, 2016; Nickloes et al., 2015).
    B. Management goals are symptom relief and treatment of the underlying disease precipitating SVCS.
    C. Chemotherapy is the treatment of choice for patients with chemosensitive malignancies, especially non-Hodgkin lymphoma, small cell lung cancer, and germ cell tumors (Drews & Rabkin, 2016; NCI, 2015; Nickloes et al., 2015). When there is venous stasis in the upper extremities and the thorax, chemotherapy may be administered through a dorsal foot vein (Drews & Rabkin, 2016) or a femoral vein (Shelton, 2013).
    D. Radiation therapy is delivered urgently to relieve SVCS obstruction when life-threatening symptoms are present. It is the standard treatment for SVCS caused by non-small cell lung cancer (NSCLC) (Escalante et al., 2015).
    E. Endovascular stent placement has been recommended as the first treatment choice to relieve severe SVCS symptoms.
        1. Agreement is lacking on the need for anticoagulation after stenting (Fagedet et al., 2013; Lanciego et al., 2009).
        2. Endovascular stenting also is recommended to palliate symptoms of SVCS related to newly diagnosed NSCLC while waiting for radiation therapy, used alone or in combination with chemotherapy, to become effective in treating the malignancy (Drews & Rabkin, 2016).
    F. Thrombolytic therapy is used to treat SVCS due to thrombosis related to the presence of intravascular devices.
        1. Therapy may include thrombectomy, with or without the use of thrombolytic agents, such as tissue plasminogen activator, streptokinase, or urokinase (NCI, 2015; National Comprehensive Cancer Network®, 2015).
        2. Thrombolysis is contraindicated in patients with absolute risk factors for bleeding, including hemorrhagic stroke, surgery, or head injury in the previous three weeks; ischemic stroke within the prior three months; or severe thrombocytopenia (National Comprehensive Cancer Network, 2015).
    G. Balloon angioplasty may be used emergently in some patients to open an SVC obstruction (Escalante et al., 2015) and in preparation for stent placement (De Raet, Vos, Morshuis, & van Boven, 2012).
    H. Surgical bypass graft or open surgical procedures usually are limited to patients with SVCS due to benign conditions (Escalante et al., 2015) but rarely may be performed in patients with unsuccessful endovascular stenting or when the malignant lesion is being resected (De Raet et al., 2012).

I. Adjunct medical management
   1. Loop diuretics such as furosemide can provide immediate relief of edema, but care must be taken to avoid dehydration and decreased blood flow. Dosage depends on the patient's fluid status and renal function (Escalante et al., 2015).
   2. Corticosteroids may be useful for treating SVCS in certain situations.
      a) To reduce the risk of respiratory inflammation in patients receiving emergency radiation therapy for severe airway obstruction. Drug dosage depends on symptom severity (Drews & Rabkin, 2016; Escalante et al., 2015).
      b) To reduce the inflammation and edema surrounding the tumor mass (Beeson, 2014)
      c) To treat SVCS caused by lymphoma or thymoma, both of which are sensitive to the effects of corticosteroids (Drews & Rabkin, 2016)
J. Evaluation and follow-up (Kaplan, 2016; Shelton, 2013)
   1. Assess cardiac, respiratory, and neurologic status and report changes.
   2. Assess for pain and anxiety, and provide pharmacologic and nonpharmacologic interventions to alleviate symptoms.
   3. Institute measures to palliate symptoms.
      a) Promote oxygenation by elevating the head of the bed or sitting the patient upright, restricting activities, allaying anxiety, and providing supplemental oxygen.
      b) Maintain fluid balance to prevent dehydration and potential clot formation and avoid fluid overload.
      c) Administer IV infusions and perform blood draws and blood pressure measurements in lower extremities when edema and elevated venous pressure are present in arms.
      d) Institute bowel regimen to avoid straining at stool, which increases venous pressure.
   4. Provide instructions about administration of anticoagulants and signs of bleeding, as appropriate.
   5. Monitor efficacy and side effects of treatments, and provide education to patients and caregivers about managing and reporting side effects.
   6. Provide emotional support to patients and caregivers who may be anxious and frightened by the symptoms produced by SVCS.
   7. Provide education about the cause and management of symptoms of SVCS.
   8. Teach patients and caregivers to recognize and report manifestations of SVCS.
   9. Support the decision to decline aggressive cancer therapies, as appropriate.
K. Referrals
   1. Thoracic surgeon
   2. Hematologist or oncologist
   3. Radiation therapist
   4. Interventional radiologist
   5. Palliative care team
   6. Home care or hospice services

Case Study

J.S. is a 78-year-old retired construction worker who has been in general good health until recent weeks. His prior medical history includes hypertension and gout. He is visiting the clinic today with his wife because he has experienced several distressing symptoms over the past several weeks that seem to be increasing in severity. The advanced practice registered nurse (APRN) meets J.S. and his wife in a quiet room to gather a detailed history and perform a physical assessment. When questioned, J.S. reports that he has become short of breath even at rest and needs to sleep on several pillows to help him breathe and to relieve a "full" feeling in his head; his nose seems always to be stuffed; and his shirt collars have become tight and uncomfortable. He had to remove his wedding ring because it was digging into his finger. He has also developed a dry cough and his voice has become hoarse. His wife has to cut his food into small pieces to make swallowing food easier. J.S.'s wife tells the APRN that her husband's personality has changed; he has become irritable and has developed headaches, which were uncommon in the past.

In conducting the physical assessment, the APRN observes J.S.'s facial features and notes that he has edema of the face, periorbital area, and neck, as well as a ruddy complexion. His neck veins are distended, his upper extremities and upper thorax are edematous, and a prominent venous circulation pattern is present. His vital signs indicate tachypnea and tachycardia, and he cannot lie flat on the examination table without becoming short of breath. Based on J.S.'s presenting symptoms and physical examination, the APRN understands that he is experiencing respiratory distress most likely due to the presence of SVCS and orders an immediate chest x-ray. The chest x-ray reveals a mass in the upper lobe of the right lung, a widened mediastinum, dilation of the SVC, and engorged collateral veins.

The APRN consults with an interventional radiologist to obtain a CT of the chest with contrast to provide more details about the SVC obstruction and to guide a concurrent percutaneous fine needle biopsy of the lung mass. A tissue sample is needed to make a definitive diagnosis of the precipitating malignancy and to formulate an appropriate treatment plan. Pathology results indicate the presence of NSCLC. Based on workup to determine the extent of disease, J.S. is diagnosed with stage IIB NSCLC.

The APRN provides J.S. and his wife with emotional support and instructions about how to help palliate his distressing symptoms at home, including elevating the head of the bed, restricting physical activities, taking supplemental oxygen, maintaining adequate fluid intake to prevent both dehydration and fluid overload, and instituting a bowel regimen to minimize straining at stool.

Prompt initiation of radiation therapy is the recommended treatment for SVCS due to NSCLC, but, because J.S. has severe symptoms, the treatment team decides to provide him with immediate symptom relief by opening the SVC obstruction with an endovascular stent. The stent placement is completed successfully, and significant symptom relief occurs in a matter of days. During this time, J.S. begins treatment with radiation therapy in combination with chemotherapy to shrink the lung tumor mass causing SVC compression. During radiation therapy, dexamethasone is prescribed to reduce the risk of airway swelling and inflammation that would lead to further respiratory distress. Steroid doses are tapered when radiation therapy is completed.

J.S. experiences relief of symptoms almost immediately, and in a few weeks, all symptoms of SVCS are resolved. J.S. is able to complete his NSCLC therapies and is being followed on a routine basis by his radiation and medical oncologists. A positron-emission tomography-CT scan done after completion of antineoplastic therapies showed minimal residual disease. J.S. is then started on targeted therapy with a tyrosine-kinase inhibitor. The APRN provides continued emotional support and teaching to J.S. and his wife about how to recognize and promptly report any signs or symptoms that may indicate recurrence of disease or SVCS.

References

Ahmann, F.R. (1984). A reassessment of the clinical implications of the superior vena caval syndrome. *Journal of Clinical Oncology, 2,* 961–969.

Beeson, M.S. (2014, December 16). Superior vena cava syndrome in emergency medicine. Retrieved from http://emedicine.medscape.com/article/760301-overview

De Raet, J.M., Vos, J.A., Morshuis, W.J., & van Boven, W.-J.P. (2012). Surgical management of superior vena cava syndrome after failed endovascular stenting. *Interactive Cardiovascular and Thoracic Surgery, 15,* 915–917. doi:10.1093/icvts/ivs316

Drews, R.E., & Rabkin, D.J. (2016, March 2). Malignancy-related superior vena cava syndrome [Literature review current through April 2016]. Retrieved from http://www.uptodate.com/contents/malignancy-related-superior-vena-cava-syndrome

Escalante, C.P., Manzullo, E., & Weiss, M. (2015, November 1). Oncologic emergencies and paraneoplastic syndromes: Superior vena cava syndrome. Retrieved from http://www.cancernetwork.com/cancer-management/oncologic-emergencies-and-paraneoplastic-syndromes

Fagedet, D., Thony, F., Timsit, J.-F., Rodiere, M., Monnin-Bares, V., Ferretti, G.R., … Moro-Sibilot, D. (2013). Endovascular treatment of malignant superior vena cava syndrome: Results and predictive factors of clinical efficacy. *Cardiovascular and Interventional Radiology, 36,* 140–149. doi:10.1007/s00270-011-0310-z

Feng, Y., & Pennell, N.A. (2012). Superior vena cava syndrome in lung cancer. *Lung Cancer Management, 1,* 309–315. doi:10.2217/lmt.12.38

Kaplan, M. (2016). Structural oncologic emergencies. In B.H. Gobel, S. Triest-Robertson, & W.H. Vogel (Eds.), *Advanced oncology nursing certification review and resource manual* (2nd ed., pp. 693–736). Pittsburgh, PA: Oncology Nursing Society.

Lanciego, C., Pangua, C., Chacón, J.L., Velasco, J., Boy, R.C., Viana, A., … García, L.G. (2009). Endovascular stenting as the first step in the overall management of malignant superior vena cava syndrome. *American Journal of Roentgenology, 193,* 549–558. doi:10.2214/AJR.08.1904

National Cancer Institute. (2015, August 31). Cardiopulmonary syndromes (PDQ®) [Health professional version]. Retrieved from http://www.cancer.gov/cancertopics/pdq/supportivecare/cardiopulmonary/HealthProfessional/page6

National Comprehensive Cancer Network. (2015). *NCCN Clinical Practice Guidelines in Oncology (NCCN Guidelines®): Cancer-associated venous thromboembolic disease* [v.1.2015]. Retrieved from http://www.nccn.org/professionals/physician_gls/pdf/vte.pdf

Nickloes, T.A., Kallab, A.M., Mack, L.O., Dunlap, A.B., Long, C., & Gandhi, S.S. (2015, September 28). Superior vena cava syndrome. Retrieved from http://emedicine.medscape.com/article/460865-overview

Shelton, B.K. (2013). Superior vena cava syndrome. In M. Kaplan (Ed.), *Understanding and managing oncologic emergencies: A resource for nurses* (2nd ed., pp. 385–410). Pittsburgh, PA: Oncology Nursing Society.

Theodore, P.R., & Jablons, D. (2010). Thoracic wall, pleura, mediastinum, and lung. In G.M. Doherty (Ed.), *Current diagnosis and treatment: Surgery* (13th ed.). Retrieved from http://www.accesssurgery.com/content.aspx?aID=5214160

Yahalom, J. (2011). Oncologic emergencies: Superior vena cava syndrome. In V.T. DeVita Jr., S. Hellman, & S.A. Rosenberg (Eds.), *Cancer: Principles and practice of oncology* (9th ed., pp. 2123–2129). Philadelphia, PA: Wolters Kluwer Health/Lippincott Williams & Wilkins.

Yu, J.B., Wilson, L.D., & Detterbeck, F.C. (2008). Superior vena cava syndrome—A proposed classification system and algorithm for management. *Journal of Thoracic Oncology, 3,* 811–814. doi:10.1097/JTO.0b013e3181804791

Section VI.

Palliative Practices and Patient and Family Communication

CHAPTER 33

Communicating With the Patient and Family

Jennifer Fournier, MSN, APRN-CNS, ACNS-BC, AOCN®, CHPN

I. Definition
   A. Effective communication is the foundation for quality palliative care (McCusker et al., 2013).
   B. The ability of advanced practice registered nurses (APRNs) to direct dialogue yields crucial information for informed decision making between the provider and patient.
   C. Effective communication is vital to patient outcomes, improves patient-centered care, and can be considered as important as the medical treatments (Baer & Weinstein, 2013; Hilaire, 2013).
II. Key aspects
   A. The Agency for Healthcare Research and Quality palliative care guidelines for adults were updated in 2013 by McCusker et al. These guidelines provide a broad overview of palliative care practices for patients with chronic conditions or life-threatening illness.
   B. The U.S. Department of Health and Human Services (U.S. DHHS, n.d.) continues its three decades of work to improve the health of the nation. Healthy People 2020 established goals to meet the directives for healthcare providers to have adequate and effective communication skills. Healthy People 2020 directs providers to:
      1. Listen to patients.
      2. Provide clinical information in an understandable manner.
      3. Show respect for patients' viewpoints.
      4. Spend adequate time with patients.
      5. Involve patients in active decision making.
   C. Families make initial judgments of their care providers quickly (Twibell et al., 2012). Initial communication from interdisciplinary team members should convey trust, respect, and support for the patient and family while affirming competence, commitment, and a caring presence.
   D. The Patient Protection and Affordable Care Act requires shared decision making as an assurance of patient-centered care (Millenson & Macri, 2012).
   E. Targeted discussions throughout the disease trajectory are essential in promoting effective communication between the patient, family, and interdisciplinary healthcare team.
   F. Realistic goals and expectations should be established through shared decision making taking into account clinical options and patient and family preferences (D'Arcy, 2012; Institute of Medicine [IOM], 2013; Twibell et al., 2012).

G. The interdisciplinary team should ensure that adequate time and attention are given to perform a thorough appraisal of all available care options (Bakitas, Lyons, Hegel, & Ahles, 2013; IOM, 2013; Strand & Billings, 2012).

H. Outcomes of shared decision making (McCusker et al., 2013)

1. Goals of care are discussed and determined by the patient, family, and interdisciplinary team.

2. The patient and family are at the center or core of the plan of care.

3. The patient and family have a working relationship with all disciplines involved in the plan of care and know whom to contact and where to go to meet specific healthcare needs in the prescribed time frame.

4. Primary care providers (PCPs) serve as the conduit in the sorting and organizing of patient care needs by recognizing what discipline to recruit to meet the established care goals.

5. The patient and family are active participants in communicating with the PCP and maintaining a current plan of care that addresses the patient's unique physiologic, psychological, social, and spiritual care needs.

6. PCPs are required to engage in active discussion surrounding advance directives and provide supportive measures to ensure that the directives are carried out according to patient preferences.

7. The patient and family are prepared and well informed about the prognosis to meet care needs and concerns.

I. Barriers to communication

1. Evidence suggests that healthcare professionals, including physicians and nurses, lack the necessary training and experience to confidently address the palliative care needs of patients and families in chronic conditions (Boyd, Merkh, Rutledge, & Randall, 2011; Cannon, Watson, Roth, & LaVergne, 2014; Cheon, Coyle, Wiegand, & Welsh, 2015; Goldsmith, Ferrell, Wittenberg-Lyles, & Ragan, 2013; Granek, Krzyzanowska, Tozer, & Mazzotta, 2013; IOM, 2013; Kuebler, 2012, 2014; Kuebler et al., 2014; Von Roenn, Voltz, & Serrie, 2013; Wittenberg-Lyles, Goldsmith, & Ferrell, 2013).

2. Palliative care nursing education is seriously limited in the United States and other developed countries (Kuebler, 2012, 2014; Kuebler et al., 2014; Lippe & Carter, 2015; Von Roenn et al., 2013; Wittenberg-Lyles et al., 2013).

   a) Studies of nursing education at the graduate and undergraduate levels in the United States specifically show that nurses are not adequately prepared to care for the aging population possessing multiple chronic conditions (Kuebler, 2012, 2014; Kuebler et al., 2014).

   b) Australia has developed a unique training opportunity for general practitioners by funding six-month study leaves so they can receive education in palliative care and obtain clinical experience (Melvin, 2010).

   c) The United Kingdom first trained Macmillan nurses in the 1970s. This program has grown to support a variety of healthcare professionals through funding and training to be Macmillan professionals with a key focus on teaching effective communication skills (www.macmillan.org.uk).

   d) Nurses often learn communication skills in less than ideal conditions as they observe others interacting with patients and families and through consultations with more experienced nurses (Clayton, Reblin, Carlisle, & Ellington, 2014; Zomorodi & Lynn, 2010).

3. A helpful mnemonic for effective communication is ABCDE (McCusker et al., 2013).
    a) Advanced preparation: Gather the facts available and consider how they can best be presented to each individual patient and family dyad. Privacy is important to avoid distractions and interruptions (McCusker et al., 2013; Svarovsky, 2013).
    b) Build a therapeutic environment and relationship: Healthcare professionals should identify family members and gain an understanding of the dynamics within the family system.
        (1) The interdisciplinary team should assess the family's strengths, weaknesses, opportunities, and threats in dealing with chronic conditions from the onset of care (IOM, 2015).
        (2) Family assessment includes understanding the relationships that exist between each family member.
        (3) Identifying the key decision maker in the family and determining family cohesion are important in establishing optimal patient and family communication (Goldsmith et al., 2013).
        (4) Assessing family communication patterns will determine whether there is openness or closedness in communication, directness or indirectness, verbal and nonverbal messages, acceptance or inhibition of emotional expression, and validation of feelings.
        (5) Humor can be used when suitable, but caution is advised because humor can be misinterpreted in the context of a patient's culture or beliefs (McCusker et al., 2013).
        (6) Communication patterns in families are difficult when family members vary in their knowledge and degree of acceptance of the patient's disease and expected outcome (Goldsmith et al., 2013).
    c) Communicate well: Family members rely on the guidance, direction, affirmation, and education provided by the interdisciplinary team.
        (1) Moments of silence can be therapeutic.
        (2) Allow needed time for the processing of unfamiliar, technical, or confusing information.
    d) Deal with patient and family reactions: Anger, blame, and denial may surface. Healthcare professionals should always remain as objective as possible to address the needs of the patient and family (McCusker et al., 2013; Svarovsky, 2013).
    e) Encourage and validate emotions: Elicit the verbalization of emotions and respond empathetically.
        (1) This is important for patients and families who do not want to openly discuss a poor prognosis (Svarovsky, 2013).
        (2) Culture can have a significant effect on communication (see Chapter 41).
4. Realistic hope is a component of positive adaptation for the patient and family (Butt, 2011; Granek et al., 2013; Svarovsky, 2013).
5. Communicate pertinent clinical information in a timely manner.

III. Current findings
    A. The Center to Advance Palliative Care conducted a study of public opinions regarding palliative care in 2011. This research showed that communication is the cornerstone of palliative care.

1. Only 8% of adult consumers had an understanding of palliative care.
2. When these consumers gained an understanding of palliative care, more than 90% stated they would consider palliative care for a loved one with a serious illness.
3. Physicians continue to equate palliative care with end-of-life care and hospice care.
4. More than 50% of consumers stated their biggest concerns for patients with serious illness involved patient–physician communication, such as the following:
    a) Physicians not providing all treatment options
    b) Physicians not talking to each other
    c) Physicians not choosing the best treatment option for the patient
    d) Patients not certain about what to do once they leave the hospital or physician office
    e) Patients not given enough control of their treatment options
    f) Physicians not spending enough time listening to and talking with patients
5. One outcome from this research was a more descriptive definition of palliative care: "Palliative care is specialized medical care for people with serious illnesses. This type of care is focused on providing patients with relief from the symptoms, pain, and stresses of a serious illness—whatever the diagnosis. The goal is to improve quality of life for both the patient and the family. Palliative care is provided by a team of doctors, nurses, and other specialists who work with a patient's other doctors to provide an extra layer of support. Palliative care is appropriate at any age and at any stage in a serious illness, and can be provided together with curative treatment" (Center to Advance Palliative Care, 2011, p. 7).
6. The IOM discussion paper, *Communicating With Patients on Health Care Evidence*, identified discordance with the communication that patients obtain from healthcare providers and the communication that they ideally desire (Alston et al., 2012).
    a) The nationally representative sample consisted of 1,068 adults who had seen a healthcare provider at least once in the last 12 months.
    b) Of the sample, 38% reported having at least one chronic condition.
    c) Of those with chronic conditions, 97% agreed that coordinated care was essential, but only 54% reported receiving coordinated care to promote effective communication within the interdisciplinary team and shared decision making with the patient.
    d) Informed medical decisions require the consolidation of provider expertise, medical evidence, and patient preference.
    e) Patients reported they were not routinely asked about their preferences, goals, and concerns, which can change over time, requiring ongoing communication between the patient and the provider.
    f) The statement that provided the highest level of confidence in presenting medical evidence to patients was *"What is proven to work best . . ."* (Alston et al., 2012).
    g) The escalating costs of care for chronic conditions demands care coordination and shared medical decision making through optimal communication.
    h) Communication will be critical in the developing process to engage patients in medical care decision making, with the result being improved popula-

tion health outcomes. More than 50% of patients strongly agreed with the following statements (Alston et al., 2012, p. 3): "I want my provider . . ."

 (1) "To listen to me."

 (2) "To tell me the full truth about my diagnosis, even though it may be uncomfortable or unpleasant."

 (3) "To tell me about the risks associated with each option."

 (4) "To explain how the options may impact my quality of life."

 (5) "To understand my goals and concerns regarding the options."

 (6) "To help me understand how much each option will cost me and my family."

 (7) "To offer me choices of options."

 i) Almost half of the patients (47%) also wanted their provider to discuss what it would mean for them if they chose not to have a test or treatment.

 j) Less than 20% of these adults wanted their provider to offer only the options that the provider feels are best (Alston et al., 2012).

7. Kennedy et al. (2014) highlighted the importance of communicating with patients and their families in late-stage decision making. This integrative literature review showed that interdisciplinary team members tend to ignore the urgency of these necessary and important conversations.

8. Elements of basic shared decision making

 a) Information exchange

 b) Discussion of options

 c) Agreement of decision

9. A review of the literature on shared decision making for patients with cancer in non-Western cultures found more emphasis on the importance of family in decision making when compared to Western cultures (Obeidat, Homish, & Lally, 2013). Also, non-Western physicians were found to be more reluctant to disclose information related to cancer (Obeidat et al., 2013).

10. Patients with cancer are taking a more proactive interest in shared decision making. Of a convenience sample of adult patients aged 60 and older with symptomatic myeloma, 95% were found to seek shared decision making (Tariman, Doorenbos, Schepp, Singhal, & Berry, 2014).

11. Wittenberg-Lyles et al. (2013) conducted a focus group of oncology nurse managers to explore barriers to patient-centered communication and pinpoint communication skills needed by oncology nurses to deliver patient-centered care.

 a) Two themes emerged as barriers to patient-centered communication.

  (1) Inconsistency among interdisciplinary team communication

  (2) Physician expectations and suppositions of nursing tasks without verifying these expectations with the oncology nurse as the liaison between the patient and family unit and the physician

 b) Two primary topics emerged as vital to patient-centered care.

  (1) Pain

  (2) Spirituality (this was a limited topic)

12. The efficacy of communication skills training in group settings was analyzed to determine oncology providers' communication behaviors and attitudes resulting from training (Barth & Lannen, 2011).

 a) The conclusion drawn in the meta-analysis of 13 controlled studies was that communication skill training was moderately effective.

      b) Oncologists were more likely to assimilate communication skills into continued behaviors when the training was in-depth and lasted three or more days.

   13. Granek et al. (2013) studied oncologists' communication about the end of life, which was described to be one of their most challenging tasks.

      a) Effective communication strategies identified

        (1) Open and honest dialogue

        (2) Ongoing, early discussions

        (3) Altering goals of care as indicated

        (4) Harmonizing reality with hope

        (5) Taking cues from the patient

      b) Barriers to effective end-of-life communication identified

        (1) Physician barriers

          (a) Difference between treating disease and palliating symptoms

          (b) Own reluctance to discuss death

          (c) Other team members not wanting to discuss death

          (d) Focus on cure, the "death-defying mode"

          (e) Lack of experience

          (f) Lack of mentoring while in training

        (2) Patient barriers

          (a) Family reluctance to discuss end of life

          (b) Patient reluctance to face death

          (c) Language barriers

          (d) Younger patients

        (3) Institutional barriers

          (a) Palliative care stigma

          (b) Lack of protocol

          (c) Lack of training and tools

      c) This study shows that oncologists recognize the importance of end-of-life discussions with their patients but need training and tools for this "communication dance" (Granek et al., 2013).

IV. Relevance to practice

  A. Spoken words may not always match the intended meaning; it is the interdisciplinary team's role to decipher discrepancies to move patients and families closer to understanding core feelings (Goldsmith et al., 2013).

  B. Interdisciplinary care of chronic conditions requires effective communication and coordination among team members to achieve the result of patient-centered care (IOM, 2013).

  C. Communication deficiencies among patients, families, nurses, and physicians were identified as the most prevalent barrier to end-of-life care in the intensive care unit (Zomorodi & Lynn, 2010).

  D. At times, healthcare providers will need to communicate bad news, and avoiding this communication may result in patients and families having false hope (Baer & Weinstein, 2013). Practice is required to do this skillfully and therapeutically (Patterson & Harmon, 2010).

    1. The professional's countenance may foretell the reluctance to be the bearer of bad news.

    2. It is helpful to preface your statements with something to the effect of "I regret that I have some bad news" (Goldsmith et al., 2013). These suggestions allow the patient and family a moment of time to prepare.

3. Ask the patient and family to verbalize their understanding of the subject and then ask them what more they want to know.
4. Use words that match the patient's level of understanding. Be honest in information sharing.
5. Brief periods of silence can give the patient and family time to process the communication and formulate additional questions.
6. Create a safe, accepting, and calm environment for the patient and family. Inquire about feelings and allow expressions of emotions. Reflective listening can validate understanding of what the patient and family have stated.

E. Baer and Weinstein (2013) identified questions that may be asked of patients and families to facilitate difficult communication (p. E48):
1. "What is the hardest part of what is going on with you and your family?"
2. "Tell me more . . . ."
3. "What bothers you most?"
4. "What is most important to you if your time is limited?"
5. "What is your life like outside of the hospital or clinic?"
6. "What do you enjoy?"
7. "How can we help you do more of this?"
8. "When you think of the future, what concerns you most?"

F. End-of-life communication strategies
1. Encouraging family members to say all the things they want and need to say to the patient is extremely valuable (Kennedy et al., 2014).
2. At times, patients and families are given the gift of the patient's "premortem surge" to have a final opportunity to communicate (Schreiber & Bennett, 2014).
3. Families should be encouraged to touch their loved one gently, even if the patient does not respond (Kanacki, Roth, Georges, & Herring, 2012).
4. Ongoing verbal and nonverbal communication benefits family members, friends, and caregivers and can have a positive, calming effect on the patient (Close & Long, 2012; Goldsmith et al., 2013).

G. The COMFORT communication curriculum (Goldsmith et al., 2013; Wittenberg-Lyles et al., 2013) is directed to oncology nurses and involves the entire interdisciplinary team. It has seven components:
1. "C"—communication, verbal, nonverbal, active listening
2. "O"—orientation and opportunity, culture, each patient and situation are unique
3. "M"—mindful presence, being there, allow expression of feelings
4. "F"—family, understand relationships and roles, honor decisions
5. "O"—openings, turning points, transitions, social support
6. "R"—relating, search for true meanings
7. "T"—team, interdisciplinary, structure, trust

V. Role of the APRN
A. APRNs play a pivotal role for patients with multiple chronic conditions and their families in understanding the comprehensive role of palliative care in the treatment plan (Del Ferraro, Ferrell, Van Zyl, Freeman, & Klein, 2014; Svarovsky, 2013).
B. The advanced educational preparation and refined communication skills of APRNs can prevent the disengagement that can occur during intense, sensitive communication sessions.
1. Transition points occur in the chronic condition disease trajectory where APRNs' communication skills are vital (Svarovsky, 2013).

2. Difficult conversations should be based on what the patient and family want to know. Determining this is the first step in the communication process (Svarovsky, 2013).
3. Silence can be useful to allow patients and families time to process and reflect.
4. Patients desire various levels of information, but the majority of patients want their APRN to be realistic, address their concerns, and make recommendations based on their specific needs (Svarovsky, 2013).

C. According to the 2011 IOM report, *The Future of Nursing: Leading Change, Advancing Health*, nurses are accepting the challenge to ensure that conversations are occurring with patients and their families throughout the disease trajectory, with APRNs being especially suited to this task.

D. Twibell et al. (2012) synthesized five important needs of families in a hospital setting:
1. Honest communication
2. Ability to "be with" the patient as desired
3. To feel cared for
4. Facts and expected outcomes
5. Emotional support

E. APRNs use the best evidence to achieve the best outcomes for patients through the synthesis of knowledge. Effective communication builds patient rapport and trust while instilling confidence in the healthcare team. Patients embrace the knowledge that the team has their best interest at stake.

VI. Interface to palliative care
A. Communication is a critical instrument for the interdisciplinary team to use in palliative care and is the foundation that supports the patient and family in understanding all aspects of the chronic condition, thereby allowing effectual decision making (Cheon et al., 2015; Goldsmith et al., 2013; Kennedy et al., 2014; Twibell et al., 2012; U.S. DHHS, n.d.).

B. Zhang, Nilsson, and Prigerson (2012) showed that a salutary relationship between the patient and physician had a positive influence on the patient's quality of life. Patients need to feel valued and treated with respect and dignity throughout their life.

C. Decision aids can be useful to help the patient and family visualize options for care with the resulting expected benefits and harms (IOM, 2013).

D. "Ask, Tell, Ask" can be a simple effective communication strategy for palliative care conversations (Svarovsky, 2013).
1. Ask what the patient and family want to know; request permission to discuss sensitive topics.
2. Tell them the information requested to answer their question based on their level of understanding and desire.
3. Ask if their question was answered satisfactorily.

E. Much of palliative care communication is intense because of the topics of discussion, such as prognosis and treatment options, which often are avoided in routine medical care (Goldsmith et al., 2013; Wittenberg-Lyles et al., 2013). Ask what each topic means to the patient and family to gain additional understanding and direction for the conversation (Svarovsky, 2013).

F. Palliative care is now expected to be available to patients and families at the time of diagnosis of a serious illness to support them through physical and psychosocial aspects of symptom management, treatment, and transitions in care as the chronic condition progresses (Goldsmith et al., 2013; U.S. DHHS, n.d.; Wittenberg-Lyles et al., 2013).

G. Culture can affect family communication, as identified by Gómez-Batiste et al. (2013). The tool used in their Spanish study included a culturally relevant question that included family members' choice for the patient, as the family has the responsibility for decision making on behalf of the patient.

Case Study

R.B. is a 67-year-old Hispanic woman who was hospitalized three days ago with a new diagnosis of hypertrophic cardiomyopathy. The hospitalist made a palliative care referral to assist with the management of R.B.'s symptoms and provide support for the patient and family regarding this unexpected event. The APRN completes a medical record review in preparation for the upcoming appointment.

The RN assigned to care for R.B. shares that the husband and oldest son have made all the medical decisions for R.B. thus far. The palliative care APRN schedules an appointment with the patient and members of the family to discuss goals of care. The patient and family have not heard of palliative care before, but once the APRN thoroughly explains the concept, they welcome the assistance of the palliative care interdisciplinary team to assist in the coordination of care.

R.B.'s cardiologist states that surgery is necessary to effectively treat the congestive heart failure, and the family does not fully understand what that would entail. The APRN spends significant time discussing the details related to the diagnosis of hypertrophic cardiomyopathy, thus building the therapeutic relationship with R.B. and her family. The APRN asks the family to request any information that they need for decision making and then answers their questions carefully. To ensure understanding, the APRN clarifies that the family understands the answers. The youngest daughter cries and states that she is scared that something might happen during the surgery. The APRN acknowledges the fear of the unknown and is able to reassure the daughter and the rest of the family that the surgery has few complications with minimal recovery pain. R.B.'s family expresses appreciation for the involvement of the palliative care APRN in the care of R.B. and helping them to understand what they need to know as they begin caring for a loved one with a chronic condition.

References

Alston, C., Paget, L., Halvorson, G., Novelli, B., Guest, J., McCabe, P., … Von Kohorn, I. (2012). *Communicating with patients on health care evidence* [Discussion paper]. Retrieved from http://nam.edu/perspectives-2012-communicating-with-patients-on-health-care-evidence

Baer, L., & Weinstein, E. (2013). Improving oncology nurses' communication skills for difficult conversations [Online exclusive]. *Clinical Journal of Oncology Nursing, 17*, E45–E51. doi:10.1188/13.CJON.E45-E51

Bakitas, M., Lyons, K.D., Hegel, M.T., & Ahles, T. (2013). Oncologists' perspectives on concurrent palliative care in a National Cancer Institute-designated comprehensive cancer center. *Palliative and Supportive Care, 11*, 415–423. doi:10.1017/S1478951512000673

Barth, J., & Lannen, P. (2011). Efficacy of communication skills training courses in oncology: A systematic review and meta-analysis. *Annals of Oncology, 22*, 1030–1040. doi:10.1093/annonc/mdq441

Boyd, D., Merkh, K., Rutledge, D.N., & Randall, V. (2011). Nurses' perceptions and experiences with end-of-life communication and care [Online exclusive]. *Oncology Nursing Forum, 38*, E229–E239. doi:10.1188/11.ONF.E229-E239

Butt, C.M. (2011). Hope in adults with cancer: State of the science [Online exclusive]. *Oncology Nursing Forum, 38*, E341–E350. doi:10.1188/11.ONF.E341-E350

Cannon, C.A., Watson, L.K., Roth, M.T., & LaVergne, S. (2014). Assessing the learning needs of oncology nurses. *Clinical Journal of Oncology Nursing, 18*, 577–580. doi:10.1188/14.CJON.577-580

Center to Advance Palliative Care. (2011). *2011 public opinion research on palliative care: A report based on research by Public Opinion Strategies.* New York, NY: Author.

Cheon, J., Coyle, N., Wiegand, D.L., & Welsh, S. (2015). Ethical issues experienced by hospice and palliative nurses. *Journal of Hospice and Palliative Nursing, 17,* 7–13. doi:10.1097/NJH.0000000000000129

Clayton, M., Reblin, M., Carlisle, M., & Ellington, L. (2014). Communication behaviors and patient and caregiver emotional concerns: A description of home hospice communication. *Oncology Nursing Forum, 41,* 311–321. doi:10.1188/14.ONF.311-321

Close, J.F., & Long, C.O. (2012). Delirium: Opportunity for comfort in palliative care. *Journal of Hospice and Palliative Nursing, 14,* 386–394. doi:10.1097/NJH.0b013e31825d2b0a

D'Arcy, Y. (2012). Managing end-of-life symptoms. *American Nurse Today, 7*(7), 22–27. Retrieved from https://americannursetoday.com/managing-end-of-life-symptoms

Del Ferraro, C., Ferrell, B., Van Zyl, C., Freeman, B., & Klein, L. (2014). Improving palliative cancer care. *Journal of the Advanced Practitioner in Oncology, 5,* 331–338. doi:10.6004/jadpro.2014.5.5.3

Goldsmith, J., Ferrell, B., Wittenberg-Lyles, E., & Ragan, S.L. (2013). Palliative care communication in oncology nursing. *Clinical Journal of Oncology Nursing, 17,* 163–167. doi:10.1188/13.CJON.163-167

Gómez-Batiste, X., Martínez-Muñoz, M., Blay, C., Amblàs, J., Vila, L., Costa, X., … Constante, C. (2013). Identifying patients with chronic conditions in need of palliative care in the general population: Development of the NECPAL tool and preliminary prevalence rates in Catalonia. *BMJ Supportive and Palliative Care, 3,* 300–308. doi:10.1136/bmjspcare-2012-000211

Granek, L., Krzyzanowska, M.K., Tozer, R., & Mazzotta, P. (2013). Oncologists' strategies and barriers to effective communication about the end of life. *Journal of Oncology Practice, 9,* E129–E135. doi:10.1200/JOP.2012.000800

Hilaire, D.M. (2013). The need for communication skills training in oncology. *Journal of the Advanced Practitioner in Oncology, 4,* 168–171. doi:10.6004/jadpro.2013.4.3.4

Institute of Medicine. (2011). *The future of nursing: Leading change, advancing health.* Washington, DC: National Academies Press.

Institute of Medicine. (2013). *Delivering high-quality cancer care: Charting a new course for a system in crisis.* Washington, DC: National Academies Press.

Institute of Medicine. (2015). *Dying in America: Improving quality and honoring individual preferences near the end of life.* Washington, DC: National Academies Press.

Kanacki, L.S., Roth, P., Georges, J.M., & Herring, P. (2012). Shared presence: Caring for a dying spouse. *Journal of Hospice and Palliative Nursing, 14,* 414–425. doi:10.1097/NJH.0b013e3182554a2c

Kennedy, C., Brooks-Young, P., Gray, C.B., Larkin, P., Connolly, M., Wilde-Larsson, B., … Chater, S. (2014). Diagnosing dying: An integrative literature review. *BMJ Supportive and Palliative Care, 4,* 263–270. doi:10.1136/bmjspcare-2013-000621

Kuebler, K.K. (2012). Implications for palliative care nursing education. *Clinical Scholars Review, 5,* 86–90. doi:10.1891/1939-2095.5.2.86

Kuebler, K.K. (2014). National graduate nursing survey: Chronic disease, symptoms and self-management. *Journal of Palliative Care and Medicine, 4.* doi:10.4172/2165-7386.1000186

Kuebler, K., Lampley, T., Shake, E., White-Hurst, E., Taggart, H., & Hagerty, D. (2014). A systematic review: A collaborative partnership on evaluating graduate nursing education in chronic symptomatic disease. *Clinical Scholars Review, 7,* 98–104. doi:10.1891/1939-2095.7.2.98

Lippe, M.P., & Carter, P. (2015). End-of-life care teaching strategies in prelicensure nursing education: An integrative review. *Journal of Hospice and Palliative Nursing, 17,* 31–39. doi:10.1097/NJH.0000000000000118

McCusker, M., Ceronsky, L., Crone, C., Epstein, H., Greene, B., Halvorson, J., … Setterlund, L. (2013, November). *Institute for Clinical Systems Improvement (ICSI) health care guideline: Palliative care for adults.* Retrieved from https://www.icsi.org/_asset/k056ab/PalliativeCare.pdf

Melvin, C.S. (2010). Patient's and families' misperceptions about hospice and palliative care: Listen as they speak. *Journal of Hospice and Palliative Nursing, 12,* 107–115. doi:10.1097/NJH.0b013e3181cf7933

Millenson, M.L., & Macri, J. (2012, March). *Will the Affordable Care Act move patient-centeredness to center stage? Timely analysis of immediate health policy issues.* Robert Wood Johnson Foundation. Retrieved from http://www.rwjf.org/content/dam/farm/reports/reports/2012/rwjf72412

Obeidat, R.F., Homish, G.G., & Lally, R.M. (2013). Shared decision making among individuals with cancer in non-Western cultures: A literature review. *Oncology Nursing Forum, 40,* 454–463. doi:10.1188/13.ONF.454-463

Patterson, K., & Harmon, H. (2010). How to deliver bad news. *American Nurse Today, 5*(1), 23–24. Retrieved from https://americannursetoday.com/how-to-deliver-bad-news

Schreiber, T.P., & Bennett, M.J. (2014). Identification and validation of premortem surge. *Journal of Hospice and Palliative Nursing, 16,* 430–437. doi:10.1097/NJH.0000000000000094

Strand, J.J., & Billings, J.A. (2012). Integrating palliative care in the intensive care unit. *Journal of Supportive Oncology, 10,* 180–187.

Svarovsky, T. (2013). Having difficult conversations: The advanced practitioner's role. *Journal of the Advanced Practitioner in Oncology, 4,* 47–52. doi:10.6004/jadpro.2013.4.1.5

Tariman, J.D., Doorenbos, A., Schepp, K.G., Singhal, S., & Berry, D.L. (2014). Older adults newly diagnosed with symptomatic myeloma and treatment decision making. *Oncology Nursing Forum, 41,* 411–419. doi:10.1188/14 .ONF.411-419

Twibell, R., Neal, A., Cox, C., Harris, D., Osborne, K., Paul, N., & Duncan, J. (2012). Puzzling over family presence: Word search at the bedside. *American Nurse Today, 7*(7), 8–10. Retrieved from https://american nursetoday.com/puzzling-over-family-presence-word-search-at-the-bedside

U.S. Department of Health and Human Services. (n.d.). Health communication and health information technology: Objectives. Retrieved from http://www.healthypeople.gov/2020/topicsobjectives2020/objectiveslist. aspx?topicId=18

Von Roenn, J.H., Voltz, R., & Serrie, A. (2013). Barriers and approaches to the successful integration of palliative care and oncology practice. *Journal of the National Comprehensive Cancer Network, 11*(Suppl. 1), S11–S16. Retrieved from http://www.jnccn.org/content/11/suppl_1/S-11.long

Wittenberg-Lyles, E., Goldsmith, J., & Ferrell, B. (2013). Oncology nurse communication barriers to patient-centered care. *Clinical Journal of Oncology Nursing, 17,* 152–158. doi:10.1188/13.CJON.152-158

Zhang, B., Nilsson, M.E., & Prigerson, H.G. (2012). Factors important to patients' quality of life at the end of life. *Archives of Internal Medicine, 172,* 1133–1142. doi:10.1001/archinternmed.2012.2364

Zomorodi, M., & Lynn, M.R. (2010). Critical care nurses' values and behaviors with end-of-life care: Perceptions and challenges. *Journal of Hospice and Palliative Nursing, 12,* 89–96. doi:10.1097/NJH.0b013e3181cf7cf6

CHAPTER 34

Preparing the Patient and Family for End of Life

Jennifer Fournier, MSN, APRN-CNS, ACNS-BC, AOCN®, CHPN

I. Definition
   A. Defining end of life (EOL) is ambiguous (Kennedy et al., 2014).
   B. Patients who are in the final stage of chronic conditions or have a life-limiting illness tolerate symptoms poorly, largely because of weakness and generalized debility.
   C. The appropriate plan of care during the final phase of life should be proactive and prevent or control distressing symptoms with the goal of honoring the patient's preferences (Boyd, Merkh, Rutledge, & Randall, 2011; D'Arcy, 2012; Gómez-Batiste et al., 2013; Kennedy et al., 2014; McCusker et al., 2013; National Cancer Institute [NCI], 2016; Zhang, Nilsson, & Prigerson, 2012).
      1. In the palliative care setting, the term *dying* or *actively dying* refers to the final weeks, days, or hours of life (McCusker et al., 2013).
      2. The pivotal first step in effective EOL care is the accurate prognosis of dying, which is said to be "part art, part science" (Kennedy et al., 2014, p. 263).
      3. Life-limiting illness can best be defined by the affirmative answer to the question, "Would you be surprised if your patient died within the next one to two years?" Thinking of a patient's prognosis in this manner clarifies a patient population that could benefit from palliative care services (Gómez-Batiste et al., 2013; McCusker et al., 2013).
II. Key aspects
   A. Palliative care should not be confused with hospice care or EOL care.
      1. Although hospice care is delivered in a palliative approach, it is limited to patients not seeking curative treatment, with an expected prognosis of six months or less to live (NCI, 2016).
      2. Palliative care is intended to be delivered concurrently with routine treatment of a chronic condition from the time of diagnosis throughout the disease trajectory (McCusker et al., 2013; Parikh, Kirch, Smith, & Temel, 2013; Von Roenn, Voltz, & Serrie, 2013).
   B. The Institute of Medicine (IOM) established goals for the provision of care to patients with cancer in its report, *Delivering High–Quality Cancer Care: Charting a New Course for a System in Crisis* (IOM, 2013). Selected goals from this report can be used to prepare patients and families for EOL care.

1. Provide patients and their families with understandable information about cancer prognosis, treatment benefits and harms, palliative care, psychosocial support, and costs.
2. Provide patients with EOL care that meets their individual needs, values, and preferences.
3. Ensure coordinated and comprehensive patient-centered care.

C. The Agency for Healthcare Research and Quality palliative care guidelines for adults were updated in 2013 by McCusker et al. These guidelines are intended as a broad overview of palliative care practices for patients with chronic conditions or life-threatening illness.

1. The palliative care team anticipates, monitors, and addresses the physical, psychological, social, and spiritual symptoms that accompany the dying process to prepare patients and families for EOL (D'Arcy, 2012; IOM, 2013).
2. Each interdisciplinary team member possesses specific abilities to provide individualized care to patients and families (Goldsmith, Ferrell, Wittenberg-Lyles, & Ragan, 2013).
3. Zhang et al. (2012) showed an increase in quality of life at EOL when hospitalized patients were visited by a pastor.
4. This study showed that patients with a strong faith base that included prayer or meditation had an improved quality EOL.

D. Attempting to normalize the dying process is important not only for patients but also for their loved ones. The manner in which a person dies will forever remain in the memories of the survivors, affecting their grief and bereavement (Kanacki, Roth, Georges, & Herring, 2012; Revier, Meiers, & Herth, 2012; Schreiber & Bennett, 2014).

1. Open communication regarding EOL can promote optimal growth through sharing, reminiscing, and closeness of the family members (NCI, 2016).
2. Approaches to provide support to family members as they are caring for their loved one at EOL include the following:
    a) Provide them with information on prognosis, treatment options and expected results, palliative care, psychosocial support, and financial information in a comprehensible manner (IOM, 2013).
    b) Help the family to acknowledge the situation and its personal magnitude to reach the point of acceptance and understanding.
    c) Clearly establish priorities in care with the patient and family as early in the process as possible (Strand & Billings, 2012).
    d) Explore the greatest concerns of the patient and family and ask what assistance they need (D'Arcy, 2012).
    e) Encourage the family to explore the meaning of their personal loss.
        (1) Providing family members the opportunity to talk about this can promote personal growth.
        (2) It is not necessary for all losses to be accepted, resolved, and forgotten.
        (3) Some are resolved and forgotten, others remain painful, and still others serve as a means of growth and change.
        (4) The Jewish perspective is that EOL continues to be a time of personal growth and a time to give and share love (Schultz & Bar-Sela, 2013).
    f) Encourage the family to have physical closeness.

         (1) Family members can reassure their loved ones of how life will go on.

         (2) They may need to be gently encouraged to say their good-byes, which may occur over a period of time.

    g) Help the family to resolve interpersonal conflicts and complete any unfinished business. Recognizing these issues and integrating psychological support can aid the family in the bereavement process (Schreiber & Bennett, 2014).

    h) Reassure the patient and loved ones that it is normal for the patient to describe vivid and emotional dreams or to have visions of loved ones who have previously died (Schreiber & Bennett, 2014). Offer a nonjudgmental presence and acceptance of any intimate thoughts and feelings.

    i) Assist family members to understand that the social isolation or "closing in on self" is an important process for the dying and not a personal rejection.

    j) Identify that the psychosocial needs of the dying are similar to those of the living. These needs include affiliation, being connected, and to love and to be loved. Interpersonal interaction occurs at one's level of physical, cognitive, and spiritual capability and provides a sense of purpose to the lives of others.

    k) Educate family members regarding the likely trajectory of the dying process and the expected physical manifestations (D'Arcy, 2012; NCI, 2016; Schreiber & Bennett, 2014).

    l) Discuss useful resources to assist families through all phases of the dying process and beyond the actual death (Cloyes, Berry, Reblin, Clayton, & Ellington, 2012; D'Arcy, 2012; Kanacki et al., 2012; Revier et al., 2012).

3. Organ systems decompensate and eventually shut down at EOL. Effective communication with patients and family concerning the physiologic signs and symptoms that may be exhibited is critical.

4. Basic knowledge about what is "normal" in the dying process is essential to communicate to patients and families in a manner in which they can understand.

    a) It is important to provide simple comfort measures in the last days of life and to educate family caregivers in their role of comforting their dying loved one.

    b) Effective management of physical symptoms takes precedence over psychosocial issues in the hierarchy of needs (Kennedy et al., 2014; McCusker et al., 2013). However, that does not diminish the importance of psychosocial needs at EOL (Kennedy et al., 2014).

    c) Patients studied by Kennedy et al. (2014) described exploring "the meaning and purpose of life" as being of great importance to them.

E. EOL has observable symptoms that need to be explored with patients and families to reduce the anxiety associated with the experience and communicate what comfort measures might best support the patient (D'Arcy, 2012).

F. Common symptoms that often occur at EOL, treatment of those symptoms, and communication suggestions

1. Dehydration

    a) Dehydration is a result of various etiologies, but, at EOL, patients are further debilitated and have diminished oral intake, thereby increasing dehydration.

    b) Symptom management should guide the use of artificial hydration.

    c) Myoclonus, agitation, hypercalcemia, and delirium can be effectively managed with artificial hydration, whereas congestion, edema, and death rattle often are increased by artificial hydration (NCI, 2016).

    d) Dehydration, if left untreated, can lead to renal failure and the body's inability to clear active metabolites that may be contributing to untoward symptoms such as delirium or agitation.

    e) Opioid metabolite accumulation as a result of dehydration can create nausea, confusion, restlessness, myoclonus, delirium, nightmares, hallucinations, and hyperalgesia (D'Arcy, 2012; Kozlov, Anderson, & Sparbel, 2011; NCI, 2016).

    f) To lessen the accumulation of toxic metabolites, patients who are not receiving hydration but are receiving opioids should have the dose titrated down when indicated.

    g) Dehydrated patients are more sensitive to the analgesic side effects associated with long-acting opioid metabolites.

2. Cognitive function decline

    a) Changes in cognition occur as life draws to an end, with the most common being somnolence, delirium, difficulty communicating, labile mood, hallucinations, agitation, or restlessness.

    b) Patients with glioma in particular have been identified as having cognitive decline at EOL (Kennedy et al., 2014).

3. Delirium

    a) Delirium frequently occurs near EOL and is distressful for the family or caregivers to observe (D'Arcy, 2012; NCI, 2016; Oligario, Buch, & Piscotty, 2015).

    b) It is important to evaluate for a reversible etiology and modify treatment when warranted (Close & Long, 2012; D'Arcy, 2012; Oligario et al., 2015).

    c) Several studies have identified the presence of delirium in as many as 88% of patients in their final weeks of life (D'Arcy, 2012; Oligario et al., 2015).

    d) Delirium generally is multifactorial and can be reversible, such as with drug toxicities, metabolic disorders, and dehydration.

    e) The importance of distinguishing delirium from dementia should not be underestimated.

        (1) The instrument evaluation by Oligario et al. (2015) showed that senior, experienced hospice and palliative nurses were not able to subjectively distinguish between delirium and dementia 40% of the time.

        (2) The use of a validated tool such as the Confusion Assessment Method was recommended to accurately assess for delirium (Oligario et al., 2015).

        (3) Determinant factors in delirium are sudden onset, inattention, restlessness, agitation, scattered thought process, and altered consciousness, whereas in dementia the onset is gradual and consciousness is unimpaired.

        (4) Delirium can occur concurrently with dementia or other cognitive impairments (Close & Long, 2012; D'Arcy, 2012; Oligario et al., 2015).

  f) All medications require a thorough investigation to determine if they
  are contributing to delirium (i.e., anticholinergics, opioids, benzodiazepines, antidepressants, antihistamines, anticonvulsants, neuroleptics, dihydropyridines, corticosteroids, metoclopramide, ranitidine, angiotensin-
  converting enzyme inhibitors, and digoxin) (McPherson, Kim, & Walker,
  2012). Haloperidol is considered to be the medication of choice to quickly
  reduce delirium but is contraindicated in patients with Parkinson disease
  or Lewy body dementia (Close & Long, 2012; D'Arcy, 2012).

4. Dysphagia
  a) Patients at EOL can develop dysphagia, or difficulty swallowing, because
  of weakness or impaired cognition.
  b) Liquid medications are easy to administer through a syringe placed in
  the back of the mouth.
  c) Customarily, the only drugs necessary in the final days of life are those
  used to control symptoms (D'Arcy, 2012; McPherson et al., 2012).

5. Urinary retention or incontinence
  a) Patients need to be assessed regularly for incontinence or urinary retention.
  b) Urinary retention can result from an enlarged prostate, anticholinergic or
  opioid medications, weakness, disinterest due to depression, lack of cognitive awareness, or a full rectal vault.
  c) It is important to recognize the underlying cause and consider possible
  indwelling catheterization when indicated.
  d) While incontinence may be manageable at EOL, it may require frequent
  linen and position changes, which may be uncomfortable for patients
  (Arenella, n.d.).

6. Anorexia
  a) Offer the patient's favorite foods. Provide family education that eating
  changes are normal, as the body has significantly less nutritional needs
  (D'Arcy, 2012).
  b) Help the family understand that force-feeding the patient will not be
  beneficial.
  c) Sips of fluids or moistened mouth sponges will keep the patient's mouth
  from becoming dry.
  d) Small amounts of ice chips may be soothing.
  e) Reassure the family that the patient is not "starving" and encourage patient
  participation in oral care (Arenella, n.d.).

7. Immobility
  a) As the patient becomes bedbound, use durable medical equipment to
  transfer the patient to reduce falls and ease caregiver lifting.
  b) Draw sheets or transfer belts can assist with moving the patient.
  c) Teach the family to perform passive range-of-motion and position changing for patient comfort.
  d) Educate and support the patient and family through changes in goals of
  care, as increasing weakness may indicate approaching death when observed
  in conjunction with a semicomatose state and ability to only take sips of
  liquid (D'Arcy, 2012; Kennedy et al., 2014).

8. Breathing changes
  a) Dyspnea, tachypnea, Cheyne-Stokes respiration, apnea, and labored
  breathing often are associated with nearing death (D'Arcy, 2012).

     b) In patients with cancer and amyotrophic lateral sclerosis, these breathing changes can be strong indicators that the patient is in the last phase of dying (Kennedy et al., 2014).

     c) Proper use of medications such as opiates, anxiolytics, or bronchodilators can ease symptoms (D'Arcy, 2012).

     d) Use patient positioning (e.g., high Fowler, 45° degree angle) to lessen distress.

     e) Minimize the patient's energy expenditure.

     f) Instruct the family in providing good oral care and communicate reassurance for the care provided.

     g) Encourage the patient to use pursed-lip breathing when indicated.

     h) Increase ventilation by opening a window or using a fan to increase air movement.

9. Noisy respirations, "death rattle"

     a) Administer anticholinergics prior to secretion presence.

     b) Modify the patient's position to side-lying or elevate the head of bed.

     c) Communicate to the family that noisy respirations are a normal occurrence at EOL (D'Arcy, 2012; NCI, 2016), particularly in patients with cardiac or lung-related chronic conditions.

     d) Secretions generally can be managed with anticholinergics.

     e) Careful assessment warrants earlier or prophylactic interventions to prevent or reduce the occurrence of excessive secretions (McPherson et al., 2012).

10. Hypoxia or cyanosis

     a) Reassure the family that peripheral cyanosis is an expected observance and that mottling of the extremities frequently progresses toward the trunk.

     b) The skin may feel cool to the touch.

11. Social withdrawal

     a) The dying process is unique for each individual.

     b) The patient may shift focus and disengage from loved ones because of lack of energy for relationships.

     c) Social withdrawal may be a hallmark of impending death (Kennedy et al., 2014).

     d) Preparing the family to expect withdrawal is important to avoid feelings of rejection as the patient turns inward.

12. Pain

     a) Pain is a frequent symptom throughout the course of chronic illnesses and often continues until the time of death.

     b) It is also the symptom that patients fear the most (D'Arcy, 2012).

     c) In a study of symptoms in patients with cancer, almost half of the patients reported a pain intensity greater than 5 on a 10-point scale (McMillan, Tofthagen, Choe, & Rheingans, 2015). Furthermore, about 75% of patients with advanced cancer have pain (D'Arcy, 2012).

     d) In this day of frequent pain assessment when guidelines are followed and protocols exist to manage pain, it is unnecessary for patients to suffer from pain (Caraceni et al., 2013; D'Arcy, 2012).

     e) Wittenberg-Lyles, Goldsmith, and Ferrell (2013) and Cannon, Watson, Roth, and LaVergne (2014) identified pain as an educational priority to ensure quality patient care.

     f) Adequate analgesia must be aggressively pursued at all times using the most efficacious route for the situation.

        g) Transmucosal fentanyl has been shown to achieve the fastest relief of breakthrough pain in patients with cancer (Caraceni et al., 2013; Zeppetella, 2103) and can decrease morphine-induced delirium (NCI, 2016).

13. Agitation or restlessness
    a) Agitation may be the predecessor of the final stage of life (Kennedy et al., 2014).
    b) Assess for a distended bladder, fecal impaction, sleep deprivation, and uncontrolled pain as physical causes of agitation (Close & Long, 2012; D'Arcy, 2012; Oligario et al., 2015).
    c) Haloperidol is the drug of choice if the restlessness is not reversible (D'Arcy, 2012) and may be titrated to effect.
    d) Help the family understand that the patient may "act out" toward them because they are a "safe" target.

14. Nearing death awareness
    a) Reassure the family that this is not confusion or hallucinations but important work for the patient at EOL.
    b) Listen to what the patient may be trying to communicate, and address any unresolved issues.
    c) Patients may request to see or talk to specific individuals to resolve unfinished business.
    d) Educate the family that the patient may have a "premortem surge" or "deathbed rally" where there can be a sudden period of 6–24 hours of increased alertness and energy during the final 24–48 hours of life (Schreiber & Bennett, 2014).
    e) Encourage family members to finalize their time with the patient and say good-bye (D'Arcy, 2012; Del Ferraro, Grant, Koczywas, & Dorr-Uyemura, 2012; Kozlov et al., 2011; McCusker et al., 2013; NCI, 2016; Schreiber & Bennett, 2014).

III. Current findings
  A. The Spanish study by Gómez-Batiste et al. (2013) noted that 75% of middle- to high-income country residents died from one or more chronic conditions.
    1. The early identification of patients with chronic conditions who would benefit from palliative care was deemed a critical responsibility for primary care to improve quality of life.
    2. The *Necesidades Paliativas* (Palliative Needs) tool was developed to identify the palliative care needs in primary care patients and identified these factors as predictive of death within 12–14 months in their Mediterranean population:
        a) Most indicative was a positive response to the question, "Would you be surprised if this patient dies within one year?"
        b) Any request to limit treatments
        c) Nutritional decline
        d) Functional decline
            (1) Advanced frailty
            (2) Infections
            (3) Dysphagia
            (4) Delirium
            (5) Pressure ulcers
            (6) Falls
        e) Severe psychological distress

    f) Two or more chronic conditions

    g) Two or more emergency admissions in the past 12 months

B. Another European study conducted in the Netherlands for early identification of palliative care needs in general practice specifically examined patients with congestive heart failure, chronic obstructive pulmonary disease (COPD), and cancer (Thoonsen et al., 2012).

  1. The RADboud indicators for PAlliative Care Needs tool developed through a three-step process of literature review, focus groups, and the modified Rand Delphi process identified six to eight indicators for each studied condition.

  2. A common indicator in the three groups was a Karnofsky score less than 50%.

  3. Weight loss was common for patients with COPD and cancer, while weight gain was seen in patients with congestive heart failure as indicators for referral to palliative care.

C. Using the theoretical framework of Bowen's value-behavior congruency, Zomorodi and Lynn (2010) interviewed intensive care unit (ICU) nurses regarding EOL care.

  1. ICU nurses are highly trained to respond to patients in an aggressive, curative mode and have difficulty identifying the time to switch gears to provide EOL comfort care only.

  2. Barriers to effective EOL care in the ICU include the following:

    a) Lack of educational preparation

    b) Focus on curative care

    c) Fragmentation of care

    d) Incongruent communication

    e) Time constraints

    f) Patient monitor screens

    g) Noise

D. Zhang et al. (2012) conducted a prospective, longitudinal cohort study of patients with cancer and their caregivers at multiple sites in the United States.

  1. The focus of the study was to look at patients' quality of life in the last week of life.

  2. Factors identified as having negative influences (listed in descending order)

    a) ICU stay

    b) Dying in the hospital

    c) Patient self-reported worry at baseline

    d) Feeding tube use

    e) Chemotherapy

  3. Factors identified as having positive influences listed in descending order

    a) Religious prayer or meditation at baseline

    b) Hospital or clinic pastoral care

    c) Patient–physician relationship with good communication

  4. Zhang et al. (2012) concluded that patients with cancer who spend their last week of life at home rather than in a hospital or ICU continue prayer or meditation and are not worried about having the best quality of life as life comes to an end.

E. Kennedy et al. (2014) completed an integrative literature review of "diagnosing dying" from 23 papers discussing chronic conditions across several continents covering the time frame of 2001–2011.

  1. The central theme of "uncertainty in diagnosing dying" appeared.

  2. Subthemes of "characteristics of dying" and "treatment orientation" also appeared in this literature review.

a) "Characteristics of dying" identified many physical symptoms and symptom clusters in specific chronic conditions that often increase as death nears.

b) "Treatment orientation" identified futile interventions as often continuing to the very end of life.

c) Cancer diagnoses were often more straightforward when determining EOL.

3. "Clinical wisdom" assists experienced clinicians in determining when patients are at EOL:

a) Assimilating patient history

b) Affecting goals of care

c) Allowing patient's preparation

F. Hui et al. (2015) identified eight observable indicators of death among patients with cancer in two inpatient palliative care units.

1. All patients who died had at least one of these indicators within three days of death.

2. Indicators with at least a 95% confidence interval and positive likelihood ratios

a) Nonreactive pupils

b) Decreased response to verbal stimuli

c) Decreased response to visual stimuli

d) Inability to close eyelids

e) Drooping of the nasolabial fold

f) Hyperextension of the neck

g) Grunting of vocal cords

h) Upper gastrointestinal bleeding

G. Boyd et al. (2011) conducted a descriptive correlational survey study of 31 oncology nurses at a Magnet® facility regarding their experiences and perceptions of EOL care and communication.

1. It would be expected that this group of nurses would have progressive attitudes regarding EOL discussions and be fairly competent to provide EOL care to their patients.

2. Findings from this study

a) Nurses rated their EOL competence as only midrange.

b) Sixty-three percent acknowledged having received some level of hospice training within the past five years.

c) Opportunities to discuss EOL were overlooked.

d) Almost 30% of these oncology nurses had never discussed hospice care with patients, and almost 20% had never discussed hospice care with family members.

e) Timely referrals to hospice were not facilitated.

f) Only about one-third of nurses discussed hospice with patients and families at EOL, but these same nurses identified that almost all of these patients would have benefited from hospice or earlier hospice referral.

g) Requesting additional pain medication plus using active and passive listening skills were the most frequent palliative care interventions.

H. Temel et al. (2010) landmark study of patients with metastatic non-small cell lung cancer showed the following benefits of early palliative care:

1. Increased quality of life

2. Improved mood

    3. Fewer symptoms of depression

    4. More days under hospice care

    5. Decreased aggressive EOL care

    6. Increased survival of approximately two months

IV. Relevance to practice

    A. When caring for patients who are living with and dying from chronic conditions, do so from the perspective of understanding and appreciating the unique experience it brings to each patient and family.

    B. Although similarities do exist in the dying process, it is important to acknowledge the differences that exist between disease pathophysiology, pharmaceutical metabolism, culture, gender, religious, and spiritual components and how all of these influence clinical decision making.

        1. Death often occurs in the presence of family or caregivers when the healthcare provider is not available.

        2. The importance of family preparation is crucial (McCusker et al., 2013; NCI, 2016).

        3. Family and caregivers who understand what to expect and how to help support their loved one are less fearful when death occurs.

        4. If a member of the interdisciplinary team is privileged to be present as EOL occurs, tremendous support can be provided to the family and caregivers during a fragile and emotional experience.

        5. Waves of grief that were mixed throughout the disease trajectory may suddenly resurface at the moment of death.

        6. The rhythm of care abruptly changes in the face of death and focuses more on the immediate needs of the family.

        7. The prepared interdisciplinary team has assessed individual rituals and activated them to promote a healthy grieving process.

        8. Rituals are social practices that facilitate and provide ways to understand and accentuate the positive aspects of the contradictory and complex nature of human existence (McCusker et al., 2013).

V. Role of the advanced practice registered nurse (APRN)

    A. APRNs providing care for patients at EOL require knowledge and skills that address the complex needs that encompass the whole person at the center of care (IOM, 2013) and includes the family.

    B. Multiple chronic conditions elicit numerous symptoms that often are interrelated, necessitating thorough assessment provided by APRNs to determine not only the intensity of each symptom but also the interference with quality of life and the distress caused by the symptom (D'Arcy, 2012; McMillan et al., 2015).

    C. Communication skills necessary for difficult discussions with patients and families are more likely to be found among APRNs (Svarovsky, 2013).

        1. The role of APRNs is to ensure that these difficult conversations take place in a therapeutic manner to allow the patient and family the opportunity to have the information they need and want for appropriate decision-making tasks (Svarovsky, 2013).

        2. Patients who are facing life's end are left with the memories of the life they have lived.

        3. These memories include past experiences, strengths, weaknesses, different degrees of spirituality, and possibly unwritten life chapters.

    D. Death is as monumental as birth, and each life is unique (D'Arcy, 2012).

    E. APRNs who are skilled in palliative care are able to provide patients and families with the tools to engage in EOL care planning and also assist in the expert management of symptoms that promote optimal quality of life (Melvin, 2010).

VI. Interface to palliative care

    A. Palliative care consultations can effectively bridge the information gap that often leads to undesirable, aggressive treatment interventions near EOL with standard acute care of chronic conditions (IOM, 2015; Melvin, 2010).

    B. EOL care is complex and requires an adequately trained interdisciplinary team to meet the fluctuating physical, emotional, spiritual, and social needs of patients and families in a coordinated fashion (IOM, 2015).

        1. Members of the interdisciplinary team include the physician, APRN, nurse, social worker, chaplain, and others as needed.

        2. The focus of palliative care is expert, aggressive symptom management to mitigate the impact of patients' symptoms on their functioning (Marchetti, Voltz, Rubio, Mayeur, & Kopf, 2013).

    C. Patients at EOL must be thoroughly assessed for a multitude of symptoms before these symptoms can be successfully managed, ideally based on evidence (D'Arcy, 2012; Klein-Fedyshin, 2015; McMillan et al., 2015). Many medical choices are not evidence based and future research should be aimed at the various components of EOL care (IOM, 2013).

    D. Patients may be receiving palliative care as they approach EOL.

        1. Hospice care should be a consideration when the patient's life expectancy is six months or less and there is no desire for curative treatment (Boyd et al., 2011; IOM, 2013).

        2. Hospice care is always delivered in a palliative manner. It is available as a Medicare benefit and often covered by private insurance (McCusker et al., 2013).

    E. Gómez-Batiste et al. (2013) noted that palliative care has been historically reserved for patients with cancer but that the mortality rate for patients with chronic conditions is 2:1 compared to patients with cancer. This study highlighted the importance of primary care screening for palliative care needs in patients with chronic conditions to allow for early integration of palliative care services to promote optimal quality of life.

    F. Palliative care involvement may result in fewer EOL hospital admissions and improved patient outcomes when adequate time is available for palliative care interventions. Palliative care involvement that is provided too late in the progression of the chronic condition, or not at all, often results in an increased burden to the patient and family and decreased quality of life for all (Melvin, 2010).

Case Study

    D.S. is an 87-year-old Caucasian man living with his wife of 13 years in an assisted living facility three hours from their nearest family member. D.S. has COPD, adult-onset diabetes, and mild renal insufficiency as chronic conditions. For the past five months, D.S. has become increasingly short of breath and more dependent on supplemental oxygen. D.S. has two sons living in different states, and his wife has a niece living in the same town as one of the sons. The decision was made to move D.S. and his wife to an assisted living facility in the town where the one son and the niece live to allow for greater family assistance with care. Soon after D.S. and his wife are settled in their new home, D.S. becomes increasingly forgetful, not taking medications as prescribed, not eating well, losing weight, and even more short of breath. Because D.S. is a veteran, an appointment is made with the APRN at the local Veterans Affairs clinic to review these symptoms. The astute APRN recognizes the symptoms of nearing EOL and initiates a discussion to identify the desires of the patient and family. D.S., his wife, and his son acknowledge the decline in D.S.'s health and accept the referral to palliative care. D.S. and his family go to the palliative care appointment later that week. The palliative care APRN discusses EOL plans and identifies that D.S. has completed an advance directive, does not want to die in the hospital "hooked up to machines," and just wants to be kept "comfortable." The APRN addresses the concerns of the son regarding his father's difficulty breathing and assures the family that managing breathing would be a priority for symptom management. The APRN suggests that D.S. use a hospital bed at home to allow for comfortable positioning to promote optimal breathing. The APRN also suggests using a fan to increase air movement and keeping the room cool to further ensure ease in breathing. D.S.'s wife expresses distress at the thought of becoming a widow for the second time. The palliative care chaplain is called in to provide additional support to the wife. Medications are reviewed, and any that are not important for symptom management are discontinued. D.S.'s blood sugar testing has been below 75 mg/dl on several occasions in the past two weeks. Therefore, the glyburide was discontinued to avoid the possibility of hypoglycemia in the setting of decreased food intake. A referral is made to the local hospice to provide comfort care. D.S. enjoys the time at home with his family, and his breathing is comfortable with continuous oxygen. D.S. begins to sleep more than half the day and is taking in little food. The hospice nurse applies a scopolamine patch behind D.S.'s ear to prevent the accumulation of secretions and lessen the anticipated "death rattle." The family notes that D.S. is not responding to them when they try to talk to him or get his attention. The son states that his dad cannot seem to close his eyes. D.S. dies comfortably three days later with his family at his bedside. The family is saddened at his death but fully appreciates the preparation provided by the interdisciplinary team that allowed D.S.'s desires to be honored and their needs for support and information to be met.

References

Arenella, C. (n.d.). Artificial nutrition and hydration at the end of life: Beneficial or harmful? Retrieved from http://americanhospice.org/caregiving/artificial-nutrition-and-hydration-at-the-end-of-life-beneficial-or -harmful

Boyd, D., Merkh, K., Rutledge, D.N., & Randall, V. (2011). Nurses' perceptions and experiences with end-of-life communication and care [Online exclusive]. *Oncology Nursing Forum, 38,* E229–E239. doi:10.1188/11.ONF. E229-E239

Cannon, C.A., Watson, L.K., Roth, M.T., & LaVergne, S. (2014). Assessing the learning needs of oncology nurses. *Clinical Journal of Oncology Nursing, 18,* 577–580. doi:10.1188/14.CJON.577-580

Caraceni, A., Davies, A., Poulain, P., Cortés-Funes, H., Panchal, S.J., & Fanelli, G. (2013). Guidelines for the management of breakthrough pain in patients with cancer. *Journal of the National Comprehensive Cancer Network, 11*(Suppl. 1), S29–S26. Retrieved from http://www.jnccn.org/content/11/suppl_1/S-29.long

Close, J.F., & Long, C.O. (2012). Delirium: An opportunity in palliative care. *Journal of Hospice and Palliative Nursing, 14,* 386–394. doi:10.1097/NJH.0b013e31825d2b0a

Cloyes, K.G., Berry, P.H., Reblin, M., Clayton, M., & Ellington, L. (2012). Exploring communication patterns among hospice nurses and family caregivers: A content analysis of in-home speech interactions. *Journal of Hospice and Palliative Nursing, 14,* 426–437. doi:10.1097/NJH.0b013e318251598b

D'Arcy, Y. (2012). Managing end-of-life symptoms. *American Nurse Today, 7*(7), 22–27. Retrieved from https://americannursetoday.com/managing-end-of-life-symptoms

Del Ferraro, C., Grant, M., Koczywas, M., & Dorr-Uyemura, L.A. (2012). Management of anorexia-cachexia in late-stage lung cancer patients. *Journal of Hospice and Palliative Nursing, 14,* 397–402. doi:10.1097/ NJH.0b013e31825f3470

Goldsmith, J., Ferrell, B., Wittenberg-Lyles, E., & Ragan, S.L. (2013). Palliative care communication in oncology nursing. *Clinical Journal of Oncology Nursing, 17,* 163–167. doi:10.1188/13.CJON.163-167

Gómez-Batiste, X., Martínez-Muñoz, M., Blay, C., Amblàs, J., Vila, L., Costa, X., … Constante, C. (2013). Identifying patients with chronic conditions in need of palliative care in the general population: Development of the NECPAL tool and preliminary prevalence rates in Catalonia. *BMJ Supportive and Palliative Care, 3,* 300–308. doi:10.1136/bmjspcare-2012-000211

Hui, D., dos Santos, R., Chisholm, G., Bansal, S., Crovador, C.S., & Bruera, E. (2015). Bedside clinical signs associated with impending death in patients with advanced cancer: Preliminary findings of a prospective, longitudinal cohort study. *Cancer, 121,* 960–967. doi:10.1002/cncr.29048

Institute of Medicine. (2013). *Delivering high-quality cancer care: Charting a new course for a system in crisis.* Washington, DC: National Academies Press.

Institute of Medicine. (2015). *Dying in America: Improving quality and honoring individual patient preferences near the end of life.* Washington, DC: National Academies Press.

Kanacki, L.S., Roth, P., Georges, J.M., & Herring, P. (2012). Shared presence: Caring for a dying spouse. *Journal of Hospice and Palliative Nursing, 14,* 414–425. doi:10.1097/NJH.0b013e3182554a2c

Kennedy, C., Brooks-Young, P., Gray, C.B., Larkin, P., Connolly, M., Wilde-Larsson, B., … Chater, S. (2014). Diagnosing dying: An integrative literature review. *BMJ Supportive and Palliative Care, 4,* 263–270. doi:10.1136/bmjspcare-2013-000621

Klein-Fedyshin, M. (2015). Translating evidence into practice at the end of life: Information needs, access, and usage by hospice and palliative nurses. *Journal of Hospice and Palliative Nursing, 17,* 24–30. doi:10.1097/NJH.0000000000000117

Kozlov, M., Anderson, M.A., & Sparbel, K.J. (2011). Opioid-induced neurotoxicity in the hospice patient. *Journal of Hospice and Palliative Nursing, 13,* 341–346. doi:10.1097/NJH.0b013e3182271932

Marchetti, P., Voltz, R., Rubio, C., Mayeur, D., & Kopf, A. (2013). Provision of palliative care and pain management services for oncology patients. *Journal of the National Comprehensive Cancer Network, 11*(Suppl. 1), S17–S27. Retrieved from http://www.jnccn.org/content/11/suppl_1/S-17.long

McCusker, M., Ceronsky, L., Crone, C., Epstein, H., Greene, B., Halvorson, J., … Setterlund, L. (2013, November). *Institute for Clinical Systems Improvement (ICSI) health care guideline: Palliative care for adults.* Retrieved from https://www.icsi.org/_asset/k056ab/PalliativeCare.pdf

McMillan, S.C., Tofthagen, C., Choe, R., & Rheingans, J. (2015). Assessing symptoms experienced by patients with cancer: Occurrence, intensity, distress, interference, and frequency. *Journal of Hospice and Palliative Nursing, 17,* 56–65. doi:10.1097/NJH.0000000000000123

McPherson, M.L., Kim, M., & Walker, K.A. (2012). 50 practical medication tips at end of life. *Journal of Supportive Oncology, 10,* 222–229.

Melvin, C.S. (2010). Patient's and families' misperceptions about hospice and palliative care: Listen as they speak. *Journal of Hospice and Palliative Nursing, 12,* 107–115. doi:10.1097/NJH.0b013e3181cf7933

National Cancer Institute. (2016, April 8). Last days of life (PDQ®) [Health professional version]. Retrieved from http://www.cancer.gov/about-cancer/advanced-cancer/caregivers/planning/last-days-hp-pdq

Oligario, G.C., Buch, C., & Piscotty, R. (2015). Nurses' assessment of delirium with underlying dementia in end-of-life care. *Journal of Hospice and Palliative Nursing, 17,* 16–21. doi:10.1097/NJH.0000000000000099

Parikh, R.B., Kirch, R.A., Smith, T.J., & Temel, J.S. (2013). Early specialty palliative care—Translating data in oncology into practice. *New England Journal of Medicine, 369,* 2347–2351. doi:10.1056/NEJMsb1305469

Revier, S.S., Meiers, S.J., & Herth, K.A. (2012). The lived experience of hope in family caregivers caring for a terminally ill loved one. *Journal of Hospice and Palliative Nursing, 14,* 438–446. doi:10.1097/NJH.0b013e318257f8d4

Schreiber, T.P., & Bennett, M.J. (2014). Identification and validation of premortem surge. *Journal of Hospice and Palliative Nursing, 16,* 430–437. doi:10.1097/NJH.0000000000000094

Schultz, M., & Bar-Sela, G. (2013). Initiating palliative care conversations: Lessons from Jewish bioethics. *Journal of Supportive Oncology, 11,* 1–7.

Strand, J.J., & Billings, J.A. (2012). Integrating palliative care in the intensive care unit. *Journal of Supportive Oncology, 10,* 180–187.

Svarovsky, T. (2013). Having difficult conversations: The advanced practitioner's role. *Journal of the Advanced Practitioner in Oncology, 4,* 47–52. doi:10.6004/jadpro.2013.4.1.5

Temel, J.S., Greer, J.A., Muzikansky, A., Gallagher, E.R., Admane, S., Jackson, V.A., … Lynch, T.J. (2010). Early palliative care for patients with metastatic non–small-cell lung cancer. *New England Journal of Medicine, 363,* 733–742. doi:10.1056/NEJMoa1000678

Thoonsen, B., Engels, Y., van Rijswijk, E., Verhagen, S., van Weel, C., Groot, M., & Vissers, K. (2012). Early identification of palliative care patients in general practice: Development of RADboud indicators for PAlliative Care Needs (RADPAC). *British Journal of General Practice, 62,* e625–e631. doi:10.3399/bjgp12X654597

Von Roenn, J.H., Voltz, R., & Serrie, A. (2013). Barriers and approaches to the successful integration of palliative care and oncology practice. *Journal of the National Comprehensive Cancer Network, 11*(Suppl. 1), S11–S16. Retrieved from http://www.jnccn.org/content/11/suppl_1/S-11.long

Wittenberg-Lyles, E., Goldsmith, J., & Ferrell, B. (2013). Oncology nurse communication barriers to patient-centered care. *Clinical Journal of Oncology Nursing, 17,* 152–158. doi:10.1188/13.CJON.152-158

Zeppetella, G. (2013). Evidence-based treatment of cancer-related breakthrough pain with opioids. *Journal of the National Comprehensive Cancer Network, 11*(Suppl. 1), S37–S43. Retrieved from http://www.jnccn.org/content/11/suppl_1/S-37.long

Zhang, B., Nilsson, M.E., & Prigerson, H.G. (2012). Factors important to patients' quality of life at the end of life. *Archives of Internal Medicine, 172,* 1133–1142. doi:10.1001/archinternmed.2012.2364

Zomorodi, M., & Lynn, M.R. (2010). Critical care nurses' values and behaviors with end of life care: Perceptions and challenges. *Journal of Hospice and Palliative Nursing, 12,* 89–96. doi:10.1097/NJH.0b013e3181cf7cf6

CHAPTER 35

Advance Care Planning

Jennifer Fournier, MSN, APRN-CNS, ACNS-BC, AOCN®, CHPN

I. Definition
   A. Advance care planning is the evolving process of goal setting and planning communication among patients, families, and the interdisciplinary healthcare team to establish and deliver care based on patient wishes (Institute of Medicine [IOM], 2015). The interdisciplinary team is prepared to communicate with patients and families regarding advance care planning (Del Ferraro, Ferrell, Van Zyl, Freeman, & Klein, 2014; McCusker et al., 2013).
   B. Advance care planning is an integral component to palliative care and is considered for every adult (McCusker et al., 2013).
   C. IOM (2015) recommended that the initiation of advance care planning be tied to a developmental milestone similar to obtaining a driver's license for the first time, turning 18, or getting married, as these events are all linked to changes in responsibility.
      1. The ideal time to inform family members of advance directives is while health is good and considerations can be equally weighed.
      2. Studies have shown that patients look to healthcare professionals to initiate the discussion of advance care planning at routine office visits (Cohen & Nirenberg, 2011; IOM, 2015; McCusker et al., 2013).
      3. Advance directives are intended to be reevaluated with annual health visits and changes in physical status (IOM, 2015).
   D. Legal terms used in advance care planning (McCusker et al., 2013)
      1. Competency: Determined by a judge at the conclusion of a hearing; a legal status imposed by a court
      2. Decisional: Patients may be deemed to have the ability to make medical decisions (decision-making capacity) regarding their own care if the healthcare professional determines they are able to receive information, process information, and express preferences based on the information provided.
      3. Healthcare agent: Individual appointed by the patient, as named in the advance directive or as permitted by law, to make healthcare decisions on behalf of the patient if the patient loses decision-making capacity
      4. Healthcare or advance directive
         a) A written document completed by the patient to make healthcare preferences known if the patient becomes unable to communicate wishes
         b) This document only becomes active when the patient no longer has decision-making capacity.
         c) Individual state laws vary.

      d) Two legal directives exist:
        (1) Living will, which is a document outlining the patient's wishes for care at the end of life
        (2) Medical power of attorney, which is a person appointed by the patient to make medical decisions on behalf of the patient
      e) Power of attorney: Person appointed by the patient to make financial or real estate transactions on behalf of the patient
      f) Surrogate: Person who by default becomes the decision maker for a patient without a designated healthcare agent (IOM, 2015)

II. Key aspects
  A. Advance care planning is acknowledged as a vital aspect of palliative care (McCusker et al., 2013).
  B. The Patient Self-Determination Act of 1990 requires that all adults be asked if they have completed advance directives before being admitted to a healthcare facility receiving Medicare or Medicaid reimbursement (IOM, 2015; McCusker et al., 2013). The intent of this law is to allow adults the opportunity to communicate individual wishes before a life-threatening event or health crisis occurs.
  C. Another component of the Patient Self-Determination Act is the requirement for community and staff education regarding advance directives (IOM, 2015; McCusker et al., 2013).
    1. National Healthcare Decisions Day (NHDD) is held each year on or about April 16 in an attempt to promote nationwide education and discussions about advance care planning (NHDD, 2016).
      a) Participation from more than 100 national organizations and 1,600 state organizations
      b) Participation of U.S. military bases worldwide
      c) Advance directive training provided to more than 3.5 million facility and organization staff
      d) Participation in local events by more than two million Americans
      e) Completion of more than 30,000 advance directives on the first seven NHDDs (2008–2014)
      f) Participation of social media sites, newspaper, radio, and television to increase public awareness
      g) Formally recognized by both houses of Congress in its inaugural year (2008)
    2. Physician orders for life-sustaining treatment (POLST) facilitates communication across settings to ensure that patients' preferences for treatment are translated into orders. It is not an advance directive nor does it replace an advance directive (IOM, 2015).
      a) POLST addresses the issues of resuscitation, interventions, antibiotics, future hospitalizations, and artificial nutrition and hydration.
      b) POLST is intended for use during the last year of life for frail patients (IOM, 2015).
      c) POLST is especially important in emergency situations because emergency medical services personnel cannot honor living wills or take direction from a family member (IOM, 2015; McCusker et al., 2013).
  D. Barriers to advance care planning (McCusker et al., 2013)
    1. Healthcare professionals fear sending the wrong message to patients who are healthy.
    2. Patients believe that the financial power of attorney covers medical decisions.

      3. A medical power of attorney is needed for medical decision making for a person not competent to make his or her own healthcare decisions.

      4. Patients fear losing control.

      5. Patients fear they will not be treated.

      6. African American, Hispanic, and Asian cultures tend to avoid advance care planning (IOM, 2015; Yu, Chae, Choi, & Kim, 2013).

      7. Common misconception exists among both patients and healthcare providers that only older adults need advance care planning.

      8. Patients who need advance care planning the most may be the least likely to complete the required documentation (Cohen & Nirenberg, 2011).

  E. For patients near death, ensure that advance directives are in place and followed (National Comprehensive Cancer Network® [NCCN®], 2015).

  F. Less than one-third of patients admitted to hospitals have completed advance care planning (Wenger, Asakura, Fink, & Oman, 2012).

III. Current findings

  A. Kennedy et al. (2014) completed an integrative literature review of diagnosing dying from 23 publications discussing chronic conditions across several continents.

      1. This review showed the importance of investigating approaching death with the patient and the family and allowing the time needed to process intense information and make critical decisions regarding advance care planning.

      2. The authors identified that trust and support of the patient and family could be strengthened by the interdisciplinary team acknowledging the uncertainty of knowing precisely when death might occur.

  B. Boyd, Merkh, Rutledge, and Randall (2011) conducted a descriptive correlational survey study of 31 oncology nurses at a Magnet® hospital to evaluate personal experiences and perceptions of end-of-life care and patient and family communication. Findings showed that 29% of nurses did not discuss advance care planning because they did not want to take away hope, and 69% of nurses believed that older patients trust the physician to develop the best plan of care.

  C. Research of 160 RNs at a university hospital showed that less than 16% of these nurses had completed advance care planning, which is less than the national average of 20%–30% (Wenger et al., 2012).

      1. An educational intervention was held with the opportunity for the RNs to complete the Five Wishes® advance directive.

      2. Of those attending the event, 58% completed the advance directive.

IV. Relevance to practice

  A. Without a clear understanding of both advance care planning and palliative care, patients and families may respond to the need to make future treatment decisions for chronic conditions with a sense of loss of hope or futility (Del Ferraro et al., 2014; Strand & Billings, 2012).

      1. Studies suggest that truthful conversations do not take away hope (IOM, 2015).

      2. A systematic review of the literature regarding hope shows a positive relationship between hope and the ability to cope with the situation (Butt, 2011).

      3. The interdisciplinary team can work toward meeting the patient's and family's sense of hope and goals for care (Baer & Weinstein, 2013).

  B. Shared decision making among the interdisciplinary healthcare team, patient, and family includes the following (Kane, Halpern, Squiers, Treiman, & McCormack, 2014; McCusker et al., 2013):

      1. All options are discussed, to include hospice when indicated.

    2. Patients and families know whom to contact.

    3. Clinicians know the key decision makers.

    4. Goals of care are discussed and determined.

    5. Optimal medical management is provided; treatment adherence is maintained.

    6. Patients and families direct the plan of care and have confidence in the plan and the interdisciplinary team.

    7. Patients and families are prepared for likely outcomes and have a sense of physical and emotional well-being.

C. Advance care planning is a fluid process and may change as the patient's condition or goals change (Cohen & Nirenberg, 2011; IOM, 2015; McCusker et al., 2013; Von Roenn, 2013).

D. Advance care planning is a process that embodies clear, honest, and thoughtful communication as the patient and family develop a trusting relationship with the interdisciplinary team that takes all aspects of their being into consideration for the plan.

    1. Respecting Choices® (Gundersen Health System, 2015) is one of the leading advance directive initiatives focused on providing patients with ongoing communication directed at ensuring that patients' end-of-life wishes are known and honored. The goal is to change professional and institutional culture and processes to facilitate comprehensive advance care planning.

    2. Five Wishes (Aging with Dignity, 2011) provides a patient- and family-friendly advance directive for adults that meet almost every U.S. state's legal requirements and allows adults to make their final wishes known. Statements listed in Five Wishes include the following:

        a) "I wish to have my favorite music played."

        b) "I wish to know about options for hospice care."

        c) "I wish to have my hand held and be talked to."

        d) "I wish to be forgiven."

        e) "I wish for my family and friends and caregivers to respect my wishes even if they don't agree with them."

        f) "I wish for my family and friends to look at my dying as a time of personal growth for everyone, including me. This will help me live a meaningful life in my final days."

V. Role of the advanced practice registered nurse (APRN)

A. APRNs are well suited to communicate with patients and families the importance of advance care planning based on clinical experience, training, and proficiency in the subject (Del Ferraro et al., 2014).

B. IOM (2015) recommends that APRNs are qualified to conduct consultations regarding advance care planning.

C. APRNs should acknowledge that end-of-life conversations can be difficult for all involved, but the rewards for the task can be increased understanding, improved quality of life, closer relationships, and honoring patient preferences (Cohen & Nirenberg, 2011; Von Roenn, 2013).

    1. Studies support that informed patients who have completed advance care planning generally prefer to forgo resuscitation, ventilator usage, and intensive care when these interventions will not result in cure of the condition (IOM, 2015; Von Roenn, 2013).

    2. Medicare beneficiaries are eligible for an initial visit within 12 months of enrolling in Medicare Part B titled, "Welcome to Medicare" preventive visit. One aspect of this visit is to discuss advance directives (Medicare.gov, n.d.).

3. This "Welcome to Medicare" preventive visit code is seldom used, however, and an opportunity to address advance care planning is lost (IOM, 2015).

4. The 2016 Medicare Physician Fee Schedule now includes two new payment codes for advance care planning (Medicare.gov, n.d.).

D. Transitions in care, such as progression of disease, allow APRNs to inquire about changes in goals of care, especially as related to end-of-life desires (Cohen & Nirenberg, 2011; IOM, 2013; Svarovsky, 2013).

E. A healthcare model utilizing APRNs resulted in a higher number of completed advance directives when compared to a model without APRNs (Cohen & Nirenberg, 2011).

F. Promotion of collaboration by APRNs may elicit earlier advance care planning through palliative care referrals (Cohen & Nirenberg, 2011).

VI. Interface to palliative care

A. Palliative care is ideally conducive to advance care planning in patients with chronic conditions.

1. The interdisciplinary team is poised to assist patients and families through this intense journey of exploration of feelings, desires, and goals.

2. The palliative care team devotes the time needed for patient autonomy in the process of examining all available treatment options and the considerations that apply to each (D'Arcy, 2012; IOM, 2013; Zalonis & Slota, 2014).

3. The patient and family are left with a clearer understanding of the goals of care and a respect for the decisions made.

B. As patients are identified as embodying the need for palliative care, the need for advance care planning is inherent (Gómez-Batiste et al., 2013).

C. Patients with multiple chronic conditions are especially prone to difficulty in advance care planning because of the fragmentation of care that frequently results from a multitude of providers with possibly conflicting or overly optimistic communication (Cheon, Coyle, Wiegand, & Welsh, 2015; Zalonis & Slota, 2014).

1. Fragmentation of care in patients with chronic conditions also can result from multiple transfers between settings of care, including potentially unwarranted hospitalizations (IOM, 2015).

2. Determining prognosis to facilitate decision making is equally problematic (D'Arcy, 2012; Kennedy et al., 2014).

3. It is especially difficult to predict overall prognosis in patients with multiple chronic conditions (IOM, 2015).

D. Ongoing communication between the interdisciplinary team and the patient and family is essential.

1. Patients need honest and complete information, including the benefits and burdens of treatment or no treatment (Von Roenn, 2013).

2. Patients do not always sense when they are nearing the end of life.

3. Physicians have been shown to overestimate life expectancy by twofold or greater in multiple studies (McCusker et al., 2013).

E. Goals of care may change as the chronic condition progresses. Reexamine goals to make any desired changes at decision points along the chronic condition continuum (Cohen & Nirenberg, 2011; IOM, 2013; McCusker et al., 2013; NCCN, 2015).

F. NCCN (2015) palliative care guidelines encourage healthcare professionals to inquire about patient preferences for organ donation, autopsy, and place of death.

G. The American Bar Association Commission on Law and Aging (n.d.) suggests that advance directives be reviewed any time one of the five D's occurs:

1. New decade in age
2. Death of a loved one
3. Divorce
4. Diagnosis of a significant medical condition
5. Decline in health

Case Study

L.L. is a 65-year-old African American woman who is seeing the APRN for her first full physical examination under Medicare. One component of this preventive visit allows for a discussion of advance care planning. L.L. is accompanied by her 64-year-old husband. Neither L.L. nor her husband had thought about advance care planning but listen intently as the APRN explains the importance of completing a personal advance directive. The APRN discusses the importance for L.L. and her husband to engage in a meaningful discussion together about their expectations of care as they age and to include family members or close friends who may be involved in their plan for care, knowing that transparent and open communication has to occur for advance care planning to be successful. The standardized Five Wishes document is provided to L.L. to complete together with her husband and family. The APRN explains that advance care planning will be discussed again from time to time, especially if changes occur in L.L.'s health or living situation. The APRN ensures that L.L. understands the components of the advance care planning discussion by asking if she has any questions. L.L. asks what she should do with the form once it is completed. The APRN states that the form has to be signed in the presence of two witnesses not affected by the choices made by L.L. and notarized to meet state requirements. The APRN informs L.L. that a copy of her advance care plan will be placed in her medical records and that she should keep the original document with other important papers in her home. The APRN asks again if L.L. understands and if there are any other questions. L.L. and her husband state that they appreciate the opportunity to learn about advance care planning and to make important decisions affecting their care at the end of life without the added pressure of dealing with a serious illness.

References

Aging with Dignity. (2011). Five Wishes® [Brochure]. Tallahassee, FL: Author.

American Bar Association Commission on Law and Aging. (n.d.). Myths and facts about health care advance directives. Retrieved from http://www.americanbar.org/content/dam/aba/migrated/Commissions/myths_fact_hc_ad.authcheckdam.pdf

Baer, L., & Weinstein, E. (2013). Improving oncology nurses' communication skills for difficult conversations [Online exclusive]. *Clinical Journal of Oncology Nursing, 17,* E45–E51. doi:10.1188/13.CJON.E45-E51

Boyd, D., Merkh, K., Rutledge, D.N., & Randall, V. (2011). Nurses' perceptions and experiences with end-of-life communication and care [Online exclusive]. *Oncology Nursing Forum, 38,* E229–E239. doi:10.1188/11.ONF.E229-E239

Butt, C.M. (2011). Hope in adults with cancer: State of the science [Online exclusive]. *Oncology Nursing Forum, 38,* E341–E350. doi:10.1188/11.ONF.E341-E350

Cheon, J., Coyle, N., Wiegand, D.L., & Welsh, S. (2015). Ethical issues experienced by hospice and palliative nurses. *Journal of Hospice and Palliative Nursing, 17,* 7–13. doi:10.1097/NJH.0000000000000129

Cohen, A., & Nirenberg, A. (2011). Current practices in advance care planning: Implications for nurses. *Clinical Journal of Oncology Nursing, 15,* 547–553. doi:10.1188/11.CJON.547-553

D'Arcy, Y. (2012). Managing end-of-life symptoms. *American Nurse Today, 7*(7), 22–27. Retrieved from https://americannursetoday.com/managing-end-of-life-symptoms

Del Ferraro, C., Ferrell, B., Van Zyl, C., Freeman, B., & Klein, L. (2014). Improving palliative cancer care. *Journal of the Advanced Practitioner in Oncology, 5,* 331–338. doi:10.6004/jadpro.2014.5.5.3

Gómez-Batiste, X., Martínez-Muñoz, M., Blay, C., Amblàs, J., Vila, L., Costa, X., ... Constante, C. (2013). Identifying patients with chronic conditions in need of palliative care in the general population: Development of the NECPAL tool and preliminary prevalence rates in Catalonia. *BMJ Supportive and Palliative Care, 3,* 300–308. doi:10.1136/bmjspcare-2012-000211

Gundersen Health System. (2015). Return on investment: Implementation of Respecting Choices® model of advance care planning. Retrieved from http://www.gundersenhealth.org/upload/docs/respecting-choices/Respecting-Choices-return-on-investment.pdf

Institute of Medicine. (2013). *Delivering high-quality cancer care: Charting a new course for a system in crisis.* Washington, DC: National Academies Press.

Institute of Medicine. (2015). *Dying in America: Improving quality and honoring individual patient preferences near the end of life.* Washington, DC: National Academies Press.

Kane, H.L., Halpern, M.T., Squiers, L.B., Treiman, K.A., & McCormack, L.A. (2014). Implementing and evaluating shared decision making in oncology practice. *CA: A Cancer Journal for Clinicians, 64,* 377–388. doi:10.3322/caac.21245

Kennedy, C., Brooks-Young, P., Gray, C.B., Larkin, P., Connolly, M., Wilde-Larsson, B., ... Chater, S. (2014). Diagnosing dying: An integrative literature review. *BMJ Supportive and Palliative Care, 4,* 263–270. doi:10.1136/bmjspcare-2013-000621

McCusker, M., Ceronsky, L., Crone, C., Epstein, H., Greene, B., Halvorson, J., ... Setterlund, L. (2013, November). *Institute for Clinical Systems Improvement (ICSI) health care guideline: Palliative care for adults.* Retrieved from https://www.icsi.org/_asset/k056ab/PalliativeCare.pdf

Medicare.gov. (n.d.). Your Medicare coverage: Preventive visit and yearly wellness exams. Retrieved from http://www.medicare.gov/coverage/preventive-visit-and-yearly-wellness-exams.html

National Comprehensive Cancer Network. (2015). *NCCN Clinical Practice Guidelines in Oncology (NCCN Guidelines®): Palliative care* [v.1.2016]. Retrieved from http://www.nccn.org/professionals/physician_gls/pdf/palliative.pdf

National Healthcare Decisions Day. (2016). Retrieved from http://www.nhdd.org

Strand, J.J., & Billings, J.A. (2012). Integrating palliative care in the intensive care unit. *Journal of Supportive Oncology, 10,* 180–187.

Svarovsky, T. (2013). Having difficult conversations: The advanced practitioner's role. *Journal of the Advanced Practitioner in Oncology, 4,* 47–52. doi:10.6004/jadpro.2013.4.1.5

Von Roenn, J.H. (2013). Advance care planning: Ensuring that the patient's voice is heard. *Journal of Clinical Oncology, 31,* 663–664. doi:10.1200/JCO.2012.46.8181

Wenger, B., Asakura, Y., Fink, R.M., & Oman, K.S. (2012). Dissemination of the Five Wishes advance directive at work. *Journal of Hospice and Palliative Nursing, 14,* 551–558. doi:10.1097/NJH.0b013e31825ebae0

Yu, S.J., Chae, Y.R., Choi, Y.S., & Kim, H.S. (2013). Patients' perceptions of advance directives and preferences for medical care near the end of life in South Korea. *Journal of Hospice and Palliative Nursing, 15,* 233–243. doi:10.1097/NJH.0b013e31827bdbc0

Zalonis, R., & Slota, M. (2014). The use of palliative care to promote autonomy in decision making. *Clinical Journal of Oncology Nursing, 18,* 707–711. doi:10.1188/14.CJON.707-711

CHAPTER 36

Preparation Versus Crisis Approach to Care

Jennifer Fournier, MSN, APRN-CNS, ACNS-BC, AOCN®, CHPN

I. Definition
   A. Preparation for optimal palliative care requires an interdisciplinary evaluation and assessment of the complex care needs of the patient and family living with and dying from multiple chronic conditions (MCCs).
   B. Palliative care requires coordinated interdisciplinary interventions that are enacted at the onset of diagnostically confirmed symptomatic MCCs. This concept is supported by the American Society of Clinical Oncology, the Center to Advance Palliative Care, the World Health Organization, and the National Comprehensive Cancer Network® (Glare, 2013).
   C. Palliative care that addresses the multidimensional needs of the family requires the support and expertise provided by the interdisciplinary healthcare team (Melvin, 2010).
   D. Meeting these complex needs requires preventing the patient and family from reaching a crisis-like situation wherein physical, emotional, and spiritual symptoms reach heightened levels that provoke anxiety and fear.
   E. Patients and families who experience a crisis situation often avoid the important preparation that is required to accept and understand the progressive nature of MCCs and how to be proactively prepared to utilize the interdisciplinary team to monitor and advise during times of uncertainty (Melvin, 2010).
II. Key aspects
   A. Of patients with advanced-stage cancer, 65%–80% erroneously believed that medical interventions will provoke a cure (Institute of Medicine [IOM], 2013). Specifically, 81% of patients with stage IV colorectal cancer and 69% of patients with stage IV lung cancer believed that chemotherapy treatments would eradicate their disease despite poor prognosis (Weeks et al., 2012).
   B. Unfortunately, the integration of an interdisciplinary team skilled in palliative interventions often is reserved for end-of-life care and not considered when patients are newly diagnosed with a chronic symptomatic condition (Glare, 2013).
      1. Palliative interventions directed by the interdisciplinary team should be included in the care plan when patients present with physical, psychosocial, or spiritual symptoms.
      2. Palliative care should be integrated throughout the disease trajectory and used to support the family into bereavement (IOM, 2013; McCusker et al., 2013; Strand & Billings, 2012; Zalonis & Slota, 2014).

C. Chronic conditions that warrant palliative care are not limited to cancer diagnoses but include advanced cardiac disease, pulmonary disorders, renal disease, hepatic disease, and neurologic conditions, all of which eventually lend to disability and reduced physical functioning (D'Arcy, 2012; Gómez-Batiste et al., 2013; McCusker et al., 2013; Melvin, 2010; Strand, Kamdar, & Carey, 2013).

D. Determining the initial integration of palliative interventions can occur in any setting, such as outpatient clinics, long-term care, private primary care practices, and acute care settings (Gómez-Batiste et al., 2013; McCusker et al., 2013).

E. Conducting patient and family meetings can be an effective preparation tool when assessing the patient and family's realistic understanding of the patient's prognosis.
1. Taking the opportunity during this time to establish mutual goals offers the interdisciplinary team an opportunity to determine literacy needs, answer questions, clarify misconceptions, provide support, and elicit pertinent referrals (Strand & Billings, 2012).
2. Patients and families who are in a time of crisis will be unable to effectively engage in a family meeting (IOM, 2015).

F. Acceptance of the inevitable final stages associated with progressive chronic conditions can lead to a sense of peace and the renewed value of life remaining when planned and thoughtful preparation has been made (Zhang, Nilsson, & Prigerson, 2012).

G. Physician orders for life-sustaining treatment (POLST) discussions are intended for the last year of life as a way to prepare and honor individual patients' end-of-life care wishes that result in a medical directive that is accepted in most states in the United States (IOM, 2015).

H. Up to one-fourth of patients admitted to an intensive care unit (ICU) have a life expectancy of months rather than years (Adolph, Frier, Stawicki, Gerlach, & Papadimos, 2011).
1. Old age and the burden from MCCs are the strongest predictors of death (Adolph et al., 2011).
2. The ICU often is a site for crisis care for patients with MCCs.
3. Family distress often is heightened when a loved one is admitted to the ICU with poorly managed symptoms, perpetuating a crisis-like situation (Strand & Billings, 2012; Zomorodi & Lynn, 2010).
4. Zhang et al. (2012) demonstrated that the quality of life of patients with cancer in the last week of life was adversely affected by admission to the ICU or an acute care setting. The researchers found that the use of feeding tubes and dying in the hospital were connected to worse patient-perceived quality of life.
5. Approaches to provide support to family members as they prepare to care for their loved one's chronic conditions are similar to those used when family members are caring for patients at the end of life (see Chapter 35). Acknowledge that caregiver support is crucial for effective, patient-centered care (IOM, 2015).

III. Current findings
A. Resolving ethical issues is vital to avoiding the crisis approach to care.
1. A survey by Cheon, Coyle, Wiegand, and Welsh (2015) showed that ethical issues often require an interdisciplinary team approach to filter conflicts and fully understand the intricacies of the situation.
2. Issues are resolved using a variety of techniques such as family meetings, inclusion of palliative medicine, ethics committee review, support for the patient and family, and clarification of goals (Cheon et al., 2015).

B. Preparation can be hampered by the individual's perception of his or her condition.
   1. This was demonstrated in a study of adult women diagnosed with late-stage all-cause cancer (Croom, Hamann, Kehoe, Paulk, & Wiebe, 2013).
   2. This cross-sectional study of 105 women demonstrated that personal beliefs about illness can have a greater impact on behavior than medical aspects of the diagnosis.
C. Patients can have a premortem surge or last-minute rally that can disturb family members if they are not prepared for this possible occurrence (Schreiber & Bennett, 2014).
   1. Families may incorrectly believe that their loved one is getting better.
   2. This swift period of increased alertness and liveliness can last for 6–24 hours and usually occurs in the last 24–48 hours of life.
D. Bakitas, Lyons, Hegel, and Ahles (2013) conducted a study of oncologists' perspectives on a concurrent palliative care model following the conclusion of the Educate, Nurture, Advise, Before Life Ends (ENABLE II).
   1. Qualitative, descriptive study of 35 oncology clinicians at a National Cancer Institute (NCI)-designated comprehensive cancer center
   2. Clinician participants included medical oncology, hematology, and radiation oncology physicians and nurse practitioners.
   3. Randomized clinical trial
   4. The studied cancer center had long-standing interdisciplinary palliative care, both inpatient and outpatient, which was a well-integrated component of the standard of care.
   5. One-half of the ENABLE II participants received nurse-led, telephonic supportive care over four structured sessions with monthly follow-up; the other half received standard care.
   6. Results showed that oncologists valued the palliative care interdisciplinary team as being "consultants and co-managers," as "sharing the load," and as taking the "extra time" available for complex patients and families.
   7. Patients who are provided a description and introduction to palliative care through skilled and sensitive communication without distraction are more likely to embrace the benefits of palliative care. This intervention helps to reduce crisis by providing the appropriate time for discussion and ultimate preparation.
E. Boyd, Merkh, Rutledge, and Randall (2011) conducted a descriptive correlational survey study of 31 oncology nurses at a Magnet® facility querying their experiences and perceptions of end-of-life care and communication.
   1. The hypothesis for this study was that these nurses would have progressive attitudes regarding the implementation and use of important palliative care discussions and would be fairly competent to provide these conversations with patients and families.
   2. Startling findings from this study include the following:
      a) Opportunities to discuss end-of-life care were overlooked.
      b) Of the nurses surveyed, 29% had never discussed advance care with patients, and almost 20% had never discussed end-of-life care with family members, often a contributing factor for development of a crisis-like situation.
      c) Providing prognostic information is critical; 90% of the nurses believed it was essential for dying patients to be informed of their prognosis. This leads to better preparation as the trajectory for chronic conditions progresses toward debility and eventual death.

   F. Strand and Billings (2012) described a proactive approach to providing palliative care in the ICU to avoid a reactive crisis mode of care.
      1. The researchers illustrate the effectiveness of an automatic consult for a family meeting with the palliative care interdisciplinary team within 72 hours of a patient's admission to ICU.
      2. This preparation resulted in collective goals of care, increased family satisfaction with communication, and shorter ICU lengths of stay (Strand & Billings, 2012).
   G. A literature review of the implementation of shared decision making with patients with cancer recommended that a shared decision-making process increases patient and family satisfaction with care and leads to improved outcomes (Kane, Halpern, Squiers, Treiman, & McCormack, 2014).
   H. Recommended steps in shared decision making
      1. Invite the patient and family to participate. Patients and families will require differing degrees of information based on literacy levels.
      2. Present all care options to the patient, including benefits and risks.
      3. Acknowledge uncertainties and allow time to process information.
      4. Ascertain the patient's preferences, values, and wishes.
      5. Involve the family as desired by the patient.
      6. Define care goals developed by the shared decision-making process. Proposed statements to facilitate the process include the following:
         a) "Sometimes things in medicine are not as clear as most people think. Let's work together so we can come up with the decision that is right for you."
         b) "People have different goals and concerns. As you think about your options, what is important to you?"
         c) "Do you want to think about this decision with anyone else—someone who might be affected by the decision or who might help sort things out?"
         d) "I want to be sure I have explained things well. Please tell me what you heard."
IV. Relevance to practice
   A. Understanding the needs of the patient and family as they prepare and make plans for care involves an appreciation of the multiple and complex aspects that make a human being more than the sum of body systems.
      1. The art of supporting the patient's needs and responding to emotions during a crisis should include recruiting resources from all members of the disciplinary team (Dunn, 2011; Kanacki, Roth, Georges, & Herring, 2012; Revier, Meiers, & Herth, 2012; Zalonis & Slota, 2014).
      2. Common emotions to evaluate
         a) Anxiety
         b) Strong emotional feelings
         c) Anger
         d) Sadness
         e) Loneliness
         f) Depression
         g) Withdrawal
   B. Revier et al. (2012) found spirituality to be important in end-of-life care as a component of instilling hope in grieving loved ones.
      1. Spiritual providers can offer regular visitation, devotional and worship activities, consultation and referral for different cultures, grief counseling, and help

to support patients and families in different settings using community support systems (Kanacki et al., 2012).

   2. Pastoral visits to patients with cancer in hospitals and clinics have been shown to have a positive effect on quality of life in the last week of life. Prayer or meditation also was shown to exhibit a positive effect (Zhang et al., 2012).

C. Uncontrolled symptoms, especially in the later stages of the disease, can easily escalate into a crisis for both the patient and family as a result of increased symptom burden and diminished resiliency (D'Arcy, 2012; NCI, 2016; Zhang et al., 2012).

D. The interdisciplinary team can help to identify unresolved emotional or spiritual issues and inform the family and caregivers about any changes in the patient's condition.

V. Role of the advanced practice registered nurse (APRN)

A. Despite the growing practice of palliative care, many physicians continue to equate palliative care with hospice care or reserve the consult to palliative care until the end of life (Bauman & Temel, 2014; Boyd et al., 2011; D'Arcy, 2012; Glare, 2013).

B. APRNs can foster earlier consults to palliative care in patients with MCCs, thereby allowing for adequate preparation and education for patients and families and avoiding a stressful, crisis experience that disrupts quality of life (D'Arcy, 2012; Del Ferraro, Ferrell, Van Zyl, Freeman, & Klein, 2014; IOM, 2013).

C. Preparation for care involves APRNs building relationships based on trust and respect with patients and families. As transition points in care occur, APRNs can communicate these changes with patients and families in a manner that works best for them to address physical, psychosocial, spiritual, and emotional needs (IOM, 2013; McCusker et al., 2013; Svarovsky, 2013).

D. Bakitas et al. (2013) conducted a qualitative randomized clinical trial to investigate oncology physician and APRN views regarding embedded palliative care in their practice at a NCI-designated comprehensive cancer center. These providers identified the value of early palliative care referrals to assist with preparing patients and caregivers for appropriate care through the ENABLE II intervention.

E. Patients with advanced cancer and their caregivers perceived palliative care provided by the interdisciplinary team as a normal part of care when it was introduced in the beginning of care, thus reducing a barrier that occurs when referrals to palliative care are delayed until later in the disease trajectory or closer to death.

VI. Interface to palliative care

A. Care conferences or family meetings are an integral component of palliative care and can be useful to prepare patients and families for the progressive course of MCCs (Cheon et al., 2015; IOM, 2013).

B. Goals of a care conference (McCusker et al., 2013)

   1. Understand patient wishes and ask the patient what he or she feels is important.
   2. Promote effective, honest communication among the interdisciplinary team, family, and patient.
   3. Develop a realistic plan that fits the needs of the moment; review goals periodically and modify course as needed.
   4. Develop an ongoing, trusting relationship with the patient and family.

C. Gómez-Batiste et al. (2013) stressed the importance of preparation versus crisis care in their study to identify primary care patients with chronic conditions who would benefit from early palliative care. Their tool was designed to identify patients within the last year of life to facilitate the use of palliative care services.

Case Study

The APRN makes a routine homecare visit on the first day of summer to C.T., a 78-year-old Caucasian man with stage IV lung cancer. A student nurse is shadowing the APRN for the day. C.T. is resting comfortably in his hospital bed on the back porch, watching his grandchildren play hide-and-seek in the back yard of their riverfront home. C.T.'s wife of 55 years is frosting a cake to celebrate their anniversary and sadly informs the APRN that she knows this will be their last anniversary. C.T. wants the student nurse to have a good understanding of his case and asks the APRN, the student, and his wife to sit down with him while he talks about their life together and his death, which will come soon. C.T. recounts his wedding day, the births of their five children, their memorable trip to the Grand Canyon, and other fond memories. He shares that these last five months have been good and he has been able to feel well enough to enjoy his time with the family without having to deal with multiple clinic visits for uncomfortable treatments. C.T. talks about the first day he went to the medical oncologist after he was diagnosed with incurable disease and expressed great appreciation for the interdisciplinary team. C.T. says that he and his wife were informed about all the available options to treat and manage his conditon in detail.

The first day of chemotherapy stands out for C.T. because of the serious reaction he had to the first dose and how the palliative care team was there for him afterward to make sure that he was well managed. C.T. explains how the palliative care team prepared him and his family for the future. He commented on how each member of the team discussed the disease process, medications for symptom management, and what to expect as the lung cancer progressed. C.T. had completed his advance care planning more than 10 years ago and he was impressed with how the palliative care team reviewed these documents to ensure his wishes had not changed. C.T. explains to the student nurse that because he was in his last year of life, the palliative care team added a bright pink POLST form to ensure that physician orders were in place to direct his care if needed.

C.T. assures the APRN, the student nurse, and his wife that he is not fearful and knows that all his needs will be promptly addressed as they arise. He says he is confident that his needs will be followed through his proactive preparation. The student nurse thanks C.T. and his wife for the time that they have shared and tells them that this personal experience will be immensely beneficial throughout her nursing career.

References

Adolph, M.D., Frier, K.A., Stawicki, S.P.A., Gerlach, A.T., & Papadimos, T.J. (2011). Palliative critical care in the intensive care unit: A 2011 perspective. *International Journal of Critical Illness and Injury Science, 1,* 147–153. doi:10.4103/2229-5151.84803

Bakitas, M., Lyons, K.D., Hegel, M.T., & Ahles, T. (2013). Oncologists' perspectives on concurrent palliative care in a National Cancer Institute-designated comprehensive cancer center. *Palliative and Supportive Care, 11,* 415–423. doi:10.1017/S1478951512000673

Bauman, J.R., & Temel, J.S. (2014). The integration of early palliative care with oncology care: The time has come for a new tradition. *Journal of the National Comprehensive Cancer Network, 12,* 1763–1771. Retrieved from http://www.jnccn.org/content/12/12/1763.long

Boyd, D., Merkh, K., Rutledge, D.N., & Randall, V. (2011). Nurses' perceptions and experiences with end-of-life communication and care [Online exclusive]. *Oncology Nursing Forum, 38,* E229–E239. doi:10.1188/11.ONF .E229-E239

Cheon, J., Coyle, N., Wiegand, D.L., & Welsh, S. (2015). Ethical issues experienced by hospice and palliative nurses. *Journal of Hospice and Palliative Nursing, 17,* 7–13. doi:10.1097/NJH.0000000000000129

Croom, A.R., Hamann, H.A., Kehoe, S.M., Paulk, E., & Wiebe, D.J. (2013). Illness perceptions matter: Understanding quality of life and advanced illness behaviors in female patients with late-stage cancer. *Journal of Supportive Oncology, 11,* 165–173.

D'Arcy, Y. (2012). Managing end-of-life symptoms. *American Nurse Today, 7*(7), 22–27. Retrieved from https://americannursetoday.com/managing-end-of-life-symptoms

Del Ferraro, C., Ferrell, B., Van Zyl, C., Freeman, B., & Klein, L. (2014). Improving palliative cancer care. *Journal of the Advanced Practitioner in Oncology, 5,* 331–338. doi:10.6004/jadpro.2014.5.5.3

Dunn, G.P. (2011). Surgical palliative care: Recent trends and developments. *Surgical Clinics of North America, 91,* 277–292. doi:10.1016/j.suc.2011.01.002

Glare, P.A. (2013). Early implementation of palliative care can improve patient outcomes. *Journal of the National Comprehensive Cancer Network, 11*(Suppl. 1), S3–S9. Retrieved from http://www.jnccn.org/content/11/suppl_1/S-3.long

Gómez-Batiste, X., Martínez-Muñoz, M., Blay, C., Amblàs, J., Vila, L., Costa, X., ... Constante, C. (2013). Identifying patients with chronic conditions in need of palliative care in the general population: Development of the NECPAL tool and preliminary prevalence rates in Catalonia. *BMJ Supportive and Palliative Care, 3,* 300–308. doi:10.1136/bmjspcare-2012-000211

Institute of Medicine. (2013). *Delivering high-quality cancer care: Charting a new course for a system in crisis.* Washington, DC: National Academies Press.

Institute of Medicine. (2015). *Dying in America: Improving quality and honoring individual patient preferences near the end of life.* Washington, DC: National Academies Press.

Kanacki, L.S., Roth, P., Georges, J.M., & Herring, P. (2012). Shared presence: Caring for a dying spouse. *Journal of Hospice and Palliative Nursing, 14,* 414–425. doi:10.1097/NJH.0b013e3182554a2c

Kane, H.L., Halpern, M.T., Squiers, L.B., Treiman, K.A., & McCormack, L.A. (2014). Implementing and evaluating shared decision making in oncology practice. *CA: A Cancer Journal for Clinicians, 64,* 377–388. doi:10.3322/caac.21245

McCusker, M., Ceronsky, L., Crone, C., Epstein, H., Greene, B., Halvorson, J., ... Setterlund, L. (2013, November). *Institute for Clinical Systems Improvement (ICSI) health care guideline: Palliative care for adults.* Retrieved from https://www.icsi.org/_asset/k056ab/PalliativeCare.pdf

Melvin, C.S. (2010). Patient's and families' misperceptions about hospice and palliative care: Listen as they speak. *Journal of Hospice and Palliative Nursing, 12,* 107–115. doi:10.1097/NJH.0b013e3181cf7933

National Cancer Institute. (2016, April 8). *Last days of life (PDQ®)* [Health professional version]. Retrieved from http://www.cancer.gov/about-cancer/advanced-cancer/caregivers/planning/last-days-hp-pdq

Revier, S.S., Meiers, S.J., & Herth, K.A. (2012). The lived experience of hope in family caregivers caring for a terminally ill loved one. *Journal of Hospice and Palliative Nursing, 14,* 438–446. doi:10.1097/NJH.0b013e318257f8d4

Schreiber, T.P., & Bennett, M.J. (2014). Identification and validation of premortem surge. *Journal of Hospice and Palliative Nursing, 16,* 430–437. doi:10.1097/NJH.0000000000000094

Strand, J.J., & Billings, J.A. (2012). Integrating palliative care in the intensive care unit. *Journal of Supportive Oncology, 10,* 180–187.

Strand, J.J., Kamdar, M.M., & Carey, E.C. (2013). Top 10 things palliative care clinicians wished everyone knew about palliative care. *Mayo Clinic Proceedings, 88,* 859–865. doi:10.1016/j.mayocp.2013.05.020

Svarovsky, T. (2013). Having difficult conversations: The advanced practitioner's role. *Journal of the Advanced Practitioner in Oncology, 4,* 47–52. doi:10.6004/jadpro.2013.4.1.5

Weeks, J.C., Catalano, P.J., Cronin, A., Finkelman, M.D., Mack, J.W., Keating, N.L., & Schrag, D. (2012). Patients' expectations about effects of chemotherapy for advanced cancer. *New England Journal of Medicine, 367,* 1616–1625. doi:10.1056/NEJMoa1204410

Zalonis, R., & Slota, M. (2014). The use of palliative care to promote autonomy in decision making. *Clinical Journal of Oncology Nursing, 18,* 707–711. doi:10.1188/14.CJON.707-711

Zhang, B., Nilsson, M.E., & Prigerson, H.G. (2012). Factors important to patients' quality of life at the end of life. *Archives of Internal Medicine, 172,* 1133–1142. doi:10.1001/archinternmed.2012.2364

Zomorodi, M., & Lynn, M.R. (2010). Critical care nurses' values and behaviors with end of life care: Perceptions and challenges. *Journal of Hospice and Palliative Nursing, 12,* 89–96. doi:10.1097/NJH.0b013e3181cf7cf6

CHAPTER 37

Identifying Team Disciplines

Suzette Walker, DNP, FNP-BC, AOCNP®

I. Definition
   A. The interdisciplinary team is composed of all disciplines who come together with the patient and family to provide supportive decision making and develop, implement, and coordinate the individualized plan of care.
   B. Each member of the interdisciplinary team offers collaborative contribution with the patient and family at the center of care without a hierarchy (World Health Organization [WHO], 2013).
   C. The interdisciplinary team comprises the following:
      1. Patient and family: Family is composed of important and significant individuals relevant to the patient and may not include the traditional definition of family (e.g., unrelated individuals).
      2. Friends, significant others, spiritual advisers, love relationships, etc.
      3. Medical disciplines
         a) Primary care providers (e.g., physicians, advanced practice providers)
         b) Medical specialists (e.g., pulmonologists, cardiologists, rheumatologists, psychiatrists)
         c) Physician assistants
      4. Nursing disciplines
         a) Doctors of nursing practice
         b) Nurse practitioners
         c) Clinical nurse specialists
         d) RNs
         e) Licensed practical nurses
         f) Nurse aides
      5. Behavioral health disciplines
         a) Psychologists
         b) Medical social workers
         c) Counselors
         d) Group therapists
      6. Spiritual disciplines
         a) Priests, pastors, reverends, rabbis, etc.
         b) Church-affiliated support groups
      7. Pharmacy disciplines

    a) Doctors of pharmacy
    b) Pharmacists
    c) Medical science liaisons
   8. Rehabilitation disciplines
    a) Physical therapists
    b) Occupational therapists
    c) Pulmonary rehabilitation teams
    d) Cardiac rehabilitation teams
   9. Registered dietitians
   10. Volunteers
 II. Key aspects
  A. The interdisciplinary team includes healthcare professionals who have received appropriate education, credentialing, and experience with the skills and knowledge to meet the physical, psychological, social, and spiritual needs of the patient and family (WHO, 2013).
   1. The interdisciplinary team and the patient and family collaborate and communicate openly to establish realistic, patient-specific goals and address a plan of care to meet these goals.
   2. The interdisciplinary team provides services to the patient and family consistent with the care plan by collaborating with appropriate and required disciplines to meet the myriad needs of patients living with and dying from multiple chronic conditions (MCCs).
   3. The interdisciplinary team should focus on specific domains of care, including the following:
    a) Structure and processes of care
     (1) Occurs throughout the disease trajectory from diagnosis of a chronic condition until death
     (2) Patient-specific plan of care that focuses on promoting the physical, psychological, social, and spiritual domains of what is perceived as quality of life pertinent to the individual patient's perspective (WHO, 2013)
     (3) Care that is provided in a safe environment, respecting the patient's and family's values, preferences, and wishes
    b) Physical aspects of care
     (1) Maintenance and promotion of ongoing physical functioning as the number-one indicator for patient-perceived quality of life
     (2) Prompt recognition of symptoms that require proactive assessment, evaluation, and monitoring
     (3) Knowledge of underlying etiology and the implications of concomitant conditions and reduction of symptom burden
     (4) Use of evidence-based interventions and less frequent reliance on expensive diagnostic measurements that do not influence the patient's medical management
    c) Psychological and emotional aspects of care
     (1) Ongoing psychological and emotional well-being assessment
     (2) Prompt recognition and management of depression, anxiety, restlessness, insomnia, or any emotional symptoms that precipitate somatic discomfort
     (3) Preparation for loss, grief, and bereavement for the patient and family

     d) Social aspects of care
       (1) Recognition that every patient and family is unique in their approach to disease, debility, and dying process
       (2) Use of supportive interventions with a specific focus on patient culture, values, strengths, goals, and personal preferences
     e) Spiritual, religious, and existential aspects of care
       (1) Evaluation and assessment of patient affiliation to church, religious relationships, or a place of spiritual or religious practice
       (2) Recruitment of key people identified by the patient to participate in the plan of care
       (3) Maintenance of open communication with religious affiliation, including information on any changes of patient condition (per patient approval)
     f) Cultural aspects of care
       (1) Awareness by interdisciplinary team members of any cultural differences that the patient and family may require
       (2) Inclusion of cultural beliefs and practices that best support the patient and family needs
       (3) Involvement of interpreters, cultural leaders, and supportive measures to assist the interdisciplinary team to ensure best patient-centered outcomes

B. The Chronic Care Model, first described by Bodenheimer, Wagner, and Grumbach in 2002, is an organized framework for improving chronic care in the primary care setting and can serve as an example of how the interdisciplinary team can support each individual patient and his or her family. The six components of this model are as follows (Bodenheimer, Wagner, et al., 2002; Improving Chronic Illness Care, n.d.):

1. Health system
   a) A culture, organization, and mechanism that promote safe, high-quality care
   b) Support for improvement at all levels of the organization, beginning with senior leaders
   c) Effective improvement strategies aimed at comprehensive system change
   d) Open and systematic handling of errors and quality problems
   e) Incentives based on care quality
   f) Agreements that facilitate care coordination within and across organizations
2. Community resources
   a) Patient participation in effective community programs
   b) Partnerships with community organizations to fill gaps in needed services
   c) Policies that improve patient care
3. Self-management support
   a) Empowerment and preparation of patients to manage their health and health care
   b) Emphasis on patients' role in managing their health
   c) Effective self-management strategies including assessment, goal setting, action planning, problem solving, and follow-up
   d) Internal and community resources for supporting patients in self-management
4. Delivery system design
   a) Delivery of effective, efficient care and self-management support
   b) Definition of team member roles and distribution of tasks
   c) Planned interactions to support evidence-based care

        d) Clinical case management services for complex patient cases

        e) Regular follow-up by the care team

        f) Care that patients understand and that fits with their cultural background

    5. Decisional support

        a) Clinical care consistent with evidence and patient preferences

        b) Use of evidence-based guidelines in daily clinical practice

        c) Sharing of evidence-based guidelines with patients to encourage participation

        d) Use of proven education methods

        e) Integration of specialist expertise and primary care

    6. Clinical information systems

        a) Organization of patient and population data to facilitate efficient and effective care

        b) Timely reminders for providers and patients

        c) Identification of relevant subpopulations for proactive care

        d) Individual patient care planning

        e) Information sharing with patients and providers to coordinate care

        f) Performance monitoring of the practice team and care system

  C. The integration of palliative care into the care and management of patients with MCCs in the primary care setting can be accomplished by the interdisciplinary team working together to provide primary care services to support the patient and family.

    1. Together, the team can discuss treatment goals and promote earlier advance planning through an established relationship with the patient and family.

    2. Primary care providers can and should rely on the skills and knowledge available to address and meet the multiple needs that patients and families face as chronic conditions progress and associated symptomatology develops.

III. Current findings

  A. WHO (2013) provided a report for strengthening the integration of palliative care into the management of MCCs. This report called for the integration of palliative care services into existing routine global healthcare services for all patients.

  B. A review of 10 years of experience using the Chronic Care Model summarized that care should be redesigned to use this model to include palliative care, as data have shown this can lead to improved patient care and better patient-centered outcomes (Coleman, Austin, Brach, & Wagner, 2009).

IV. Relevance to practice

  A. The patient–healthcare provider relationship has changed over time from being a dictatorship to being a partnership.

  B. This partnership is collaborative care in which the provider and patient make healthcare decisions together. Collaborative care allows for providers to have the expertise on management of the illness, while at the same time allowing patients to be the expert regarding their own values and preferences.

  C. Patients should be informed and active in their own care with the providers. Self-management is essential in empowering patients to achieve their own established goals of care.

    1. Self-management practices allow patients to be proactive in their own care and can be used to reduce symptoms, prevent disease exacerbations, and seek appropriate resources to address escalating problems.

    2. Self-management education can improve clinical outcomes and reduce healthcare costs (Bodenheimer, Lorig, Holman, & Grumbach, 2002).

V. Role of the advanced practice registered nurse (APRN)

    A. A significant need exists for more primary care providers in the United States. APRNs are ideal members of the interdisciplinary team to ensure appropriate clinical management and integration of the interdisciplinary team in patients living with symptomatic MCCs (Horrocks, Anderson, & Salisbury, 2002; Laurant et al., 2005; Newhouse et al., 2011).

    B. Other studies have shown that APRNs are effective in providing palliative care in in various disease states and settings, including inpatient units, outpatient services, long-term facilities, and home care (Carlson, Lim, & Meier, 2011; Deitrick et al., 2011; Kaasalainen et al., 2013; Lowery et al., 2012; Lukas, Foltz, & Paxton, 2013; Owens et al., 2012).

    C. The role of the APRN will depend on the model and setting of care. Traditionally, three common models are used in palliative care.

        1. The first model, which represents most of what is done in chronic illness, has the primary care provider both approaching the need of palliative care with the patient as well as providing this care.

        2. The second model is the palliative care team as a consult team.

            a) In some programs, the primary care team then chooses what suggestions to use.

            b) In other programs, the consult team implements suggestions.

        3. The third model is the concept that the primary care team would integrate palliative care into its disease management program, and palliative care would act as a consultant to the team and provide more specialized palliative services as needed.

    D. The majority of patients do not receive care in a tertiary care center where specialized palliative care teams practice.

        1. The first model is where the majority of patients will receive care and is the realm that APRNs excel in.

        2. The Chronic Care Model is congruent with the traditional palliative care model, making it possible for all patients to benefit.

VI. Interface to palliative care

    A. In 2014, the National Center for Health Statistics reported that almost half of adults in the country died from cardiovascular disease or cancer.

    B. Palliative care improves the life of patients and their families, as well as provides benefits to the health system as a whole by reducing the use of healthcare services (Heinle, McNulty, & Hebert, 2014).

    C. WHO (2013) estimates that 20 million people worldwide need palliative care services every year and just as many people need palliative care in the year of their death, bringing the total to 40 million people annually who will use these services.

    D. The Center to Advance Palliative Care (2015) provides a comprehensive definition of palliative care.

        1. Palliative care is specialized medical care for people with serious illnesses that is focused on providing relief from the symptoms, pain, and stress of living with a chronic condition.

        2. Palliative care improves healthcare quality in the following three ways:

            a) Relieves physical and emotional suffering

            b) Strengthens communication and decision making among patients, families, and physicians

            c) Ensures coordination of care across all healthcare settings

Case Study

L.N. is a 62-year-old woman who presents to her primary care provider for a six-month medication review. She is accompanied by her 16-year-old granddaughter. Her past medical history includes stage 3 chronic obstructive pulmonary disease, hypertension, and hyperlipidemia. Current medications include albuterol inhaler every four to six hours as needed for dyspnea, tiotropium dry powder inhalation once daily, lisinopril 20 mg daily, and simvastatin 40 mg at bedtime.

L.N. believes she is doing all right with her medications. She describes having an increase in dyspnea and has been using her albuterol rescue inhaler every three to four hours. She is using the albuterol before climbing the steps to her bedroom. She describes her cough as productive and is easily fatigued. She has lost 15 pounds since her last clinic visit six months ago. She denies loss of appetite or nausea. L.N. is concerned about her physical decline. She is worried about her granddaughter, whom she has raised. She has not communicated with her daughter in 15 years and does not have legal custody of her granddaughter. She fears falling in the shower and takes a shower only when she knows her granddaughter is home. She believes that the weight loss is due to anxiety and not eating. It takes her until noon most days to complete her morning care and come downstairs. She is eating once a day in the evening with her granddaughter.

The APRN's assessment findings include stage 3 chronic obstructive pulmonary disease worsening, weakness, weight loss, and fall risk. After conversation with the APRN, L.N. states that although she has been reluctant to talk about advance planning for her health care, she believes it is now time to meet with the social worker. She identifies her best friend and her sister-in-law as her support system and will ask them to be at this meeting. She would also like to meet with the social worker to talk about options for the care of her granddaughter. She agrees to pulmonary rehabilitation and a visit with the dietitian. Although she is reluctant, as she fears what her granddaughter will think, she agrees to a home safety evaluation with a home nursing agency.

At her follow-up appointment three weeks later, she and her provider discuss the recommendations of the other team members. L.N. is very pleased with the dietitian referral and has implemented the changes advised. She has increased her protein intake and now keeps high-protein snacks and drinks in her upstairs bedroom so that she can have nutrition without going downstairs.

She believes she is doing better with pulmonary rehabilitation and says she looks forward to continuing therapy. The provider shares with L.N. that she agrees with the desire of the pulmonary therapist to perform an overnight home pulse oxygen study to see if night use of oxygen helps her. L.N. is worried about what this will look like to her granddaughter.

The provider reviews with L.N. the home safety report, and L.N. confirms the delivery of a shower chair and installation of grip bars in the upstairs and downstairs bathrooms. However, she says she is not sure she will be able to afford to have a railing installed for the stairway.

She is meeting weekly with the social worker but feels she is still not ready to have a heart-to-heart with her granddaughter. She says she has requested her best friend to speak to her pastor for support. L.N. asks whether the APRN agrees with the social worker that a medication for depression or anxiety may help her. After discussion, she agrees to start a low dose of an antidepressant.

Two weeks later, the social worker reports to the APRN that L.N. has made great progress. She has completed the advance directives, and a copy is within the medical record. She has made her sister-in-law her patient advocate and power of attorney for health care. This will ensure that her healthcare wishes will be met. Although L.N. does not think that the new medication for depression is helping, both the social worker and the respiratory therapist believe they see an improvement in her anxiety level.

L.N. met with her pastor to discuss her granddaughter. Together, the pastor, L.N., and her sister-in-law met with L.N.'s granddaughter to discuss the decline in L.N.'s health. The granddaughter will now be receiving counseling from the youth pastor at the church in which she grew up. As an added bonus, the men's group in the church volunteered to finance and install the railing on L.N.'s stairway.

The respiratory therapist reports that the sleep PO_2 readings were concerning, with a low of 79% during sleep and an average of 84%. The therapist obtains an order for home O_2 at 2 L per nasal cannula. At this point, L.N. has agreed to wear it at night and during her personal care. She is uneasy about using it downstairs.

The dietitian reports a three-pound weight gain for L.N. since her first visit and was also able to encourage L.N.'s best friend to arrange for a girls' afternoon with several of their friends. The focus was on cooking, packaging, and labeling meals for L.N.'s freezer with high-protein nutritious foods from recipes provided by the dietitian and L.N.'s friends. These will be used on L.N.'s bad days.

The home nursing service is sending an RN weekly with an aide visiting twice a week to help with personal care. L.N. was hesitant to accept this much care but has agreed. Home nursing will continue to assess and increase care as needed. The nurse shares that L.N. did not pick up her long-acting inhaler at the pharmacy this morning because the co-pay had increased from $20 to $325. L.N. called and spoke to the pharmacist, who confirmed with the insurance company that the preferred long-acting inhaler has changed. The pharmacist stated that once the order arrived, the pharmacy would deliver the new inhaler to the home. The APRN immediately sent a new prescription electronically to the pharmacy with the now-approved inhaler.

At L.N.'s next visit with the APRN, she states that she has improved. She says she did not realize she was depressed until she started to feel better. She states that with the work she is doing with the pastor and the social worker, she feels at peace. She has learned that it is all right to lean on family and friends when she needs to. She feels stronger and feels like she is even thinking better. She relays that she and her sister-in-law have met with a lawyer to ensure that provisions and care are provided for her granddaughter. She says the lawyer thinks this could take a few months. However, L.N. states that she is sure that with "her team" helping her, she will be able to obtain this goal as well.

References

Bodenheimer, T., Lorig, K., Holman, H., & Grumbach, K. (2002). Patient self-management of chronic disease in primary care. *JAMA, 288,* 2469–2475. doi:10.1001/jama.288.19.2469

Bodenheimer, T., Wagner, E.H., & Grumbach, K. (2002). Improving primary care for patients with chronic illness. *JAMA, 288,* 1775–1779. doi:10.1001/jama.288.14.1775

Carlson, M.D.A., Lim, B., & Meier, D.E. (2011). Strategies and innovative models for delivering palliative care in nursing homes. *Journal of the American Medical Directors Association, 12,* 91–98. doi:10.1016/j.jamda.2010.07.016

Center to Advance Palliative Care. (2015). The growth of palliative care in U.S. hospitals: 2015 snapshot (2000–2013). Retrieved from https://media.capc.org/filer_public/34/77/34770c03-a584-4079-a9ae-edb98dab6b20/growth_snapshot_2016_final.pdf

Coleman, K., Austin, B.T., Brach, C., & Wagner, E.H. (2009). Evidence on the Chronic Care Model in the new millennium. *Health Affairs, 28,* 75–85. doi:10.1377/hlthaff.28.1.75

Deitrick, L.M., Rockwell, E.H., Gratz, N., Davidson, C., Lukas, L., Stevens, D., ... Sikora, B. (2011). Delivering specialized palliative care in the community: A new role for nurse practitioners. *Advances in Nursing Science, 34,* E23–E36. doi:10.1097/ans.0b013e318235834f

Heinle, R., McNulty, J., & Hebert, R.S. (2014). Nurse practitioners and the growth of palliative medicine. *American Journal of Hospice and Palliative Medicine, 31,* 287–291. doi:10.1177/1049909113489163

Horrocks, S., Anderson, E., & Salisbury, C. (2002). Systematic review of whether nurse practitioners working in primary care can provide equivalent care to doctors. *BMJ, 324,* 819–823. doi:10.1136/bmj.324.7341.819

Improving Chronic Illness Care. (n.d.). Steps for Improvement (1): Models. Retrieved from http://www.improvingchroniccare.org/index.php?p=1:_Models&s=363

Kaasalainen, S., Ploeg, J., McAiney, C., Martin, L.S., Donald, F., Martin-Misener, R., ... Sangster-Gormley, E. (2013). Role of the nurse practitioner in providing palliative care in long-term care homes. *International Journal of Palliative Nursing, 19,* 477–485. doi:10.12968/ijpn.2013.19.10.477

Laurant, M., Reeves, D., Hermens, R., Braspenning, J., Grol, R., & Sibbald, B. (2005). Substitution of doctors by nurses in primary care. *Cochrane Database of Systematic Reviews, 2005*(2). doi:10.1002/14651858.cd001271.pub2

Lowery, J., Hopp, F., Subramanian, U., Wiitala, W., Welsh, D.E., Larkin, A., ... Vaitkevicius, P. (2012). Evaluation of a nurse practitioner disease management model for chronic heart failure: A multi-site implementation study. *Congestive Heart Failure, 18,* 64–71. doi:10.1111/j.1751-7133.2011.00228.x

Lukas, L., Foltz, C., & Paxton, H. (2013). Hospital outcomes for a home-based palliative medicine consulting service. *Journal of Palliative Medicine, 16,* 179–184. doi:10.1089/jpm.2012.0414

National Center for Health Statistics. (2014). *Health, United States, 2014: With special feature on adults aged 55–64.* Retrieved from http://www.cdc.gov/nchs/data/hus/hus14.pdf

Newhouse, R.P., Stanik-Hutt, J., White, K.M., Johantgen, M., Bass, E.B., Zangaro, G., ... Weiner, J.P. (2011). Advanced practice nurse outcomes 1990–2008: A systematic review. *Nursing Economics, 29,* 230–250.

Owens, D., Eby, K., Burson, S., Green, M., McGoodwin, W., & Isaac, M. (2012). Primary Palliative Care Clinic Pilot Project demonstrates benefits of a nurse practitioner-directed clinic providing primary and palliative care. *Journal of the American Academy of Nurse Practitioners, 24,* 52–58. doi:10.1111/j.1745-7599.2011.00664.x

World Health Organization. (2013, December 20). Strengthening of palliative care as a component of integrated treatment throughout the life course (Report by the Secretariat). Retrieved from http://apps.who.int/gb/ebwha/pdf_files/EB134/B134_28-en.pdf

CHAPTER 38

Patient and Family Goal Setting

Janice Firn, PhD, LMSW

I. Definitions

    A. Shared decision making (SDM) "occurs when a health care provider and a patient work together to make a health care decision that is best for the patient. The optimal decision takes into account evidence-based information about available options, the provider's knowledge and experience, and the patient's values and preferences" (Agency for Healthcare Research and Quality, 2014).

    B. SDM opportunities can occur in any setting and may arise over a variety of situations (Minnesota Shared Decision-Making Collaborative, n.d.).

        1. Onetime treatment or testing decisions (e.g., transesophageal echocardiogram, bronchoscopy)

        2. Possible serial treatments (e.g., chemotherapy)

        3. Preventive care or screening (e.g., prostate-specific antigen test, colorectal cancer screening)

        4. Lifestyle decisions (e.g., exercise, diet changes, smoking cessation)

        5. Chronic care decisions (e.g., heart disease, anticoagulation)

        6. Life stage decisions (e.g., moving into a skilled care facility)

    C. *Goals of care* are the intended purposes of healthcare interventions as agreed upon by the patient or substitute decision maker, family, and healthcare team (Reuben & Tinetti, 2012). Goals of care decisions take into account but are not limited to the following features:

        1. All parties' understanding of the disease and what to realistically expect based on the trajectory of disease and disability

        2. Physical, emotional, spiritual, social, and financial implications, resources, and limitations

        3. Physical functioning of the patient and informal caregivers

        4. Cognitive intactness of the patient and informal caregivers

        5. Family and caregiver availability to participate in care and to what degree

        6. Location and level of care needed now and how that may change over the course of the illness

        7. Insurance benefits, financial considerations, transportation requirements, and other practical and tangible needs

        8. Timing, frequency, and location of interventions

        9. Specific patient or family events (e.g., travel, anniversaries, wedding, birth of a grandchild)

D. *Patient decision aids* are tools that help patients participate in their own healthcare decisions in ways of their own choosing (International Patient Decision Aid Standards Collaboration, 2012).

   1. Decision aids are implemented when more than one medically reasonable option to diagnose or treat a problem exists.

   2. Each option has positive and negative features that individuals may value differently.

   3. Decision aids prepare patients to make decisions by providing facts about the condition and the risks and benefits of the intervention options, helping patients to clarify what matters to them most (values and wishes) and to share their thoughts with their healthcare providers.

E. *Informed consent* is defined as consent obtained from a competent person to whom adequate information was provided in a manner that facilitates understanding of the risks and benefits of an intervention tailored to the individual and is without coercion, manipulation, or undue influence on the person's choice (Ploug & Holm, 2015). Informed consent shares similar values to SDM in that it protects personal autonomy by allowing an individual the chance to reflect, identify, and act upon his or her own wishes by having been informed about a potential intervention (Ploug & Holm, 2015).

II. Key aspects

A. Understanding and defining patient and family wishes, preferences, and goals for health care is central to the delivery of comprehensive and coordinated care for patients with multiple chronic conditions (MCCs).

B. When several different disease processes are occurring at the same time, there is even greater need to achieve clarity about goals.

C. Patients with MCCs and their families will experience a number of changes over the course of an illness.

D. As an illness progresses, the patient, family, and interdisciplinary team work together to identify patient-centered goals based on the patient's situation, priorities, and healthcare wishes.

   1. The interdisciplinary team is responsible for offering patients and families opportunities to engage in conversations about values, priorities, and goals.

   2. Discussions with the interdisciplinary team prepare patients and families for the ongoing changes brought about by MCCs and establish priorities for care as conditions continue to change over time.

   3. These discussions occur throughout the trajectory of an illness and are part of routine care. More formal discussions may occur as part of care conferences if the patient's status has changed and current disease-focused treatments or options for symptom management need to be reassessed (Billings, 2011a; Weissman, Quill, & Arnold, 2010d).

E. Once goals are identified, a patient-centered plan of care can be established that will allow the patient and family to realize their defined goals (Weissman, Quill, & Arnold, 2010b).

   1. The Institute of Medicine identified patient-centered care as "care that is respectful of and responsive to individual patient preferences, needs, and values" and that ensures patients' values guide all healthcare decisions (Institute of Medicine, 2001, p. 6).

      a) This patient-centered approach to care allows for identification of goals and development of a mutually agreed-upon plan of care between the patient and provider.

> *b)* The patient defines meaning and quality, and the healthcare team provides information about expectations for and ability of a specific healthcare intervention to meet the goal.
>
> *c)* Patient-centered care allows patients, families, and the healthcare team to come to agreement on what steps to take and how to monitor progress to meet patient-specific goals (Reuben & Tinetti, 2012).
>
> > (1) Determining patient preferences, needs, and values requires accurate medical information, good communication of options and choices, advocacy, and encouragement, as well as, at times, negotiation (Billings, 2011b; Elwyn et al., 2012).
> >
> > (2) This approach to care ensures that the patient is not abandoned.
> >
> > (3) The clinician remains a partner with the patient and provides education, recommendations, and guidance about what is possible for the entire disease trajectory (You, Fowler, & Heyland, 2014).
>
> 2. Values underpinning a patient-centered approach
>
>   *a)* Healthcare providers hold individual self-determination—the ability of patients to protect and preserve their own well-being—in high regard.
>
>   *b)* Healthcare providers support patients' self-determination by respecting patients' individual competence and interdependence on others.
>
>   *c)* Healthcare providers support patient autonomy through good provider–patient relationships (Elwyn et al., 2012).
>
>   *d)* The process that patients and providers enter into to reach this objective of patient-centered care is SDM (Elwyn et al., 2012).

F. The SDM approach to care is best achieved when providers establish and maintain a balanced relationship with patients and families and appreciate the ways patients' decisions about care are influenced by what matters most to them (Minnesota Shared Decision-Making Collaborative, n.d.). When patients' preferences are sought, they are able to consider the risks and benefits for all care options, including "doing nothing," and are able to reach an informed decision about what is best for their own lives (Minnesota Shared Decision-Making Collaborative, n.d.).

G. SDM differs from and takes place prior to the informed consent process, before the patient and family commit to an intervention (Minnesota Shared Decision-Making Collaborative, n.d.).

1. SDM includes the gathering of information to gain the knowledge needed to shape decisions about the goals and plan of care.
2. SDM helps to facilitate informed consent.

H. The SDM process (Coulter & Collins, 2011; Légaré et al., 2014; Stacey et al., 2014)

1. Recognition from an involved party (provider, patient, family or caregiver) that a decision needs to be made
2. Knowledge transfer and exchange between the provider and patient
3. Expression of values and preferences
4. Deliberation
5. The decision
6. Documentation and implementation of the decision
7. Establishment of a timeline for follow-up and review

I. SDM is tailored to the situation and involves the patient, provider or providers, and other interested parties (e.g., family members, caregivers) as indicated by the decision being made and whose involvement is needed to obtain the information necessary and reach a decision.

J. Facilitators of the SDM process (Légaré et al., 2014; Stacey et al., 2014; Stacey, Légaré, Pouliot, Kryworuchko, & Dunn, 2010)
   1. Relationship between patient, provider, and others involved in the SDM process
   2. Access to health information
   3. Availability of decision-making aids (e.g., pamphlets, videos, web-based tools) that describe options available and risks and benefits in an unbiased manner
   4. Access to healthcare services and resources
K. The Agency for Healthcare Research and Quality (2014) has developed a five-step process for SDM, called SHARE, that includes exploration and comparison of the benefits, harms, and risks for each option through conversations with patients about what matters most to them.
   1. Step 1: Seek the patient's participation.
   2. Step 2: Help the patient explore and compare treatment options.
   3. Step 3: Assess the patient's values and preferences.
   4. Step 4: Reach a decision with the patient.
   5. Step 5: Evaluate the patient's decision.
L. Goals of care discussions in the context of SDM go beyond reviewing the risks or benefits of specific treatment options to facilitating the patient's maintenance of all the aspects that make up his or her life: relationships, function, hopes, fears, spiritual beliefs, emotional well-being, physical health, and practical or financial needs (Mansel, 2014; Reuben & Tinetti, 2012).
M. To holistically assess for and address these needs, an interdisciplinary team approach is needed. Each discipline brings knowledge and expertise to outline possible interventions, burdens and benefits of specific interventions, and supports available to help reach each goal.
N. With the implementation of the Centers for Medicare and Medicaid Services' new primary payment structure for chronic care management, the primary care clinic and the primary interdisciplinary care team are responsible for having these conversations and reaching these goals (Centers for Medicare and Medicaid Services, 2015).
   1. The relationship among the patient with MCCs, the family, and the interdisciplinary team is the basis from which goals and plans of care are developed.
   2. Conversations that set the stage for SDM and goal setting flow from this relationship and, when done in a compassionately truthful manner, can help reduce patient or family distress and meet their needs (Bernacki & Block, 2014).
O. Care conference
   1. Prior to the care conference
      a) Different members of the interdisciplinary team may attend the care conference to address different components of goal setting, depending on their role and expertise.
      b) Decisions about which members of the interdisciplinary healthcare team should participate in care conference discussions will depend on the needs of the patient, which members have relationships with the patient, and the topics that need to be covered during the meeting (i.e., tangible needs, resources, emotional support, disease trajectory).
      c) For example, the social worker may attend to discuss community resources, and the physical therapist may attend to discuss function and options for home safety modification.
   2. Conference components (Billings & Block, 2011)

   a) Exploring what the patient and family understand about the situation and options

   b) Filling in gaps in knowledge

   c) Identifying an individualized care plan with the patient and family that is dynamic and meets their needs and expectations

3. Ideally, goals of care discussions include information about debility and progressive weakness or changes in physical functioning and how to prepare for anticipated changes and challenges (Bernacki & Block, 2014; You et al., 2014).

4. Phases in the care conference

   a) The phases involved in care conference meetings are preparation for the meeting, the meeting itself, and making plans for how to continue care (Billings & Block, 2011; Weissman, Quill, & Arnold, 2010a; Weissman et al., 2010b; Weissman, Quill, & Arnold, 2010c; Weissman et al., 2010d; Weissman, Quill, & Arnold, 2010e) (see Figure 38-1).

   (1) Hold a pre-meeting with the healthcare team to determine who will lead the meeting, the goals for the meeting (to share information versus need for specific decision), consensus among healthcare

---

Figure 38-1. Language for Goals of Care Discussions

Assessing Understanding and Values (Bernacki & Block, 2014; Peereboom & Coyle, 2012; You et al., 2014)
- "What is your understanding of your disease?"
- "What have the doctors told you about what is happening and what to expect?"
- "Tell me about your mom—what does she like to do? What is important to her for quality of life?"
- "What did you like to do before you became ill?"
- "What questions do you have about your illness?"

Determining Information Preferences (Bernacki & Block, 2014)
- "Some patients like to know how much time they have, whereas others would prefer to take it a day at a time and have the hospice team alert them to changes as they arise. What do you prefer?"
- "Would you like to hear all of the details, or would you prefer we talk to your family in another room and come back to summarize?"
- "How much information do you want today?"
- "Who else do you want to have be part of decision making?"

Using Exploratory Prompts (Peereboom & Coyle, 2012)
- "Tell me more about that . . . ."
- "Help me understand . . . ."
- "How can we help?"
- "You said you're worried about having your grandchildren see you; can you say more about that?"
- "What else are you hoping for or worried about?"

Ascertaining Coping and Support Mechanisms (Peereboom & Coyle, 2012)
- "What helps you cope?"
- "What sustains you?"
- "How have you dealt with difficult situations in the past?"
- "Who helps you make decisions?"
- "How is your family coping?"
- "What does your family know about your illness and what to expect?"

(Continued on next page)

Figure 38-1. Language for Goals of Care Discussions *(Continued)*

Defining Patient's and Family's Goals of Care (Bernacki & Block, 2014; Peereboom & Coyle, 2012)
- "What is important to you right now?"
- "What are your goals?"
- "What level of physical function is important to you?"
- "If your condition were to worsen, what would be important then?"
- "What does 'quality of life' mean to you?"
- "What relationships are most important to you?"

Exploring Fears and Worries (Bernacki & Block, 2014; Weissman et al., 2010b)
- "What worries you about the future?"
- "What are you afraid of?"

Exploring Hopes (Weissman et al., 2010b)
- "Given what we just talked about, what are you hoping for?"
- "What are you hoping for in the time you have left?"
- "Tell me what you're hoping for in the future."

Discussing Trade-Offs (Bernacki & Block, 2014)
- "If your condition worsens, how much suffering are you willing to go through to extend the length of your life?"
- "Some patients are willing to be less alert in order to be comfortable, whereas others prioritize alertness over comfort. What would you like to do?"
- "Some patients don't mind coming back and forth to the emergency department; others want to prioritize other things. What would you like to do?"

Addressing Life and Event Goals (Weissman et al., 2010b)
- "What events are you hoping to attend?"
- "What relationships are important to you now?"
- "Who do you need to see or speak to?"
- "Would speaking to someone from spiritual care be helpful?"

---

providers where possible, and how differences of opinion between providers will be managed if consensus is not possible (Billings & Block, 2011; Weissman et al., 2010d).

(2) The members of the interdisciplinary team who will attend the meeting then review the medical record, current treatments, all treatment options being proposed, and any previous goals of care discussions or family meetings and what transpired (Billings & Block, 2011; Weissman et al., 2010d).

(3) Determine which members of the interdisciplinary team need to review specific pieces of information and who is responsible for addressing each topic during the meeting.

(4) Prior to starting the meeting, determine which tests and interventions will improve, worsen, or have no impact on the patient's function, quality of life, and longevity (Weissman et al., 2010d).

(5) Review information from other treatment providers and specialists involved in the patient's care to prepare to answer questions and fill in missing information (Billings & Block, 2011; Fineberg, Kawashima, & Asch, 2011; Weissman et al., 2010d).

(6) Have an awareness of psychosocial information, family dynamics, and financial or practical concerns that may affect how decisions are made, as well as cultural or spiritual beliefs that may inform decision making (Billings & Block, 2011; Weissman et al., 2010d).

5. During the care conference
   a) Determine who takes the leadership role in the family, who is considered the primary caregiver, who is the durable power of attorney, and how these people will interface in SDM or patient-centered goal setting.
   b) Pay attention to the number of people involved so as to not overwhelm the patient or family. For patients without decision-making capacity, decide how much they are able to participate in the meeting or whether having the meeting in another room and giving a summary to the patient may make more sense.
   c) Solicit from the patient and family what they already know, their understanding of the patient's medical condition and how things are going, and changes they have seen over time (for example, the last three to six months) (Edmonds, Ajayi, Cain, Yeung, & Thornberry, 2014).
   d) When what the patient and family understand is known, confirm their understanding, fill in gaps in knowledge or provide new information, and correct misinformation (Weissman et al., 2010c).
   e) Review existing advance directives or specific wishes previously expressed by the patient, and identify the named surrogate decision maker as needed (Weissman et al., 2010d).
      (1) This information can aid in guiding the conversation and should be updated and reviewed periodically throughout the illness to help guide future discussions.
      (2) Regular review ensures the wishes and desires can be updated as needed based on progression of the disease (i.e., interventions that may have been desirable for their effectiveness at diagnosis may no longer be desired or effective in the setting of advanced disease).
      (3) Any changes to advance directives should be communicated to the proxy decision maker.
      (4) The choice of proxy decision maker also should be reviewed periodically to ensure the person is still able and willing to serve in that capacity.

6. Discussing the disease trajectory
   a) Delivering honest information about what to expect over the course of an illness helps patients and families maintain hope, identify realistic goals, and develop a plan of care that best fits their values and preferences (Bernacki & Block, 2014; Smith et al., 2010).
   b) Patients and families vary greatly in the amount of information and level of detail they desire regarding the disease trajectory (Bernacki & Block, 2014; Campbell et al., 2010; Innes & Payne, 2009).
      (1) Some patients and families may prefer to discuss information that relates to the more-near future, finding longer-term information overwhelming.
      (2) Clinicians should seek permission from the patient and family before sharing prognostic information (Campbell et al., 2010; Weissman et al., 2010b).

    (3) Although there is great benefit to patients and families when they realistically understand how a disease will progress over time, they may not want all of the information at one time (Bernacki & Block, 2014; Campbell et al., 2010; Smith et al., 2010).

    (4) Asking how much information they want and at what level of detail shows respect and maintains trust.

    (5) Being able to receive information on their own terms is empowering and reassuring for patients and families (Innes & Payne, 2009; You et al., 2014).

  c) Patients' and families' goals will change as the disease becomes more advanced and physical functioning changes. Continued discussion about place of care, formal and informal caregiver availability, and other resources within the community will need to take place over the course of the illness.

7. Maximizing the value of the meeting

  a) Efforts to minimize information gaps can reduce the chance that patients and families will misunderstand information about the medical condition and can help them remain realistic about the disease trajectory, what to expect, and overall prognosis.

  b) Clear and consistent information sharing among and from all the healthcare providers involved in the patient's care is paramount for reducing confusion.

  c) Many medical situations have a high degree of uncertainty, and healthcare providers may not be able to provide clear recommendations until more time has passed.

  d) Acknowledging and addressing uncertainty can help reassure patients and families and assist with decision making.

  e) Using nonmedical language to describe diagnosis, treatment options, and risks and burdens, as well as providing a recommendation based on the values and preferences of the patient, can reduce confusion and help with decision making.

  f) Striking a balance with regard to the amount of information shared at one time with the patient and family will decrease the likelihood of them being overwhelmed. These conversations take time and happen over time.

  g) Being aware of cultural or language issues that also may affect how and with whom information is shared can guide preparation for the meeting and assist with moving forward in goal identification and decision making.

  h) These conversations can be emotionally intense.

    (1) Heightened emotions can greatly influence decision making.

    (2) Common emotions are grief, fear, anxiety, guilt, anger, and hope.

    (3) Identifying and addressing the emotions elicited during the conversation can aid in moving toward resolution.

  i) To increase the success of the meeting and enhance decision making, be aware of, manage, and support patients and families who may have internal disagreements among themselves or differ in their perceptions of the situation.

  j) Be aware of previous encounters or a cultural history of mistreatment from the medical team that could influence the current patient–provider relationship.

III. Current findings

    A. Patients and families expect healthcare providers to initiate conversations about care planning in the setting of MCCs (Bernacki & Block, 2014).

        1. The most frequently stated goals of patients and families are to be cured; to live longer; to improve or maintain function, quality of life, or independence; to be comfortable; to achieve life goals; and to provide support for family or caregivers (Kaldjian, Curtis, Shinkunas, & Cannon, 2009).

        2. Patients with MCCs who have conversations with their healthcare providers about their goals of care throughout the disease trajectory and who, with guidance from the medical team, thoughtfully create advance care plans are more likely to receive care that meets their individual needs and priorities (Bernacki & Block, 2014).

    B. Models of communication

        1. "Ask, Tell, Ask" communication strategy (Gaster, Edwards, Trinidad, Gallagher, & Braddock, 2010; Peereboom & Coyle, 2012) (see Chapter 33)

           a) This model is conversational in style.

           b) First, the clinician uses open-ended questions to assess the patient's and family's understanding of the situation, diagnosis, and current treatment or symptom management options (ask).

           c) Second, the clinician provides information to address the patient's needs and clarify any misunderstandings (tell).

           d) Third, the clinician asks another open-ended question to clarify the patient's and family's understanding of the information shared and to elicit additional concerns (ask).

        2. SPIKES six-step protocol for delivering emotionally difficult information such as a new diagnosis, progression of disease, or approaching end of life (Nakajima, Kusumoto, Onishi, & Ishida, 2015; Peereboom & Coyle, 2012; You et al., 2014) (see Figure 38-2)

        3. PERSON communication model (Edmonds et al., 2014)

           a) The PERSON model was designed to be used throughout the illness trajectory and serves as a tool for exploration and advocacy.

           b) Using open-ended questions and avoiding assumptions, explore the patient's and family's perception (P) of present health status.

           c) Explore (E) the patient's life before the current illness, listening to the narrative of the patient's story.

           d) Provide medical information and relate (R) the patient's story to the medical reality of the situation.

           e) Assess sources (S) of worry for the patient using hope and worry statements.

           f) Outline (O) the next steps for moving forward, time-limited trials, and timing for assessment of progress or next meeting.

           g) Notify (N) anyone else who needs to know what was shared, including other family members, consulting teams, and other members of the multidisciplinary team.

        4. Words that work

           a) As the disease trajectory progresses, goals should be reevaluated often.

           b) Patients and families can benefit from clear language about where they are along the disease trajectory, what has changed about the patient's health status, and why previously mentioned treatment options may no longer be effective (Back, Trinidad, Hopley, & Edwards, 2014).

Figure 38-2. SPIKES Mnemonic for Sharing Bad News

SET up the care conference (Bernacki & Block, 2014; Weissman et al., 2010d; You et al., 2014)
- Consider setting, including the time, location, lighting, privacy, and seating.
- Include everyone who should participate from the family and healthcare team.
- Make sure the healthcare team is in agreement or make a plan for how differences of opinion will be managed.
- Determine if a decision needs to be made or if this is an information-sharing meeting only.
- Gather necessary medical information and understand treatment options and their anticipated effectiveness and outcomes.

Assess the patient's and family's PERCEPTION (Edmonds et al., 2014; Weissman et al., 2010c; You et al., 2014)
- "What have you heard about your diagnosis from the medical team?"
- "Tell me what the past six months have been like for you?"
- "How has your health changed in the past year?"
- "What events led up to this hospitalization?"

Obtain the patient's and family's INVITATION (Bernacki & Block, 2014; You et al., 2014)
- "I'd like to share some information with you about your prognosis; is that okay?"
- "Would it be OK if I give you some additional information about your diagnosis?"
- "Is it OK if I talk a bit more about the treatment options and what we expect them to do?"
- "That was a good summary. I have new information to add; is that OK?"
- "Some patients want a lot of detail about prognosis; what would you like?"

Give information and KNOWLEDGE (Weissman et al., 2010c; You et al., 2014)
- Provide information in small amounts using nonmedical language, stopping periodically for the patient and family to ask questions.
- Recognize uncertainty and acknowledge what can be controlled and influenced and what cannot.
- Use the word "dying" when relevant; speak plainly and avoid euphemisms.
- Clearly indicate that the situation has changed and things are different now.
- Make recommendations about how to continue care in light of the new information.

Empathically address EMOTIONS (Weissman et al., 2010c; You et al., 2014)
- Allow time for silence.
- Invite the patient and family to express emotions (e.g., "Were you surprised to hear this information?").
- Identify the emotions behind statements or questions.
- Normalize emotional responses (e.g., "This information is really hard to hear").

SUMMARIZE and strategize (Edmonds et al., 2014; Weissman et al., 2010b; You et al., 2014)
- Summarize what was discussed and what decisions were reached.
- Plan a time to meet again if relevant.
- Communicate results of meeting to other healthcare providers.
- Document conversation and any decisions in medical record.

---

c) Strong cues from the clinician are needed to convey that things have changed (Weissman et al., 2010c).

d) The clinician should indicate disruption from the previous plan and that the status quo cannot continue (Back et al., 2014).

e) To decrease feelings of abandonment, clinicians should communicate that although the situation has changed, there are still aggressive and active things to do now (van Vliet, van der Wall, Plum, & Bensing, 2013).

f) These actions may no longer be focused at the reversing or slowing of the underlying disease, but care continues (van Vliet et al., 2013).

       g) Communicating clear options for the next steps guides patients and families from uncertainty to give them back some control (Back et al., 2014).

       h) Whether meeting with a patient newly diagnosed with a life-limiting illness or an individual nearing the end of life, clinicians can help patients and families identify how they want to live now that death is known to be closer (Back et al., 2014).

    5. Religious beliefs, hope, and miracles

       a) Responding well to statements of religious belief or hope for a miracle can be an important part of patient-centered goals of care discussions.

       b) Clinicians understandably have different comfort with and skill levels for responding to and addressing these expressions of faith (Ernecoff, Curlin, Buddadhumaruk, & White, 2014).

       c) Respectfully exploring patients' and families' religious beliefs and involving health system spiritual care staff or their own clergy can assist with reaching decisions about goals of care (Billings, 2011b).

IV. Relevance to practice

  A. To provide patient-centered care, clinicians need to be versed in exploring and discussing patient goals and values (Houben, Spruit, Groenen, Wouters, & Janssen, 2014).

  B. These types of discussions are dynamic and can be facilitated by a therapeutic relationship with the interdisciplinary team (Peereboom & Coyle, 2012).

V. Role of the advanced practice registered nurse (APRN)

  A. APRNs advocate for their patients by understanding patient wishes and communicating these to the physician, other members of the healthcare team, and the patient's family (Adams, Bailey, Anderson, & Docherty, 2011).

  B. APRNs often receive information from a number of sources and can help synthesize and summarize it for patients and families (Adams et al., 2011). They may mediate on behalf of patients, getting multiple providers or family members together to share information, provide continuity, and develop a holistic plan.

  C. APRNs are well positioned to have long-term relationships with patients and have the skills necessary to communicate compassionately, honestly, and empathically with patients and families (Hospice and Palliative Nurses Association, 2013; Peereboom & Coyle, 2012; Samanta & Samanta, 2010). Through the relationship and trust they build with patients and families, nurses support the ongoing discussion of goals (Peereboom & Coyle, 2012).

  D. APRNs provide emotional support, witness and address suffering, are able to act as translators for medical jargon to increase patient and family understanding, and are able to see the "big picture" (Adams et al., 2011).

  E. APRNs are able to demonstrate empathy and compassion through valuing patients' narratives (Mansel, 2014; Peereboom & Coyle, 2012).

    1. Patients and families may feel more comfortable being vulnerable, sharing openly, and asking personal questions of nurses with whom they have a long-term relationship.

    2. Nurses can be a source of accurate information for patients and families about their medical condition to help apply that information holistically to situations based on the patient's values (Hospice and Palliative Nurses Association, 2013).

  F. APRNs who have had long-term relationships with patients and families are able to reflect the reality of the situation, deterioration over time, and the impact of worsening disease in order to give guidance and recommendations about treatments or symptom management.

1. They coach and encourage patients and families as they make care decisions over the course of an illness.
2. At the end of life, nurses can gently and realistically inform patients and families about death and the dying process and what to expect.

VI. Interface to palliative care

A. The use of palliative care in chronic illness has increased over the past several years (Meier, 2011). Unfortunately, referrals to palliative care continue to occur late in the disease process (Beernaert et al., 2013; Bernacki & Block, 2014). Patients and families desire to have these conversations earlier in and throughout the disease process (Bernacki & Block, 2014). Delaying conversations about goals of care until the end of life is detrimental, leading to poor quality of life, anxiety, family distress, prolonged dying process, undesired hospital admissions, mistrust of the healthcare system, and high costs (Bernacki & Block, 2014; Meier, 2011).

B. Working collaboratively, the interdisciplinary team has the skills to provide guidance and advocacy to help patients and families identify their values and define their goals of care.
   1. As medical technology, treatment options, and interventions become more complex, conversations about goals of care also increase in complexity.
   2. All clinicians have a responsibility to provide primary palliative care services, to address goals, and to give recommendations about the plan of care.

C. Palliative care has rich resources for guiding these conversations as well as educational materials for patients and families about future choices they may face.

D. Identifying palliative care as an active and aggressive form of care and integrating palliative care services into patients' care early in the disease trajectory can help assure them that care is continuing, reduce feelings of abandonment, and aid them in achieving other goals that they are hoping to reach, even when cure is no longer possible (Meier, 2011).

Case Study

N.J., a 72-year-old woman, has been dealing with congestive heart failure and type 2 diabetes for many years. She now has a new diagnosis of pulmonary hypertension. At a clinic visit with her primary care physician the week after she received the diagnosis, N.J. and her husband sit down with the physician, APRN, and social worker to discuss the anticipated disease trajectory, the options for palliative management of her symptoms, and what her caregiving needs would be in the short term. At that first meeting, the APRN elicits from N.J. what is important to her about her level of function, hobbies, activities, and the things that make life meaningful for her. She identifies that her faith is important to her and helps her cope with difficult situations. Spending time with her husband, visiting her grandchildren, and being able to garden are also important. Her goals at this time are to be able to travel to Arizona in three months to visit her daughter, son-in-law, and grandchildren; she also hopes to go on an Alaskan cruise in the fall. This summer she has big plans for her garden. She reports feeling short of breath and expresses concern about not being able to enjoy these events if she continues to feel this way. Together the interdisciplinary team and N.J. review the clinical practice guidelines for pulmonary hypertension and congestive heart failure and discuss which portions of the guidelines to prioritize based on her goals. In addition, they identify specific strategies for managing N.J.'s primary symptom: shortness of breath. N.J. also asks questions about the role of the intensive care unit and artificial life supports and says she does not think she wants to be on a ventilator or to be resuscitated. The conversation is documented in her electronic health record.

Over the course of several years, the pulmonary hypertension continues to progress, as does her congestive heart failure. With each change in her medical status, the primary care interdisciplinary team revisits their previous conversations, exploring again what function, activities, and hobbies bring meaning to N.J., the changes she has experienced over time, how her different illnesses are affecting each other, and what to anticipate about the disease trajectory given these interactions and the changes she is experiencing. N.J. requires more O_2 at home but with good symptom management is still able to enjoy visiting with her family, attending church, and spending time in her garden. As her functional status declines, she now requires a wheeled walker for short distances and sometimes uses a wheelchair for longer distances. With continued review of N.J.'s priorities and wishes about quality of life, the interdisciplinary team is able to make recommendations for what palliative treatments to pursue to continue meeting N.J.'s goals.

Over the past three months, N.J. has been hospitalized with exacerbation of her disease three times. Her functional status continues to decline. N.J. and her husband are willing for her to temporarily stay in a nursing home for rehabilitation but do not want her to remain in a facility long term. Caring for her at home has become increasingly difficult for N.J.'s husband, as he has MCCs as well. Their children live out of state. She is receiving home nursing and needs to use the wheelchair all of the time. At the follow-up visits after each hospitalization, in addition to reviewing N.J.'s medical status, anticipated trajectory, and symptom management needs, the interdisciplinary team discusses with her and her husband possible resources for additional caregiver support in the home, whether or not further readmissions are something she would want, and, if she is readmitted, different options for approaching her care in the hospital.

References

Adams, J.A., Bailey, D.E., Jr., Anderson, R.A., & Docherty, S.L. (2011). Nursing roles and strategies in end-of-life decision making in acute care: A systematic review of the literature. *Nursing Research and Practice, 2011*, Article 527834. doi:10.1155/2011/527834

Agency for Healthcare Research and Quality. (2014, July). The SHARE approach—Essential steps of shared decision making: Quick reference guide. Retrieved from http://www.ahrq.gov/professionals/education/curriculum-tools/shareddecisionmaking/tools/tool-1/index.html

Back, A.L., Trinidad, S.B., Hopley, E.K., & Edwards, K.A. (2014). Reframing the goals of care conversation: "We're in a different place." *Journal of Palliative Medicine, 17*, 1019–1024. doi:10.1089/jpm.2013.0651

Beernaert, K., Cohen, J., Deliens, L., Devroey, D., Vanthomme, K., Pardon, K., & Van den Block, L. (2013). Referral to palliative care in COPD and other chronic diseases: A population-based study. *Respiratory Medicine, 107*, 1731–1739. doi:10.1016/j.rmed.2013.06.003

Bernacki, R.E., & Block, S.D. (2014). Communication about serious illness care goals: A review and synthesis of best practices. *JAMA Internal Medicine, 174*, 1994–2003. doi:10.1001/jamainternmed.2014.5271

Billings, J.A. (2011a). The end-of-life family meeting in intensive care—Part I: Indications, outcomes, and family needs. *Journal of Palliative Medicine, 14*, 1042–1050. doi:10.1089/jpm.2011.0038

Billings, J.A. (2011b). The end-of-life family meeting in intensive care—Part II: Family-centered decision making. *Journal of Palliative Medicine, 14*, 1051–1057. doi:10.1089/jpm.2011.0038-b

Billings, J.A., & Block, S.D. (2011). The end-of-life family meeting in intensive care—Part III: A guide for structured discussions. *Journal of Palliative Medicine, 14*, 1058–1064. doi:10.1089/jpm.2011.0038-c

Campbell, T.C., Carey, E.C., Jackson, V.A., Saraiya, B., Yang, H.B., Back, A.L., & Arnold, R.M. (2010). Discussing prognosis: Balancing hope and realism. *Cancer Journal, 16*, 461–466. doi:10.1097/PPO.0b013e3181f30e07

Centers for Medicare and Medicaid Services. (2015, February 18). Payment of chronic care management services under CY 2015 Medicare PFS [Press release]. Retrieved from http://www.cms.gov/Outreach-and-Education/Outreach/NPC/National-Provider-Calls-and-Events-Items/2015-02-18-Chronic-Care-Management-new.html

Coulter, A., & Collins, A. (2011). Making shared decision-making a reality: No decision about me, without me. Retrieved from http://www.kingsfund.org.uk/sites/files/kf/Making-shared-decision-making-a-reality -paper-Angela-Coulter-Alf-Collins-July-2011_0.pdf

Edmonds, K.P., Ajayi, T.A., Cain, J., Yeung, H.N., & Thornberry, K. (2014). Establishing goals of care at any stage of illness: The PERSON mnemonic. *Journal of Palliative Medicine, 17,* 1087. doi:10.1089/jpm.2014.0253

Elwyn, G., Frosch, D., Thomson, R., Joseph-Williams, N., Lloyd, A., Kinnersley, P., … Barry, M. (2012). Shared decision making: A model for clinical practice. *Journal of General Internal Medicine, 27,* 1361–1367. doi:10.1007/s11606-012-2077-6

Ernecoff, N.C., Curlin, F., Buddadhumaruk, P., & White, D.B. (2014). How do clinicians respond to religious statements by surrogates during goals of care discussions? [Meeting abstract]. A24. End of Life and Stressors in the ICU. *American Journal of Respiratory and Critical Care Medicine, 189,* Abstract No. A1147. doi:10.1164/ ajrccm-conference.2014.189.1_MeetingAbstracts.A1147

Fineberg, I.C., Kawashima, M., & Asch, S.M. (2011). Communication with families facing life-threatening illness: A research-based model for family conferences. *Journal of Palliative Medicine, 14,* 421–427. doi:10.1089/ jpm.2010.0436

Gaster, B., Edwards, K., Trinidad, S.B., Gallagher, T.H., & Braddock, C.H., III. (2010). Patient-centered discussions about prostate cancer screening: A real-world approach. *Annals of Internal Medicine, 153,* 661–665. doi:10.7326/0003-4819-153-10-201011160-00010

Hospice and Palliative Nurses Association. (2013). HPNA position statement: The nurse's role in advance care planning. Retrieved from https://www.hpna.org/filemaintenance_view.aspx?ID=23

Houben, C.H.M., Spruit, M.A., Groenen, M.T.J., Wouters, E.F.M., & Janssen, D.J.A. (2014). Efficacy of advance care planning: A systematic review and meta-analysis. *Journal of the American Medical Directors Association, 15,* 477–489. doi:10.1016/j.jamda.2014.01.008

Innes, S., & Payne, S. (2009). Advanced cancer patients' prognostic information preferences: A review. *Palliative Medicine, 23,* 29–39. doi:10.1177/0269216308098799

Institute of Medicine. (2001). *Crossing the quality chasm: A new health system for the 21st century.* Washington, DC: National Academies Press.

International Patient Decision Aid Standards Collaboration. (2012, June 20). What are patient decision aids? Retrieved from http://ipdas.ohri.ca/what.html

Kaldjian, L.C., Curtis, A.E., Shinkunas, L.A., & Cannon, K.T. (2009). Review article: Goals of care toward the end of life: A structured literature review. *American Journal of Hospice and Palliative Medicine, 25,* 501–511. doi:10.1177/1049909108328256

Légaré, F., Stacey, D., Turcotte, S., Cossi, M.J., Kryworuchko, J., Graham, I.D., … Donner-Banzhoff, N. (2014). Interventions for improving the adoption of shared decision making by healthcare professionals. *Cochrane Database of Systematic Reviews, 2014*(9). doi:10.1002/14651858.CD006732.pub3

Mansel, J.K. (2014). The diagnostic and healing qualities of story: Goals of care. *JAMA Internal Medicine, 174,* 1037. doi:10.1001/jamainternmed.2014.1800

Meier, D.E. (2011). Increased access to palliative care and hospice services: Opportunities to improve value in health care. *Milbank Quarterly, 89,* 343–380. doi:10.1111/j.1468-0009.2011.00632.x

Minnesota Shared Decision-Making Collaborative. (n.d.). Defining shared decision-making. Retrieved from http://msdmc.org/sdm-explained/definition-of-sdm

Nakajima, N., Kusumoto, K., Onishi, H., & Ishida, M. (2015). Does the approach of disclosing more detailed information of cancer for the terminally ill patients improve the quality of communication involving patients, families, and medical professionals? *American Journal of Hospice and Palliative Medicine, 32,* 776–782. doi:10.1177/1049909114548718

Peereboom, K., & Coyle, N. (2012). Facilitating goals-of-care discussions for patients with life-limiting disease—Communication strategies for nurses. *Journal of Hospice and Palliative Nursing, 14,* 251–258. doi:10.1097/NJH.0b013e3182533a7f

Ploug, T., & Holm, S. (2015). Routinisation of informed consent in online health care systems. *International Journal of Medical Informatics, 84,* 229–236. doi:10.1016/j.ijmedinf.2015.01.003

Reuben, D.B., & Tinetti, M.E. (2012). Goal-oriented patient care—An alternative health outcomes paradigm. *New England Journal of Medicine, 366,* 777–779. doi:10.1056/NEJMp1113631

Samanta, A., & Samanta, J. (2010). Advance care planning: The role of the nurse. *British Journal of Nursing, 19,* 1060–1061. doi:10.12968/bjon.2010.19.16.78208

Smith, T.J., Dow, L.A., Virago, E., Khatcheressian, J., Lyckholm, L.J., & Matsuyama, R. (2010). Giving honest information to patients with advanced cancer maintains hope. *Oncology, 24,* 521–525. Retrieved from http:// www.cancernetwork.com/oncology-journal/giving-honest-information-patients-advanced-cancer-maintains -hope

Stacey, D., Légaré, F., Col, N.F., Bennett, C.L., Barry, M.J., Eden, K.B., … Wu, J.H.C. (2014). Decision aids for people facing health treatment or screening decisions. *Cochrane Database of Systematic Reviews, 2014*(1). doi:10.1002/14651858.CD001431.pub4

Stacey, D., Légaré, F., Pouliot, S., Kryworuchko, J., & Dunn, S. (2010). Shared decision making models to inform an interprofessional perspective on decision making: A theory analysis. *Patient Education and Counseling, 80,* 164–172. doi:10.1016/j.pec.2009.10.015

van Vliet, L.M., van der Wall, E., Plum, N.M., & Bensing, J.M. (2013). Explicit prognostic information and reassurance about nonabandonment when entering palliative breast cancer care: Findings from a scripted video-vignette study. *Journal of Clinical Oncology, 31,* 3242–3249. doi:10.1200/JCO.2012.45.5865

Weissman, D.E., Quill, T.E., & Arnold, R.M. (2010a). The family meeting: Causes of conflict #225. *Journal of Palliative Medicine, 13,* 328–329. doi:10.1089/jpm.2010.9862

Weissman, D.E., Quill, T.E., & Arnold, R.M. (2010b). The family meeting: End-of-life goal setting and future planning #227. *Journal of Palliative Medicine, 13,* 462–463. doi:10.1089/jpm.2010.9846

Weissman, D.E., Quill, T.E., & Arnold, R.M. (2010c). The family meeting: Starting the conversation #223. *Journal of Palliative Medicine, 13,* 204–205. doi:10.1089/jpm.2010.9878

Weissman, D.E., Quill, T.E., & Arnold, R.M. (2010d). Preparing for the family meeting #222. *Journal of Palliative Medicine, 13,* 203–204. doi:10.1089/jpm.2010.9879

Weissman, D.E., Quill, T.E., & Arnold, R.M. (2010e). Responding to emotion in family meetings #224. *Journal of Palliative Medicine, 13,* 327–328. doi:10.1089/jpm.2010.9863

You, J.J., Fowler, R.A., & Heyland, D.K. (2014). Just ask: Discussing goals of care with patients in hospital with serious illness. *CMAJ, 186,* 425–432. doi:10.1503/cmaj.121274

CHAPTER 39

Interdisciplinary Team Collaboration, Continuity, and Communication

Janice Firn, PhD, LMSW

I. Definitions
  A. Interdisciplinary team: A dynamic group of diverse people with common objectives and different responsibilities who provide services to patients (Blackmore & Persaud, 2012) (see Chapter 37)
  B. Teamwork: A complex process where different types of staff (professionals and other ancillary healthcare personnel) share expertise, knowledge, and skills to collectively meet the needs of patients and families (Nancarrow et al., 2013)
  C. Continuity of care for chronic conditions: The integration of services and therapies across settings and providers that support the individual needs of patients, addressing self-management, clinical information systems, delivery systems, clinical disease guidelines, healthcare organizations, and community resources (Nici & ZuWallack, 2012)
  D. Collaboration
    1. Successful collaboration is accomplished when team members cooperate to achieve a common goal, are willing to participate, share care plan development and decision making, contribute from their expertise, share responsibility, and share power based on knowledge and expertise (Nancarrow et al., 2013).
    2. Collaboration occurs when team members are willing to work together in an atmosphere of trust, mutual respect, and communication (Blackmore & Persaud, 2012).
  E. Integrated care: The continuum of organized and coordinated holistic, patient-centered services for patients with chronic conditions, with the goal of realizing the optimal daily functioning and health status for individuals (Nici & ZuWallack, 2012)
  F. Transitions of care: Actions designed to ensure safe and effective coordination and continuity of care within, between, and across settings as patients experience a change in health status, care needs, healthcare providers, or location (Dusek, Pearce, Harripaul, & Lloyd, 2014)
  G. Handoffs: Transitions in patient care that occur between members of the patient's healthcare team (Solan, Yau, Sucharew, & O'Toole, 2014)

II. Key aspects
  A. Patients with multiple chronic conditions (MCCs) are followed by many health-care providers and receive care in a number of settings over the course of their illness (see Figure 39-1).
  B. Until recently, many healthcare systems in the United States were a loose assortment of physician groups, hospitals, specialty clinics, subacute care centers, and community agencies, leading to many providers operating in isolation and fragmented care for many patients (Nici & ZuWallack, 2012).
    1. To remedy the fragmented approach to care, the Patient Protection and Affordable Care Act of 2010 has initiated several new payment models for both Medicare, Medicaid, and private payers to comprehensively meet the needs of patients with MCCs with an economical, efficient, and effective chronic disease management approach that reaches across healthcare settings and continues cohesively throughout the trajectory of a disease (U.S. Department of Health and Human Services [DHHS], 2015).
    2. To expand alternative payment models beyond Medicare to private payers, employers, consumers, providers, states, and state Medicaid programs, a new network has been created, the Health Care Payment Learning and Action Network (U.S. DHHS, 2015).
    3. These new models, which will be tied 90% to Medicare payments by 2018, include accountable care organizations, primary care medical homes, and new models of bundling payments for episodes of care (U.S. DHHS, 2015).

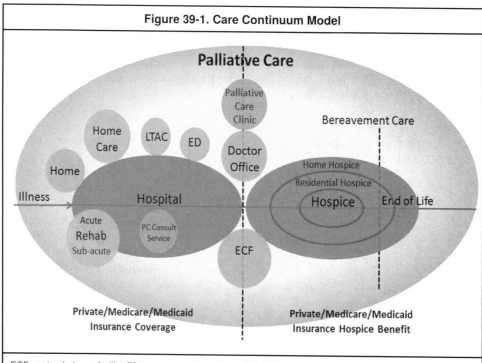

Figure 39-1. Care Continuum Model

ECF—extended care facility; ED—emergency department; LTAC—long-term acute care; PC—palliative care

Note. Figure courtesy of Jamie Frey and Kelly Ingerly. Used with permission.

    a) These alternative payment models hold healthcare providers accountable for the cost and quality of the care they provide to patients.

    b) In addition to collaborative care across settings being the best way to provide care to patients, there is now a financial incentive to coordinate care as well.

    c) To fully realize this high level of collaborative care, good communication within and among settings and within and among healthcare teams is needed.

    d) Implementation and use of health information technology allows for the sharing of healthcare data needed to track patient care efforts and ensures efficient use of resources for optimal patient outcomes.

C. In the largest change made to date for primary care payments, the Centers for Medicare and Medicaid Services (CMS) began making separate payments under the Medicare Physician Fee Schedule for chronic care management services in 2015 (CMS, 2015).

    1. Chronic care management services include non–face-to-face care management and coordination services for certain Medicare beneficiaries with two or more chronic conditions (CMS, 2015).

    2. Healthcare providers are required to use a certified electronic health record; provide 24/7 access to staff who have access to the electronic health record; maintain a designated provider for each patient; and coordinate care through transitions to and from the hospital, specialists, or other providers in order to bill for this fee (CMS, 2015).

    3. Additionally, chronic care management requires collaboration with the patient to create and maintain a comprehensive care plan, including a list of health issues, medication management instructions, and a record of involved social and community services (CMS, 2015).

D. Medical management of patients with one or more chronic medical conditions uses 86% of every healthcare dollar spent in the United States (Agency for Healthcare Research and Quality [AHRQ], 2014).

    1. MCCs require an interdisciplinary team–based approach, given the complexity of patient needs (Nancarrow et al., 2013).

    2. Care should be planned and managed across the disease trajectory from diagnosis until the end of life and between settings (Nici & ZuWallack, 2012).

    3. Care transitions between settings are complex and, if they are to happen well, need to be patient centered and involve the coordination and management of multiple components of patient care (Coleman, 2015; Dusek et al., 2014).

    4. Elements of successful transition programs (Coleman, 2015)

        a) The patient is knowledgeable about medications and has a medication management system.

        b) A patient-centered record is managed by the patient or informal caregiver to facilitate communication and allow for continuity of care across and between providers and settings.

        c) The patient or informal caregiver are empowered to be active participants in scheduling and completing follow-up visits and interacting with the primary care physician or specialist physician.

        d) The patient or informal caregiver is well informed on signs that indicate the condition is worsening and how to respond.

E. Effective communication, coordination of care, and communication among healthcare providers and patients reduces healthcare costs, decreases hospitalizations, increases patient satisfaction, and improves quality of life (Coleman, 2015; Courtenay, Nancarrow, & Dawson, 2013; Menefee, 2014; Popejoy et al., 2014).

F. Interdisciplinary teams promote cost-effective, safe, and comprehensive care for patients with MCCs throughout the disease trajectory and across the continuum of care (Albert et al., 2015; Boult & Wieland, 2010; Nici & ZuWallack, 2012).

G. Vital to managing MCCs well is the provision of wide-ranging team-based care; an orientation toward the whole person, which extends to supporting and caring for caregivers as well; care that is coordinated across healthcare settings and into the patient's community; and access to care that allows for multiple modes of communication (Shaw et al., 2013). Interdisciplinary palliative care services, beginning in the early stage of the illness and continuing through the end of life, are an effective approach to manage the symptoms associated with MCCs.

H. To reach this high standard of care, a multilevel, multifaceted approach is needed.
   1. Patients and informal caregivers need information about which care options may work best, given their individual conditions, situations, and preferences.
   2. Healthcare providers need evidence-based information about the daily problems they face in practice.
   3. Insurers need information that can help them make the best decisions on how to improve health outcomes for their members.
   4. To provide information to patients, caregivers, healthcare providers, and insurers, further research is needed and is being funded to gather the evidence needed to inform decision making and help to improve outcomes in high-burden, high-impact conditions (Patient-Centered Outcomes Research Institute, 2014).

I. Interdisciplinary teams work together to address the needs described previously, to minimize the symptoms caused by MCCs, and to help patients and families maintain as normal a lifestyle as possible (Giladi, Manor, Hilel, & Gurevich, 2014).
   1. Interdisciplinary teams are able to comprehensively address the quality of life of patients, families, and caregivers throughout the course of a disease (Nici & ZuWallack, 2012).
   2. Partnership is improved with trust; the more harmonious and unified the partnerships among team members, the better the cohesion of the group and the desire to support one another (Blackmore & Persaud, 2012; Burroughs & Bartholomew, 2014).
   3. Cooperation among team members allows for the standardization, optimization, and economization of care, which in turn improves the quality of care and lowers costs (Burroughs & Bartholomew, 2014; Pannick, Beveridge, Wachter, & Sevdalis, 2014).
   4. Features for successful interdisciplinary teamwork include the following (Nancarrow et al., 2013) (see Table 39-1):
      a) Leadership and management: The team has a clearly identified leader who provides good direction and management, listens and acts, takes a democratic approach toward team participation in decision making, is willing to share power, and provides support and supervision to all members of the team (Blackmore & Persaud, 2012; Canadian Interprofessional Health Collaborative, 2010; Giladi et al., 2014; Nancarrow et al., 2013).

Table 39-1. Characteristics of a Good Interdisciplinary Team	
Themes	**Description**
1. Leadership and management	Having a clear leader of the team, with clear direction and management; democratic; shared power; support/supervision; personal development aligned with line management; leader who acts and listens.
2. Communication	Individuals with communication skills; ensuring that there are appropriate systems to promote communication within the team.
3. Personal rewards, training and development	Learning; training and development; training and career development opportunities; incorporates individual rewards and opportunity, morale and motivation.
4. Appropriate resources and procedures	Structures (for example, team meetings, organizational factors, team members working from the same location). Ensuring that appropriate procedures are in place to uphold the vision of the service (for example, communication systems, appropriate referral criteria, and so on).
5. Appropriate skill mix	Sufficient/appropriate skills, competencies, practitioner mix, balance of personalities; ability to make the most of other team members' backgrounds; having a full complement of staff, timely replacement/cover for empty or absent posts.
6. Climate	Team culture of trust, valuing contributions, nurturing consensus; need to create an interprofessional atmosphere.
7. Individual characteristics	Knowledge, experience, initiative, knowing strengths and weaknesses, listening skills, reflexive practice; desire to work on the same goals.
8. Clarity of vision	Having a clear set of values that drive the direction of the service and the care provided. Portraying a uniform and consistent external image.
9. Quality and outcomes of care	Patient-centered focus, outcomes and satisfaction, encouraging feedback, capturing and recording evidence of the effectiveness of care and using that as part of a feedback cycle to improve care.
10. Respecting and understanding roles	Sharing power, joint working, autonomy.

Note. From "Ten Principles of Good Interdisciplinary Team Work," by S.A. Nancarrow, A. Booth, S. Ariss, T. Smith, P. Enderby, and A. Roots, 2013, *Human Resources for Health, 11*, p. 9. Copyright 2013 by Nancarrow et al. This is an Open Access article distributed under the terms of the Creative Commons Attribution License (http://creativecommons.org/licenses/by/2.0), which permits unrestricted use, distribution, and reproduction in any medium, provided the original work is properly cited.

(1) The leader may change depending on the situation, task, and type of expertise required to address the need (Canadian Interprofessional Health Collaborative, 2010).

(2) Leadership skills consists of both task orientation, where the leader is responsible for keeping the team members moving toward completion of a goal, and relationship orientation, where the leader helps team members work more effectively together (Canadian Interprofessional Health Collaborative, 2010).

b) Communication: In an interdisciplinary environment, verbal, written, and nonverbal communication takes place between team members and is demonstrated through listening, negotiating, consulting, interacting, discussing, or debating with each other (Canadian Interprofessional Health Collaborative, 2010).

(1) Team members have good communication skills and are given regular, formal opportunities to communicate, as well as informal opportunities for communication (Blackmore & Persaud, 2012; Giladi et al., 2014; Nancarrow et al., 2013).

(2) Communication (written and verbal) is done in a timely manner and is clear, concise, and information rich (Albert et al., 2015; Blackmore & Persaud, 2012; Giladi et al., 2014; Nancarrow et al., 2013).

(3) Information is relayed in a nonconfrontational manner (Blackmore & Persaud, 2012).

(4) Team members are able to address conflict in a constructive manner because they are comfortable with differing opinions and styles (Blackmore & Persaud, 2012).

(5) Individual team members do not dominate the conversation or decision making and less vocal members' opinions are intentionally sought, ensuring everyone participates (Blackmore & Persaud, 2012).

(6) Positive feedback is given (Blackmore & Persaud, 2012; Nancarrow et al., 2013).

(7) Consensus is fostered as contributions are recognized and valued (Blackmore & Persaud, 2012; Giladi et al., 2014; Nancarrow et al., 2013).

c) Common team goal: The team's goal is congruent with the mission of the organization and team and is agreed upon by all team members (Blackmore & Persaud, 2012; Interprofessional Education Collaborative Expert Panel, 2011; Nancarrow et al., 2013).

d) Ability and willingness to work together: Having the right mix of team members with the right skills facilitates working effectively together, as well as results in high-quality patient care (Blackmore & Persaud, 2012; Giladi et al., 2014; Interprofessional Education Collaborative Expert Panel, 2011).

(1) Effective teams are action oriented, assist each other, and are committed to the team as a whole (Blackmore & Persaud, 2012; Nancarrow et al., 2013). These attributes help the team to remain intact.

(a) Requires the capacity and desire for continued cooperation necessary to maintain group cohesion and meet goals, which includes regularly reflecting on team process and identifying areas for improvement (Canadian Interprofessional Health Collaborative, 2010; Interprofessional Education Collaborative Expert Panel, 2011; Nancarrow et al., 2013)

(b) Requires a diverse yet complementary array of roles to meet goals (Giladi et al., 2014; Interprofessional Education Collaborative Expert Panel, 2011; Nancarrow et al., 2013)

(2) Team members need the necessary skills, knowledge, and attitudes to complete tasks and meet team goals (Blackmore & Persaud, 2012; Interprofessional Education Collaborative Expert Panel, 2011).

(3) Attitudes of effective team members (Blackmore & Persaud, 2012)

(a) Help each other be right.

> *(b)* Look for ways that new ideas can work.
> *(c)* Do not make negative assumptions about others.
> *(d)* Help each other win.
> *(e)* Speak positively about each other and the organization.
> *(f)* Do everything with enthusiasm.
> *(g)* Maintain positive mental outlook even in stressful times.

e) Decision making

(1) Team decision making is aided when a decision-making process is agreed upon(Blackmore & Persaud, 2012; Canadian Interprofessional Health Collaborative, 2010; Nancarrow et al., 2013).

(2) Decisions need to be patient focused and in line with the organization's and team's goals and mission (Blackmore & Persaud, 2012; Canadian Interprofessional Health Collaborative, 2010; Interprofessional Education Collaborative Expert Panel, 2011; Nancarrow et al., 2013).

(3) Decisions are both timely and collaborative; all team members participate in decision making (Blackmore & Persaud, 2012; Canadian Interprofessional Health Collaborative, 2010).

(4) Different ideas, views, and perspectives of team members are freely and openly expressed in the decision-making process (Blackmore & Persaud, 2012; Canadian Interprofessional Health Collaborative, 2010).

f) Relationships

(1) Relationships are professional in high-functioning teams (Blackmore & Persaud, 2012).

(2) Professionalism includes mutual respect for fellow team members and the ability to trust that all team members are working for the common good of the patient and family, the team, and the organization (Canadian Interprofessional Health Collaborative, 2010; Giladi et al., 2014; Interprofessional Education Collaborative Expert Panel, 2011; Nancarrow et al., 2013).

(3) When feedback is given, it is provided in a respectful, sensitive way with the goal of protecting the reputation of the person receiving the feedback, and the focus is on issues or processes, not on the person (Blackmore & Persaud, 2012; Interprofessional Education Collaborative Expert Panel, 2011).

(4) The person receiving the feedback responds in a respectful manner (Interprofessional Education Collaborative Expert Panel, 2011).

g) Formal, clear roles and processes

(1) For collaboration to occur, teams need clear roles and responsibilities for their members, which contribute to accomplishing the team's goals (Blackmore & Persaud, 2012; Canadian Interprofessional Health Collaborative, 2010; Interprofessional Education Collaborative Expert Panel, 2011; Nancarrow et al., 2013).

(2) Well-defined processes and infrastructures are needed to uphold the provision of services (i.e., referral process, handoffs, and communication infrastructure), including good documentation in the medical record (Albert et al., 2015; Canadian Interprofessional Health Collaborative, 2010).

    (3) Role interdependency exists between team members while individual roles and autonomy are still respected (Blackmore & Persaud, 2012; Interprofessional Education Collaborative Expert Panel, 2011; Nancarrow et al., 2013).

  h) Attention to growth and skill attainment: Team effectiveness and collaboration are improved when the team values and promotes professional development through training, rewards, recognition, and other opportunities for skill building for everyone on the team (Interprofessional Education Collaborative Expert Panel, 2011; Nancarrow et al., 2013).

  i) Knowledge sharing: Invariably, multiple disciplines are involved in addressing complex patient problems, making knowledge sharing across disciplines foundational to effective care.

    (1) The Institute of Medicine (IOM, 2011) has called for systematic reviews to guide practice, skills to translate evidence into practice, and interdisciplinary education.

    (2) Providers from all disciplines must be able to collaborate effectively to narrow the gap between knowledge generation and knowledge translation.

    (3) The future includes healthcare providers who are educated to deliver patient-centered care in interdisciplinary teams and are knowledgeable about evidence-based policy and care, as well as have the expertise necessary to address quality improvement and skills to work efficiently with informatics solutions (Newhouse & Spring, 2010).

III. Current findings

  A. Gaps in care exist across settings and throughout the disease trajectory (Schoen et al., 2011).

    1. These gaps consist of a lack of communication about test results, duplication of tests because information was not shared, and a lack of consistent discharge planning, clear follow-up plans, or written instructions (Schoen et al., 2011).

    2. Additional areas where collaboration falls short include the outpatient physician not being informed of inpatient care, failures to review medications, and preventable errors caused by a lack of communication (Schoen et al., 2011).

    3. Patients also lack someone whom they can easily contact between visits (Schoen et al., 2011).

  B. For patients with MCCs, clinical practice guidelines fail to adequately address the complexity of their situations (National Quality Forum, 2012; Nici & ZuWallack, 2012).

    1. Current standards do not require guideline developers to address differences in treatment response or competing disease or treatment interactions in patients with MCCs, and they fail to prioritize recommendations within a single disease, let alone among diseases (National Quality Forum, 2012; Nici & ZuWallack, 2012).

    2. When multiple clinical practice guidelines are used, challenges arise regarding how to establish goals.

      a) To appropriately meet the mounting needs of patients with MCCs, the U.S. healthcare system is working to transform from a disease-specific model to a patient-centered one (AHRQ, 2014).

        b) A whole-person, patient-centered approach to care allows patients to identify and choose the health goals important to them and to prioritize the implementation of clinical practice guidelines (Reuben & Tinetti, 2012).

  C. Previously, most healthcare professionals had not been trained to work in teams to provide complex chronic care, which posed challenges to continuity and collaboration (Boult & Wieland, 2010).

    1. With the support of IOM, CMS, AHRQ, and other agencies, a greater emphasis on interdisciplinary education and evidence-based practice behaviors has become the standard of care (AHRQ, 2014).

    2. Limitations and challenges still exist. Not every outpatient setting has access to the full array of interdisciplinary team members (e.g., social work, dietitian, physical therapy), and expansion of sophisticated health information technologies continues to grow slowly (Boult & Wieland, 2010).

    3. However, strides are being made in reimbursement and care delivery, such as CMS's recognition of care management for MCCs as one of the critical components of primary care that contributes to better well-being for individuals, as well as reduced spending (CMS, 2015).

  D. Issues of quality, safety, services, and cost must be addressed in an interdisciplinary manner or they will not effectively translate to sustainable initiatives (AHRQ, 2014; Newhouse & Spring, 2010).

  E. Collaboration across settings allows for the integration of community resources to enhance the traditional medical services for patients with MCCs and can reduce the burden and stress of the illness; however, many patients are unaware of community resources and need advocacy and encouragement from the interdisciplinary team to access them (Nici & ZuWallack, 2012).

IV. Relevance to practice

  A. The IOM (2011) report *The Future of Nursing: Leading Change, Advancing Health* called for interdisciplinary collaboration among all healthcare providers.

  B. Nurses are encouraged to build a strong knowledge base and be change agents to improve the healthcare system (Menefee, 2014).

  C. CMS has targeted chronic disease management and specifically called for an interdisciplinary management approach led by primary care practice (CMS, 2015; Menefee, 2014).

  D. Section 3001 of the Affordable Care Act calls for patient-centered care models that efficiently and effectively deliver improved outcomes. An interdisciplinary team approach to chronic disease management is necessary to meet the legislation's requirements (Menefee, 2014).

  E. The Joint Commission asks for healthcare providers to develop a standardized approach to communicating about transitions of care, including opportunities for healthcare providers to ask and respond to one another's questions (Solan et al., 2014).

  F. The majority of care for patients with MCCs occurs in the outpatient setting (Shaw et al., 2013).

  G. A shortage of 56,000 primary care physicians is expected by 2020 (Shaw et al., 2013).

    1. To meet the needs of patients with MCCs, the roles of other members of the interdisciplinary team must be expanded (Shaw et al., 2013).

    2. Advanced practice nurses are well positioned to meet this need and are accustomed to working in interdisciplinary teams and have training necessary to manage the care of patients with MCCs (Shaw et al., 2013).

V. Role of the advanced practice registered nurse (APRN)

   A. APRNs are well suited to provide care for patients with MCCs (Albert et al., 2015; Shaw et al., 2013).

      1. APRNs provide care that is global, patient focused, and part of the interdisciplinary team to address MCCs (Shaw et al., 2013).

      2. APRNs act as role models and coaches for patients as they educate, encourage, and guide self-care behaviors, as well as provide direct communication between the patient, caregiver, and other healthcare providers (Albert et al., 2015).

      3. APRNs prepare patients, families, and caregivers on self-management, medication reconciliation, and anticipation of what challenges may arise for the patient given the disease course and care setting, and identify options for addressing those challenges (Albert et al., 2015; Shaw et al., 2013).

      4. APRNs' interactions with other team members encompass formal, scheduled meetings; informal, daily, face-to-face interactions; and both formal and informal written communication (Giladi et al., 2014).

      5. APRNs often are present for patient visits, ensuring that patients' and families' most important concerns are identified and helping them to develop a plan of action to address needs (Giladi et al., 2014).

      6. APRNs make sure that the appropriate appointments are scheduled, resources are identified, and follow-up plans are put in place (Giladi et al., 2014).

   B. APRNs are knowledgeable about all aspects of each chronic condition, including who the appropriate specialists are and the indications and timing for when to involve them in the treatment plan, not only for patients but for families and caregivers as well (Albert et al., 2015; Giladi et al., 2014; Nici & ZuWallack, 2012).

   C. Elements incorporated into high-quality care provided by APRNs include the following (Giladi et al., 2014; Nici & ZuWallack, 2012):

      1. Disease prevention

      2. Promotion of a healthy lifestyle

      3. Early identification of a disease

      4. Treatment of the disease through optimization of pharmacologic and non-pharmacologic therapies

      5. Use of clinical practice guidelines that are adapted to the individual needs of patients, families, and caregivers

      6. Coordination of hospital, outpatient, subacute, and community services

      7. Self-management education

      8. Crisis management

   D. Self-management: APRNs educate and advocate for patients, families, and caregivers to be successful at self-management. A comprehensive approach to self-management encompasses symptom management and creatively addresses the changes or limitations to patients' lifestyle and function, as well as the changes in roles and relationships that result from disease progression (Rijken et al., 2014).

   E. Crisis management: APRNs are essential in assisting with crisis management for patients with MCCs and their families and caregivers, as these conditions affect patients for many years, are progressive, and are characterized by multiple crises (Boult & Wieland, 2010; Giladi et al., 2014).

      1. Crisis prevention, preparation, and intervention are important across the disease continuum (Boult & Wieland, 2010; Giladi et al., 2014).

    2. Crises can be emotional and psychosocial, practical, or medical, and the type may change throughout the disease process (Boult & Wieland, 2010; Giladi et al., 2014).

    3. The number of possible crises requires a large group of professionals to address the needs of patients, families, and caregivers, as well as a team member to lead the coordinated response. APRNs play an important role in coordinating these professionals and ensuring a comprehensive crisis response (Giladi et al., 2014).

    4. APRNs alert other team members that the crisis is occurring by communicating with the relevant providers based on the type of crisis, arranging a meeting between providers if needed, and collaborating to design and deliver the intervention (Giladi et al., 2014).

F. APRNs are situated to recognize when a patient is approaching a transition between settings or from one level of care to another and prepare the patient for what to anticipate before, during, and after the transition (Dusek et al., 2014).

    1. APRNs participate in transition planning meetings, identifying patient needs and goals for care, and coordinating and communicating with other healthcare providers on both the sending and receiving ends of the transition to minimize system barriers (Dusek et al., 2014).

    2. APRNS are key providers of information to healthcare teams within and between settings (Dusek et al., 2014).

G. APRNs help with assessing and identifying which team members and types of interventions are needed for a specific patient or family and help connect them to these services, which is especially important for systems or clinics that do not have all of the necessary team members in one place at all times (Dusek et al., 2014; Giladi et al., 2014). Such a personalized approach is only possible with coordination and clear communication among all team members and the direction of a team leader (Giladi et al., 2014; Nancarrow et al., 2013).

VI. Interface to palliative care

A. Palliative care approaches patients and families from an interdisciplinary holistic viewpoint.

B. Palliative care teams regularly collaborate with other interdisciplinary teams to address the needs of patients with MCCs and their families or caregivers.

C. Important steps when multiple interdisciplinary teams are involved in a patient's care include the following:

    1. Identify who is leading the care (i.e., primary care team member versus palliative care team member).

    2. Identify roles and responsibilities of the primary team and what the palliative care team will be assisting with to avoid role conflict and duplication of services.

    3. Identify clear processes for communication between teams.

    4. Identify whom the patient and family should contact, when that particular team member should be contacted, and for what symptom.

Case Study

    M.M. is an 82-year-old man with MCCs of congestive heart failure, prostate cancer, Parkinson disease, and dementia. His cancer is slow growing and he is not currently undergoing cancer therapy. M.M. has not seen a primary care physician in several years because of the number of specialty clinics he is involved in. M.M. most frequently has appointments with his APRN in the cardiology clinic and the APRN in the neurology clinic.

M.M. is admitted to the hospital with an exacerbation of congestive heart failure. His care in the hospital is managed by the APRN on the heart failure team. During the hospitalization, the APRN communicates with both clinics. At the request of M.M. and his wife, they are visited by the APRNs from each clinic while he is in the hospital.

Prior to the admission, he was living at home with 24/7 supervision from his wife, who is also elderly. She has reported that caring for him at home was becoming more difficult, especially in the month before the admission. Given his level of deconditioning and difficulties with function at home, M.M. is discharged to a subacute rehabilitation center two weeks after being admitted. The heart failure APRN coordinates the discharge.

While in the rehabilitation center, he is cared for by the APRN at the facility. This stay is his first admission to a rehabilitation center. Both he and his wife are reluctant to transition to the rehabilitation setting and need encouragement and education to feel more comfortable with the discharge plan.

During his stay, M.M. has follow-up appointments at both the cardiology and neurology clinics. The APRNs from each clinic communicate with the APRN at the rehabilitation center about medication management. They also begin discussions about whether M.M. could go home and what care may need to look like once he does return home. He is more functional than when he left the hospital but, given the progression of his MCCs, he has not returned to his preadmission baseline and is not expected to do so. Both he and his wife express the desire to have him home; however, his wife indicates concern that she still may not be able to care for him well at home.

After three weeks at the rehabilitation center, M.M. is cleared for discharge home with ongoing homecare services. The APRN from the rehabilitation facility assists with coordinating between the facility and the homecare agency regarding the plan of care. M.M. will receive home physical and occupational therapy, and a home palliative care consult is placed for continued symptom management as well as to limit the number of clinic appointments, as these were becoming burdensome for M.M. and his wife because of M.M.'s poor functional status. A social work consult also is placed for ongoing emotional support to M.M.'s wife because she has expressed a high level of caregiver stress. The APRN also contacts both the cardiology and neurology care teams to provide updates.

A week after M.M. returns home, his wife contacts the neurology clinic to report that she was not able to care for him at home but is unsure how to have him transition into another level of care, what it will cost, or how the change to long-term care will affect their relationship as a couple or M.M.'s coping. The APRN from the home palliative care team works with the clinic APRNs and the homecare social worker to address the couple's concerns and needs.

M.M. transitions to a long-term care setting where he continues to be followed by the APRN from the home palliative care team. Given the progression of his disease, he and his wife, along with his cardiology and neurology teams, have decided to take a more comfort-focused approach to his care. He has the option of returning to the clinics if desired, but the team would like to limit the number of visits if possible. The APRN from the palliative care team will now take the leadership role in his care.

Author's note: The Agency for Healthcare Research and Quality has developed TeamSTEPPS®: Strategies and Tools to Enhance Performance and Patient Safety, a federal initiative to improve patient safety using a team approach. Visit www.ahrq.gov/professionals/education/curriculum -tools/teamstepps/index.html for information about this program.

References

Agency for Healthcare Research and Quality. (2014, April). *Multiple chronic conditions chartbook: 2010 Medical Expenditure Panel Survey data* (AHRQ Pub. No. 14-0038). Retrieved from http://www.ahrq.gov/sites/default/files/wysiwyg/professionals/prevention-chronic-care/decision/mcc/mccchartbook.pdf

Albert, N.M., Barnason, S., Deswal, A., Hernandez, A., Kociol, R., Lee, E., … White-Williams, C. (2015). Transitions of care in heart failure: A scientific statement from the American Heart Association. *Circulation: Heart Failure, 8,* 384–409. doi:10.1161/HHF.0000000000000006

Blackmore, G., & Persaud, D.D. (2012). Diagnosing and improving functioning in interdisciplinary health care teams. *Health Care Manager, 31,* 195–207. doi:10.1097/HCM.0b013e3182619d48

Boult, C., & Wieland, G.D. (2010). Comprehensive primary care for older patients with multiple chronic conditions: "Nobody rushes you through." *JAMA, 304,* 1936–1943. doi:10.1001/jama.2010.1623

Burroughs, J., & Bartholomew, K. (2014). New ways for physicians and nurses to work together. *Physician Executive, 40*(3), 60–62, 64.

Canadian Interprofessional Health Collaborative. (2010, February). *A national interprofessional competency framework.* Vancouver, Canada: College of Health Disciplines, University of British Columbia.

Centers for Medicare and Medicaid Services. (2015, February 18). Payment of chronic care management services under CY 2015 Medicare PFS [Press release]. Retrieved from http://www.cms.gov/Outreach-and-Education/Outreach/NPC/National-Provider-Calls-and-Events-Items/2015-02-18-Chronic-Care-Management-new.html

Coleman, E.A. (2015). The Care Transitions Program®. Retrieved from http://caretransitions.org

Courtenay, M., Nancarrow, S., & Dawson, D. (2013). Interprofessional teamwork in the trauma setting: A scoping review. *Human Resources for Health, 11,* 57. doi:10.1186/1478-4491-11-57

Dusek, B., Pearce, N., Harripaul, A., & Lloyd, M. (2014). Care transitions: A systematic review of best practices. *Journal of Nursing Care Quality, 30,* 233–239. doi:10.1097/NCQ.0000000000000097

Giladi, N., Manor, Y., Hilel, A., & Gurevich, T. (2014). Interdisciplinary teamwork for the treatment of people with Parkinson's disease and their families. *Current Neurology and Neuroscience Reports, 14,* 493. doi:10.1007/s11910-014-0493-1

Institute of Medicine. (2011). *The future of nursing: Leading change, advancing health.* Washington, DC: National Academies Press.

Interprofessional Education Collaborative Expert Panel. (2011). *Core competencies for interprofessional collaborative practice: Report of an expert panel.* Washington, DC: Author.

Menefee, K.S. (2014). The Menefee model for patient-focused interdisciplinary team collaboration. *Journal of Nursing Administration, 44,* 598–605. doi:10.1097/NNA.0000000000000132

Nancarrow, S.A., Booth, A., Ariss, S., Smith, T., Enderby, P., & Roots, A. (2013). Ten principles of good interdisciplinary team work. *Human Resources for Health, 11,* 19. doi:10.1186/1478-4491-11-19

National Quality Forum. (2012, May). *Multiple chronic conditions measurement framework.* Retrieved from http://www.qualityforum.org/Publications/2012/05/MCC_Measurement_Framework_Final_Report.aspx

Newhouse, R.P., & Spring, B. (2010). Interdisciplinary evidence-based practice: Moving from silos to synergy. *Nursing Outlook, 58,* 309–317. doi:10.1016/j.outlook.2010.09.001

Nici, L., & ZuWallack, R. (2012). An official American Thoracic Society workshop report: The integrated care of the COPD patient. *Proceedings of the American Thoracic Society, 9,* 9–18. doi:10.1513/pats.201201-014ST

Pannick, S., Beveridge, I., Wachter, R.M., & Sevdalis, N. (2014). Improving the quality and safety of care on the medical ward: A review and synthesis of the evidence base. *European Journal of Internal Medicine, 25,* 874–887. doi:10.1016/j.ejim.2014.10.013

Patient-Centered Outcomes Research Institute. (2014, September 10). Why PCORI was created. Retrieved from http://www.pcori.org/content/why-pcori-was-created

Patient Protection and Affordable Care Act, 42 U.S.C. § 18001 et seq. (2010). Retrieved from http://www.hhs.gov/healthcare/about-the-law/read-the-law/index.html

Popejoy, L.L., Khalilia, M.A., Popescu, M., Galambos, C., Lyons, V., Rantz, M., … Stetzer, F. (2014). Quantifying care coordination using natural language processing and domain-specific ontology. *Journal of the American Medical Informatics Association, 22,* e93–e103. doi:10.1136/amiajnl-2014-002702

Reuben, D.B., & Tinetti, M.E. (2012). Goal-oriented patient care—An alternative health outcomes paradigm. *New England Journal of Medicine, 366,* 777–779. doi:10.1056/NEJMp1113631

Rijken, M., Bekkema, N., Boeckxstaens, P., Schellevis, F.G., De Maeseneer, J.M., & Groenewegen, P.P. (2014). Chronic disease management programmes: An adequate response to patients' needs? *Health Expectations, 17,* 608–621. doi:10.1111/j.1369-7625.2012.00786.x

Schoen, C., Osborn, R., Squires, D., Doty, M., Pierson, R., & Applebaum, S. (2011). New 2011 survey of patients with complex care needs in eleven countries finds that care is often poorly coordinated. *Health Affairs, 30,* 2437–2448. doi:10.1377/hlthaff.2011.0923

Shaw, R.J., McDuffie, J.R., Hendrix, C.C., Edie, A., Lindsey-Davis, L., & Williams, J.W., Jr. (2013, August). *Effects of nurse-managed protocols in the outpatient management of adults with chronic conditions.* Retrieved from http://www.hsrd.research.va.gov/publications/esp/rn-protocols.pdf

Solan, L.G., Yau, C., Sucharew, H., & O'Toole, J.K. (2014). Multidisciplinary handoffs improve perceptions of communication. *Hospital Pediatrics, 4,* 311–315. doi:10.1542/hpeds.2014-0005

U.S. Department of Health and Human Services. (2015, January 26). Better, smarter, healthier: In historic announcement, HHS sets clear goals and timeline for shifting Medicare reimbursements from volume to value. Retrieved from http://www.hhs.gov/about/news/2015/01/26/better-smarter-healthier-in-historic-announcement-hhs-sets-clear-goals-and-timeline-for-shifting-medicare-reimbursements-from-volume-to-value.html

CHAPTER 40

Cultural Considerations

*Christine Estabrook, DNP, MSN, ANP-BC, AOCNP®,
and Ami K. Goodnough, DNP, NP-C, ACHPN*

I. Definitions
  A. *Culture* is a collective group of ideas and values assimilated by members of society that directly affect and influence the way those individuals respond to real-world situations (Evans & Ume, 2012; Long, 2011).
    1. A set of attitudes, beliefs, behaviors, and policies to which people identify and adhere
    2. The sum total ways of living, including behavioral norms, language, communication style, patterns of thinking, beliefs, and values (Guide to Community Preventive Services, 2015)
    3. The way a person self-identifies according to ethnicity, race, religion, sexual orientation, socioeconomic status, or age
  B. *Cultural rituals* are a recognized set of predictable behaviors or actions that are derived from social or cultural beliefs or values that go beyond the formalized action (Mohammed & Peter, 2009).
  C. The term *culture* should not be used interchangeably with the terms *race* or *ethnicity*.
    1. *Race* is biologic and refers to a person's physical appearance, such as skin color, eye color, hair color, bone or jaw structure, etc.
    2. *Ethnicity* refers to cultural factors such as nationality, heritage, ancestry, language, and beliefs (Clark, 2012).
    3. An individual's approach to mortality is derived from specific customs, traditions, and core beliefs (Hiruy & Mwanri, 2014).
  D. *Cultural competence* is the attempt of healthcare providers to become aware of cultural predisposition and preferences of the individuals for which they care.
    1. Part of individualized patient care that demonstrates respect for a patient's healthcare beliefs and acknowledges that these beliefs play a role in effective healthcare delivery
    2. Recognition that illness occurs within a biopsychosocial construct in response to health beliefs and practices, which is essential for delivering efficient and effective healthcare (Evans et al., 2012; Saccomano & Abbatiello, 2014)
    3. Referring patients to resources that are culturally appropriate, including the use of medical interpreters, spiritual or religious services, and providers who have received specialty training in cross-cultural practices based on evidence-based practice (Saccomano & Abbatiello, 2014)
  E. *Cultural diversity* is the acceptance of individual characteristics such as skin color, religion, income, gender, and geographical location and facilitating equal access to

culturally competent care (Lowe & Archibald, 2009; Saccomano & Abbatiello, 2014). Cultural beliefs, practices, and values are learned initially at home, in social organizations where people gather, and then, ultimately, at educational institutions (Purnell, 2013).

II. Key aspects

    A. Awareness of self and others

        1. Understanding culture is vital in managing multiple chronic conditions (MCCs).

            a) Culture informs how a person understands health and makes decisions for managing chronic illness.

            b) It acts as a touchstone, or road map, for navigating health, illness, and times of trial.

            c) Diagnosis of chronic illness can trigger feelings of loss, grief, and decreased sense of control (Kagawa-Singer & Blackhall, 2011).

            d) Learned behaviors and perceptions provide meaning in life as well as a protocol for managing adversities (Kagawa-Singer & Blackhall, 2011).

        2. Theoretical models help guide healthcare practice and provide a framework for understanding broad concepts such as culture.

            a) The Purnell Model for Cultural Competence (PMCC) is an organized and comprehensive framework that provides a succinct method of understanding concepts of culture.

            b) This model takes into account situations that influence an individual's worldview in the setting of historical experiences.

            c) The PMCC links specific characteristics of culture to develop a road map that can facilitate culturally sensitive and competent patient care (Purnell, 2013) (see Figure 40-1).

                (1) The PMCC is displayed as a circle with four perimeters (Purnell, 2013; Sagar, 2012):

                    (a) Global society (outside perimeter)

                    (b) Community (second perimeter)

                    (c) Family (third perimeter)

                    (d) Individual (fourth perimeter)

                  (2) Purnell designed a saw-toothed line at the bottom of the circle designated as "nonlinear concept of cultural competence," which delineates four levels of cultural competence, specifically, unconsciously incompetent, consciously incompetent, consciously competent, and unconsciously competent (Sagar, 2012, p. 21).

                (3) The cultural domains of the model are reflected as 12 pie-shaped wedges within the circle of the PMCC.

                    (a) The domains are concepts that are interconnected and transferable to various cultures.

                    (b) The interconnectedness of the domains has a direct impact on an individual's health and healthcare decision making (Purnell, 2013; Sagar, 2012).

    B. Needs assessment for the patient and family

        1. Every culture has specific values or practices that can influence or dictate healthcare treatment. Understanding a patient's culture can allow healthcare providers to develop an effective treatment strategy for chronic health conditions derived from the cultural preferences and practices of each individual and family.

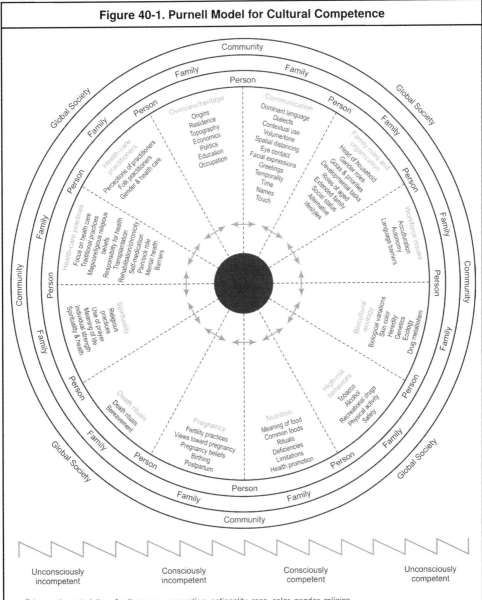

Figure 40-1. Purnell Model for Cultural Competence

Unconsciously incompetent

Consciously incompetent

Consciously competent

Unconsciously competent

Primary characteristics of culture: age, generation, nationality, race, color, gender, religion

Secondary characteristics of culture: educational status, socioeconomic status, occupation, military status, political beliefs, urban versus rural residence, enclave identity, marital status, parental status, physical characteristics, sexual orientation, gender issues, and reason for migration (sojourner, immigrant, undocumented status)

Unsconsciously incompetent: not being aware that one is lacking knowledge about another culture
Consciously incompetent: being aware that one is lacking knowledge about another culture
Consciously competent: learning about the client s culture, verifying generalizations about the client s culture, and providing culturally specific interventions
Unsconsciously competent: automatically providing culturally congruent care to clients of diverse cultures

Note. Figure courtesy of Larry D. Purnell, PhD, RN, FAAN. Used with permission.

2. In 2010, the Joint Commission mandated standards for culturally competent patient care that focused on various aspects of cultural issues, including religious beliefs, perceptions of health status, nutritional needs, and modesty issues (Saccomano & Abbatiello, 2014). These assessments can be broad based with a specific focus on chronic disease conditions.

3. Performing a thorough patient and family assessment allows for a comprehensive understanding of individual cultural preferences related to healthcare decision making, creating the foundation for culturally sensitive, patient-centered healthcare interventions (Frost, Cook, Heyland, & Fowler, 2011). The DIVERSE mnemonic (see Figure 40-2) is an example of a tool to guide assessment of cultural preferences.

4. Healthcare providers can meet the needs of patients across varying cultures by cultivating a rapport with patients and families based on their cultural preference. A focus should be placed on fostering an environment with the patient and family that provides the following (Kagawa-Singer & Blackhall, 2011):
   a) A sense of safety and security
   b) A sense of integrity and meaningfulness of life
   c) A sense of belonging

5. Self-assessment and reflection is a process for gaining insight into an individual's beliefs, attitudes, and values. It is vital for healthcare providers to perform a reflective self-assessment to determine preexisting prejudice and bias. One such tool is Mazanec and Panke's (2016) self-assessment, Cultural Knowledge and Beliefs, which assesses information on culture while allowing individuals to reflect on their perspective of cultural facts and beliefs.

6. When approaching conversations with patients from varying cultures, it is useful to consider styles in conversation to enhance communication. The Industry Collaboration Effort provides useful tips to enhance communication (see Figure 40-3).

III. Current findings
   A. African Americans
      1. Facts
         a) According to the U.S. Census Bureau (2015), African Americans comprise approximately 12.6% of the U.S. population.
         b) The African American community constitutes more than 30 million people and is expected to increase to close to 35 million people by 2050 (U.S. Census Bureau, 2015).
         c) It is important for healthcare providers to understand the cultural considerations that influence healthcare decisions for the African American community.
         d) Finding an effective way to integrate cultural concerns to reduce barriers to care is essential to decrease the morbidity and mortality rates from chronic illnesses in the African American population.
      2. Approach to health care
         a) Several barriers have been identified that prohibit African Americans from pursuing health care.
            (1) These barriers include socioeconomic status, masculinity, prejudice, not recognizing the need to seek health care, peer and family influences, and religious beliefs.

Figure 40-2. DIVERSE Mnemonic for Patient Encounters

A mnemonic will assist you in developing a personalized care plan based on cultural/diversity aspects. Place in the patient's chart or use the mnemonic when gathering the patient's history on a SOAP progress note.

	Assessment	Sample Questions	Assessment Information/ Recommendations
D	Demographics: Explore regional background, level of acculturation, age, and sex as they influence healthcare behaviors.	Where were you born? Where was "home" before coming to the United States? How long have you lived in the United States? What is the patient's age and sex?	
I	Ideas: Ask the patient to explain his/her ideas or concepts of health and illness.	What do you think keeps you healthy? What do you think makes you sick? What do you think is the cause of your illness? Why do you think the problem started?	
V	Views of healthcare treatments: Ask about treatment preference, use of home remedies, and treatment avoidance practices.	Are there any healthcare procedures that might not be acceptable? Do you use any traditional or home health remedies to improve your health? What have you used before? Have you used alternative healers? Which? What kind of treatment do you think will work?	
E	Expectations: Ask about what your patient expects from his/her doctor.	What do you hope to achieve from today's visit? What do you hope to achieve from treatment? Do you find it easier to talk with a male/ female? Someone younger/older?	
R	Religion: Ask about your patient's religious and spiritual traditions.	Will religious or spiritual observances affect your ability to follow treatment? How? Do you avoid any particular foods? During the year, do you change your diet in celebration of religious and other holidays?	
S	Speech: identify your patient's language needs, including health literacy levels. Avoid using a family member as an interpreter.	What language do you prefer to speak? Do you need an interpreter? What language do you prefer to read? Are you satisfied with how well you read? Would you prefer printed or spoken instructions?	

(Continued on next page)

	Figure 40-2. DIVERSE Mnemonic for Patient Encounters *(Continued)*		
E	Environment: Identify patient's home environment and the cultural/diversity aspects that are part of the environment. Home environment includes the patient's daily schedule, support system, and level of independence.	Do you live alone? How many other people live in your house? Do you have transportation? Who gives you emotional support? Who helps you when you are ill or need help? Do you have the ability to shop or cook for yourself? What times of day do you usually eat? What is your largest meal of the day?	

Note. From *Better Communication, Better Care: Provider Tools to Care for Diverse Populations* (p. A-05-04), by Industry Collaboration Effort (ICE) Cultural and Linguistics Workgroup, 2004. Retrieved from https://www.iceforhealth.org/library/documents/ICE_C&L_Provider_Toolkit_7.10.pdf.

  (2) In addition, slavery and the Tuskegee Syphilis Experiment have made some in the African American population distrustful of physicians and healthcare institutions (Osher et al., 2011).
 b) Decision making regarding care is based on a collectivist approach, meaning that the family is interdependent and all decisions for health care are made by the family or group based on past history, culture, and ethical issues (Hiruy & Mwanri, 2014).
 c) African Americans have strong feelings of spirituality, and infusing spiritual elements with the treatment planning improves healthcare outcomes (Tanyi & Werner, 2007).
 d) African Americans tend to focus on living and sustaining life with a more aggressive approach to life-sustaining interventions. Many reasons exist for this approach to health care by African Americans, including education level and access to health care, historical mistrust of physicians and the healthcare system, and religious beliefs (Wicher & Meeker, 2012).
 e) Healthcare providers need to consider the influences of distrust of medical systems, the importance of family involvement in healthcare decisions, and the role of religious beliefs and the faith community when considering end-of-life care and discussions and decisions (Mazanec, Daly, & Townsend, 2010).
 f) Healthcare providers should provide tailored education and counseling for African American patients while paying attention to cultural issues to determine treatment interventions for patients with chronic diseases (Lenz et al., 2005; Nzerue, Demissochew, & Tucker, 2002).
 B. Asian Americans and Pacific Islanders
  1. Basic principles
   a) The basic principles behind Eastern medicine are founded on a belief system based on a state of balance between the physical, social, and supernatural environment.
   b) The Eastern medicine approach to health care is based on the assumption that the body is whole, with each organ affected by both mental and

physical function. This approach often counters the Western medicine approach, which assumes that disease stems from external forces such as viruses, bacteria, or degeneration of functional ability.

Figure 40-3. Working With Diverse Patients: Tips for Successful Patient Encounters

To enhance patient–provider communication and to avoid being unintentionally insulting or patronizing, be aware of the following:

Styles of speech: People vary greatly in length of time between comment and response, the speed of their speech, and their willingness to interrupt.
• Tolerate gaps between questions and answers; impatience can be seen as a sign of disrespect.
• Listen to the volume and speed of the patient's speech as well as the content. Modify your own speech to more closely match that of the patient to make them more comfortable.
• Rapid exchanges, and even interruptions, are a part of some conversational styles. Don't be offended if no offense is intended when a patient interrupts you.
• Stay aware of your own pattern of interruptions, especially if the patient is older than you are.

Eye contact: The way people interpret various types of eye contact is tied to cultural background and life experience.
• Most Euro-Americans expect to look people directly in the eyes and interpret failure to do so as a sign of dishonesty or disrespect.
• For many other cultures, direct gazing is considered rude or disrespectful. Never force a patient to make eye contact with you.
• If a patient seems uncomfortable with direct gazes, try sitting next to them instead of across from them.

Body language: Sociologists say that 80% of communication is nonverbal. The meaning of body language varies greatly by culture, class, gender, and age.
• Follow the patient's lead on physical distance and touching. If the patient moves closer to you or touches you, you may do the same. However, stay sensitive to those who do not feel comfortable, and ask permission to touch them.
• Gestures can mean very different things to different people. Be very conservative in your own use of gestures and body language. Ask patients about unknown gestures or reactions.
• Do not interpret a patient's feelings or level of pain just from facial expressions. The way that pain or fear is expressed is closely tied to a person's cultural and personal background.

Gently guide patient conversation: English predisposes us to a direct communication style; however, other languages and cultures differ.
• Initial greetings can set the tone for the visit. Many older people from traditional societies expect to be addressed more formally, no matter how long they have known their physician. If the patient's preference is not clear, ask how they would like to be addressed.
• Patients from other language or cultural backgrounds may be less likely to ask questions and more likely to answer questions through narrative than with direct responses. Facilitate patient-centered communication by asking open-ended questions whenever possible.
• Avoid questions that can be answered with "yes" or "no." Research indicates that when patients, regardless of cultural background, are asked, "Do you understand," many will answer, "yes" even when they really do not understand. This tends to be more common in teens and older patients.
• Steer the patient back to the topic by asking a question that clearly demonstrates that you are listening. Some patients can tell you more about their health through story telling than by answering direct questions.

Note. From *Better Communication, Better Care: Provider Tools to Care for Diverse Populations* (p. A-02-04), by Industry Collaboration Effort (ICE) Cultural and Linguistics Workgroup, 2004. Retrieved from https://www.iceforhealth.org/library/documents/ICE_C&L_Provider_Toolkit_7.10.pdf.

    c) Blending these two approaches is essential for success when treating patients of Asian or Pacific Islander descent.

  2. Approach to health care

    a) In many Asian and Middle Eastern cultures, the concept of autonomy changes to a more collective decision-making approach.

      (1) Family members believe that patients need to be protected from any unnecessary stress or worry.

      (2) In many cases, the families do not want patients to know their diagnosis and will make treatment decisions without the patient's consent (de Pentheny O'Kelly, Urch, & Brown, 2011; Tang et al., 2006).

    b) Often, it is believed that patients will lose hope if told the truth, and this is discouraged or alternate vocabulary is used. Furthermore, many Asian cultures view end-of-life decisions as family-centered activities because the death affects all those close to the dying person (Searight & Gafford, 2005).

    c) Direct communication regarding terminal conditions is considered rude or cruel. Asian patients believe that Western medicine is too strong and will dose reduce or discontinue treatment when symptoms begin to resolve.

    d) Appropriate medications and dosing are essential for successful supportive care patient interventions. Research regarding drug metabolism in the Asian population supports decreased metabolism rates with drugs used in palliative care settings (Kuebler, Varga, & Mihelic, 2003).

    e) Consideration of patients' beliefs and values is essential when providing care for Asians and Pacific Islanders.

    f) Asian families tend to exemplify stoicism in the face of chronic health issues, which is an approach that does not often complement the approach of Western medicine.

    g) Healthcare providers need to identify the family decision maker and acknowledge family roles when determining healthcare decisions, as patients may defer all decisions to other family members.

C. Hispanic Americans and Latinos

  1. Facts

    a) Approximately 50.5 million Latinos were living in the United States in 2010, representing 16% of the total population (U.S. Census Bureau, 2015).

    b) An increase occurred from 2000 to 2010, which accounted for more than 50% of the population growth during that time (U.S. Census Bureau, 2015).

    c) Hispanic culture places a great deal of emphasis on relationships with immediate and extended family members.

    d) Family members, rather than professional healthcare providers, are expected to care for loved ones who are sick or dying.

  2. Approach to health care

    a) In general, Hispanic and Latino patients look toward religion and spirituality for guidance in challenging times, especially in instances of healthcare interventions.

    b) Prayer is extremely important, with families holding prayer vigils over ill members and lighting candles for sick and dying patients. Hispanic families believe that members who have died oversee the living. For this reason, families pray for the members to provide guidance and support during crisis (Davila, Reifsnider, & Pecina, 2011; Shuster, Clough, Higgins, & Klein, 2009).

     c) Cultural traditions are used for prevention and treatment of disease, including the use of candles, statues, and medals. Folk healers within the community treat disease with the use of prayer, herbs, counseling, and supernatural forces (Davila et al., 2011).

     d) Family approval and religious practices often affect healthcare decision making. Latino patients will forgo decision making regarding health care and defer to family members regarding treatment interventions (Davila et al., 2011).

     e) Hispanic Americans view illness as a family issue and involve family members in almost all healthcare decisions.

     f) Healthcare providers should recognize the importance of family-centered decision making and offer patients the opportunity to make decisions together with their families when possible (Kelley, Wenger, & Sarkisian, 2010). Healthcare providers should consider the patient, family, and Hispanic community when interacting with patients to determine treatment planning (Thomson & Hoffman-Goetz, 2009).

IV. Relevance to practice

  A. Healing, curing, and management of MCCs must exist within the mosaic of the cultural backgrounds of both the patients and the clinicians (Kagawa-Singer & Blackhall, 2011).

  B. Because culture informs life, health, and death on physical, spiritual, and metaphysical levels, it must be addressed on a regular basis (Kagawa-Singer & Blackhall, 2011).

  C. Culture influences the verbal and physical expression of pain and discomfort; it can be seen as a trial, test, or punishment (Kagawa-Singer & Blackhall, 2011).

  D. Drug metabolism is influenced by genetics and genetic polymorphism (Kagawa-Singer & Blackhall, 2011) (see Chapter 8).

  E. Culture influences emotional response to diagnosis (Kagawa-Singer & Blackhall, 2011).

  F. Consider and be aware of whom to address and who makes decisions (Kagawa-Singer & Blackhall, 2011).

  G. Be aware of dependency and provision of support—who gives and receives (Kagawa-Singer & Blackhall, 2011).

  H. Consider and be aware of specific etiquette of communication patterns (Kagawa-Singer & Blackhall, 2011).

  I. Each culture has a different perception of truth telling, including how much should be revealed and to whom (Kagawa-Singer & Blackhall, 2011).

  J. The American Nurses Association (as cited in Saccomano & Abbatiello, 2014) advocates for advancement of cultural diversity so that all patients can receive culturally competent care.

  K. Specialty training in cross-cultural practice supports cultural diversity and assists practitioners in determining culturally sensitive clinical interventions (Saccomano & Abbatiello, 2014).

    1. Determine cultural rituals.

    2. Identify the decision maker in the family.

    3. Understand views of pain management, such as the use of opioids or antidepressants.

    4. Ascertain how to manage declining performance status and affect of family.

V. Role of the advanced practice registered nurse (APRN)

    A. Introspection for every APRN or clinician is important while engaging patients to determine the best responses to patients based on individual, family, and cultural aspects.

    B. Ethical dilemmas may occur if cultural values and traditions are not considered.

    C. Because many factors influence cultural views, end-of-life care and advance directives should be explored individually with each patient, regardless of ethnicity.

        1. APRNs must become self-aware and demonstrate a willingness to set aside biases and beliefs to develop cultural competence.

        2. APRNs must become familiar with frequently encountered cultural customs to cultivate a knowledge base from which to initiate conversations and determine appropriate interventions.

    D. Identification of patient goals through direct, open-ended questions based on patients' and families' beliefs and preferences is most effective when discussing advance directives and end-of-life topics.

    E. The role of APRNs is one of an intermediary for patients and physicians. APRNs can mediate between these two groups to provide culturally sensitive decisions for patient care (Mohammed & Peter, 2009).

    F. APRNs must develop skills for assessing cultural rituals to effectively enable communication while identifying cultural needs. This is completed by asking culturally sensitive questions regarding beliefs and practices of patients and families when determining medical decisions and healthcare delivery (Douglas et al., 2014).

    G. The use of patient cultural assessments, derived through covert or overt interventions, can create opportunities for determining specific knowledge, leading to a culturally competent APRN (Evans et al., 2012).

    H. The role of APRNs is to facilitate the communication between clinicians, patients, and patients' social support.

        1. Who is family? The smallest unit of analysis of fulfillment of human need.

        2. Western culture places family lower than patient.

        3. Other more sociocentric cultures focus on family needs and suppress individual needs.

        4. Who is involved in decision making; how is the burden shared (Kagawa-Singer & Blackhall, 2011)?

    I. To effectively manage MCCs, awareness of the cultural background of each patient is especially important.

        1. People receive and process information based on their previous experiences, which is intricately informed by their culture.

        2. Culture is a pervasive conglomeration of all that a person is, and it must be addressed when providing comprehensive, holistic care.

    J. Figure 40-4 lists websites with additional resources for delivering culturally competent care.

VI. Interface to palliative care

    A. Goals of palliative care are improved health outcomes, increased quality of life, and decreased suffering of the patient and family until death. Providers must be aware that this may look different in each culture (Kagawa-Singer & Blackhall, 2011).

    B. If the goal is quality care, each patient must be treated individually and uniquely, not simply as a member of a homogenous group.

    C. Culturally competent care cannot be replicated across people groups. Each person and family must be assessed for their unique needs.

Figure 40-4. Additional Resources for Delivering Culturally Competent Care

Agency for Healthcare Research and Quality (AHRQ) and U.S. Department of Health and Human Services
- AHRQ Spanish website, "Healthcare 411": http://healthcare411.ahrq.gov/defaultes.aspx
- Better Communication, Better Care: Provider Tools to Care for Diverse Populations: https://innovations.ahrq.gov/qualitytools/better-communication-better-care-provider-tools-care-diverse-populations
- Continuing Education for Culturally Competent Care (free online educational programs for physicians, advanced practice providers, nurses, social workers, crisis workers, mental health and oral health providers): www.thinkculturalhealth.hhs.gov/Content/ContinuingEd.asp
- Cultural and Linguistic Competence: www.ahrq.gov/health-care-information/topics/external/Cultural-and-Linguistic-Competence.html#clinicians
- Culturally Tailored Programs: https://innovations.ahrq.gov/issues/2012/01/18/culturally-tailored-programs
- Industry Collaboration Effort (ICE) training for culturally competent care: www.iceforhealth.org/messagedetail.asp?mid=5427

Addressing Linguistic Needs in Diverse Cultures
- Guide to Providing Effective Communication and Language Assistance Services: https://hclsig.thinkculturalhealth.hhs.gov
- INTERPRET Tool: www.thinkculturalhealth.hhs.gov/pdfs/InterpretTool.pdf
- Working With an Interpreter: www.thinkculturalhealth.hhs.gov/pdfs/WorkingWithAnInterpreter.pdf
- CLAS Clearinghouse: Results for "Clinical & Mental Health": www.thinkculturalhealth.hhs.gov/CloudSearch/KeywordSearch_RightNav.asp?id=2

National Committee for Quality Assurance and Eli Lilly and Company
- *Multicultural Health Care: A Quality Improvement Guide*: www.ncqa.org/Portals/0/HEDISQM/CLAS/CLAS_toolkit.pdf

---

Case Study

B.W. is a 26-year-old woman of Arab origin with metastatic pancreatic cancer who now resides in the United States. She has recently entered a prearranged marriage to an accountant from India. She has received treatment with two different chemotherapy agents, with poor response to treatment. Today, she is hospitalized with a biliary obstruction. The surgical team has deemed her a poor surgical candidate and has placed a biliary drain for palliative management of the obstruction. The medical oncology team does not recommend further chemotherapy based on her poor performance status and is referring her to supportive care and hospice.

The patient's older brother-in-law is a dentist and has been selected to make all medical decisions for the patient, though he resides in another state and is not present for these conversations. Males in the family Arab origin may be considered to have more authority with regard to medical decisions than females. He does not support the recommendations of the medical team and encourages B.W. and her husband to travel out of state for a second opinion. The patient is in severe pain, rated as a 9 out of 10, but her brother-in-law does not want opioids to be used for pain control. He does not understand why the patient cannot be treated with further chemotherapy. He does not believe the patient is too unstable to travel to another state for a second opinion and chemotherapy.

As a healthcare provider, it is important to identify patients with Arab ancestry to determine their preferences regarding their own healthcare decisions and whether they would prefer to involve or defer to other family members in their decision-making process. The healthcare team needs to provide a clear description of the treatment regimens, including the use of long-term medications, so that the patient and family members can make informed decisions. This may require some negotiating with the patient or family to promote adherence to long-term drug regimens. A gentle approach regarding these issues allows for better understanding of the patient and family perspective and the importance of traditional remedies in the overall care plan. Also, if there is a terminal or serious diagnosis, identify the patient's preferences concerning the disclosure of clinical findings and continue to address these wishes periodically throughout the treatment regimen.

References

Clark, D. (2012). Cultural considerations in planning palliative and end of life care. *Palliative Medicine, 26*, 195–196. doi:10.1177/0269216312440659

Davila, Y.R., Reifsnider, E., & Pecina, I. (2011). Familismo: Influence on Hispanic health behaviors. *Applied Nursing Research, 24*, e67–e72. doi:10.1016/j.apnr.2009.12.003

de Pentheny O'Kelly, C., Urch, C., & Brown, E.A. (2011). The impact of culture and religion on truth telling at the end of life. *Nephrology Dialysis Transplantation, 26*, 3838–3842. doi:10.1093/ndt/gfr630

Douglas, M.K., Rosenkoetter, M., Pacquiao, D.F., Callister, L.C., Hattar-Pollara, M., Lauderdale, J., ... Purnell, L. (2014). Guidelines for implementing culturally competent nursing care. *Journal of Transcultural Nursing, 25*, 109–121. doi:10.1177/1043659614520998

Evans, B.C., & Ume, E. (2012). Psychosocial, cultural, and spiritual health disparities in end-of-life and palliative care: Where we are and where we need to go. *Nursing Outlook, 60*, 370–375. doi:10.1016/j.outlook.2012.08.008

Evans, N., Meñaca, A., Koffman, J., Harding, R., Higginson, I.J., Pool, R., & Gysels, M. (2012). Cultural competence in end-of-life care: Terms, definitions, and conceptual models from the British literature. *Journal of Palliative Medicine, 15*, 812–820. doi:10.1089/jpm.2011.0526

Frost, D.W., Cook, D.J., Heyland, D.K., & Fowler, R.A. (2011). Patient and healthcare professional factors influencing end-of-life decision-making during critical illness: A systematic review. *Critical Care Medicine, 39*, 1174–1189. doi:10.1097/CCM.0b013e31820eacf2

Guide to Community Preventive Services. (2015, October 13). Promoting health equity: Culturally competent health care. Retrieved from http://www.thecommunityguide.org/healthequity/healthcare/ccc.html

Hiruy, K., & Mwanri, L. (2014). End-of-life experiences and expectations of Africans in Australia: Cultural implications for palliative and hospice care. *Nursing Ethics, 21*, 187–197. doi:10.1177/0969733012475252

Kagawa-Singer, M., & Blackhall, L.J. (2011). Negotiating cross-cultural issues at the end of life: "You got to go where he lives." In S.J. McPhee, M.A. Winker, M.W. Rabow, S.Z. Pantilat, & A.J. Markowitz (Eds.), *Care at the close of life: Evidence and experience* (pp. 417–430). Columbus, OH: McGraw-Hill.

Kelley, A.S., Wenger, N.S., & Sarkisian, C.A. (2010). Opiniones: End-of-life care preferences and planning of older Latinos. *Journal of the American Geriatrics Society, 58*, 1109–1116. doi:10.1111/j.1532-5415.2010.02853.x

Kuebler, K.K., Varga, J., & Mihelic, R.A. (2003). Why there is no cookbook approach to palliative care: Implications of the P450 enzyme system. *Clinical Journal of Oncology Nursing, 7*, 569–572. doi:10.1188/03.CJON.569-572

Lenz, O., Mekala, D.P., Patel, D.V., Fornoni, A., Metz, D., & Roth, D. (2005). Barriers to successful care for chronic kidney disease. *BMC Nephrology, 6*, 11. doi:10.1186/1471-2369-6-11

Long, C.O. (2011). Cultural and spiritual considerations in palliative care. *Journal of Pediatric Hematology/Oncology, 33*(Suppl. 2), S96–S101. doi:10.1097/MPH.0b013e318230daf3

Lowe, J., & Archibald, C. (2009). Cultural diversity: The intention of nursing. *Nursing Forum, 44*, 11–18. doi:10.1111/j.1744-6198.2009.00122.x

Mazanec, P.M., Daly, B.J., & Townsend, A. (2010). Hospice utilization and end-of-life care decision making of African Americans. *American Journal of Hospice and Palliative Medicine, 27*, 560–566. doi:10.1177/1049909110372087

Mazanec, P.M., & Panke, J. (2016). Cultural considerations in palliative care. In B.R. Ferrell (Series Ed.) & N. Coyle (Vol. Ed.), *HPNA Palliative Nursing Manuals: Vol. 6. Social aspects of care* (pp. 99–118). New York, NY: Oxford University Press.

Mohammed, S., & Peter, E. (2009). Rituals, death and the moral practice of medical futility. *Nursing Ethics, 16*, 292–302. doi:10.1177/0969733009102691

Nzerue, C.M., Demissochew, H., & Tucker, J.K. (2002). Race and kidney disease: Role of social and environmental factors. *Journal of National Medical Association, 94*(Suppl. 8), 28S–38S.

Osher, T., Garay, L., Jennings, B., Jimerson, D., Markus, S., & Martinez, K. (2011, September). *Closing the gap: Cultural perspectives on family-driven care.* Retrieved from http://www.tapartnership.org/docs/ClosingThe Gap_FamilyDrivenCare.pdf

Purnell, L.D. (2013). *Transcultural health care: A culturally competent approach.* Philadelphia, PA: F.A. Davis.

Saccomano, S.J., & Abbatiello, G.A. (2014). Cultural considerations at the end of life. *Nurse Practitioner, 39*(2), 24–31. doi:10.1097/01.NPR.0000441908.16901.2e

Sagar, P.L. (2012). *Transcultural nursing theory and models: Application in nursing education, practice, and administration.* New York, NY: Springer.

Searight, H.R., & Gafford, J. (2005). Cultural diversity at the end of life: Issues and guidelines for family physicians. *American Family Physician, 71,* 515–522. Retrieved from http://www.aafp.org/afp/2005/0201/p515.html

Shuster, G.F., Clough, D.H., Higgins, P.G., & Klein, B.J. (2009). Health and health behaviors among elderly Hispanic women. *Geriatric Nursing, 30,* 18–27. doi:10.1016/j.gerinurse.2008.03.002

Tang, S.T., Liu, T.-W., Lai, M.-S., Liu, L.-N., Chen, C.-H., & Koong, S.-L. (2006). Congruence of knowledge, experiences, and preferences for disclosure of diagnosis and prognosis between terminally-ill cancer patients and their family caregivers in Taiwan. *Cancer Investigation, 24,* 360–366. doi:10.1080/07357900600705284

Tanyi, R.A., & Werner, J.S. (2007). Spirituality in African American and Caucasian women with end-stage renal disease on hemodialysis treatment. *Health Care for Women International, 28,* 141–154. doi:10.1080/07399330601128486

Thomson, M.D., & Hoffman-Goetz, L. (2009). Defining and measuring acculturation: A systematic review of public health studies with Hispanic populations in the United States. *Social Science and Medicine, 69,* 983–991. doi:10.1016/j.socscimed.2009.05.011

U.S. Census Bureau. (2015). QuickFacts United States. Retrieved from http://www.census.gov/quickfacts/table/PST045215/00

Wicher, C.P., & Meeker, M.A. (2012). What influences African American end-of-life preferences? *Journal of Health Care for the Poor and Underserved, 23,* 28–58. doi:10.1353/hpu.2012.0027

Section VII.

Spiritual Support and Self-Care for Professionals

CHAPTER 41

Spiritual and Religious Care

Rebecca Lichwala, MSN, ARNP, AOCNP®, NP-C

I. Definitions
   A. Spirituality (Edwards, Pang, Shiu, & Chan, 2010; Puchalski, Ferrell, Otis-Green, & Handzo, 2014)
      1. An individual's search for life meaning and finding a purpose to life
      2. Has no boundaries
      3. Associated with an individual's relationship with a Higher Power
      4. Can be associated with or separate from a religion
   B. Religion (Edwards et al., 2010)
      1. An organized group of individuals who believe in the same practices and customs
      2. Often share same moral and ethical beliefs
   C. Spiritual care (Puchalski et al., 2014)
      1. Providing interventions that promote relationships between individuals and a Higher Power
      2. Helping to provide a union of mind, body, and spirit
      3. Providing compassionate care
      4. Fostering positive and supportive thinking and being present with another through challenging times
   D. Spiritual coping (Puchalski et al., 2014)
      1. Adapting to stress by focusing on spiritual or religious beliefs and practices
      2. Use of ritual, prayer, songs, and readings that promote personal reflection to seek a balance and understanding of specific events
II. Key aspects
   A. Importance of addressing spirituality (Moritz, Kelly, Xu, Toews, & Rickhi, 2011)
      1. Relationship between spirituality and health: Recent data suggest that spiritual well-being can be used to help prevent the occurrence or progression of depression.
      2. The use of spirituality or religion lessens symptoms of depression and results in improved outcomes and a quicker recovery.
      3. In a survey of 400 people diagnosed with emotional instability, 48% of the participants relied on the use of religion to cope with their symptoms. Those participants were found less likely to be hospitalized (Baetz & Toews, 2009).
      4. In a qualitative study of semi-structured interviews, the integration of spiritual teaching programs was demonstrated to improve mood in depressed patients (Moritz et al., 2011).

B. Importance of defining spirituality and religion with the patient (Edwards et al., 2010)
   1. Allows the provider to explore the patient's use of spirituality and religion in difficult situations
   2. Provides a multidimensional perspective of the patient and family to include spiritual and religious preferences and practices, which can create a richer relationship between the patient and the interdisciplinary team
C. National Consensus Project for Quality Palliative Care (Puchalski et al., 2009)
   1. Recognizes inclusion of spirituality in palliative care as one of eight domains of care
   2. Recommendations for improving spiritual care in seven areas
      a) Developing specific spiritual care models
      b) Ongoing use of spiritual assessment
      c) Spiritual care inclusion in the development of patient-specific care planning
      d) Implementation of the interdisciplinary team to support all dimensions of individual patients
      e) Requirement for spiritual and religious providers to undergo appropriate training and certification when interfacing with patients with life-limiting disease
      f) Personal and professional development in spiritual and religious aspects of care for interdisciplinary team members, which allows providers to facilitate empathetic care and develop meaningful relationships with patients
      g) Quality improvement projects to ensure appropriate integration of spirituality and religion in the comprehensive care management of patients living with and dying from advanced chronic conditions
III. Current findings
   A. Evidence has shown that spirituality is a major priority for almost all patients and families who are faced with a life-limiting condition (Edwards et al., 2010).
   B. Asking patients and families about the value and importance of religion was found to be beneficial in 51%–77% of patients with advanced disease (Edwards et al., 2010).
   C. Reliance on spirituality and religion can affect how well patients can cope with their condition (Puchalski et al., 2014).
      1. Spiritual coping can be used to increase patient-perceived satisfaction and quality of life.
      2. Spiritual well-being interfaces with all areas of the patient and family life.
         a) Overall acceptance and appreciation of life experiences
         b) Emotional health
         c) Physical health
         d) Socialization that reduces isolation and loneliness
      3. Patients and families who rely on spirituality and religion have a sense of inner strength that comes from individualized practices of faith, prayer, and religious rituals.
      4. The interdisciplinary team should evaluate and assess for the presence of negative religious coping that can interfere with effective symptom management.
         a) Patients may have hidden or deep-seated emotions that can create feelings of guilt, anger, anxiety, and fear, to name a few. These triggers can elicit somatic pain without a significant pathophysiologic etiology.
         b) The interdisciplinary team will be required to investigate causes of spiritual discomfort and to engage the appropriate spiritual adviser or religious leader to support individualized patient needs.

D. Patients should be allowed to define spirituality in their own terms. This can occur through the following (Edwards et al., 2010):
  1. Sharing meaningful stories about his or her own life
  2. Reviewing relationships and having served a purpose in life
  3. Reviewing relationships with others—what is meaningful and important versus what is no longer regarded as a priority
  4. Reviewing personal relationship with nature, music, and the arts and how these are used to support meaning and understanding of life purpose
  5. Reviewing personal and private relationship with God or higher being
  6. Gaining ongoing hope, meaning, and purpose in life
E. Barriers to spiritual care (Edwards et al., 2010)
  1. Time: Providers may not have enough time to properly assess spirituality.
     a) Inadequate staffing
     b) Large number of patients scheduled in the clinic setting
     c) Lack of appropriate funding or reimbursement
     d) Disinterest in considering this aspect of patient care
  2. Environment: Patients may not be comfortable discussing their spiritual or religious preferences in an acute or emergent care setting or in openly discussing with a busy medical provider.
  3. Lack of training for healthcare professionals
     a) Listening skills
     b) Awareness of patients' spiritual and religious needs
     c) Cultural beliefs that are unfamiliar or different
     d) Lack of confidence in assessing patients for spiritual distress
  4. Personal beliefs
     a) The interdisciplinary team recognizes the value and expertise of each member of the team. Spiritual advisers and religious leaders are used to address and support the spiritual dimensions of patients and families.
     b) The interdisciplinary team should remain open-minded and accepting of any specific beliefs and practices used by patients and families to define meaning and loss.
IV. Relevance to practice
  A. All healthcare disciplines are provided information in basic training on multidimensional aspects of individuals and how each dimension interfaces with one another—for example, spirituality or the use of religion cannot be excluded from the physical, emotional, and social dimensions that create wholeness and determine patient-specific quality of life.
  B. All interventions that target symptoms should consider spiritual distress because this can be physically manifested into somatic discomfort. This requires keen assessment and use of spiritual advisers or religious leaders.
  C. Patients who are not provided spiritual or religious support can become isolated and fearful, which begins a chain of emotional events that trigger depression, anxiety, agitation, insomnia, and other physical and emotional symptoms (Puchalski et al., 2014).
V. Role of the advanced practice registered nurse (APRN)
  A. Assessment
    1. Can be completed by a trained healthcare provider or a certified chaplain, priest, pastor, rabbi, etc.
    2. All patients should receive a spiritual screening when entering into a healthcare system.

3. Healthcare professionals should be trained to complete a spiritual screening and a patient-specific spiritual history.

4. Spiritual screening usually consists of one or two questions to triage spiritual practices and potential needs and identify patients who need urgent spiritual intervention (Puchalski et al., 2009). Common screening questions include:

   a) Is spirituality or religion an important part of your life?

   b) How have you used spirituality or religion in the past to cope with difficult situations? What do you need now?

5. Spiritual history

   a) Encourage patients to facilitate their own spiritual or religious measures to support or cope with the challenges associated with the burden of symptomatic disease.

   b) Facilitate appropriate referrals based on patient preferences, beliefs, and practices.

   c) FICA spiritual history tool (Borneman, Ferrell, & Puchalski, 2010)

      (1) Validated tool created in 1996 used to take a spiritual history

      (2) Open-ended questions that help providers address patients' spiritual needs

      (3) Four domains used to collect data for a spiritual assessment

         (a) Faith and belief: Do you consider your life spiritual or religious? Do you have spiritual beliefs that help you cope with stress? What gives your life meaning?

         (b) Importance and influence: What importance does your faith or belief have in your life? On a scale of 0 (not important) to 5 (very important), how would you rate the importance of your faith in your life? Have your beliefs influenced you in how you handle stress? What role do your beliefs play in your healthcare decision making?

         (c) Community: Are you part of a spiritual or religious community? Is there a group of people you really love or who are important to you?

         (d) Address in care: How would you like your healthcare providers to use this information about your spirituality as they care for you?

   d) HOPE questions (Anandarajah & Hight, 2001)

      (1) A teaching tool created to help providers address spirituality during a medical history

      (2) In contrast to the FICA spiritual history tool, the HOPE questions are not validated by research but allow providers to examine patients' spiritual beliefs and potential support systems.

      (3) The mnemonic HOPE is used to help providers ask open-ended questions:

         (a) H: Where do you find your source of hope, meaning, comfort, strength, and peace?

         (b) O: Do you find importance and meaning in organized religion?

         (c) P: What are your personal practices that are important to you?

         (d) E: What effect do your beliefs have on medical care and end of life?

      (4) After using this tool, providers can incorporate spirituality into the patient's care plan.

B. Interventions aimed for patients and families
1. Remain open-minded, accepting, and understanding about the myriad differences among patients, families, and cultures.
2. Recognize appropriate referral sources based on individual patient preferences and needs.
3. Never assume that personal spirituality and religion fit the needs and goals of patients and families.
4. Provide the resources required to support patients and families in their need to be spiritual or religious.
5. Assist patients and families in developing the plan of care to include spiritual and religious dimensions.

VI. Interface to palliative care
A. National Consensus Project for Quality Palliative Care recommends palliative care programs to provide spiritual care (Puchalski et al., 2014).
1. Palliative care programs should provide and document spiritual care.
2. A standardized assessment tool should be used to assess spirituality.
3. Quality improvement frameworks should be initiated.
4. Research that includes spiritual care should be supported.
5. Funding should be provided to continue research in spiritual care.
B. APRNs' role is to help patients identify end-of-life goals.
C. Aggressive treatment and end-of-life decisions often are navigated by patients' or their families' beliefs (Puchalski et al., 2014).

Case Study

S.M. is a 53-year-old woman with stage III breast cancer being treated with chemotherapy and surgery, followed by radiation therapy. She is tolerating treatment well, with minimal and manageable side effects. When first diagnosed, she described being religious and prayed often to get her through the initial diagnosis. During follow-up visits in the beginning of her diagnosis, she would frequently make references to prayer and God. During her past few visits, she has not mentioned her religion and says she is mad at God for giving her cancer.

The APRN recognizes the change in S.M. and is able to associate her abrupt change in mood of being withdrawn and agitated to her anger with God. The APRN takes the time to sit down next to S.M. and quietly asks her what has changed—she had previously been reliant on prayer and made frequent comments about how her faith had gotten her through her treatments.

S.M. begins to cry and informs the APRN that everything has become overwhelming and she does not know how to communicate her fears with her family. The APRN sits with S.M. while she regains her composure and asks if she could contact her priest. S.M. is grateful for the opportunity to allow herself to hear what she has been keeping from her family and agrees that speaking to her priest would help to regain the faith that she needed to help her get through the remainder of her radiology treatments.

References

Anandarajah, G., & Hight, E. (2001). Spirituality and medical practice: Using the HOPE questions as a practical tool for spiritual assessment. *American Family Physician, 63,* 81–89. Retrieved from http://www.aafp.org/afp/2001/0101/p81.html

Baetz, M., & Toews, J. (2009). Clinical implications of research on religion, spirituality, and mental health. *Canadian Journal of Psychiatry, 54,* 292–301.

Borneman, T., Ferrell, B., & Puchalski, C.M. (2010). Evaluation of the FICA tool for spiritual assessment. *Journal of Pain and Symptom Management, 40,* 163–173. doi:10.1016/j.jpainsymman.2009.12.019

Edwards, A., Pang, N., Shiu, V., & Chan, C. (2010). Review: The understanding of spirituality and the potential role of spiritual care in end-of-life and palliative care: A meta-study of qualitative research. *Palliative Medicine, 24,* 753–770. doi:10.1177/0269216310375860

Moritz, S., Kelly, M.T., Xu, T.J., Toews, J., & Rickhi, B. (2011). A spirituality teaching program for depression: Qualitative findings on cognitive and emotional change. *Complementary Therapies in Medicine, 19,* 201–207. doi:10.1016/j.ctim.2011.05.006

Puchalski, C.M., Ferrell, B., Otis-Green, S., & Handzo, G. (2014, October 7). Overview of spirituality in palliative care [Literature review current through April 2016]. Retrieved from http://www.uptodate.com/contents/overview-of-spirituality-in-palliative-care

Puchalski, C.M., Ferrell, B., Virani, R., Otis-Green, S., Baird, P., Bull, J., … Sulmasy, D. (2009). Improving the quality of spiritual care as a dimension of palliative care: The report of the Consensus Conference. *Journal of Palliative Medicine, 12,* 885–904. doi:10.1089/jpm.2009.0142

CHAPTER 42

Hope and Loss

Rebecca Lichwala, MSN, ARNP, AOCNP®, NP-C

I. Definition
   A. Hope is an emotion that is identified by positive feelings about the future, short and long term.
   B. Hope is associated with increased motivation, optimism, and an upbeat mood and spirit ("Hope," 2016).
   C. Hope can guide toward the future.
   D. Hope is both universal and specific.
      1. *Universal hope* is a broad acceptance of the future. It is a safeguard for patients by illuminating life itself (Kavradim, Özer, & Bozcuk, 2013).
      2. *Specific hope* is connected to time and a certain event in the patient's life, such as hoping a treatment cures a disease or that disease is stabilized in order to carry out future events (e.g., to see a birth of a grandchild, a son's wedding, or a daughter's graduation) (Kavradim et al., 2013).
      3. When hope is made vulnerable, universal hope can aid in helping the patient to not surrender hope to a specific situation or personal experience.
   E. Hopelessness (Sachs, Kolva, Pessin, Rosenfeld, & Breitbart, 2013)
      1. The inability to maintain a good feeling and to develop self-soothing responses to a disappointment, leading to feelings of disheartenment or disappointment
      2. Experiencing negative feelings and pessimistic expectations when thinking about the future
      3. When hope has been lost or the patient has nothing to look forward to
II. Key aspects
   A. When a patient is faced with the diagnosis of a chronic medical condition, a sense of hope should be instilled by the patient's medical team. A sense of hope can be used to support individualized patient coping skills and ease the patient's feelings of fear or loss.
   B. Effects of hope (Mattioli, Repinski, & Chappy, 2008; McLean, 2011)
      1. Hope provides patients with a reason for living and for interfacing with people and events important and personal to them.
      2. Hope can be used to maintain self-esteem.
      3. Hope can help patients to develop a sense of meaning and understanding about their diagnosis.
      4. Patients who have high levels of hope are more likely to develop meaningful coping strategies that assist the family and loved ones to have a healthier perspective of the impact of disease and disability.

C. Hope can be used to provide a positive impact on the patient, family, and interdisciplinary team providing care and management of a chronic condition (Kavradim et al., 2013).

1. Helps patients cope with the disabilities of their disease by identifying meaningful coping strategies and facilitating these strategies to prevent negative emotions, such as depression and anxiety

2. Increases sense of well-being and provides a positive outlook and a reason for living

3. Provides the opportunity for patients and families to adapt to abrupt changes associated with symptomatic disease

D. Threats or consequences that can interfere with hope (Landmark, Bøhler, Loberg, & Wahl, 2008)

1. Being diagnosed with a serious advanced disease that predisposes the patient and family to a life-limiting prognosis

2. Experiencing an aggressive progression of disease that affects the patient's physical functioning

3. Experiencing any change in the treatment or management of the disease state that may precipitate untoward side effects or generate symptoms of fatigue or lethargy

4. Recognizing that the progressive nature of the disease has progressed into the end of life

5. Providing false hope: When healthcare personnel offer false hope to a patient with a chronic disease or a terminal illness, this can raise expectations for the patient and family and can promote a disappointment and loss if the expectation is not met.

E. Hopelessness (Sachs et al., 2013)

1. Places patients at risk for detachment, depression, and giving up

   a) Associated with eagerness for an accelerated death and interferes with patient-perceived quality of life

   b) Can be the result of poorly managed symptoms and disease exacerbations or side effects from interventions

2. Hopelessness should be evaluated when considering the symptom of depression. If not appropriately evaluated and managed, prolonged hopelessness can lead to suicide ideation.

F. Patients' emotional status can decline and precipitate additional symptoms, such as anxiety, anger, agitation, and insomnia, to accompany the underlying depression.

III. Current findings: Positive effects on hope (Mattioli et al., 2008; Sachs et al., 2013)

A. Strong family relationships: Family can help facilitate acceptance with a poor prognosis of an advanced disease or condition.

B. Strong support systems can help with coping.

IV. Relevance to practice

A. A gap exists between evidence and practice. Hope is not evaluated or assessed, and interventions to increase hope are not routinely considered or included in patients' care plans.

B. Side effects of treatment and relationship to hope (Kavradim et al., 2013)

1. Managing side effects is a part of the scope of practice of advanced practice registered nurses (APRNs).

2. Negative side effects can lower hope scores (see Section IV.A).

   a) Pain

       b) Anxiety

       c) Nausea and vomiting

       d) Mucositis

       e) Peripheral neuropathy

  C. Positive interactions between patients and the interdisciplinary team can help increase hope levels and decrease anxiety.

  D. Building relationships with patients and families can also increase quality of life.

V. Role of the APRN

  A. Assessment of hope: Herth Hope Index (Herth, 2000)

    1. Scale used to assess levels of hope and is widely used in clinical practice

    2. Designed for patients who are critically ill

    3. Has 12 questions that use a four-point Likert scale

    4. Scores range from 12 to 48; higher scores show a higher level of hope.

    5. APRNs can use the Herth Hope Index to evaluate patients at various points in the disease trajectory.

      a) Time of diagnosis

      b) During treatment

      c) After treatment

  B. Maintain or build hope (Rosenblatt & Meyer, 2016)

    1. Face diagnosis, prognosis, and symptoms directly.

    2. Provide a caring attitude and environment.

    3. Help patients make realistic short-term goals.

    4. Allow patients to have an active role in their care and treatment plan.

    5. Have conversations with patients about what brings meaning to their life.

    6. Respect patients' dignity at all times.

    7. Help patients establish a meaning to their life and the time they have left.

    8. Assist with helping patients reestablish past relationships that would help provide them support.

    9. Help patients find importance in their life.

    10. Help patients remember and acknowledge their past accomplishments.

  C. Interventions

    1. Interventions can be implemented to help enhance hope levels.

    2. Interventions can be patient guided or nurse guided.

      a) Patient-guided interventions

        (1) Multimedia intervention (Oh & Kim, 2010)

          (a) CD-ROMs given to patients during their appointment, which they can use at home

          (b) Self-paced

          (c) The focus of the intervention is to increase hope by developing coping skills, learning stress management, enhancing symptom management, strengthening social relationships, and practicing hopeful goal setting.

          (d) Hope levels are evaluated prior to and after the intervention.

          (e) APRNs can set up a follow-up appointment to evaluate level of hope.

        (2) Benefits of patient-guided interventions include the ease of delivery and cost-effectiveness.

      b) Nurse-guided interventions (Rustøen, Cooper, & Miaskowski, 2011)

        (1) Support groups led by nurses

(2) Each group meeting has a topic of discussion that assists in facilitating hope.

VI. Interface to palliative care (Philip et al., 2012; Sachs et al., 2013)

A. Palliative care in chronic illnesses

1. Patients with an advanced chronic condition have an increase in physical and psychological morbidity.
2. Palliative care is recommended for patients with chronic conditions to help them manage the signs and symptoms of their illness.
3. Healthcare providers can maintain patients' hope by helping them to create attainable goals and making them feel as though they have a purpose in their life.
4. For healthcare providers, helping patients find the meaning in life—creating hope—is an important responsibility.

B. Hope helps patients live with meaning and purpose. High levels of hope can reduce psychological stress.

Case Study

T.B. is a 67-year-old man who has a history of chronic obstructive pulmonary disease (COPD). He requires 2 L of oxygen greater than 15 hours/day. He rarely goes out anymore because he cannot "catch his breath." He has been hospitalized with COPD exacerbations four times in the past year. He is widowed but has two children who live locally and frequently come to check on him. He is seeing his primary care provider in the office for a routine checkup. He says he feels depressed because his dyspnea has taken over his life. His daughter is pregnant, and he wants to be able to greet his new grandchild in the next six months. The APRN reviews T.B.'s recent spirometry of forced expiratory volume in one second, which was less than 50%, and understands that his symptoms are directly correlated with his pulmonary function. She sits down with T.B. and develops a realistic plan for reducing the incidence of exacerbation and improving his symptoms through adherence to the appropriate medications. The APRN makes a referral to the clinical psychologist to offer ongoing discussions with T.B. to evaluate for depression and set realistic goals that T.B. can achieve. The APRN makes a referral to a pulmonary specialist for a review of T.B.'s medications and ability to endure a six-minute walk test. T.B. has recently been introduced to the adult day center in his community, and the APRN helps recruit transportation to assist T.B. in maintaining social interactions to improve his mood and engage him in activities.

References

Herth, K. (2000). Enhancing hope in people with a first recurrence of cancer. *Journal of Advanced Nursing, 32,* 1431–1441. doi:10.1046/j.1365-2648.2000.01619.x

Hope. (2016, January 21). Retrieved from http://www.goodtherapy.org/blog/psychpedia/what-is-hope

Kavradim, S.T., Özer, Z.C., & Bozcuk, H. (2013). Hope in people with cancer: A multivariate analysis from Turkey. *Journal of Advanced Nursing, 69,* 1183–1196. doi:10.1111/j.1365-2648.2012.06110.x

Landmark, B., Bøhler, A., Loberg, K., & Wahl, A.K. (2008). Women with newly diagnosed breast cancer and their perceptions of needs in a health-care context. *Journal of Clinical Nursing, 17,* 192–200. doi:10.1111/j.1365 -2702.2008.02340.x

Mattioli, J.L., Repinski, R., & Chappy, S.L. (2008). The meaning of hope and social support in patients receiving chemotherapy. *Oncology Nursing Forum, 35,* 822–829. doi:10.1188/08.ONF.822-829

McLean, P. (2011). Balancing hope and hopelessness in family therapy for people affected by cancer. *Australian and New Zealand Journal of Family Therapy, 32,* 329–342. doi:10.1375/S0814723X00001923

Oh, P.J., & Kim, S.H. (2010). Effects of a brief psychosocial intervention in patients with cancer receiving adjuvant therapy [Online exclusive]. *Oncology Nursing Forum, 37,* E98–E104. doi:10.1188/10.ONF.E98-E104

Philip, J., Gold, M., Brand, C., Douglass, J., Miller, B., & Sundararajan, V. (2012). Negotiating hope with chronic obstructive pulmonary disease patients: A qualitative study of patients and healthcare professionals. *Internal Medicine Journal, 42,* 816–822. doi:10.1111/j.1445-5994.2011.02641.x

Rosenblatt, L., & Meyer, F.L. (2016, February 5). Psychosocial issues in advanced illness [Literature review current through May 2016]. Retrieved from http://www.uptodate.com/contents/psychosocial-issues-in -advanced-illness

Rustøen, T., Cooper, B.A., & Miaskowski, C. (2011). A longitudinal study of the effects of a hope intervention on levels of hope and psychological distress in a community-based sample of oncology patients. *European Journal of Oncology Nursing, 15,* 351–357. doi:10.1016/j.ejon.2010.09.001

Sachs, E., Kolva, E., Pessin, H., Rosenfeld, B., & Breitbart, W. (2013). On sinking and swimming: The dialectic of hope, hopelessness, and acceptance in terminal cancer. *American Journal of Hospice and Palliative Medicine, 30,* 121–127. doi:10.1177/1049909112445371

Compassionate Self-Care: An Interdisciplinary Approach

*Nancy Jo Bush, RN, MN, MA, AOCN®, FAAN,
and Debi Boyle, MSN, RN, AOCNS®, FAAN*

I. Definition
  A. Florence Nightingale (1969) was the first to identify essential self-care in nursing by encouraging nurses to not "undermine your own health" (p. 16). This advice is salient then and now, for nurses and all interdisciplinary team members.
  B. Compassionate self-care is exemplified by a synergy and balance among physical, emotional, spiritual, intellectual, social, personal, and professional well-being that results in a healthy nurse (Kushner & Ruffin, 2015).
  C. Self-care is essential to health and healing.
    1. An essential job requirement is caring for oneself (Kushner & Ruffin, 2015).
    2. The relationship between self-care and self-compassion has been investigated as it affects patient care.
    3. If there is a deficit in self-care, nurses' therapeutic use of self can be compromised in the provision of compassionate care (Mills, Wand, & Fraser, 2015).
    4. Work–life balance is an important strategy to optimize overall well-being (Gillman et al., 2015).
  D. Research has shown that when nurses do not attend to their own needs, the quality of patient care suffers (Hooper, Craig, Janvrin, Wetsel, & Reimels, 2010).
    1. Abernethy (2012) stated that self-care is often neglected in the medical professions, and may "contribute to medical errors, disinterest in or depersonalization of patient care, and lower quality of care" (p. e9).
    2. Health systems should routinely measure the wellness of care providers as an indicator of the quality of the health system such that suboptimum caregiver wellness adversely affects system performance (Wallace, Lemaire, & Ghali, 2009).
  E. All professionals on the interdisciplinary team should work together in a supportive and collegial manner to ensure self-care practices that, in turn, ensure quality patient care.
    1. Provision 5 of the American Nurses Association's *Code of Ethics for Nurses* (2015) states, "The nurse owes the same duties to self as to others, including responsibility to promote health and safety, preserve wholeness of char-

acter and integrity, maintain competence, and continue personal and professional growth" (p. 19).

2. The code advises nurses to carry out the same health maintenance measures and promotion activities as they teach to patients.

3. Interventions to combat compassion fatigue are outlined in the code.

4. These include following a healthy diet, exercising, engaging in relationships with family and friends, carrying out leisure and recreational activities, and attending to spiritual and religious needs.

5. The code requires nurse leaders to recognize the importance of promoting healthy work environments that support self-care.

6. A balance between personal and professional life is viewed as the goal of compassionate self-care.

F. The American Holistic Nurses Association (2013) incorporates self-care and healing in the organization's standards of practice for holistic nurses.

1. Holistic nursing recognizes the interconnectedness of mind, body, spirit, and environment in both personal and professional activities.

2. Nurses are seen as responsible to model health-promoting behaviors and are challenged to achieve harmony in their own lives as well as for their patients.

G. The Oncology Nursing Society's (2012) leadership competencies define self-care as personal health maintenance incorporating components of physical, mental, emotional, and spiritual well-being. Nurse leaders are viewed as role models of self-care and thus are encouraged to set personal priorities and boundaries necessary to protect work–life balance.

H. The American Association of Critical-Care Nurses (2016) identified six standards essential to healthy work environments: skilled communication, true collaboration, effective decision making, appropriate staffing, meaningful recognition, and authentic leadership. These guidelines provide a framework to prevent risks for burnout and compassion fatigue and to guide intervention planning in the workplace.

I. Nurses spend more time with patients and families than any other healthcare professionals, predisposing them to both physical and emotional distress (Melvin, 2015).

1. Melvin (2015) stated, "Nurses play a critical role in caring for patients who are suffering . . . it is *this very work* that predisposes nurses to distress" (p. 66).

2. Nurses should recognize their own distress and rely on a range of self-care strategies that enable them to not only survive but to thrive.

3. Work settings that foster an environment of support, promote civil working relationships, and instill a sense of empowerment are ideal to counter the distress of professional caregivers (Melvin, 2015).

J. The National Association of Social Workers (NASW) recognizes and supports the practice of professional self-care for social workers as a means of maintaining their competence, strengthening the profession, and preserving the integrity of their work with clients. NASW approved a policy statement to address professional self-care and social work and suggested the following self-care initiatives (NASW, 2008):

1. Development of continuing education programs on professional self-care

2. Development of innovative support services for social workers

3. Recognition by social work educators of the importance of self-care in the profession

4. Training of social work students on self-care

5. Further research and publications addressing the issue of professional self-care and social work and provision of tools and strategies for successful social work practice

    K. The American Society of Clinical Oncology (2015) has begun to recognize the need for physician self-care. Although the organization has not developed a formal policy statement, its annual meetings have been addressing the untoward effects of physician burnout coupled with interventions for recognition, prevention, and self-care.

II. Key aspects
    A. Core challenges in compassionate caregiving (Boyle, 2010; Halifax, 2011)
       1. Lack of anticipatory guidance in basic education about the personal toll of professional caregiving and need for self-care
       2. Cumulative work demands and stress resulting in burnout
       3. Caregiver grief or dysfunction caused by the exposure to the pain and suffering of others resulting in secondary traumatic stress or compassion fatigue
       4. Caregiver understanding of the right thing to do in a situation but inability to act upon it (i.e., moral distress)
       5. Horizontal hostility, which is behavior that controls, devalues, disrespects, or diminishes another peer or group (i.e., bullying)
       6. Structural violence, which is defined as the systematic discrimination against an individual or group
       7. Absence of work setting interventions and antidotes to minimize the consequences of compassionate caring
    B. In the absence of optimum self-care, professionals become vulnerable to these professional stressors.
    C. **Burnout** occurs within the interpersonal context of one's job (Sabo, 2011).
       1. Unhealthy work environments (i.e., low staff ratios, lack of job recognition, paternalistic leadership, feelings of powerlessness, and a mismatch between the caregiver and environment in relation to shared goals and vision) promote chronic, psychologically taxing job stressors that result in feelings of exhaustion, cynicism, and inefficacy.
       2. A professional experiencing burnout can suffer physical and psychological symptoms, including behavioral changes. Hallmark signs include anger, frustration, negativity, and withdrawal.
       3. Coworkers might notice symptoms of burnout before the person experiencing it does.
       4. Certain personality characteristics, work-related attitudes, and work or organizational characteristics have been postulated to contribute to the burnout syndrome (Cañadas-De la Fuente et al., 2015).
       5. Type A personalities, escape-avoidance coping styles, idealistic work-related expectations, and organizational stressors such as high acuity and a lack of social support services may contribute to burnout (Sabo, 2011).
       6. The organizational consequences of burnout include poor job performance and effectiveness, staff turnover, and impaired personal and social functioning. The three dimensions of the burnout continuum have been characterized as components ranging within exhaustion–energy, cynicism–involvement, and inefficacy–efficacy experiences (Melvin, 2015).
    D. **Compassion fatigue** (CF) is a consequence of professional exposure to pain, suffering, and trauma (Sabo, 2011).
       1. CF emanates from relationships between the healthcare provider and patient.
       2. CF is relational in nature (Boyle, 2015; Potter et al., 2010).
       3. The ability to be empathic and to enter into a therapeutic relationship with a patient is foundational to CF.

4. Individuals with high levels of empathy to patients' pain and trauma are vulnerable to CF (Sabo, 2011).

5. Individuals at highest risk for CF are often self-sacrificing and prone to neglecting their own self-care.

6. Individuals with unresolved grief are at equally high risk for CF.

7. Hallmark signs include feelings of sadness and grief, avoidant or withdrawal behaviors, somatic complaints, and feelings of weariness and exhaustion (Sabo, 2011).

8. CF can result in the loss of one's sense of self, meaning and purpose, feelings of compassion, or ability to be empathic (Melvin, 2015).

9. The cumulative result of CF is physical, emotional, and spiritual depletion (Lombardo & Eyre, 2011).

E. **Secondary traumatic stress** (STS) is frequently used interchangeably with CF.

1. It is exemplified by trauma symptoms of clinical significance that result from exposure to, or awareness of, significant distress in others (Watts & Robertson, 2015).

2. People with STS may experience distinct definitional corollaries to post-traumatic stress disorder.

3. These include recalling unwanted memories, having nightmares of a witnessed trauma, and experiencing increased psychological arousal (Sabo, 2011).

4. Like CF, this often occurs when boundaries between caregiver and patient become blurred and the caregiver takes on the distress experienced by the patient.

5. STS is described as an outcome of countertransference experienced by empathic caregivers when they indirectly experience the trauma of their patients (Boyle, 2010).

6. When doctors, nurses, social workers, and other members of the interdisciplinary team report symptoms related to reexperiencing the client's trauma, "wishing to avoid both the client and reminders of the client's trauma, and feeling persistent arousal due to intimate knowledge about the client's traumatic experiences, they are likely suffering from secondary trauma" (Adams, Buscarino, & Figley, 2006, p. 104).

F. **Vicarious traumatization** is a form of psychological and spiritual distress experienced by healthcare professionals when caring for the ill and traumatized.

1. Vicarious traumatization is distinguished as a negative transformation of the caregiver's inner self that results from empathic engagement with the traumatized patient (Sabo, 2011).

2. As a result of taking on the patient's trauma, the professional has difficulty in relationships with others, is unable to respond appropriately to stressful situations, experiences intrusive memories, and may suffer from an altered belief system.

3. Essentially, the caregiver integrates the patient's suffering and trauma experience as his or her own (Sabo, 2011).

4. Characteristics that predispose healthcare professionals to vicarious trauma include empathy, a nonjudgmental attitude, sensitivity, hypersensitivity to injustice, and a self-sacrificing mentality (Greville, 2015).

G. **Cumulative grief** is a risk for all healthcare professionals.

1. In specialties where death and dying are prominent, caregivers must be assertive in acknowledging grief responses and how they are affecting one's personal and professional lives.

2. The grieving process of nurses following patient death has not been investigated extensively, nor have programs been implemented to help nurses cope with loss (Gerow et al., 2010).
3. Nurses often are forced to repress their feelings on the death of a patient, making them more vulnerable to burnout and CF.
4. In the absence of proactive self-care, grief responses may be exaggerated.
5. Numerous barriers to nurses' resolution of grief exist (e.g., time constraints, staffing shortages, lack of administrative support, stoicism).
6. However, a supportive work environment with programs that address nurse grief augments nurses' ability to recognize and properly manage personal bereavement as a part of self-care (Wenzel, Shaha, Klimmek, & Krumm, 2011).

H. **Moral distress** is the emotional suffering that occurs when constraints (internal or external) prevent professionals from following the course of action they believe is appropriate (Huffman & Rittenmeyer, 2012).
   1. Moral distress is pervasive and seldom recognized, and it impedes healthcare professionals' ability to deliver optimal patient care (Cavaliere, Daly, Dowling, & Montgomery, 2010).
   2. Moral distress results in physical and emotional strain that accumulates and contributes to feelings of dissatisfaction, a sense of failure, and a loss of integrity.
   3. Moral residue is long-standing distress when personal ethical beliefs are compromised (Sauerland, Marotta, Peinemann, Berndt, & Robichaux, 2014).
   4. Nurses experiencing moral distress in the work environment risk burnout and may withdraw from relationships with patients or leave the nursing profession altogether (Cavaliere et al., 2010).

I. **Horizontal hostility** and **structural violence** are additional challenges that negatively affect well-being in the work setting.
   1. Horizontal hostility has been defined as behaviors that control, devalue, disrespect, or diminish another peer or group.
   2. Structural violence is the systemic discrimination against an individual or group and is often referred to as "bullying" (Halifax, 2011).
      a) Bullying can be in the form of verbal abuse or being ignored or ostracized from groups or conversations.
      b) A hostile work environment may support bullying or bullying behaviors that contribute to a negative workplace atmosphere.
      c) Aggressive bulling behaviors can cause psychological and physical harm to staff, disrupt nursing care, and threaten patient safety and quality outcomes (Gaffney, DeMarco, Hofmeyer, Vessey, & Budin, 2012).
      d) All interdisciplinary team members are responsible for identifying and rectifying hostile and bullying behaviors.

III. Current findings
   A. Early detection of burnout, CF, STS, vicarious traumatization, grief, moral distress, and bullying is recommended.
   B. Nurses often neglect taking care of themselves until they find themselves in crisis (Hooper et al., 2010).
      1. Engaging in self-care strategies and having supportive resources available can enable nurses to cope with constant exposure to trauma and suffering.
      2. Seminal work by Figley (1995) described nurses as being at risk to be "wounded by their work" because empathy and compassion are core values of the nursing role (Melvin, 2015).

C. Recent studies have shown that physicians managing seriously ill patients are at high risk for diminished personal well-being, including high rates of burnout; moral distress, defined as the inability to act in a manner consistent with one's personal and professional values; and compassion fatigue, in which physicians experience diminished emotional energy to care for patients (Shanafelt et al., 2014).

   1. All of these constructs are true for all interdisciplinary team members, such as social workers (Kanter, 2007), oncologists (Shanafelt & Dyrbye, 2012), and physician assistants and advanced practice nurses (Hylton, 2015).

   2. A cross-sectional survey investigated compassion satisfaction, burnout, and CF among emergency department nurses compared with nurses in other inpatient specialties (Hooper et al., 2010).

      a) The Professional Quality of Life: Compassion Satisfaction and Fatigue Subscales, R-IV (ProQOL R-IV) was completed by emergency nurses and three other specialties: oncology, nephrology, and intensive care unit (ICU) nurses.

      b) This scale tests for compassion satisfaction, CF, and burnout.

      c) Results indicated that 82% of emergency nurses had moderate to high levels of burnout, with 86% demonstrating moderate to high levels of CF.

      d) Differences between the nursing specialties did not reach significance, yet ICU nurses showed a higher risk for burnout and oncology nurses reflected a risk for higher CF.

      e) This research revealed that regardless of specialty, all nurses are at risk for burnout and CF (Hooper et al., 2010).

      f) The prevalence of burnout and CF could pose barriers to recruitment and retention of staff, optimal patient safety, and high-quality care (Hooper et al., 2010; Melvin, 2015).

   3. Yoder (2010) investigated the prevalence of CF and identified situations that led to CF and the coping mechanisms nurses used.

      a) Nurses with less than 10 years of experience reported higher levels of compassion satisfaction than nurses with longer experience.

      b) Nurses who reported interpersonal fulfillment such as "being happy," "being me," and "being connected to others" had higher compassion satisfaction scores.

   4. In a nonexperimental, descriptive, correlational study, Neville and Cole (2013) examined the relationships between nurses' utilization of health promotion behaviors and CF, burnout, and compassion satisfaction.

      a) The Health-Promoting Lifestyle Profile II and the ProQOL R-V were administered.

      b) An unexpected finding was a higher rate of CF as compared to normative data and previous research by the researchers.

      c) The data analysis supported a moderate positive association between nurses engaging in health promotion activities and compassion satisfaction.

      d) The authors also noted a positive association between health promotion behaviors and a reduction in burnout.

      e) The researchers postulated that strong affiliations with others and one's spiritual self can support compassion satisfaction and potentially reduce the risks of burnout and CF.

   5. Research by Hinderer et al. (2014) investigated burnout, CF, compassion satisfaction, and STS in a cross-sectional, descriptive study of trauma nurses.

a) A demographic and behavioral instrument (which assessed demographics, personal and environmental characteristics, coping strategies, and exposure to traumatic events), the Penn Inventory (which examined STS), and the ProQOL (which assessed burnout, CF, and compassion satisfaction) were administered.

b) In the sample of 128 trauma nurses, 35.9% of nurses had ProQOL scores indicative of burnout or risk of burnout.

c) CF was reported by 27.3% of the nurses, and 21.1% had scored low on the compassion satisfaction subscale.

d) Using the Penn Inventory, 7% demonstrated STS.

e) The use of self-medicating, negative coworker relationships, and working more hours per shift translated to higher burnout, CF, and STS scores.

6. The majority of research on moral distress has been conducted on nurses; however, the experience of moral distress is a significant phenomenon among many healthcare disciplines.

   a) An institutionwide survey investigated moral distress among healthcare professionals at a large healthcare system (Whitehead, Herbertson, Hamric, Epstein, & Fisher, 2015).

   b) The authors noted that the etiology of moral distress in direct care providers was most often the aggressive, prolonged, futile care of patients.

   c) Providers working in adult units or adult ICUs had higher levels of moral distress than clinicians in pediatric and non-ICU settings.

   d) Other findings contributing to moral distress included poor team communication and a lack of provider continuity in both ICU and non-ICU settings.

   e) Providers who left or considered leaving a position had significantly higher levels of moral distress than those who never considered leaving; therefore, moral distress was associated with burnout and the intention to leave a position.

7. Allen et al. (2013) performed another study of moral distress among healthcare professionals at a health system.

   a) Moral Distress Surveys (MDS-R) were completed by 323 healthcare professionals from disciplines including pediatric hospitalists, cardiologists, neurologists, nephrologists, pulmonologists, oncologists, intensivists, and neonatologists; adult and pediatric nurses; social workers and case managers; and respiratory therapists.

   b) All disciplines experienced moderate to high levels of moral distress.

   c) Triggers for moral distress included, "Follow the family's wishes to continue life support even though I believe it is not in the patient's best interest," and "Watch patient care suffer because of a lack of provider continuity."

   d) The number-one reason for moral distress for social workers and case managers was, "Provide less than optimum care due to pressure from administration or insurers to reduce cost."

   e) A major reason for moral distress among RNs and RTs was, "Provide less than optimum care due to pressure from administration or insurers to reduce cost."

   f) Nurses and physicians with more years of experience did not demonstrate higher moral distress, but those clinicians who had previously considered or actually left a position (versus those who had not) and those currently considering leaving a position (versus those who had not) experienced higher levels of moral distress.

D. Interventions promoting self-care

　1. In a study by Shanafelt and Dyrbye (2012), interventions to combat burnout included recommendations for practitioners to make purposeful, ongoing attempts to find meaning in work and incorporating a philosophy of work–life balance. Efforts to increase personal awareness with mindfulness-based meditation were recommended, as well as making a concerted effort to characterize work-setting variables causing distress.

　2. In a research study to determine the self-care needs of oncologists, Granek, Mazzotta, Tozer, and Krzyzanowska (2013) identified four categories: training, grief acknowledgment, institutional support, and sabbaticals.

　　a) Within training, the study participants desired information and education to be emphasized during fellowship training and grand rounds addressing the emotional distress of professionals.

　　b) To have grief acknowledged, the study participants wanted validation and normalization of their grief, forums, regular debriefings, and supportive mentorship.

　　c) Psychosocial support from the institution and access to professional help were desired along with sabbaticals and vacations for time away and nourishment.

　3. Jasperse, Herst, and Dungey (2014) made recommendations to enhance job satisfaction and engagement: increased social support and team building, ongoing education (especially stress-reduction workshops), clinical supervision, psychosocial support (individual and peer support groups), and ideally, an interdisciplinary nature for all interventions.

　4. To aid in self-care against moral distress, Houston et al. (2013) recommended use of ethics consultation teams as a resource and participation in interdisciplinary forums such as Schwartz Center Rounds.

　　a) Prevention of burnout is more effective than treatment (Guest & Bajorin, 2014).

　　b) Self-care activities for interdisciplinary professionals includes the development of skills for self-awareness, and self-care; mindfulness intervention practices; communications skills training; exercise; and "early recognition of depression from personal and family conflict as well as substance abuse and alcohol to solve the stressors" (Guest & Bajorin, 2014, p. 1102).

IV. Relevance to practice

A. The "wear and tear" of emotion work on nurses can affect professional longevity, job turnover, and retention (Erickson & Grove, 2008; Sumner & Townsend-Rocchiccioli, 2003).

B. Significant nurse caregiving experiences can result in moral residue where ongoing reflections of patient care decisions plague the nurse with potential blame, existential questioning, and ultimately, self-doubt (Gunther & Thomas, 2006).

C. Nurse burnout, as measured by emotional exhaustion and lack of personal accomplishment, is a significant factor influencing how satisfied patients are with their care (Vahey, Aiken, Sloane, Clarke, & Vargas, 2004).

　1. Across countries, high levels of nurse burnout are associated with lower ratings of care quality (Poghosyan, Clarke, Finlayson, & Aiken, 2010).

    2. Concerted efforts to optimize numerous elements of the work setting can result in greater team functioning, increased personal satisfaction with care, increased staff retention, and the reduction of nurse stressors (Blake, Leach, Robbins, Pike, & Needleman, 2013; Li, Early, Mahrer, Klaristenfeld, & Gold, 2014; Stichler, 2009; Yu, Jiang, & Shen, 2016).

V. Role of the advanced practice registered nurse (APRN)

    A. As role models, APRNs should engage in ongoing self-care and emulate this practice to staff nurses and other disciplines.

    B. APRNs in leadership positions have the ability to articulate unmet needs of nursing staff and lobby for the creation of new support programs and personnel to assist staff with the rigors of their emotionally charged specialty practice.

    C. The consequences of stress inherent within the specialty should be the target of quality improvement initiatives and formal research.

VI. Interface to palliative care

    A. Common risk factors for burnout in palliative care include workload; lack of self-confidence in communication skills; insufficient time to vent emotions and grieve patient deaths; time pressures (especially to provide emotional support); being responsible for the transmission of bad news; constant exposure to pain, suffering, and the dying trajectory; inadequate training in palliative care; and extended length of service (Pereira, Fonseca, & Carvalho, 2011; Vachon, Huggard, & Huggard, 2015).

    B. Professional affiliation and characteristics of the organizational work culture significantly affect burnout (Slocum-Gori, Hemsworth, Chan, Carson, & Kazanjian, 2013).

    C. This includes aspects of team dynamics and collegiality, presence of emotional support resources, and the caliber of leadership.

        1. Personal indices, such as having meaning and purpose in one's life and exhibiting a healthy attitude toward death, may serve as protective measures to burnout in end-of-life care (Gama, Barbosa, & Vieira, 2014).

        2. The protective effects of palliative care units in decreasing burnout require further research. Training to counter burnout could be implemented at the specialty entry-into-practice level.

    D. Self-care requires self-compassion (Vachon et al., 2015). Caring for oneself while addressing the challenges of palliative and hospice nursing can present numerous impositions, as well as opportunities to the enactment of self-care.

    E. Benefits of nursing expertise in advanced care promote realization of the ultimate brevity of existence and the need to enjoy life in the moment, which affect personal family decision making (Luxardo, Padros, & Tripodoro, 2014).

    F. Relying on team or collegial support, coming to closure following the death of patients, and the conscious creation of life balance are strategies that foster necessary self-care (Seed & Walton, 2012).

    G. Taking time away from work and having meaningful relationships outside of work are interventions associated with positive self-care (Malloy, Thrane, Winston, Virani, & Kelly, 2013).

Case Study

Marcie is an experienced oncology nurse who has practiced for 10 years on the inpatient oncology unit. She flourished and excelled at taking care of patients and their families at the end of life. This was noted by the frequent commentary of families in notes to administration about the exceptional care Marcie provided during the dying experience. Now pregnant with her third child, Marcie decided she would not return to full-time work in the acute care setting but would pursue part-time employment with more flexible hours. One of the hospice homecare coordinators approached Marcie about applying for a position with the coordinator's agency when she was ready to return to work. Marcie subsequently did such and was immediately hired.

Marcie's third child was born premature with cystic fibrosis. The baby required extra care, but Marcie's husband helped so that she could return to work. At the second month of her new job, Marcie was assigned the case of a 30-year-old man with end-stage colorectal cancer. The patient's wife had a six-month-old infant with Down syndrome who required extra care. Upon assessing the case, Marcie identified that the patient was obstructed and could not tolerate oral intake in addition to being in severe pain.

Marcie, being accustomed to the inpatient environment, was overwhelmed. She was not prepared to feel isolated from a "team," and, finding minimal resources in the home in contrast to the hi-tech hospital environment, she felt slightly panicked. Marcie was also finding the need to respond to intensive family anxiety from both the patient's wife and his mother. Despite the challenge, Marcie was able to focus on the case, tend to the patient's dehydration and pain, and even talk to the wife about her bravery caring for both a sick infant and a dying husband in the home.

Marcie found herself identifying with the young mother when she herself would return home to an infant who required supportive care. She identified with the patient because her husband was also in his thirties. Marcie found herself thinking about the patient and family even during her off hours. She began to have sleep disturbances and dreams about different scenarios and would wake up frantic and think she was not helping them as much as she could. Marcie found herself tearful both at home and at work, easily distracted, and even waking up in the mornings exhausted and ill-prepared to face the day.

Entering the hospice office one morning, Marcie's nursing administrator commented on her sad affect and irritability. To Marcie's surprise, she burst into tears describing the case to her administrator. The administrator immediately pulled her aside and took the time to listen and support Marcie's feelings and emotions.

The administrator offered advice on how Marcie could meet the challenges of the case and on the need for Marcie to practice self-care measures during this stressful time. This brief intervention by the administrator immediately brought relief to Marcie and she no longer felt guilty or ashamed of her feelings. Marcie cared for the patient and family for two weeks until the patient died quietly one evening when she was present. She was able to debrief about the case at a weekly staff meeting and was able to integrate positive feelings about how she handled a very challenging case.

References

Abernethy, A.P. (2012). A balanced approach to physician responsibilities: Oncologists' duties toward themselves. *American Society of Clinical Oncology 2012 Educational Book*, pp. e9–e14. Retrieved from http://meetinglibrary.asco.org/content/82-114

Adams, R.E., Buscarino, J.A., & Figley, C.R. (2006). Compassion fatigue and psychological distress among social workers: A validation study. *American Journal of Orthopsychiatry, 76,* 103–108. doi:10.1037/0002-9432.76.1.103

Allen, R., Judkins-Cohn, T., deVelasco, R., Forges, E., Lee, R., Clark, L., & Procunier, M. (2013).Moral distress among healthcare professionals at a health system. *JONA's Healthcare Law, Ethics, and Regulation, 15,* 111–118. doi:10.1097/NHL.0b013e3182a1bf33

American Association of Critical-Care Nurses. (2016). *AACN standards for establishing and sustaining healthy work environments: A journey to excellence* (2nd ed.). Retrieved from http://www.aacn.org/wd/hwe/docs/hwestandards.pdf

American Holistic Nurses Association. (2013). *Holistic nursing: Scope and standards of practice* (2nd ed.). Silver Spring, MD: American Nurses Association.

American Nurses Association. (2015). *Code of ethics for nurses with interpretive statements.* Retrieved from http://www.nursingworld.org/MainMenuCategories/EthicsStandards/CodeofEthicsforNurses/Code-of-Ethics-For-Nurses.html

American Society of Clinical Oncology. (2015, May 22). ASCO takes initial steps in developing interventions to improve physician wellness. Retrieved from http://am.asco.org/asco-takes-initial-steps-developing-interventions-improve-physician-wellness

Blake, N., Leach, L.S., Robbins, W., Pike, N., & Needleman, J. (2013). Healthy work environments and staff nurse retention: The relationship between communication, collaboration, and leadership in the pediatric intensive care unit. *Nursing Administration Quarterly, 37,* 356–370. doi:10.1097/NAQ.0b013e3182a2fa47

Boyle, D.A. (2010). Countering compassion fatigue: A requisite nursing agenda. *Online Journal of Issues in Nursing, 16*(1), Manuscript 2. doi:10.3912/OJIN.Vol16No01Man02

Boyle, D.A. (2015). Compassion fatigue: The cost of caring. *Nursing, 45*(7), 48–51. doi:10.1097/01.NURSE.0000461857.48809.a1

Cañadas-De la Fuente, G.A., Vargas, C., San Luis, C., García, I., Cañadas, G.R., & De la Fuente, E.I. (2015). Risk factors and prevalence of burnout syndrome in the nursing profession. *International Journal of Nursing Studies, 52,* 240–249. doi:10.1016/j.ijnurstu.2014.07.001

Cavaliere, T.A., Daly, B., Dowling, D., & Montgomery, K. (2010). Moral distress in neonatal intensive care unit RNs. *Advances in Neonatal Care, 10,* 145–156. doi:10.1097/ANC.0b013e3181dd6c48

Erickson, R.J., & Grove, W.J.C. (2008). Why emotions matter: Age, agitation, and burnout among registered nurses. *Online Journal of Issues in Nursing, 13*(1).

Figley, C.R. (1995). Compassion fatigue as secondary traumatic stress disorder: An overview. In C.R. Figley (Ed.), *Compassion fatigue: Coping with secondary traumatic stress disorder in those who treat the traumatized* (pp. 1–20). New York, NY: Brunner/Mazel.

Gaffney, D.A., DeMarco, R.F., Hofmeyer, A., Vessey, J.A., & Budin, W.C. (2012). Making things right: Nurses' experiences with workplace bullying—A grounded theory. *Nursing Research and Practice, 2012,* Article 243210. doi:10.1155/2012/243210

Gama, G., Barbosa, F., & Vieira, M. (2014). Personal determinants of nurses' burnout in end of life care. *European Journal of Oncology Nursing, 18,* 527–533. doi:10.1016/j.ejon.2014.04.005

Gerow, L., Conejo, P., Alonzo, A., Davis, N., Rodgers, S., & Domian, E.W. (2010). Creating a curtain of protection: Nurses' experiences of grief following patient death. *Journal of Nursing Scholarship, 42,* 122–129. doi:10.1111/j.1547-5069.2010.01343.x

Gillman, L., Adams, J., Kovac, R., Kilcullen, A., House, A., & Doyle, C. (2015). Strategies to promote coping and resilience in oncology and palliative care nurses caring for adult patients with malignancy: A comprehensive systematic review. *JBI Database of Systematic Reviews and Implementation Reports, 13*(5), 131–204. doi:10.11124/jbisrir-2015-1898

Granek, L., Mazzotta, P., Tozer, R., & Krzyzanowska, M.K. (2013). Oncologists' protocol and coping strategies in dealing with patient loss. *Death Studies, 37,* 937–952. doi:10.1080/07481187.2012.692461

Greville, L. (2015). Self-care solutions: Facing the challenge of asking for help. *Social Work Today, 15*(3), 14. Retrieved from http://www.socialworktoday.com/archive/051815p14.shtml

Guest, R.S., & Bajorin, D.F. (2014). Take care of yourself: We need you. *Journal of Clinical Oncology, 32,* 1101–1103. doi:10.1200/JCO.2013.54.5319

Gunther, M., & Thomas, S.P. (2006). Nurses' narratives of unforgettable patient care events. *Journal of Nursing Scholarship, 38,* 370–376. doi:10.1111/j.1547-5069.2006.00129.x

Halifax, J. (2011). The precious necessity of compassion. *Journal of Pain and Symptom Management, 41,* 146–153. doi:10.1016/j.jpainsymman.2010.08.010

Hinderer, K.A., VonRueden, K.T., Friedmann, E., McQuillan, K.A., Gilmore, R., Kramer, B., & Murray, M. (2014). Burnout, compassion fatigue, compassion satisfaction, and secondary traumatic stress in trauma nurses. *Journal of Trauma Nursing, 21,* 160–169. doi:10.1097/JTN.0000000000000055

Hooper, C., Craig, J., Janvrin, D.R., Wetsel, M.A., & Reimels, E. (2010). Compassion satisfaction, burnout, and compassion fatigue among emergency nurses compared with nurses in other selected inpatient specialties. *Journal of Emergency Nursing, 36,* 420–427.

Houston, S., Casanova, M.A., Leveille, M., Schmidt, K.L., Barnes, S.A., Trungale, K.R., & Fine, R.L. (2013). The intensity and frequency of moral distress among different healthcare disciplines. *Journal of Clinical Ethics, 24,* 98–112.

Huffman, D.M., & Rittenmeyer, L. (2012). How professional nurses working in hospital environments experience moral distress: A systematic review. *Critical Care Nursing Clinics of North America, 24,* 91–100. doi:10.1016/j.ccell.2012.01.004

Hylton, H.M. (2015, May 31). Professional burnout and the oncology workforce: A perspective on physician assistants and nurse practitioners. *ASCO Daily News.* Retrieved from http://am.asco.org/professional -burnout-and-oncology-workforce-perspective-physician-assistants-and-nurse-practitioners

Jasperse, M., Herst, P., & Dungey, G. (2014). Evaluating stress, burnout and job satisfaction in New Zealand radiation oncology departments. *European Journal of Cancer Care, 23,* 82–88. doi:10.1111/ecc.12098

Kanter, J. (2007). Compassion fatigue and secondary traumatization: A second look. *Clinical Social Work Journal, 35,* 289–293. doi:10.1007/s10615-007-0125-1

Kushner, J., & Ruffin, T. (2015). Empowering a healthy practice environment. *Nursing Clinics of North America, 50,* 167–183. doi:10.1016/j.cnur.2014.10.013

Li, A., Early, S.F., Mahrer, N.E., Klaristenfeld, J.L., & Gold, J.I. (2014). Group cohesion and organizational commitment: Protective factors for nurse residents' job satisfaction, compassion satisfaction, and burnout. *Journal of Professional Nursing, 30,* 89–99. doi:10.1016/j.profnurs.2013.04.004

Lombardo, B., & Eyre, C. (2011). Compassion fatigue: A nurse's primer. *Online Journal of Issues in Nursing, 16*(1), Manuscript 3. doi:10.3912/OJIN.Vol16No01Man03

Luxardo, N., Padros, C.V., & Tripodoro, V. (2014). Palliative care staff perspectives: The challenges of end-of-life care on their professional practices and everyday lives. *Journal of Hospice and Palliative Nursing, 16,* 165–172. doi:10.1097/NJH.0000000000000036

Malloy, P., Thrane, S., Winston, T., Virani, R., & Kelly, K. (2013). Do nurses who care for patients in palliative and end-of-life settings perform good self-care? *Journal of Hospice and Palliative Nursing, 15,* 99–106. doi:10.1097/NJH.0b013e31826bef72

Melvin, C.S. (2015). Historical review in understanding burnout, professional compassion fatigue, and secondary traumatic stress disorder from a hospice and palliative nursing perspective. *Journal of Hospice and Palliative Nursing, 17,* 66–72.

Mills, J., Wand, T., & Fraser, J.A. (2015). On self-compassion and self-care in nursing: Selfish or essential for compassionate care? *International Journal of Nursing Studies, 52,* 791–793. doi:10.1016/j.ijnurstu.2014.10.009

National Association of Social Workers. (2008). *Professional self-care and social work.* Retrieved from http://www.compassionstrengths.com/uploads/NASW.ProfesionalSelf-Care.pdf

Neville, K., & Cole, D.A. (2013). The relationships among health promotion behaviors, compassion fatigue, burnout, and compassion satisfaction in nurses practicing in a community medical center. *Journal of Nursing Administration, 43,* 348–354. doi:10.1097/NNA.0b013e3182942c23

Nightingale, F. (1969/1860). *Notes on nursing: What it is, and what it is not.* New York, NY: Dover Publications.

Oncology Nursing Society. (2012). *Oncology Nursing Society leadership competencies.* Retrieved from https://www.ons.org/sites/default/files/leadershipcomps.pdf

Pereira, S.M., Fonseca, A.M., & Carvalho, A.S. (2011). Burnout in palliative care: A systematic review. *Nursing Ethics, 18,* 317–326. doi:10.1177/0969733011398092

Poghosyan, L., Clarke, S.P., Finlayson, M., & Aiken, L.H. (2010). Nurse burnout and quality of care: Cross-national investigation in six countries. *Research in Nursing and Health, 33,* 288–298. doi:10.1002/nur.20383

Potter, P., Deshields, T., Divanbeigi, J., Berger, J., Cipriano, D., Norris, L., & Olsen, S. (2010). Compassion fatigue and burnout: Prevalence among oncology nurses [Online exclusive]. *Clinical Journal of Oncology Nursing, 14,* E56–E62. doi:10.1188/10.CJON.E56-E62

Sabo, B. (2011). Reflecting on the concept of compassion fatigue. *Online Journal of Issues in Nursing, 16*(1), Manuscript 1. doi:10.3912/OJIN.Vol16No01Man01

Sauerland, J., Marotta, K., Peinemann, M.A., Berndt, A., & Robichaux, C. (2014). Assessing and addressing moral distress and ethical climate, part 1. *Dimensions of Critical Care Nursing, 33,* 234–245. doi:10.1097/DCC.0000000000000050

Seed, S., & Walton, J. (2012). Caring for self: The challenges of hospice nursing. *Journal of Hospice and Palliative Nursing, 14,* E1–E8. doi:10.1097/NJH.0b013e31825c1485

Shanafelt, T.D., & Dyrbye, L. (2012). Oncologist burnout: Causes, consequences, and responses. *Journal of Clinical Oncology, 30,* 1235–1241. doi:10.1200/JCO.2011.39.7380

Shanafelt, T.D., Gradishar, W.J., Kosty, M., Satele, D., Chew, H., Horn, L., … Raymond, M. (2014). Burnout and career satisfaction among US oncologists. *Journal of Clinical Oncology, 32,* 678–686. doi:10.1200/JCO.2013.51.8480

Slocum-Gori, S., Hemsworth, D., Chan, W.W.Y., Carson, A., & Kazanjian, A. (2013). Understanding compassion satisfaction, compassion fatigue and burnout: A survey of the hospice palliative care workforce. *Palliative Medicine, 27,* 172–178. doi:10.1177/0269216311431311

Stichler, J.F. (2009). Healthy, healthful, and healing environments: A nursing imperative. *Critical Care Nursing Quarterly, 32,* 176–188. doi:10.1097/CNQ.0b013e3181ab9149

Sumner, J., & Townsend-Rocchiccioli, J. (2003). Why are nurses leaving nursing? *Nursing Administration Quarterly, 27,* 164–171. doi:10.1097/00006216-200304000-00010

Vachon, M.L.S., Huggard, P.K., & Huggard, J. (2015). Reflections on occupational stress in palliative care nursing: Is it changing? In B.R. Ferrell, N. Coyle, & J. Paice (Eds.), *Oxford textbook of palliative nursing* (4th ed., pp. 969–986). New York, NY: Oxford University Press.

Vahey, D.C., Aiken, L.H., Sloane, D.M., Clarke, S.P., & Vargas, D. (2004). Nurse burnout and patient satisfaction. *Medical Care, 42*(Suppl. 2), II57–II66. doi:10.1097/01.mlr.0000109126.50398.5a

Wallace, J.E., Lemaire, J.B., & Ghali, W.A. (2009). Physician wellness: A missing quality indicator. *Lancet, 374,* 1714–1721. doi:10.1016/S0140-6736(09)61424-0

Watts, J., & Robertson, N. (2015). Selecting a measure for assessing secondary trauma in nurses. *Nurse Researcher, 23*(2), 30–35. doi:10.7748/nr.23.2.30.s7

Wenzel, J., Shaha, M., Klimmek, R., & Krumm, S. (2011). Working through grief and loss: Oncology nurses' perspectives on professional bereavement [Online exclusive]. *Oncology Nursing Forum, 38,* E272–E282. doi:10.1188/11.ONF.E272-E282

Whitehead, P.B., Herbertson, R.K., Hamric, A.B., Epstein, E.G., & Fisher, J.M. (2015). Moral distress among healthcare professionals: Report of an institution-wide survey. *Journal of Nursing Scholarship, 47,* 117–125. doi:10.1111/jnu.12115

Yoder, E.A. (2010). Compassion fatigue in nurses. *Applied Nursing Research, 23,* 191–197. doi:10.1016/j.apnr.2008.09.003

Yu, H., Jiang, A., & Shen, J. (2016). Prevalence and predictors of compassion fatigue, burnout and compassion satisfaction among oncology nurses: A cross-sectional survey. *International Journal of Nursing Studies, 57,* 28–38. doi:10.1016/j.ijnurstu.2016.01.012

Index

The letter f indicates that relevant content appears in a figure; the letter t, in a table.

A